Krestel Imaging Systems for Medical Diagnostics

Authors	Sections
Ernst Ammann	7.1.4
Hansjörg Bittorf	7.1.1
Eduard David	1
Peter Durlak	7.2.3
Hans-Immo Friel	9
Ernst Geldner	3.1
Jörg Haendle	7.1.6.2, 7.1.6.4–7.1.6.6
Wolfgang Härer	4.2
Dietrich Hassler	6
Hans Heinrich	3.2
Gert Hetzel	11.2.2, 11.2.3
Bernd Heuchemer	7.2.9
Fritz-Walter Hofmann	7.1.5
Wolfango Jann	7.1.6.2
Wolfgang Knüpfer	7.1.3.1, 7.1.3.2
Rolf Koch	7.2.5–7.2.8
Peter Kraus	7.2.1
Herbert Kuhn	2, 7.1.2
Gerhard Laub	10.3.4
Reiner Liebetruth	8.1
Gerhard Linke	4.1, 7.3
Wilfried Loeffler	5
Anton Nekovar	7.1.6.7
Arnulf Oppelt	5
Rolf Pfeifer	7.2.4
Helmut Reichenberger	12
Hans-Erich Reinfelder	7.1.3.3
Heinz Runge	7.1.6.1, 7.1.6.3
Günter Schwierz	2, 4.2
Richard Soldner	11.2.1
Eckart Stetter	10.1–10.3.3
Wolf-Dieter Weckesser	8.2
Oliver Zimmermann	7.2.2
Viktor Zurinski	11.1

Imaging Systems for Medical Diagnostics

Fundamentals and technical solutions

X-ray diagnostics
Computed tomography
Nuclear medical diagnostics
Magnetic resonance imaging
Sonography
Biomagnetic diagnostics

Editor: Erich Krestel

Siemens Aktiengesellschaft

Deutsche Bibliothek Cataloguing-in-Publication Data

Imaging systems for medical diagnostics: fundamentals and technical solutions; X-ray diagnostics, computed tomography, nuclear medical diagnostics, magnetic resonance imaging, sonography, biomagnetic diagnostics / ed.: Erich Krestel. – Berlin; Munich: Siemens-Aktienges., [Abt. Verl.], 1990
Einheitssacht.: Bildgebende Systeme für die medizinische Diagnostik ⟨engl.⟩
ISBN 3-8009-1564-2
NE: Krestel, Erich [Hrsg.]; EST

Title of German original edition:
Bildgebende Systeme für die medizinische Diagnostik
Herausgeber: Erich Krestel, Siemens Aktiengesellschaft, 1988
ISBN 3-8009-1505-7

ISBN 3-8009-1564-2

Published by Siemens Aktiengesellschaft, Berlin and Munich

Printed in the Federal Republic of Germany

Preface

This book first appeared in German in 1980. As a result of the considerable improvements made to medicotechnical diagnostic systems through the innovations of microelectronics, it has been necessary to completely revise the second edition of 1988. The book was well received by university lecturers, technical colleges and technical schools. It has also proved to be a valuable reference for medical physicists in a clinical environment, medical assistants, physicians and engineers in the research and development area.

The favorable reception of the book on the part of this range of specialists fully justifies the English translation of the second edition.

The aim of the book is to present a survey of the principles and designs of diagnostic imaging systems, encompassing x-ray diagnostics, x-ray computed tomography, nuclearmedical diagnostics, magnetic resonance tomography, sonography and biomagnetic diagnostics. Also included is a treatment of lithotripsy, the diagnosis and subsequent destruction of stones in the human body, as an interventional procedure.

Specific demands are made on medical technology in developing each type of medicotechnical system. Furthermore, the development of such systems is a dynamic process, which must also take into account continuing developments originating in the hospital. The book is of particular value for the physician and the clinical researcher by pointing the way to the procedures best suited to performing the required medical diagnoses and by simplifying the choice of the required or the optimal system for the purpose envisioned.

Since the individual systems entail different types of irradiation and these in turn occur in different form (e.g. both superposition images, in x-ray diagnostics, and sectional images, in CT, are possible by means of x-rays), each system offers its particular advantages. By way of illustration: good image quality for bone presentations, good image quality for soft-tissue presentations, emphasis on the presence of pathological occurrences, non-ionizing radiation, high spatial resolution and the possibility of functional diagnosis.

It is my sincere hope that this book will also prove to be of value in the English-speaking countries for physicians, physicists, engineers and technicians.

Werner Maly

Member of the Board, Siemens AG

Foreword

Imaging systems, which with the aid of different types of radiation and supported by modern microelectronics produce images of the living organism, are today a permanent feature of medical diagnostics. Different forms of medicotechnical systems have been developed to meet the needs of different diagnostic techniques. It is the purpose of this book to present a comprehensive overview of the range of these systems (with the exception of endoscopy) from the point of view of physics and engineering.

With the advent of a number of new procedures in the last few decades, x-ray diagnostics as originally developed by Wilhelm Conrad Röntgen in the year 1895 has undergone major changes. With the invention of the camera known by his name, in 1958 H.O. Anger made possible the present form of the total image. The first total image unit for ultrasound diagnoses appeared in 1966. In 1972 followed the development of computed tomography by G.N. Hounsfield. In 1973, P.C. Lauterbuhr introduced magnetic resonance tomography, which was followed by the introduction of such systems to the market in 1982.

The rapid developments in microelectronics of the last ten years have contributed significantly to improvements in medicotechnical systems. These include improved image quality, made possible by the introduction of microchips, greatly simplified system operation, a considerable extension of the range of applications, and a substantial reduction in size and weight.

The book comprises two parts. In the first part, Fundamentals, the physiology of sight, the characterization of image quality, the effect of gamma radiation and x-radiation, the principles of x-ray computed tomography imaging and magnetic resonance tomography imaging, and ultrasonic techniques are treated in detail. The second part, Technical Solutions, deals with the special procedures of x-ray diagnoses, computed tomography, diagnoses in nuclear medicine, magnetic resonance tomography, sonography and biomagnetic diagnostics.

It is left to the discretion of those using imaging systems for medical diagnoses to select the procedure best suited to the application required from the range of possibilities offered. For this purpose, suggestions are presented. The book can serve as supporting material for lecturing and also as a useful reference. It is also intended as information for those employed in the electromedical industry. The book therefore addresses physicians, physicists, engineers in a clinical environment and lecturers, as well as those involved with research and development and sales activities for electromedical systems.

The numbering of equations, images and literature references is according to chapter. The literature references are found at the end of the book. These serve to reconstruct the historical developments of the individual methods and also to indicate sources of further information. Since the primary aim of this book is to present the most recent technological state of the systems discussed, it would be inappropriate to treat the historical aspects in greater detail.

That it is necessary to observe safety and equipment regulations, as well as the general principles of good engineering practice, goes without saying.

I would like to express my appreciation to the authors, the Siemens Technical Translation Department and the publisher for their cooperation in translating the original German version of the book.

Erlangen, September 1990 Erich Krestel

Contents

Part 1 Fundamentals

Part 2 Technical solutions

Part 1 Fundamentals

1 Physiology of vision

1.1 General considerations regarding sensory physiology

Over the last few decades great strides have been made in the area of imaging systems for use in medical diagnostics. New techniques, for example magnetic resonance tomography, have been developed, opening up new avenues in diagnosis. However, enormous improvements have also been made in conventional techniques, e.g. those using x-rays, in particular by the application of microelectronics: the amount of radiation to which the patient is exposed has been drastically reduced, and the quality of the images considerably enhanced.

Today industry is able to produce imaging systems which are to a large extent technically compatible with the biological needs of the human eye. In order to give a full account of these systems, it therefore seems appropriate to begin by giving some idea of the function of the eye as a sense organ.

The *sense organs* allow the organism to perceive its constantly changing environment. Depending on the physical dimension of the environmental change, the various sense organs are specialized for quite specific, adequate *stimuli*. Different *sensory perceptions* [1.1], also known as *sensory modalities*, arise in this way.

The amount of information received by all the sensory organs together is immense. It has been estimated at around 10^9 bits/s [1.2]. This flood of information, cannot, however, be transmitted by the nerves to the brain in its entirety. The nervous system therefore needs to select the most important information at any particular moment. This selection procedure cuts down the information received in the ratio of 10000000:1. People vary greatly in the selection they make so that the same pattern of stimuli will be perceived and assessed differently from one person to another. In principle this information selection takes place in the nervous system by means of the *excitation and inhibition of nerve cells*. Thus the nervous system has the task of comparing information in terms of the degree of neural excitation and, where necessary, of passing it on to higher decision-making centers. In order to perform this task, the nervous system has two separate functional elements: *nerve cell bodies* for converting information and *nerve fibers* for stimulus conduction. Collections of nerve cells in the brain and in the spinal cord are known as gray matter and the fibers as white matter. The neuron is the basic working unit of the central nervous system (CNS). It consists of a cell body with several projections which increase its surface area, and a long fiber, the axon, which establishes the contacts (synaptic junctions) with other nerve cells. Figure 1.1 shows a diagram of such a neuron.

This method of transforming and transmitting information applies equally to all the sensory organs, including the *eye*. In this process, specific sensory perception is not generated by the nature of the impulse, but by the anatomy of the nerve connections between the relevant sensory organs and particular areas of the brain. Thus a distinction is made anatomically between a visual pathway, an auditory pathway, an olfactory pathway, a gustatory pathway and a pain pathway. Even the quality of sensory perception, which in the case of the eye constitutes the difference between color perception and light-dark perception, is governed by the finely-structured connections between individual nerve fibers and relevant sensory cells.

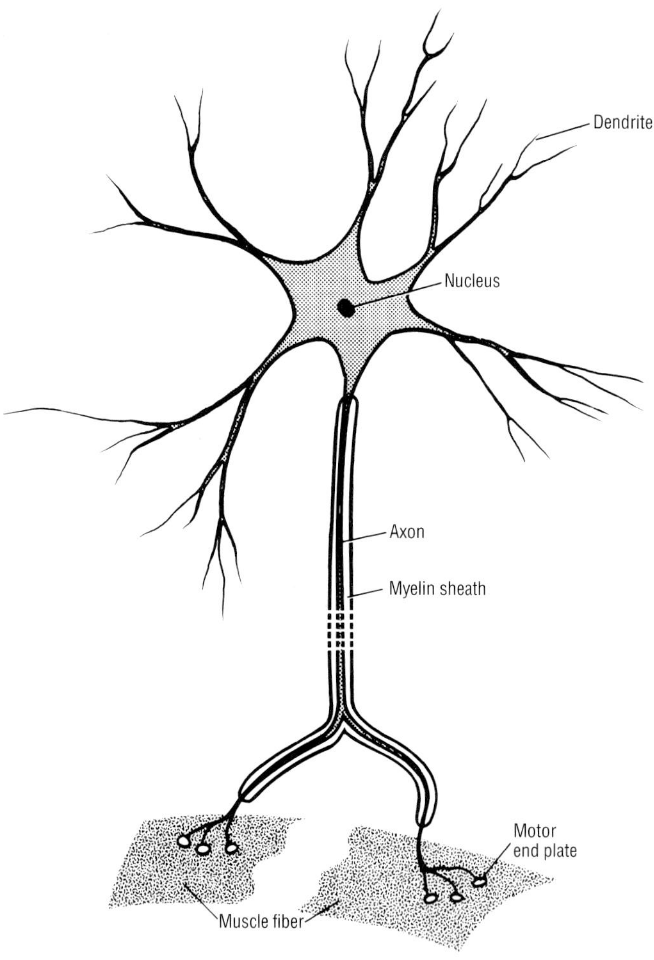

Fig. 1.1
The neuron, the basic working unit of the central nervous system

1.2 The eye

1.2.1 Adequate stimulus

The eye is sensitive to certain electromagnetic waves. These waves can be divided up into various regions [1.3] which have quite different effects on the organism. As can be seen from Fig. 1.2, the *sensitivity range of the eye* barely covers one octave (400 to 780 nm) of the electromagnetic spectrum. The frequency corresponds to the color (see Fig. 1.17), the amplitude to the degree of brightness perceived.

In addition, the sense of vision can perceive objects in three dimensions. This is because of the parallactic shift of the image seen by the right eye relative to that seen by the left eye.

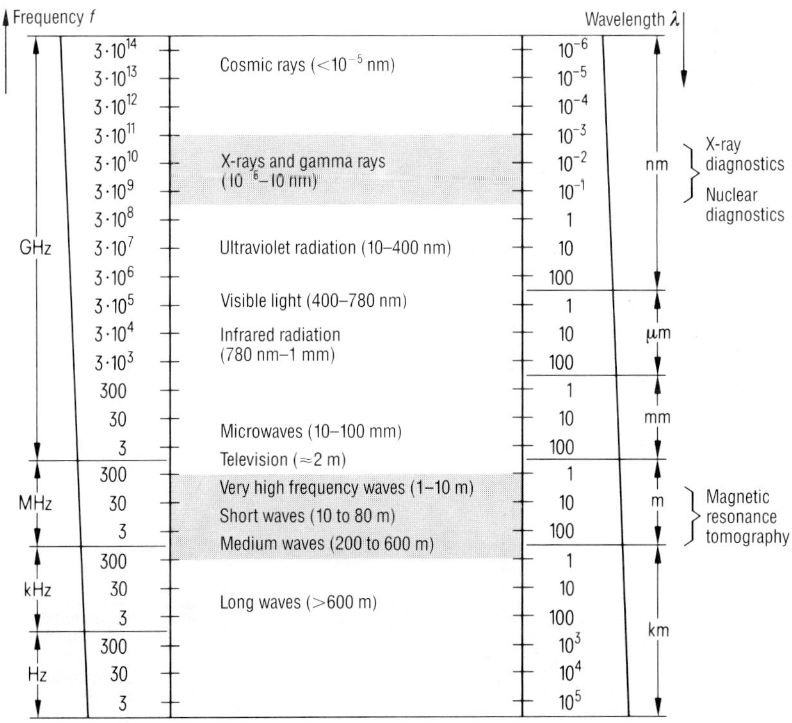

$$f = \frac{c}{\lambda} = \frac{300000}{\lambda}$$

▭ Spectral regions used in imaging systems

Fig. 1.2 Regions of the electromagnetic spectrum

1.2.2 Anatomy

Like the camera, the eye has an optical imaging system. It consists of the cornea and the lens. In order to reduce chromatic aberration (color distortion), the lens is made up of several layers, like an onion, each with a different refractive index. Anatomical details are shown in Fig. 1.3 [1.4]. The space between the cornea and the lens (anterior chamber) is filled by the crystal-clear aqueous humor. The interior of the eye is occupied by the jelly-like vitreous body, which in common with all the other transparent parts of the eye does not contain any blood vessels, receiving nutrients by diffusion. Inside the sclera (the firm white outer membrane) lies the choroid (the brownish vascular membrane), followed by the retina. The retina contains the light-sensitive elements, the rods and the cones, which convert the electromagnetic waves into nerve impulses. The retina also contains nerve cells which carry out a preliminary processing of the information on the spot. This is also where the fibers of the optical nerve start. The lens is suspended in the ring-shaped muscle of the ciliary body. The iris, which covers the front of the lens, leaves only a small aperture (the pupil) open. Six muscles, stemming from the bone wall of the eye socket and attached to the outside of the sclera, are capable of moving and turning the eyeball in all directions.

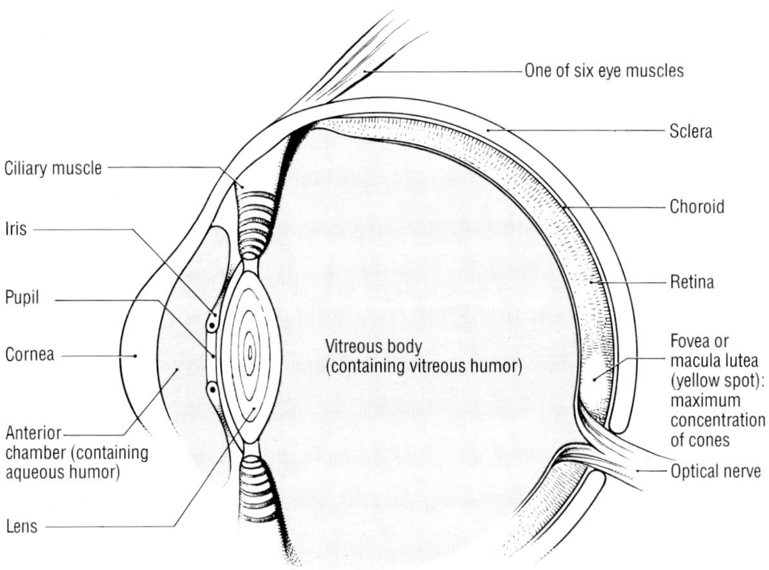

Fig. 1.3 Anatomy of the eye

1.3 Functioning of the eye

1.3.1 The imaging mechanism

The projection of an image of the environment through the cornea onto the retina obeys the laws of geometrical optics [1.5, 1.1], as shown in Fig. 1.4. The various optical media of the eye have the following refractive indices: cornea 1.38, aqueous humor 1.34, lens 1.44. Since the density of the eye roughly corresponds to that of water, the critical angle for total reflection can be calculated to be 48° 40′. In principle an image can be produced by the outer surface of the cornea alone. However, the lens in the eye permits light to be refracted to varying degrees, which in turn permits focusing on near and distant objects. The total refracting power of the healthy eye is about 48 diopters, and the capacity to vary this by means of the lens is known as the *amplitude of accommodation.* In young people the amplitude of accommodation is around 12 diopters; with increasing age (usually between 50 and 60) it approaches one diopter [1.6].

1.3.2 Aberrations in image production

As is generally the case in optics, the eye suffers from certain common lens aberrations. Spherical aberration, which leads to peripheral rays being more powerfully refracted than central rays resulting in a barrel-shaped distortion, is corrected to a large extent by the diaphragm action of the pupil. Chromatic aberration (color distortion), due to more powerful refraction of blue rays than red rays, is mitigated by the effect of the onion-like structure of the lens with

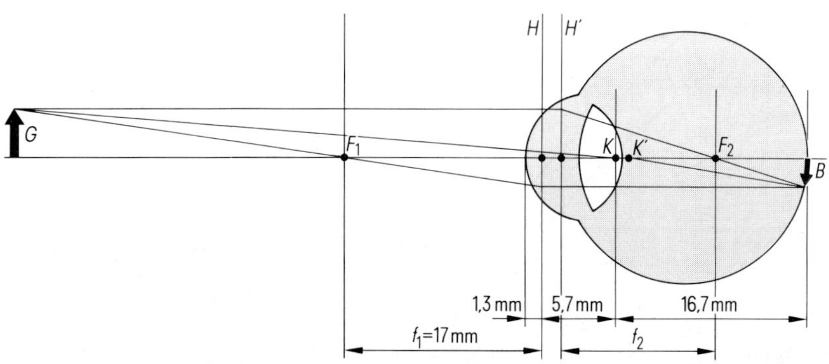

G object size
B size of image on retina
F_1 primary focal point
F_2 secondary focal point
H primary principal plane
H' secondary principal plane
K primary nodal point
K' secondary nodal point
f_1 primary focal length
f_2 secondary focal length

Fig. 1.4 Geometrical optics of the eye

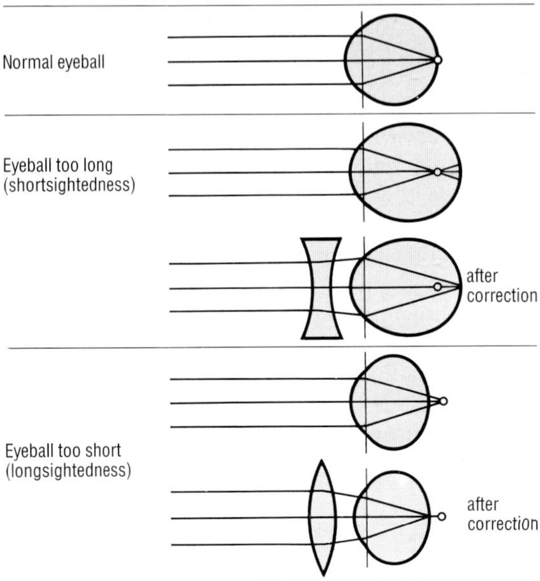

Fig. 1.5
Visual defects produced when eyeball is too long or too short, and means of correction

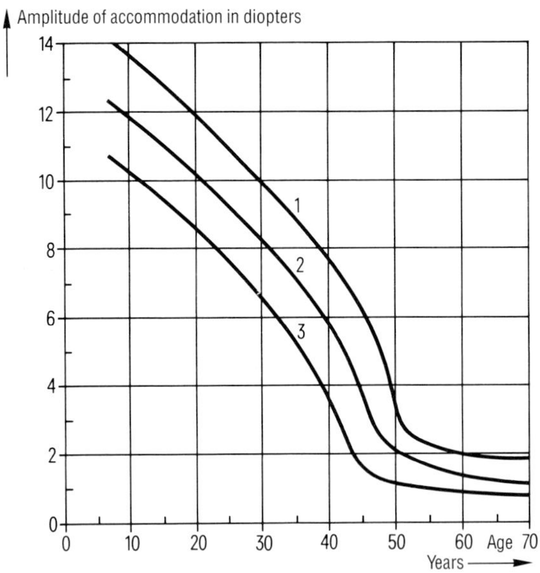

1 Upper limit
2 Mean
3 Lower limit (in case of normal vision)

Fig. 1.6
Age-dependence of the amplitude of accommodation (difference between the refracting power of the lens when looking at near and distant objects) according to GRAFF

Refractive power $= \frac{1}{\text{focal length}}$

(Unit: $m^{-1} = \text{dptr}$)

its layers of different refractive index (the inner layers refract more powerfully than the outer layers). When colored objects are observed, difficulties in accommodation can occur if the object lies in a plane close to the eye, because the eye tries to accommodate in turn to the colors with shorter or longer wavelengths. When the object is further away, this effect does not arise because of the greater depth of field.

1.3.3 Eye defects

Figure 1.5 shows that a sharp image is formed on the retina of an eye with normal vision.

In the case of an eyeball which is too long (shortsighted) or too short (longsighted), the image is formed in a plane in front of or behind the retina. A sharp image can therefore only be achieved by means of correction with appropriate lenses (glasses or contact lenses). Apart from the decrease in amplitude of accommodation due to the loss of lens elasticity associated with increasing age (as illustrated in Fig. 1.6), clouding of the lens or of the aqueous humor can cause sight to deteriorate.

1.3.4 The accommodation process

Focusing an image on the retina is achieved by changing the refractive power of the lens. This is done by contraction or relaxation of the ring-shaped ciliary muscle (see Fig. 1.3) so that the lens is compressed or stretched radially. The process is controlled by the nerve cells of the oculomotor center in the brain which adjusts the refractive power of the lens until the *size of the image reaches a minimum.*

1.3.5 Eye movements

With the help of the eye muscles shown in Fig. 1.7, the eye is moved until the image of the object to be observed is located at the point of *maximum resolving power* (smallest spatial resolution) on the retina (viz. the fovea: see Fig. 1.3). As can be seen from Fig. 1.10 (p. 29), this point has the highest cone density. The process is subject to continuous control, because the eye moves its optical axis in relation to the object observed until the *number of stimulated cones* reaches a maximum. As in any control process, there is permanent adjustment towards an optimum value, i.e. the axis of the eye is moving constantly to and fro. In order to maintain this maximum stimulation, the eye continually makes oscillatory movements (saccades) in all directions. Such movements are also carried out in a resting state (with the eyes open) at a frequency of approximately 10 Hz.

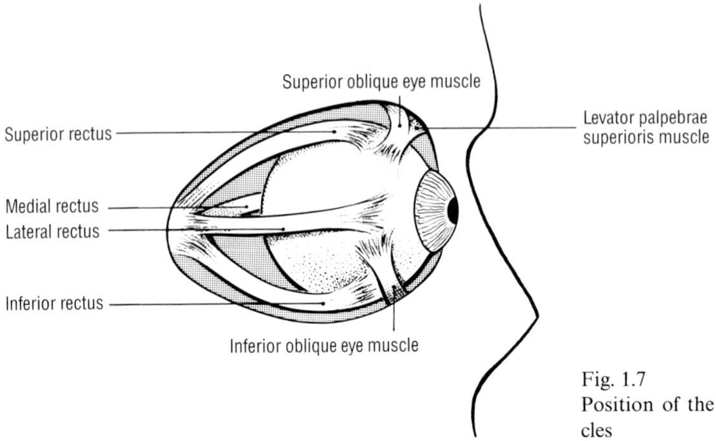

Fig. 1.7
Position of the eye muscles

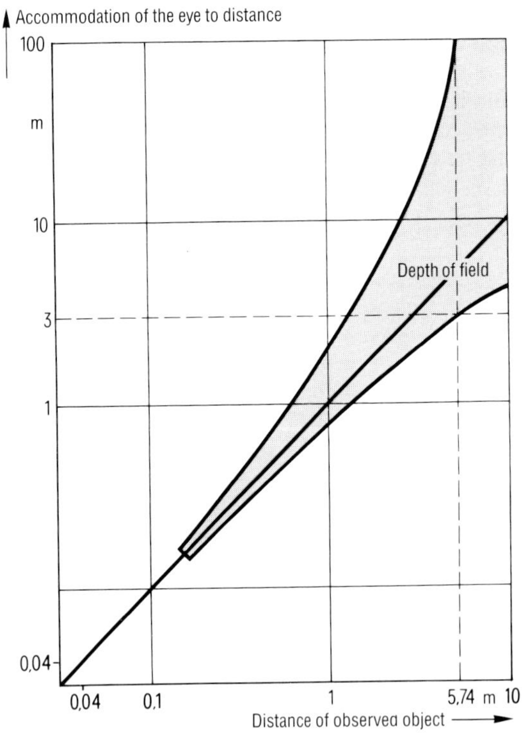

Fig. 1.8
Depth of field in relation to accommodation (depth of field of the human eye with medium pupil diameter). Accommodation to a distance of 5.74 m gives the ability to see in focus at distances between 3 m and infinity: fixed-focus setting (according to Ranke in [1.1])

1.3.6 Depth of field

The eye's depth of field depends on the same parameters as does any ordinary optical apparatus. That is, it depends on the diameter of the pupil (aperture) and on the degree of accommodation (depth adjustment). As Fig. 1.8 shows, in the case of medium pupil diameter and accommodation to a distance of 5.74 m, everything from 3 m to infinity is seen in focus [1.1].

1.4 Conversion of light into neural impulses

1.4.1 Anatomy of the retina

As Fig. 1.3 shows, the retina lines the inside of the rear half of the eyeball. It contains the photosensitive rods and cones as well as the nerve cells [1.4] which preprocess optical information. Figure 1.9 shows a diagram of a microscopic portion of the retina with all the optically active elements. From the

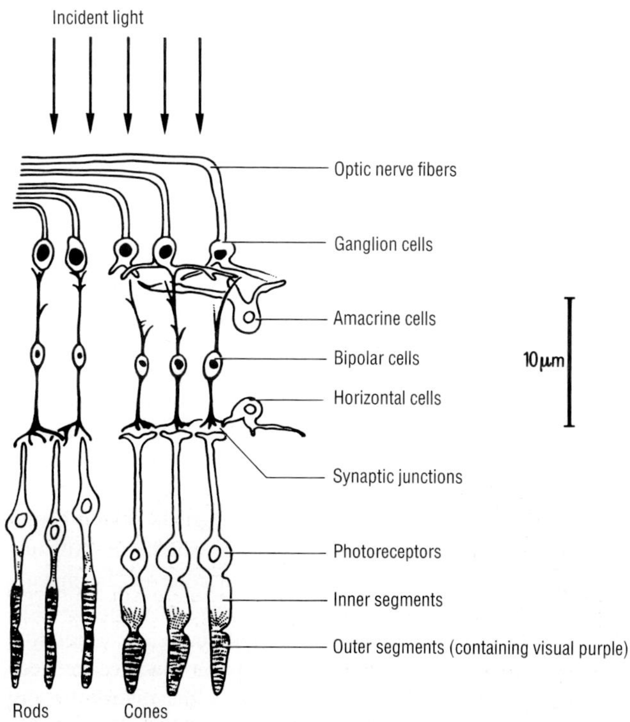

Fig. 1.9
Diagrammatic representation of the structure and relative position of the active elements of the retina

diagram it is clear that the photosensitive outer segments of the rods and cones which contain the visual purple [1.7] are turned away from the light and are partially submerged in the pigment layer (not shown). This means that the effect of scattered light is reduced and that the sensitive elements are protected from overexposure to light by creeping into the pigment layer.

The visual purple (1.8), derived as it is from vitamin A, is stored in the outer segments of the cones; it is decomposed by the absorption of light, the cleavage molecules producing an impulse which is passed on by the photoreceptors to the bipolar cells via synaptic junctions. The connection of several photoreceptors to one bipolar cell forms the *receptive field* [1.9]. Every ray of light that hits one of the receptor cells in such a group stimulates the nerve cells connected to them in such a way that those at the edge have an inhibitory effect whilst those at the center have an excitatory effect (or more rarely, the other way round). With increasing light intensity, however, the activity changes in that the amount of inhibition becomes greater. In this way the difference between light (excitation) and dark (inhibition) is reinforced. The impulses travel from the bipolar cells via further synaptic junctions to the ganglion cells and optic nerve fibers, which transmit them to the brain.

1.4.2 Spatial resolution

Visual acuity

Two points are only recognized as being separate entities when the images on the retina are so far apart that an unstimulated cone or receptive field happens to be located between the two. The bigger the receptive elements, therefore, the greater will be the distance required between the two images in order for them still to be seen separately, and the spatial resolution of the eye will be correspondingly worse. In medicine this is called the visual acuity [1.1] and is related to the angle between two light rays which can still just be told apart. As is clear from Fig. 1.10, the width of a cone in the macula lutea is about 3 μm, so that taking into account the laws governing image formation in the eye, there is a maximum possible visual acuity corresponding to 50 arc seconds. From Fig. 1.10 it is also clear that the distance between cones in the outer regions of the retina increases giving the distribution of visual acuity over the retina shown. Only in a narrow range of 5°, corresponding to the extent of the macula lutea, can the maximal visual acuity therefore be achieved.

Vernier acuity

Whilst the visual acuity of the eye is already very high, an even greater resolving power is possible under certain conditions, namely when lines, rather than two points, have to be distinguished. As shown in Fig. 1.10, the eye detects the break in a line due to a slightly offset continuation because the cones (or rather, the nerve cells connected to them) are all interlinked and can tell if on average more cones are being stimulated after the break (from the other half of the image) than before the break. By means of statistical evaluation of the distribution of the stimulated cones, the nervous system can recognize distances between lines which are even smaller than the distances detected in conditions of maximum visual acuity. This fact has long been known in the engineering workshop and is used when reading the Vernier scale on measuring instruments, which has led to the name 'Vernier acuity'. In summary it should be emphasized that the nature of the neural processing mechanisms means that visual acuity also depends on the shape of the object perceived.

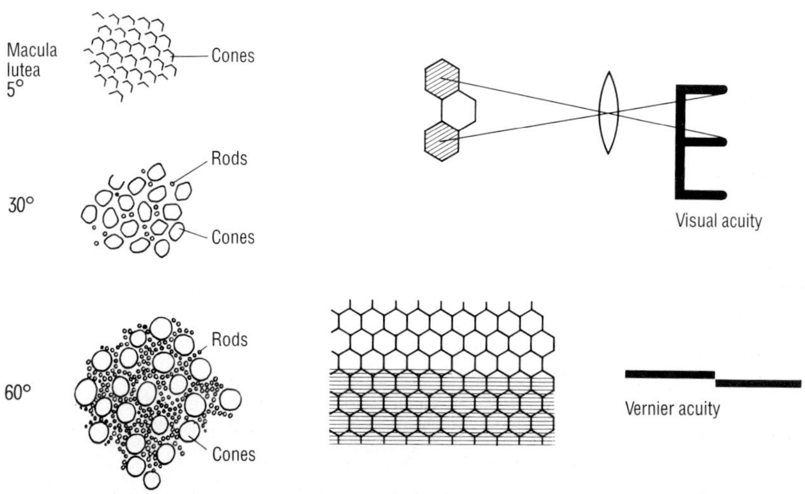

Fig. 1.10 Diagram of the rods and cones at the fovea (macula lutea) and in sections of the retina separated by an arc of 30 degrees and 60 degrees respectively from the macula. In the macula lutea there are only cones; towards the periphery both rods and cones are found, with cones becoming progressively less numerous and rods more numerous. The diagram is copied from a microphotograph. Next to it are shown the mechanisms for visual acuity and Vernier acuity. See text for details

1.4.3 Contrast resolution

Differential sensitivity

In principle one might expect that a minimum increase can be found in the brightness of an object which will produce a minimum increase in the magnitude of the eye's sensory experience. This assumption has proved to be correct, with one qualification: the minimal increase in the magnitude of the sensory experience depends upon the level of background illumination at the time. According to the Weber-Fechner law, the magnitude of the sensory experience E increases logarithmically with the stimulus intensity R according to the equation

$$E = K \ln R/R_0$$

in which, according to Fechner [1.1], K is a constant and R_0 the original stimulus intensity. If, following the practice in technical fields [1.10], the logarithmic value of the light intensity is plotted on the ordinate and the magnitude of the sensory experience is plotted on the abscissa, the graph shown in

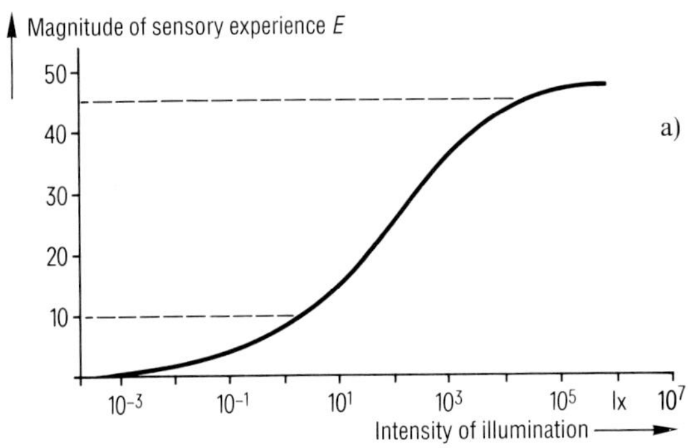

a) The magnitude of sensory experience E is represented along the ordinate as the function $K \ln^{R}/R_0$ for the example of the eye. According to the graph, the eye can distinguish 50 equally-spaced levels of sensory experience. Of these, roughly 35 lie in the linear region

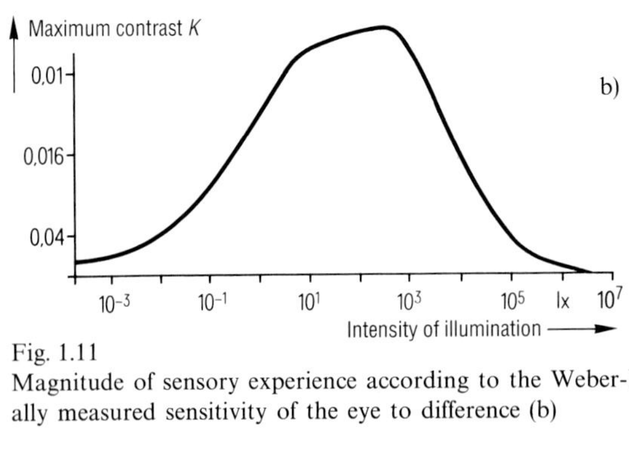

b) This graph shows the actual sensitivity of the eye to difference as measured by experiment. If the Weber-Fechner law were to hold exactly (rising straight line in a)) this curve (taken from Ranke [1.1]) would be parallel to the x-axis

Fig. 1.11
Magnitude of sensory experience according to the Weber-Fechner law (a) and the actually measured sensitivity of the eye to difference (b)

Fig. 1.11a is obtained. At the point where the graph climbs most steeply, the contrast sensitivity is high; where the graph is flat, the contrast sensitivity is low. In the top area glare is said to occur whilst in the bottom area the stimulus is said to be below threshold. Fig. 1.11b shows the differential quotient, i.e. the contrast sensitivity.

Glare

As explained in the last paragraph, the term glare [1.11] means the reduction to zero of the contrast sensitivity as a consequence of being exposed to such great light intensity that one no longer sees anything but 'brightness'. This definition, however, fails to encompass all the phenomena and causes of glare. Glare also occurs locally, if next to a brightly lit portion of the retina the strongly stimulated cones there inhibit their weakly stimulated neighbors. In this way this area of the retina falls beneath the stimulus threshold and can no longer detect any differences in brightness. Such an effect is reinforced even more by the scattered light [1.12] emanating from a bright ray of light in the not completely clear media of the eye, especially of the vitreous body. This scattered light obscures the tiny differences in brightness of the weakly illuminated surroundings of a bright spot on the retina.

Simultaneous contrast

The mutual coupling of the rods and cones described previously, which is associated with a mutual promotion or inhibition of stimulation, is known as lateral enhancement or inhibition, as the case may be. It is the cause of the fact that a brightly illuminated spot on the retina inhibits the cells around it; by so doing the difference in brightness of the stimulus, and with it the sensory experience, is reinforced. The end result is therefore always a neural enhancement in the perceived contrast, an effect which is demonstrated in Fig. 1.12.

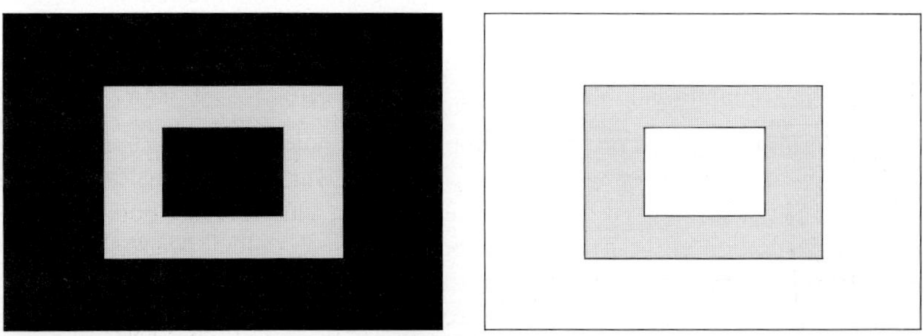

Fig. 1.12
An example of simultaneous contrast. The same gray rectangle appears darker on a white background and lighter on a black background

Successive contrast

Since in the case of pictures presented one after another the neural enhancement in the perceived contrast cannot occur because of the lack of inhibition, the contrast sensitivity is less than in the case of simultaneous contrast.

Contrast gradient (definition)

The transition from a bright to a dark area of a picture normally takes place gradually so that a contrast gradient can be defined as the decrease in brightness over the appropriate distance in the image. Should this distance reach dimensions comparable to those of the diameter of a cone, it will lie beneath visual acuity and the physical contrast gradient can be ignored. In such a case it is only the physiological mechanisms for the perception of contrast which are involved, so that any further improvement in definition using technical means does not make sense. Besides these considerations, the problems mentioned in connection with glare play an important role, especially when the change in the level of brightness is very large.

1.4.4 Adaptation

Spatial resolution, the detection of contrast and the perception of definition i.e. the mechanisms which are necessary for producing image quality, are extremely dependent on the eye's adjustment to brightness, known as adaptation [1.13]. This process can be described as follows: when bright light hits the eye, the visual purple in the cones is decomposed. The breakdown products give rise to stimulation. At the same time, however, the visual purple is reconstituted at a quite specific rate and is once more available for the visual process. When illumination starts, the breakdown process predominates, so that there is intense stimulation. With the onset of the reconstitution processes, a situation of equilibrium develops in which breakdown and reconstitution are exactly in balance. The breakdown products available at this stage are naturally smaller in number than during the initial illumination of the eye, which leads to a decrease in stimulation as shown in Fig. 1.13.

This description is based on the assumption that a potential (the receptor potential) arises at the sensory receptors (see Fig. 1.9) which is proportional to the intensity of the stimulus, if there is no adaptation. This receptor potential triggers the formation of the nerve action potential. Such potentials are temporary fluctuations in the electric potential of the nerve cell membrane with a duration of 1 ms and a constant amplitude of around 90 mV. The mechanism by which this potential is produced can be explained by the change in permeability of the membrane to sodium ions. These migrate from the region outside the cell into it, leaving behind a negative charge. This negative charge is, however,

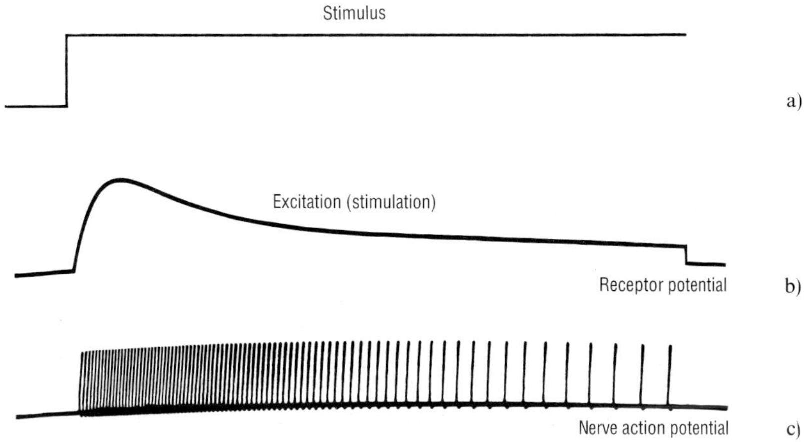

Fig. 1.13
The receptor potential (b) and the number of nerve action potentials (c) as a result of stimulation (a)

very quickly compensated by the exchange of potassium ions. Energy-consuming processes (sodium – potassium ion pump) finally ensure that the previous ion distribution is restored. By these means the intensity of the simulation is encoded into the frequency of the impulse train. The greater the stimulation, the more frequently action potentials are produced. This is the form in which the stimulation is conducted over long distances by individual nerve fibers.

The decrease in this stimulation is called adaptation. In this process the eye adapts itself to the average brightness of its surroundings. The process of adaptation is additionally reinforced by the mechanism of cone migration, by which cones which have been overexposed to light bury themselves in the pigment epithelium of the retina. These two processes take place in a time span of minutes, whereas the pupil reaction leads to fast adjustment. Here, depending on the total combined brightness of the retina, the amount of contraction in the sphincter muscle in the iris is varied so that the pupil narrows in bright light and dilates in darkness. Since when looking at nearby objects only a portion of the total brightness of the surroundings is observed, the amount of light which enters the eye is reduced. The pupil then dilates automatically, in conjunction with the process of accommodation. As previously indicated, adaptation must be understood as the eye's adjustment to the available brightness. Thus if one plots the intensity of nervous excitation as a function of the logarithm of the light intensity, the set of graphs shown in Fig. 1.14 is obtained. It shows the relevant function as a function of brightness without adaptation and with adaptation (the latter is illustrated by the unbroken lines). The eye's contrast sensitivity is greatest where the curves are steepest. The figure shows clearly that by means of adaptation the contrast sensitivity is

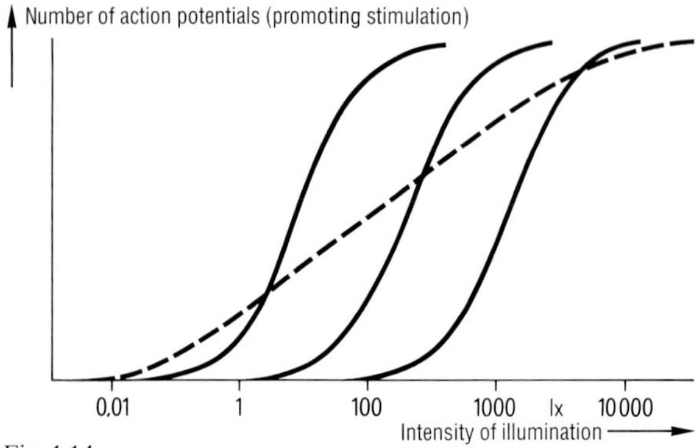

Fig. 1.14
If one enters the value of the initial overshoot as a function of the stimulus strength, one obtains the dynamic characteristics (intensity functions) of the receptor (non-adapted state). Entering the steady-state values gives the static characteristics (adapted state). These are identical to the measurements of KÖNIG and BRODHUHN. It can be seen that at the beginning of the adaptation process the characteristics slope steeply upwards, i.e. the contrast sensitivity improves. In this way the eye is able to detect 485 difference steps as opposed to 35 originally. This improvement shows the real importance of adaptation (from Ranke [1.1])

adjusted to the average brightness. The transition from one level of adaptation to another follows a particular pattern in time. This is illustrated in Fig. 1.15 and shows that at least two processes must be involved. The first part of the curve corresponds to the adaptation of the rods, the second to that of the cones. The two together result in the shape of the curve. As already shown, visual acuity depends on the grid size of the photosensitive cells on the retina. Only at the spot where vision is sharpest, the so-called macula lutea, does every sensory cell have a nerve fiber leading away from it, and thus only here is the maximum visual acuity found. At all other places on the retina several sensory cells are connected to one nerve cell in order to improve the light yield. This group of sensory cells is called a receptive field. The field's peripheral elements generally have an inhibitive function, with the result that a stimulated central part comes to be surrounded by an inhibiting ring, enhancing the contrast. As the intensity of light diminishes the inhibiting ring gets narrower and narrower, i.e. the receptive field becomes larger and thus visual acuity progressively deteriorates. A very great decrease in visual acuity also occurs during the transition from cone vision to rod vision as a consequence of dark adaptation, caused by the lack of rods in the macula lutea. Thus the birghtness of an object is also determined by its diameter. Figure 1.16 illustrates this relationship between light intensity and object diameter.

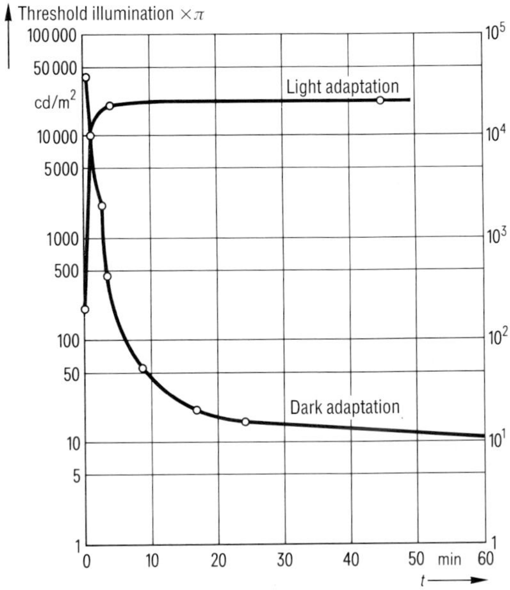

Fig. 1.15
Dark-adaptation and light-adaptation curves of the human eye measured with the Engelking adaptometer, with the threshold illumination (threshold stimulus intensity) along the y axis and the time elapsed after the initial change in illumination along the x axis. Notice the break in the dark-adaptation curve which is determined by the completion of the cones' adaptation (extra curve plotted). Evidence for the Duplicity Theory of Vision

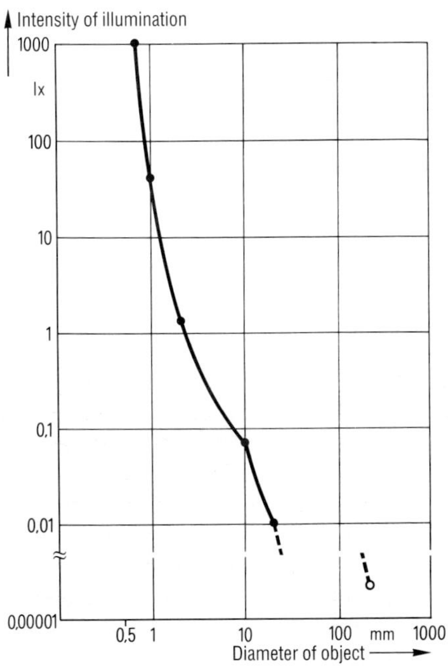

Fig. 1.16
Curve of equal sensation of brightness. According to Ricco's Law, in the area of low illumination the same experience of brightness corresponds not to radiation intensity but to the product of intensity and test field size. This dependence on the test field diameter has a strong effect on visual acuity, as shown in the figure. The break in the curve again corresponds to the transition from cone to rod vision. Distance of object 6 m, diameter of object in mm

1.4.5 Sensitivity to color

It is known empirically that the rods are responsible for the monochromatic light-dark sensitivity whilst the cones are responsible for color perception [1.14, 1.8]. The perception thresholds for the various colors can be read off from the graph in Fig. 1.17, which shows the spectral sensitivity of individual rods and cones. The threshold energy indicated in Fig. 1.17 is necessary in order to bring about the process of chemical decomposition of the visual purple. This relationship is consistent with the theory of color vision proposed by Helmholtz. This describes the presence of three different kinds of color receptors having maximum sensitivity in the red, yellow-green and green-blue bands of the light spectrum respectively. The individual color components are mixed

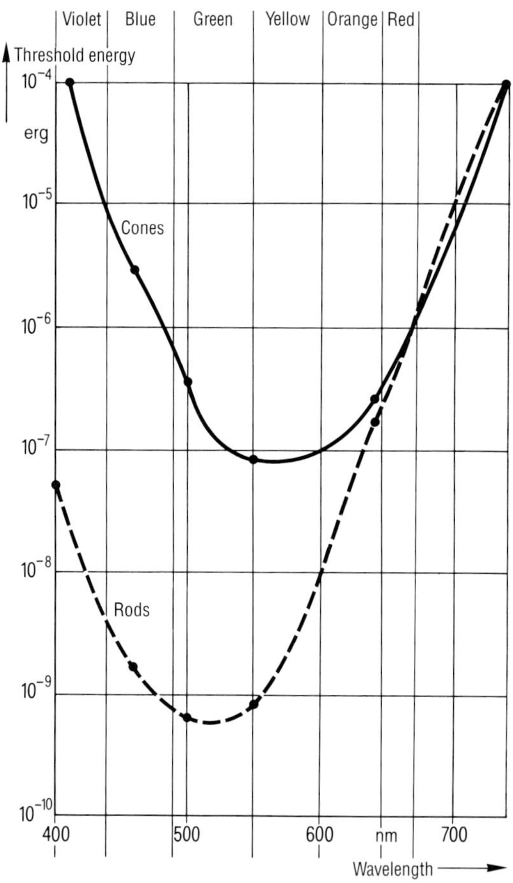

Fig. 1.17
Graphs of threshold intensities of monochromatic light for the human eye. The lower graph relates to scotopic (rod) vision, the upper graph to photopic (cone) vision. The absolute threshold (with the eye completely adapted, at a wavelength of 507 nanometers in the yellow-green region) has a value of 1.3 to 2.6×10^{-10} erg (plotted according to measurements by Trendelenburg [1.1])

in various ways to produce the familiar experiences of color. About 10 million shades of color can be distinguished. It should also be mentioned that equally intense stimulation of all three color components leads to the experience of white – or, if the stimulation is less, the various shades of gray. Following on from this, Granit has developed a second hypothesis of color perception in which he proposes that the experience of color is due to both stimulation and inhibition of the particular color receptors. Thus, inhibition will always yield the complementary color of the color receptors stimulated. This has a great impact on color contrast, since lateral enhancement and inhibition also apply to color perception. The eye's spectral sensitivity as shown in Fig. 1.18 therefore only applies to large illuminated areas of the retina, in which the neural connections to neighboring cells do not play a role.

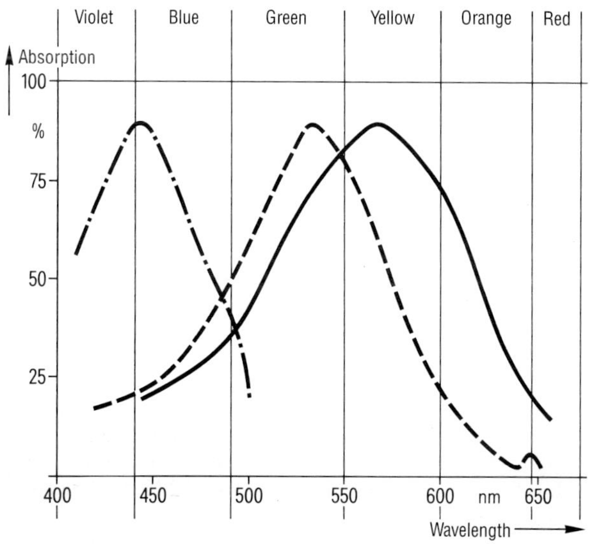

Fig. 1.18
Young-Helmholtz three component theory of color vision. This assumes that there are three receptor substances which exhibit the displayed rates of absorption (y axis) for various wavelengths of light (x axis). The strongest evidence for this theory is the clinical observation of protanopia (malfunction of the first receptor – red-green blindness or red-green deficiency), deuteranopia (second receptor) and tritanopia (third receptor). The spectral sensitivity of the human eye is in agreement with this representation

1.4.6 Temporal resolution

Absence of flicker (fusion frequency)

TALBOT was able to establish that two flashes of light lead to a single sensory experience if the time period between them is so short that the impulses provoked by the first stimulus have not decreased by more than 10 percent by the time the second stimulus is given. Because of this, it is possible to show the eye series of individual pictures which are experienced as continuously moving pictures, as in the cinema. The necessary frequency is about 16 to 26 pictures a second; it depends on the overall level of brightness and on the angle made with the optical axis. This is because the sensory cells on the periphery of the retina react more quickly to stimulation than the ones in the center. In addition, as Fig. 1.19 shows, the delayed response to brightness is determined by the state of adaptation, which means that even fairly slow series of pictures merge into a smoothly moving picture if seen in a state of dark adaptation. Such a dependence of the temporal resolving power of the eye on the average intensity of the surrounding light is of great importance in the presentation of cinematographic images.

Integration time (response time) τ

Electrophysiological investigations have shown that, when the eye is illuminated, the neural excitation E caused by the decomposition of visual purple (see Sect. 1.4.1) [1.8] increases exponentially according to the formula $E=1-e^{-t/T}$ [1.13] and decreases according to the formula $E=e^{-t/T'}$. The time constants T and T' are of the same order of magnitude. After the time $t=3\,T$, the degree of excitation reaches 95% of its final value, a value at which perception is practically complete. In about the same length of time $t=3\,T'$ the stimulation has decayed. The integration time $\tau\approx 3\,T\approx 3\,T'$ is the length of time from the start of the stimulation up to attaining full perception, or alternatively from the termination of the light stimulus up to the cessation of the perception. The integration time τ depends upon the state of adaptation, the intensity of the light stimulus and the amount of visual purple available. The latter can be assumed to be constant in the healthy eye. τ can take values from 100 to 300 ms in the dark-adapted (scotopic) eye and from 15 to 100 ms in the light-adapted (photopic) eye.

Movement threshold

Closely connected with the response time and the decay time is the ability of the eye to perceive motion. For the experience of motion to occur the stimulation of a cone must have decreased by more than 10% of its total by the time the stimulation of the neighboring cone reaches its maximum. Apart from the decay rate of the degree of stimulation (which depends on the intensity of the illumination), the spatial threshold naturally plays an important role in relation to the movement threshold.

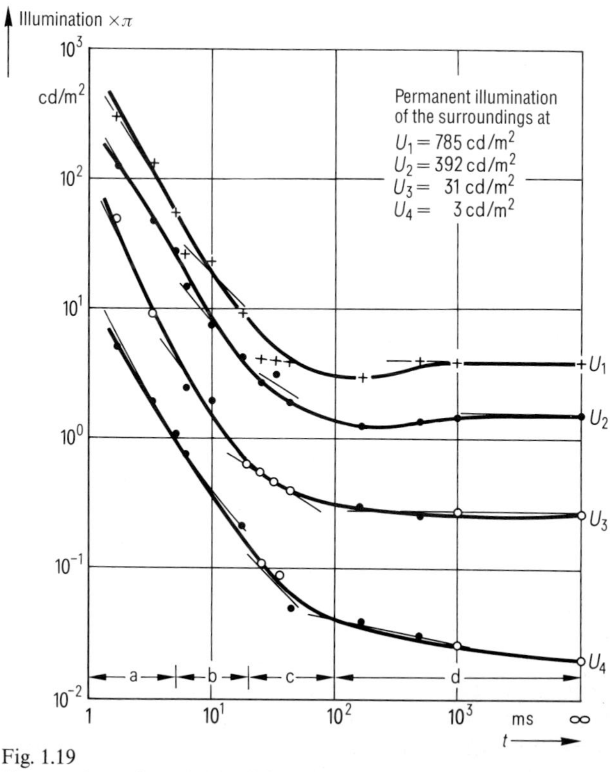

Fig. 1.19
Curves of equal sensation of brightness as a consequence of the human eye's delayed response to brightness. The curves represent equal intensity of sensation corresponding to permanent illumination with the specified luminances of the surroundings (3 to 785 cd/m²). If the period of illumination is reduced (x axis), the intensity of illumination must be increased. The relationship is nonlinear. In region a) the quantities are related by $Lt^2 = k$, in region b) by $Lt = k$, in region c) for higher values of the luminance of the surroundings the relationship is $Lt_0 = L = k$, for lower values this only holds in region d). Generally one has $Lt = f(t)$. Taking the average one arrives at a value of 50 ms for the response time of the human eye at average illumination intensities (according to Commichau [1.15])

1.5 Neural processing

1.5.1 Anatomy of the visual pathway

Impulses from the retinal photoreceptors are led to the cerebral cortex by way of the path shown in Fig. 1.20 (which includes several switching centers). Corresponding connections between the nerve fibers result in the above-mentioned receptive fields, which become more and more complex as the visual pathway progresses. The receptive field neurons located in the cortex are finally able to recognize objects independently of their location and orientation in space (constancy of visual objects). All these mechanisms provide the neural basis for the "perception of form".

1.5.2 Three-dimensional vision

The visual pathways of both eyes reach the visual centers in the cerebral cortex both directly and crossed over. Impulses from both eyes therefore enter both halves of the cerebral cortex. The image is of course somewhat different in the two eyes according to whether an object lies in front of the observed point object (fixation point) or behind it. As can be seen from the diagram (Fig. 1.21), near points on an object give rise to a bitemporally displaced image (displaced

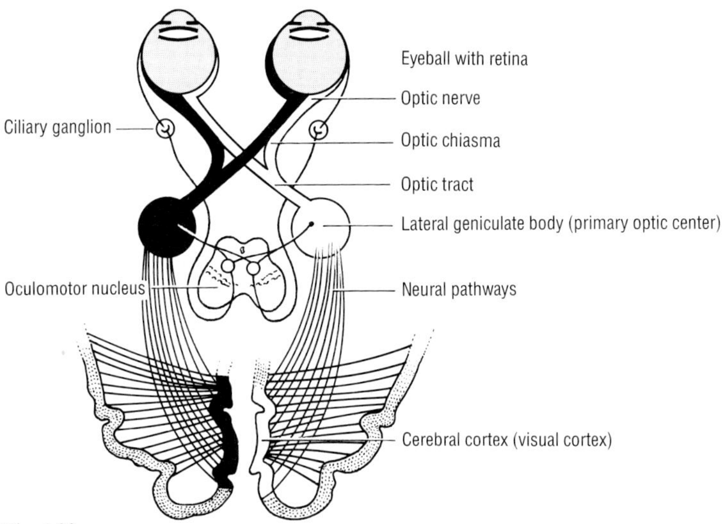

Fig. 1.20
Diagram of the visual pathway. Left visual field black, right visual field white. The nerve pathways are indicated by lines

on both sides towards the temples). Points further away on the other hand produce binasally displaced image points (i.e. displaced on both sides towards the nose). Information about the displacement (binocular disparity) [1.1] is processed by the nerve cells in the visual cortex to give an impression of distance. Such an impression always relates to the point object actually focussed on. The point object lies on the horopter plane, the geometrical locus of all point objects which, given a constant degree of accommodation, form a sharp image in the eye.

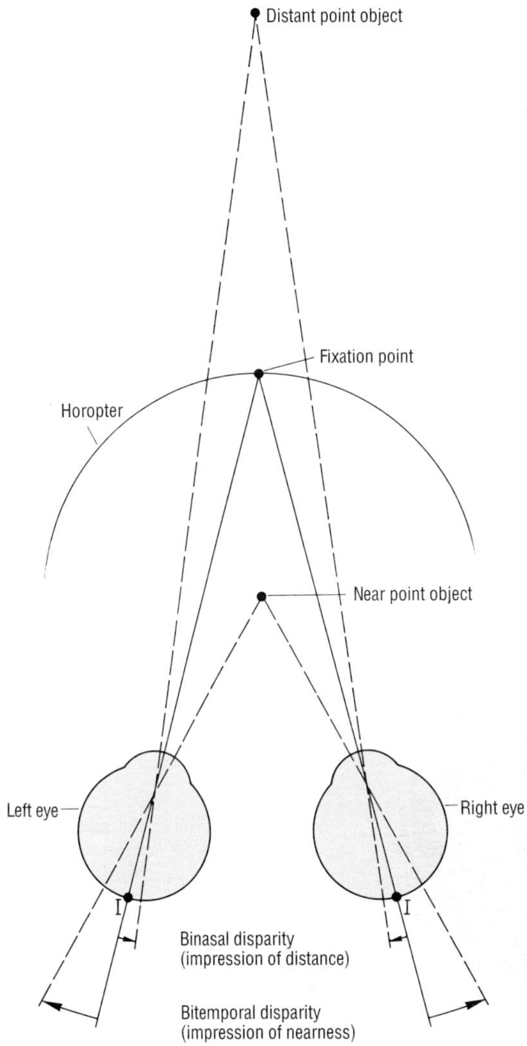

Fig. 1.21
Principle of three-dimensional vision. Whilst convergence and accommodation of the eyes are trained on a point on the horopter, the light rays from a near or distant object also form images which are laterally displaced in relation to the identical points I in the eye. This displacement (binocular disparity) is binasal in the case of distant objects and bitemporal in the case of near objects and is interpreted in the brain so as to give three-dimensional perception

1.5.3 Depth perception

In the previous section the horopter plane for a fixed degree of accommodation was described. This corresponds to a fixed convergence angle, i.e. a fixed angle between the two optical axes. What two-dimensional shape the horopter plane takes at varying distances from the eye has not yet been established. Investigations by Kienle [1.19] and Hensel [1.20] indicate that the perception of size and the related constancy of visual objects depend on the shape of the horopter plane. In physiology, the constancy of visual objects means the recognition of the size of known objects irrespective of their distance from the eye. In the case of three-dimensional vision this causes the difficulty that on a two-dimensional surface a spatial image is produced in which the individual image points are no longer in accordance with the natural proportions.

1.5.4 Optical illusions

Neuronal connection and visual memory play an important role in image processing. Thus the eye is able to recognize known image patterns quickly and to classify them correctly irrespective of their size, position and intensity of illumination. Even in the case of incomplete information patterns, it is always complete pictures which are seen. Such complementary neural processes can lead to considerable illusions [1.17] and mistaken interpretations of reality. Fig. 1.22 gives an example of this; it shows in particular how the interpretation of the observed object is influenced by information about its surroundings [1.18].

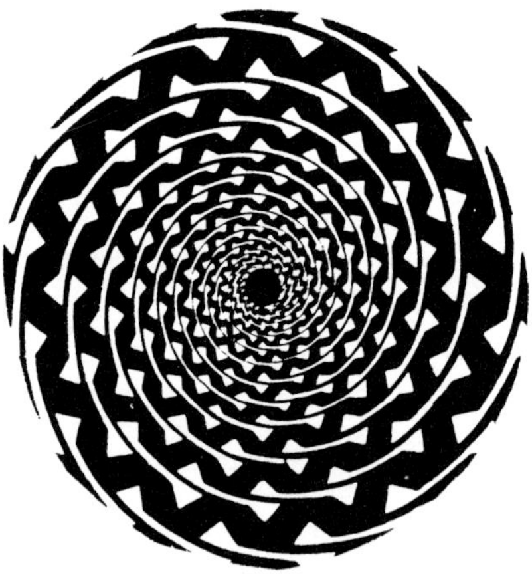

Fig. 1.22
An optical illusion of the second kind. The concentric circles are seen as arithmetic spirals. This is a consequence of the oblique shading of the circles themselves and the sloping of the shading in relation to the radially-orientated background pattern. The example shows the influence of the surroundings on perception

1.5.5 Visual memory

Afterimages

When a bright ray of light stimulates an area of the retina, visual purple is broken down at that point. When the illumination has finished the impulses produced die away gradually because of the prolonged decay time leaving behind a positive afterimage. On the other hand, fewer impulses are produced at the retina by the breakdown products of the visual purple when looking at a white wall, and the afterimage is therefore a negative one. Such afterimages are also features of color perception; in this case a negative afterimage always appears in the complementary color.

Short-term memory

Inside the higher processing centers there also exists an after-excitation (postexcitation effect) or continuation of the pattern of impulses, so that pictures can still be perceived up to several seconds later. This phenomenon, which is very marked in persons with photographic memory, is the short-term visual memory. It disappears after a short time but in certain circumstances causes the generation of memory contents which are distinctive in that they can, if necessary, be transformed into a consciously recognizable picture. The whole process is based upon a re-coding of impulse patterns into chemical changes located in the brain (long-term memory).

Recognition

In ways which still have not been investigated, the representation of an image causes the corresponding image pattern (stored in the long-term memory) to be transformed into a pattern of stimulation which, when compared with the new image, is recognized as being identical to it. Such recognition of images from the past is possible irrespective of other environmental parameters.

The nature of the images thus formed in the imagination has not yet been elucidated even though they appear to correlate with electrophysiological measurements [1.21].

2 Quantitative assessment of image quality

In order to produce images of the human body, medical technology employs almost all kinds of radiation capable of penetrating different types of tissue and at the same time interacting with it to an extent that can be measured. The radiation field modulated by the object is measured by a sensor which usually has a large area and as a rule undergoes a series of transformation processes. The end result of this process always produces a gray tone or color tone distribution, i.e. an image capable of being viewed. This transformation of physically different primary variables into a physically uniform representation represents the ideal of finding a uniform description of the properties of an image or imaging system.

The concept "image quality" can only be defined within the framework of medical diagnostics. Thus, for example, purely from the technical point of view, the brightened area behind a cyst in an ultrasound image is dismissed as image distortion or an artifact whereas for the doctor, it provides valuable diagnostic information. Therefore, from the technical point of view, at best, it is possible to quantify the assessment of individual image quality characteristics such as spatial resolution (image definition), image contrast, image noise and distortion; however, the relative value of each characteristic must be determined by the user.

The user of an imaging system is primarily interested in a method for evaluating the image quality which can be achieved with his system. However, the system designer, in addition to this, is interested in a comparison of the transfer characteristics of the successive stages of his imaging system. Such a comparison of different links in the imaging chain, often based on different physical effects, should help him to find the weakest link in this chain since in the process of continuous technical optimization, improving the weakest link in the chain holds out most promise of success.

The following considerations show that the two key characteristics for image quality "spatial resolution" and "image contrast", can both be derived from the modulation transfer function MTF. On the other hand, other criteria must be used to assess other characteristics such as distortion or image noise.

Recently, methods which attempt to evaluate the perceptibility of predefined test structures in the image (ROC curves, contrast detail diagram) are making a comeback. They make it possible to evaluate the system from medically relevant points of view, involving the observer and depart from the above-mentioned abstract and non-specific equipment characteristics. It is especially clear here, how important it is for the doctor to be already involved in the design of the evaluation procedure, since, if inappropriate test objects are used, the wrong criteria would be used for evaluating the system. However, the experimental costs of these methods prevent them from being applied on a large scale. In addition, they are only suitable for comparing similar imaging systems. They do not allow the designer to make the important comparison of the individual consecutive elements in the imaging chain.

2.1 Description of image quality in the borderline case of negligible image noise

In an abstract and idealized sense, an imaging system transfers a given spatial function $G(x, y)$ lying in a plane, the object plane, more or less error-free to an image plane.

We shall denote the image function by $B(x', y')$, in brief $B = A(G)$. G stands for the object and B for the image. Examples of object and image are the x-ray intensity distribution (ray relief) in front of a fluorescent screen, the light density distribution behind the screen, the electron density distribution behind the photocathode of an x-ray image intensifier, etc. (In order to take a specific example, it will always be assumed, however, that $G(x, y)$ and $B(x', y')$ are light densities. For the sake of simplicity, the imaging scale factor should always be taken as 1).

If image distortions due to noise are largely absent, the image quality can be given a complete description using the MTF in many cases. For this, two conditions should be required of the system: linearity and spatial invariance.

Linearity condition

For every real number $\alpha \geq 0$, we must have

$$A(\alpha G) = \alpha A(G). \tag{2.1}$$

If, for instance, an object $\tilde{G}$ is α times as bright as a given object G, its image $A(\tilde{G})$ too, should be α times as bright as $A(G)$.

In addition, for two objects G_1 and G_2, which are superimposed in the object plane, the image $A(G_1 + G_2)$ is produced as the superimposition of the images.

$A(G_1)$ and $A(G_2)$:

$$A(G_1+G_2)=A(G_1)+A(G_2) \tag{2.2}$$

Spatial invariance condition (displacement invariance)

If the object G is shifted in the object plane without deforming its object function, the image must be shifted in the same way.

The linearity and spatial invariance conditions are only approximately satisfied in real systems. Thus, the linearity condition is always only valid within certain modulation limits. For example, in photographic imaging, it can only be regarded as given when the signal fluctuations are small compared to the modulation range of the film. Here, the imaging quality is also influenced by the steepness of the characteristic, the fog as the lower limit and the shoulder as the upper limit, i.e. by the system dynamics. The spatial invariance condition is already permanently violated because all imaging systems only represent a limited area, the object field. Thus, at best, the MTF can be used without any restrictions to assess an imaging system in the central image area; it fails at the edge of the image. However, geometrical imaging errors, such as distortion, astigmatism or coma, also represent violations of the spatial invariance condition.

2.2 Mathematical introduction of the MTF

In order to introduce the MTF mathematically, we have chosen a method which is easy to understand, is based on practical measurement procedures and which avoids the concept of the Fourier transformation, although only at a superficial level. The relationship with the Fourier transformation will be briefly shown in the appendix.

If we think of a sinusoidal light density distribution in the object plane, therefore an ideal sine lattice (Fig. 2.1), then this lattice with suitable orientation of the system of coordinates in the object plane can be described as

$$g(x)=1+K_0 \sin(2\pi\nu x) \tag{2.3}$$

with $0 \leq K_0 \leq 1$. $1/\nu$ is the distance between two adjacent maxima. Therefore, ν is denoted as the spatial frequency of the lattice. Fig. 2.1 shows in addition the so-called line image of a single "line" of width Δx of the light density profile. This line image is represented in the image plane in the vicinity of the point x' with the light density

$$g(x)\, L(x'-x)\, \Delta x. \tag{2.4}$$

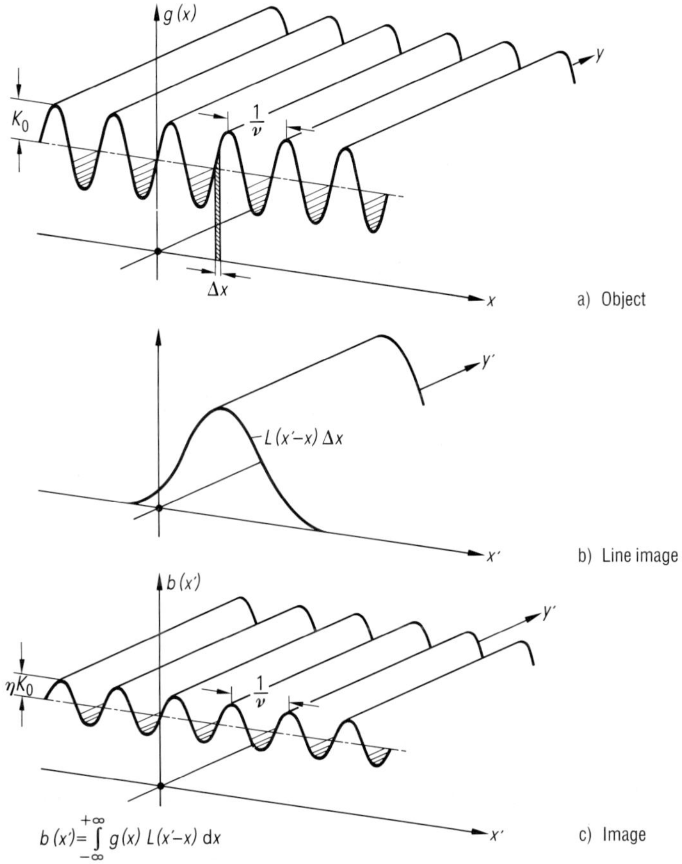

Fig. 2.1
Imaging of an object lattice $g(x)$ onto the image lattice $b(x')$; $L(x)$ describes the blurring produced by the imaging system

Since now every "line" of the lattice makes such a contribution to the image, the image $b(x')$ of $g(x)$ is given as

$$b(x') = \int_{-\infty}^{+\infty} g(x)\, L(x' - x)\, \mathrm{d}x,$$

which can also be rearranged to give

$$b(x') = \int_{-\infty}^{+\infty} g(x' - x)\, L(x)\, \mathrm{d}x.$$

If we substitute $g(x'-x)$ from equation (2.3), then we obtain

$$b(x')=\int_{-\infty}^{+\infty} L(x)\,\mathrm{d}x+K_0 \sin 2\pi\nu x' \int_{-\infty}^{+\infty} \cos 2\pi\nu x L(x)\,\mathrm{d}x$$
$$-K_0 \cos 2\pi\nu x' \int_{-\infty}^{+\infty} \sin 2\pi\nu x L(x)\,\mathrm{d}x.$$

This expression can be transformed to (2.4). For this, we set

$$\eta=\left(\left(\int_{-\infty}^{+\infty} L(x) \cos 2\pi\nu x\,\mathrm{d}x\right)^2+\left(\int_{-\infty}^{+\infty} L(x) \sin 2\pi\nu x\,\mathrm{d}x\right)^2\right)^{1/2} \tag{2.5}$$

and introduce a phase angle φ by

$$\cos\varphi=\frac{1}{\eta}\int_{-\infty}^{+\infty} L(x) \cos 2\pi\nu x\,\mathrm{d}x,$$
$$\sin\varphi=\frac{1}{\eta}\int_{-\infty}^{+\infty} L(x) \sin 2\pi\nu x\,\mathrm{d}x. \tag{2.6}$$

Taking into account the arbitrarily defined normalization

$$\int_{-\infty}^{+\infty} L(x)\,\mathrm{d}x=1$$

$b(x')$ can be represented as

$$b(x')=1+\eta K_0 \sin(2\pi\nu x'-\varphi).$$

The image $b(x')$ therefore has great similarity with the object $g(x)$ in equation (2.3): it again represents a sine lattice.

However, two differences should be noted:

1. Instead of the amplitude K_0 for g, the amplitude ηK_0 appears.
2. The image lattice appears phase-shifted compared to the object lattice.

It can be immediately seen that the factor η always lies between 0 and 1 under the condition $L(x)\geq 0$, i.e. in agreement with the assumption that $B(x', y')$ can be regarded as light density.

This follows from the estimate:

$$1=\left(\int_{-\infty}^{+\infty} L(x)\,\mathrm{d}x\right)^2=\left(\int_{-\infty}^{+\infty} |L(x)\,e^{j\,2\pi\nu x}|\,\mathrm{d}x\right)^2$$

$$\geq\left|\int_{-\infty}^{+\infty} L(x)\,e^{j\,2\pi\nu x}\,\mathrm{d}x\right|^2=\eta^2.$$

According to equation (2.5), η depends on the lattice frequency. This function η is called the modulation transfer function MTF(ν).

Because $0\leq \mathrm{MTF}(\nu)\leq 1$ and, as can be seen from equation (2.5), $\mathrm{MTF}(0)=1$, the typical course of the MTF is as shown in Fig. 2.2.

It is easy to understand its meaning. If we denote the contrast of the object lattice $g(x)$ by the expression

$$\frac{\max.\, g(x)-\min.\, g(x)}{\max.\, g(x)+\min.\, g(x)}=K_0 \tag{2.7}$$

and correspondingly, the contrast of the image grid $b(x')$ by

$$\frac{\max.\, b(x')-\min.\, b(x')}{\max.\, b(x')+\min.\, b(x')}=K_0\,\mathrm{MTF}(\nu), \tag{2.8}$$

then we simply obtain the modulation transfer function MTF as the (frequency-dependent) quotient of the image contrast of equation (2.8) and the object contrast of equation (2.7).

Because $\mathrm{MTF}(0)=1\geq\mathrm{MTF}(\nu)$ (under the assumption that $L(x)\geq 0$), the frequency $\nu=0$ is therefore never transferred more badly than any frequency $\nu\neq 0$. In the normal case, the MTF decreases monotonically with increasing frequency

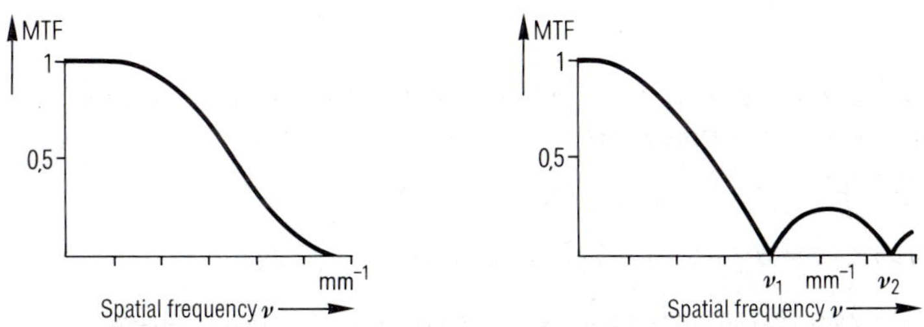

Spatial frequency
a) without pseudo resolution
b) with pseudo resolution

Fig. 2.2
Typical evolution of the modulation transfer function (MTF)

and finally decays to 0 for a certain limiting frequency ν_g. Fine structures of the object which require spatial frequencies $\geq \nu_g$, can therefore no longer be imaged. (As a practical limiting frequency, the frequency is taken for which the MTF has decreased to 4%).

If the line image function $L(x)$ is not symmetrical, so that the condition $L(x) = L(-x)$ is violated, then the phase angle $\varphi = \varphi(\nu)$ according to equation (2.6) can take any values between 0 and 2π. In many cases, however, there is symmetry at least in the central part of the image. Then, according to equation (2.6), $\sin\varphi = 0$ and consequently $\cos\varphi = +/-1$. The angle can then be 0 or π. The case $\varphi = \pi$ certainly occurs in practice. It means that the image lattice $b(x')$ has been shifted compared to $g(x)$ so that a wave peak of $b(x')$ always coincides with a wave valley of $g(x)$. In this way, dark object structures become light and light structures become dark! This phenomenon which is called pseudo resolution can be recognized from the shape of the MTF curve by noting that it becomes 0 for a certain frequency ν_1 but then rises again in order to finally become 0 at $\nu_2 > \nu_1$ (Fig. 2.2b). The frequency range $\nu_1 < \nu < \nu_2$ is then imaged phase-shifted. This phenomenon can reoccur at higher frequencies.

2.3 The MTF as a criterion for the quality of an imaging system

Obviously, it is possible to use the MTF to compare similar, competing systems. The MTF of the system is plotted as a function of ν and the best system is then the system whose MTF approximates best to the ideal curve $\mathrm{MTF}(\nu) \equiv 1$. However, it is more difficult to make the evaluation when the two MTF curves intersect. Then, the user has to decide himself on the basis of the object structures he is interested in, which of the two MTF curves is best suited to these structures.

However, what is the possibility of comparing the elements of an imaging chain with each other?

If a sine lattice $g(x)$ is brought into the object plane, the first imaging stage A_1 leads to an image

$$b_1(x') = 1 + K_0\,\mathrm{MTF}_1(\nu)\sin(2\pi\nu x' - \varphi_1)$$

in the image plane. Now, $b_1(x')$ represents in its turn an object in the image plane which is taken as object plane in the next imaging stage A_2 in the chain. The sine lattice

$$b_2(x'') = 1 + K_0\,\mathrm{MTF}_1(\nu)\,\mathrm{MTF}_2(\nu)\sin(2\pi\nu x'' - \varphi_1 - \varphi_2).$$

arises in the image plane of the imaging stage A_2. On the other hand, we expect the image of g under the combined imaging process A_{12} to be:

$$b_2(x'')=1+K_0\,\mathrm{MTF}_{12}(\nu)\sin(2\pi\nu x''-\varphi_{12}).$$

We can derive the following simple rules from this:

1. $\mathrm{MTF}_{12}(\nu)=\mathrm{MTF}_1(\nu)\,\mathrm{MTF}_2(\nu).$

The MTF of an imaging chain is simply the product of the MTFs of the chain elements.

2. $\varphi_{12}(\nu)=\varphi_1(\nu)+\varphi_2(\nu).$

The phase shifts which occur at each imaging stage are added.

This makes it possible to make a "longitudinal comparison" in an imaging chain using the MTF. After normalizing the successive chain elements to the same imaging scale, the MTFs of the chain elements can be displayed in a single graph and compared.

An example of the application of the MTF concept is the film-screen system of conventional radiography. The MTF of the overall imaging system is the product of the MTF of the receiver, i.e. the film-screen combination, the MTF of the imaging geometry characterized by the focus dimensions and the imaging scale and the MTF of the blurring caused by movement of the organ during exposure. Motion blurring can therefore also be quantitatively described using a MTF concept that contains a new variable "time multiplied by object speed".

This imaging chain is still relatively short; for example, the total MTF of x-ray image intensifier television chains is formed from a far greater number of MTF factors corresponding to the large number of chain elements (cf. Sect. 7). The development of the high-resolution television chain can be regarded as an illustrative example of the fact that finding the transfer element which has the fastest decreasing MTF is an effective optimization principle.

2.4 Practical aspects of MTF measurement

According to the above definition of the MTF, it is necessary to introduce into the beam path a grid which sinusoidally modulates the radiation intensity. However, it is known that, for example, the attenuation of x-ray radiation as a function of the irradiated material thickness follows a complicated law which is determined by the x-ray spectrum concerned. The intensity distribution behind the grid therefore still depends on the radiation quality used. This difficulty is overcome using an artificial device. The sinusoidal grid is replaced by a grid consisting of rods and spaces of equal thickness. The approximately 50 μm thick rods made of lead modulate the incident radiation intensity in a meandering manner (Fig. 2.3). However, at the output of the imaging system, we now obtain an unsharply defined, no longer meandering light density distribution so that it may not be regarded as the object grid for the next imaging process.

Formally, we can of course once again form the quotients of the image and object contrast and obtain the function $R(v)$ similar to the MTF but decreasing more slowly which is still dependent on the properties of the measuring arrangement and from which the MTF still has to be determined in any event.

Altar and Coltman [2.4, 2.5] have given a corresponding conversion formula in the form of an infinite series which obeys a remarkable generation law. We shall not go into any more detail into this generation law which requires the order of the square-wave harmonic frequencies to be decomposed into prime numbers. We shall just write down the first terms:

$$\mathrm{MTF}(v)=\frac{\pi}{4}\left|R(v)+\frac{R(3v)}{3}-\frac{R(5v)}{5}+\frac{R(7v)}{7}+\frac{R(11v)}{11}\dots\right|.$$

Every measuring device has itself to be regarded as an element of an imaging chain. It must therefore have an MTF assigned to it, the so-called inherent MTF. A measuring device is only of use if the first zero point of its inherent MTF lies higher than the highest frequency which is transferred by the system to be measured. Only then can the inherent MTF of the measuring process be extracted from the measured MTF.

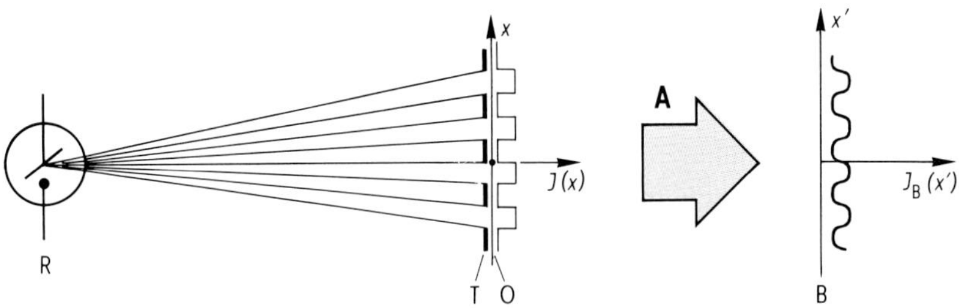

R x-ray tube
A Imaging system
T Test grid
O Object plane
B Image plane
J, J_B Intensities

Fig. 2.3
Imaging of an actual test grid made of thin lead

2.5 Determination of image disturbances due to noise

The intensity of the radiation field is constantly subject to fluctuations, so-called quantum noise. In addition, the imaging system itself contributes noise, in particular when it contains amplifying elements.

In a linear, spatially invariant imaging system, the noise transfer behaviour can in principle also be evaluated with the help of the MTF. If we call the noise power related to a spatial frequency interval the spectral noise power density, then the noise power density in the image, the so-called Wiener spectrum $W(\nu)$ (Fig. 2.4) is obtained as the product of the object noise power density and the square of the MTF.

For example, in film-screen systems with a homogeneous background, the noise spectrum imprinted on the film is given by

$$W(\nu) = \text{const.} \cdot G^2 \cdot |\text{MTF}(\nu)|^2 / N$$

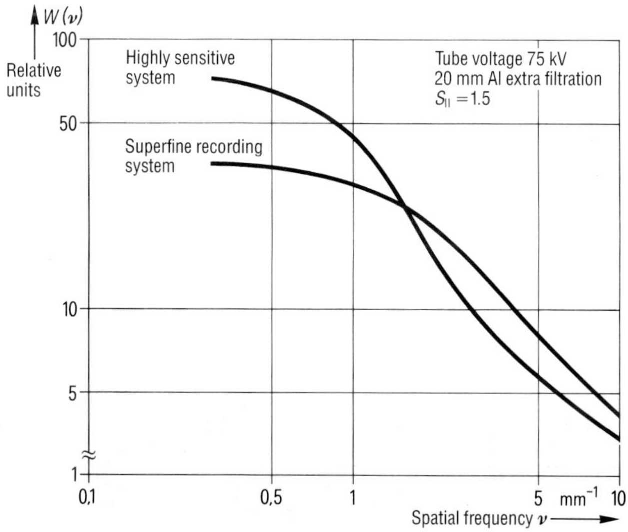

Fig. 2.4
Wiener spectrum of a highly sensitive film-screen system: it begins at a higher noise power because of the smaller number of quanta (for a certain optical density) and rapidly falls off because of the unfavorable MTF. Very high-definition film-screen system: the Wiener spectrum starts at a low noise power value and because of the more favorable MTF at high spatial frequencies runs above the spectrum for the highly sensitive system

[2.7]. G is the gradient of the characteristic. In distinction to the noise-free case, the quantum nature of the information carrier now has to be taken into consideration in the imaging theory. Here, if we assume Poisson noise, this can be done in a simple manner by means of the expectation N of the number of absorbed quanta per unit area.

This description of the noise is incomplete to the extent that the internal noise sources of the system have not yet been considered. Depending on the position of these sources within the imaging chain their noise contributions should be evaluated with the transfer factors of the next chain elements and then added (Fig. 2.5).

In the case of x-ray imaging, the experimental determination of the Wiener spectrum represents a considerable problem because on the one hand, with inhomogeneous objects, the noise overlaps the object structure so that it can hardly be separated and, on the other hand, because the noise characteristics are themselves modulated by the object structures. The noise is not stationary. Laboratory experiments for determining image noise are therefore carried out

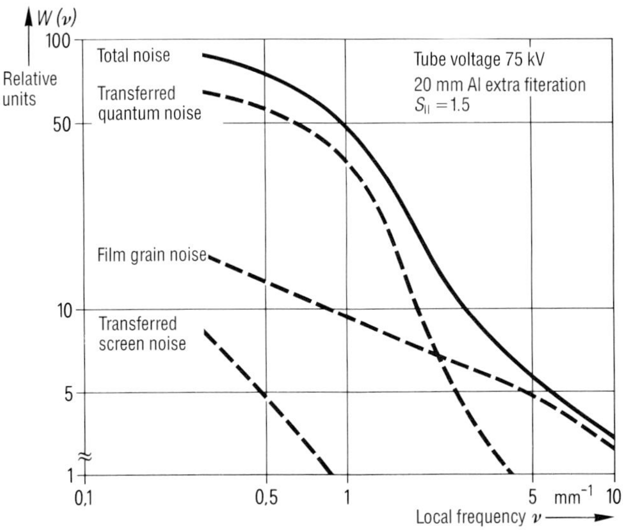

Fig. 2.5
Wiener spectrum of a highly sensitive film-screen system (FSS) and its components
Transferred quantum noise means:
quantum noise multiplied by $|MTF_{FSS}|^2$
Transferred screen noise means:
screen noise, which is based only on foil granularity, multiplied by $|MTF_{film}|^2$

to a large extent with homogeneous test phantoms in which structures of such weak contrast are inserted that the stationary behavior ensured for homogeneous objects remains practically undisturbed. Examples of such investigations can be found in section 4 (Fig. 4.11). Only if the homogeneity condition is satisfied can the noise characteristics which describe the intensity of the noise (standard deviation) or the type of "graininess" (correlations) be derived from a single image.

2.6 Image quality assessment taking into account all influencing variables at the same time

Since image noise can mask fine image structures with weak contrast, the recognizability limit always lies below the limiting frequency v_g mentioned in 2.2 and all the more, the greater the noise power. From the user's point of view (not however the designer's point of view), separate determination of the noise-independent and the noise-dependent characteristics of the image is only a stopgap. The radiologist is only interested to know whether an imaging system allows diagnostically relevant structures to be recognized.

This user requirement is satisfied by assessing the image quality in terms of ROC (receiver operating characteristic) curves and contrast-detail diagrams. A carefully worked-out test plan must be produced before beginning any investigation of this kind. Test structures have to be specified whose images will subsequently be presented to a group of expert observers. The image quality is then assessed by the relative frequencies of the correctly or incorrectly recognized test objects. Fig. 2.6 shows the image of a typical test phantom with 100 fields of which 50% are occupied statistically with test objects.

ROC curves

The observer has the job not only of correctly recognizing as many test objects as possible which are statistically scattered in an image containing noise but also of erroneously establishing the presence of such objects as seldom as possible. Therefore, the "hit probability" p (probability for true-positive statements) and the probability q for "false alarm" (probability for false-positive statements) are determined approximately [2.8].

If we plot p against q, we obtain a measurement point in the ROC diagram (Fig. 2.7). The observer group are now given different tasks which are geared on the one hand to the sensitivity and on the other hand to the specificity

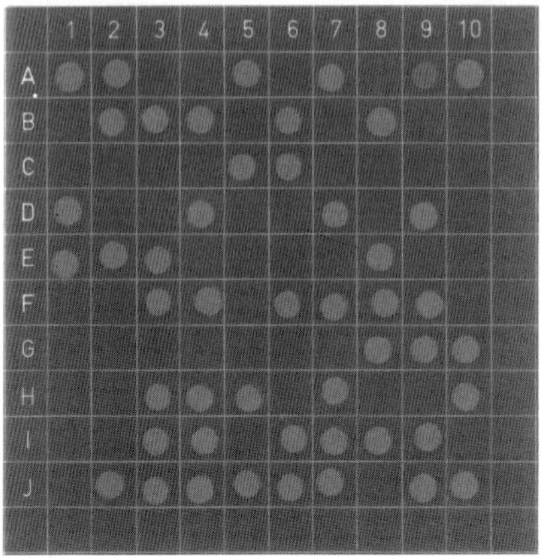

Fig. 2.6
Image of an ROC phantom. 50% of the fields have details (Al disks of 6 mm diameter)

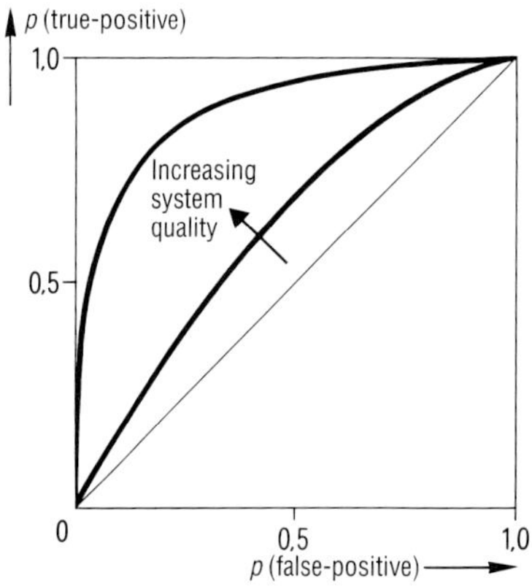

Fig. 2.7
ROC (Receiver Operating Characteristic) curves

of the diagnostic statement and result in the observers shifting their personal decision thresholds. The high sensitivity requirement leads to measurement points in the top right-hand area and the high specificity requirement leads to measurement points in the bottom left-hand area of the ROC curve.

In the extreme case, the group can consist of a single observer. Even in this case, the experimental effort is considerable since the result can only be regarded as reliable when a sufficient length of the measurement series replaces the above probabilities by relative frequencies. Obviously, the observer himself has to be regarded as part of the imaging system in every case.

Contrast detail diagrams

Assessment methods using contrast detail diagrams are based on test details of uniform structure, for example pairs of homogeneous disks of different diameter and different contrast which have a defined distance from each other. The observer has to decide what detail he can still just recognize. The minimum contrast of the detail compared to the environment which is then required for recognizability is then plotted as a function of the size of the detail (Fig. 2.8). The usefulness of the system for displaying fine bone structures can be seen from the top left-hand part of the curve. Equivalent information can be taken from the MTF in the form of its first zero point. The usefulness for differentiating large areas of soft tissue can be seen from the top right-hand part.

Similar to the ROC method, the methods of the contrast detail diagrams are subjective because they involve the physiology of vision. The first approaches are being made to automate the contrast detail diagram method so that the costs can be kept within reasonable limits by dispensing with the observer's evaluation [2.9].

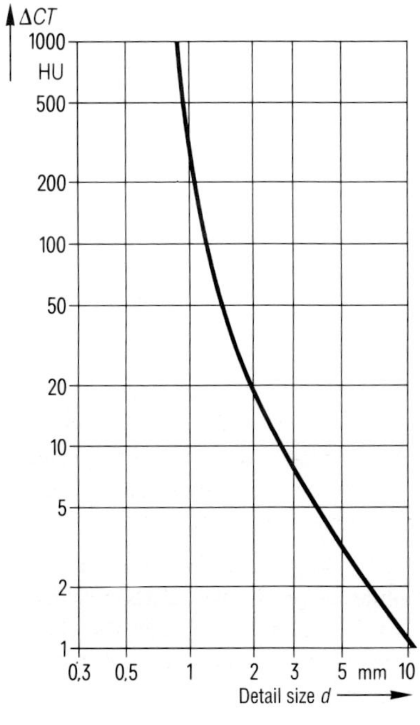

HU Hounsfield units

Fig. 2.8
Contrast detail diagram, automatically produced for a CT system and a specific phantom

2.7 Final remarks

ROC and contrast detail diagram methods meet the user's needs for a method for evaluating an imaging system because they make it possible to quantify the recognizability of given test structures without resorting to auxiliary criteria such as resolution, noise power or MTF. However, they are of limited benefit for the system developer because they do not make it possible to detect which element in a complicated imaging chain is responsible for any unfavorable behavior of the overall system. The ROC method of special interest to the user typically involves considerable experimental effort which consequently must be provided by the user himself, i.e. the radiologist. Attempts to automate such methods must be seen as an unpleasant compromise between meeting the needs of the user and economic viability. The great advantage, in particular of the ROC methods, that the system is suitable for testing specific diagnostic features, represents at the same time a great danger, the danger of faulty assessment when test objects which are diagnostically inappropriate are used. This danger is also present, although to a lesser extent, in classical seemingly objective assessment methods because here as well, the MTF of the transfer system has to be adapted to the diagnostically relevant spatial frequency range.

2.8 Relationship between the MTF and the Fourier transformation

In the literature, the MTF is often introduced by means of the Fourier transformation.

If a "light point" lies in the object plane at the point (x, y), mathematically described by a δ function, the imaging system generates an "image point of the light density" $P(x'-x, y'-y)$ (see Fig. 2.9). It is called the point image. Under the assumptions of linearity and spatial invariance of the imaging system, the Fourier transform

$$T(\nu_x, \nu_y) = \iint\limits_{-\infty}^{+\infty} P(x, y)\, e^{j\,2\pi(x\nu_x + y\,\nu_y)}\,\mathrm{d}x\,\mathrm{d}y$$

is called the transfer function and its absolute value the modulation transfer function.

$$\mathrm{MTF}(\nu_x, \nu_y) = |T(\nu_x, \nu_y)|.$$

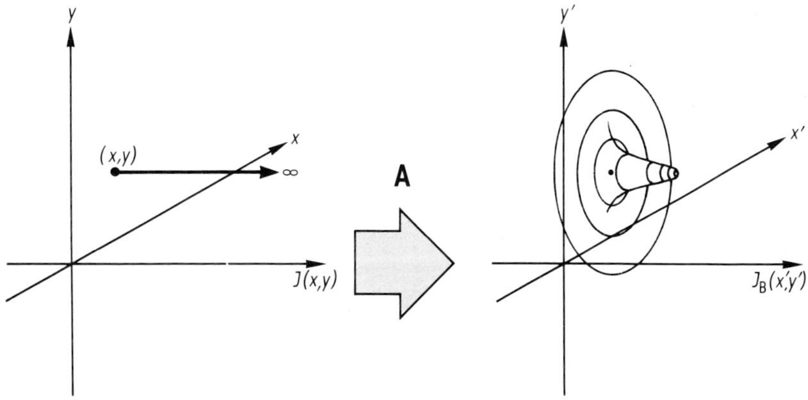

Fig. 2.9 Imaging of an object point in the image plane

Here, for the first time we have a component representation of the frequency. While, until now, the wave normal always pointed in the x direction, arbitrarily orientated plane waves are now used. The vector (v_x, v_y) points in the direction of the wave normals; its magnitude is the frequency which was previously used:

$$v = (v_x^2 + v_y^2)^{\frac{1}{2}}.$$

It can now be easily shown that for $v_y = 0$, we exactly obtain the above definition of the MTF:

$$T(v, 0) = \iint\limits_{-\infty}^{+\infty} P(x, y)\, e^{j\,2\pi v x} \mathrm{d}x\,\mathrm{d}y$$

$$= \iint\limits_{-\infty}^{+\infty} \left(\int\limits_{-\infty}^{+\infty} P(x, y)\,\mathrm{d}y \right) e^{j\,2\pi v x} \mathrm{d}x.$$

Here, the inner integral represents the line image function $L(x)$, namely the superimposition of the point images of all object points which lie on the straight line.

$$\{(x, y) | -\infty < y < +\infty\}.$$

We can therefore write

$$|T(v, 0)| = \left| \int_{-\infty}^{+\infty} L(x)\, e^{j\,2\pi v x}\, \mathrm{d}x \right|$$

and after an elementary transformation, we obtain the expression which was denoted by MTF (v).

At the same time, it can be seen that the MTF can be defined as the absolute value of the one-dimensional Fourier transform of the line image function. This definition is also common in the literature.

3 X-ray and gamma radiation

3.1 Generation of x-ray and gamma radiation

X-rays and gamma rays (wavelengths from 30 to 10^{-5} nm) are created when fast electrons collide with matter (3.1). When this happens, the kinetic energy of the electrons is mainly converted into heat energy, but some is also converted into electromagnetic energy in the form of photons. The following sequence of energy transformations is involved in the generation of x-rays and gamma rays:

The potential energy of an electron, that is, the product of the unit of electrostatic charge e and applied high tension U (Fig. 3.1) between cathode and anode

$$E_{pot} = eU, \tag{3.1}$$

is transformed into kinetic energy along its path of acceleration between the emitting filament (cathode) and the target material (anode):

$$E_{kin} = \frac{m_{el}}{2} v^2. \tag{3.2}$$

As a result of interactions between the penetrating electron and the atoms of the target material, about 99% of the energy is converted into heat and about 1% into X-ray energy with

$$E = h\nu \tag{3.3}$$

where

$h = 6.6252(\pm 0.0002) \cdot 10^{-34}\, J\,s$

(Planck's constant)

and

ν = frequency.

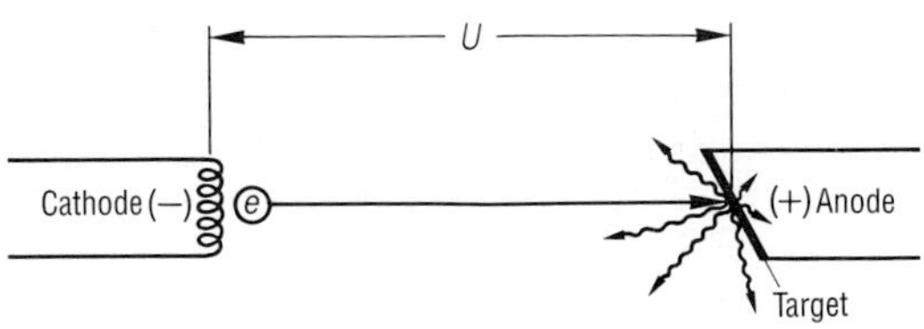

Fig. 3.1
Energy transformation in the generation of x-radiation

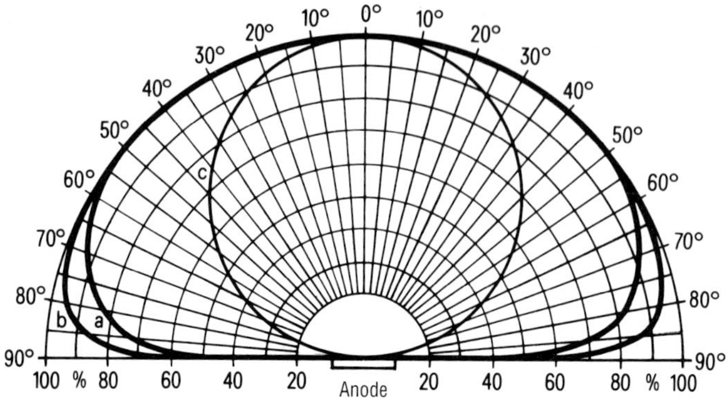

a Unfiltered radiation at 70 kV
b Filtered radiation (10 mm aluminum plate) at 70 kV
c Distribution according to the Lambert law

Fig. 3.2 Intensity distribution in various directions

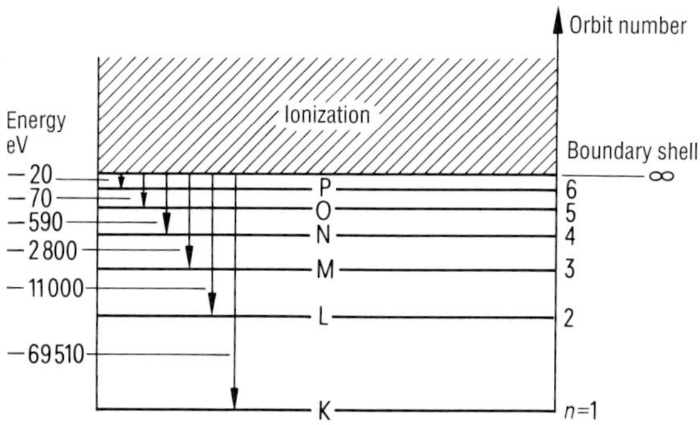

Fig. 3.3
Simplified energy level diagram of a tungsten atom with electron transitions, which lead to the emission of characteristic radiation

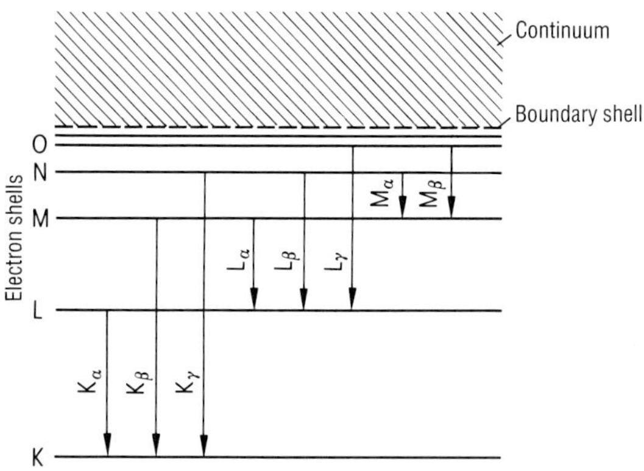

Fig. 3.4
Energy level diagram for tungsten

The slowing down of the electrons in matter takes place along their path of penetration into the target material by means of the stepwise loss of kinetic energy through interactions with the electrons in the atomic shells, and through slowing down of the electrons in the electric field of the atomic nuclei. They travel through several layers of atoms until all their energy has been lost. Hence only some of the x-rays are created at the surface of the target [3.2]. The distribution of x-rays, therefore, does not obey the Lambert Cosine Law as does the distribution of light rays. By means of the inherent absorption of the x-rays in the deeper atomic layers, the semispherical distribution in the impact plane of the electrons is compressed as in Fig. 3.2.
This drop in intensity, which increases strongly as the angle between the target surface and the electron beam decreases, is called the anode heel effect.

3.1.1 Characteristic radiation

If an electron penetrates the target atom and ionizes it in the L or K shell (in terms of the Bohr model of the atom), that is, if it knocks an electron which is strongly bound to the nucleus out of its orbit, then the primary electron loses an amount of energy which is used as ionization energy for the secondary electron (e.g. for tungsten 70 keV in the K shell) and as kinetic energy for the secondary electron. The empty position in the K shell is immediately (10^{-8} s) filled by an electron from the L, M or N shells. In this process the energy difference as, for example, in the equation

$$h\nu = E_M - E_N \qquad (3.4)$$

is liberated and is emitted in the form of a photon of characteristic frequency ν. The x-rays have a characteristic wavelength corresponding to the difference in energy of the energy levels (e.g. as in Fig. 3.3) between which the transition occurred. This is called *characteristic radiation*. The x-ray quanta, whose common final states are the K, L or M shells, are called the K, L or M series of the element in question (Fig. 3.4). As a part of the total x-ray spectrum, the characteristic x-ray spectrum is superimposed on the bremsstrahlung spectrum and is element-specific.

3.1.2 X-ray bremsstrahlung

If a primary electron penetrates the whole of the atomic shell and passes extremely close to an atomic nucleus, it is deflected from its path by the Coulomb field of the nucleus depending on the number of protons (atomic number). It undergoes an "acceleration"; in this process x-ray bremsstrahlung is created. A theoretical treatment of the process is given in [3.3].

The closer the path of the electron to the nucleus and the more energy the primary electron has, the greater the energy of the x-ray quantum generated. In the most extreme case, all the kinetic energy of the electron is transformed into radiation energy in the braking process. In such a rare case the photon created has the greatest energy possible with the *limiting frequency* $\nu_{\text{lim}} = eV/h$ and correspondingly the shortest wavelength possible (*limiting wavelength*).

$$\lambda_{\text{lim}} = \frac{c}{\nu_{\text{lim}}} = c\,\frac{h}{eU}. \tag{3.5}$$

The energy transformation usually occurs in several stages because the electron orbits lie at varying distances from the nucleus. The energies of the quanta from all the multi-stage braking processes therefore take arbitrary values below the maximum energy. Thus x-ray quanta of every possible frequency (or wavelength) are generated. They form a *continuous spectrum.*

From equation (3.1) it follows that the energy of the x-ray quanta is directly proportional to the tube voltage. Increasing the tube voltage (peak voltage) shifts the limiting frequency according to equation (3.5) to higher energies.

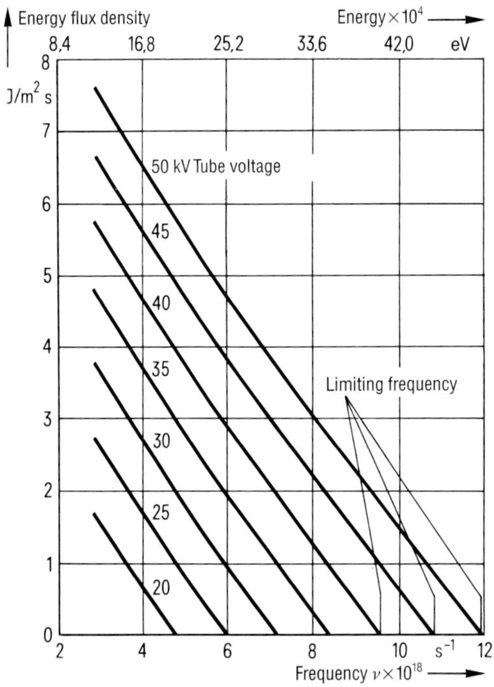

Fig. 3.5
Spectral intensity distribution. The energy flux density is shown, using a relative measure, as a function of the frequency

An increase in the current through the tube means an increase in the number of electrons and hence an increase, proportional to the current, of the energy flux. Thus when the anode voltage is higher, the x-rays generated differ both in their spectral composition (quality) and in the energy flux (quantity) [3.4] as is shown in Fig. 3.5.

3.1.3 Tungsten as a target material

Figure 3.6 depicts the continuous bremsstrahlung spectrum and the characteristic radiation of tungsten. A peak voltage of 150 kV of the x-ray generator yields x-rays up to the maximum photon energy of 150 keV. The unfiltered bremsstrahlung spectrum (in vacuum) would climb linearly in its energy flux up to zero photon energy (dashed line). As a result of the filtering effect of the glass bulb of the x-ray tube, any extra filters that there might be, and the air filtration between the radiation emitter and the measuring device, a smallest measurable photon energy is found, being the long wavelength limit of the graph. The intensities of the tungsten lines $K_{\alpha 1}$, $K_{\alpha 2}$, $K_{\beta 1}$, $K_{\beta 2}$, etc., have been superimposed provided that they still lie above the long wavelength limit.

These characteristic peaks of tungsten come about in the following way: the binding energy of an electron in the K shell is about 70 keV. An electron which has been accelerated between cathode and anode must therefore possess a kinetic energy of more than 70 keV in order to knock out an electron which is bound to the nucleus in the K shell. In the collision with such a K shell electron, the electron loses at least these 70 keV of its energy. This amount is used to release the K shell electron bound to the nucleus. The K shell is then no longer completely filled by electrons. The atom is said to be in an

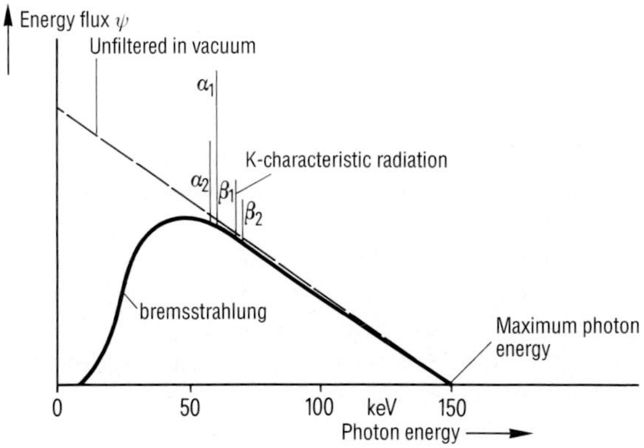

Fig. 3.6
The bremsstrahlung spectrum and the K-characteristic radiation for tungsten

ionized state. This unstable situation is resolved by the transition of an electron from the L shell. Transitions of electrons from more outlying shells are also possible. On the transition of an electron into the K shell, the electron emits the difference in energy between the energy levels in the form of a photon. In the case of tungsten, the energy difference between the L and K shell is about 59 keV. This is the difference between the binding energies in the K shell (70 keV) and in the L shell (11 keV). For tungsten the amount of energy released in the case of an L−K transition is always the same (characteristic radiation), irrespective of the energy of the free electron which knocked out the K shell electron. As a result of an electron's change of location from the L shell to the K shell, a vacant space is created in the L shell. This is filled by an electron from the M shell, and so on. In the case of tungsten the binding energy in the L shell is 11 keV and in the M shell 2 keV. Thus the energy difference of 9 keV is equal to the energy of the x-ray photon which is emitted in an electron transition from the M to the L shell. The characteristic radiation from shells further removed from the nucleus, e.g. N, O or P, has so little energy that the ionization of these outer shells only leads to very soft x-rays, and these are absorbed by inherent filtration.

The energy levels of the L, M and N shells, on the other hand, are in themselves differentiated. Thus in the transition of electrons from the L shell there are two characteristic x-ray photons of energy $K_{\alpha 1} = 59.3$ keV and $K_{\alpha 2} = 57.9$ keV respectively. Further high-intensity characteristic radiation is produced in the transition of an electron from the M to the K shell with $K_{\beta 1} = 67.2$ keV and $K_{\beta 2} = 69$ keV respectively. The contribution of characteristic radiation to the total radiation spectrum of an x-ray tube with tungsten target is negligible below 70 keV. Between 70 and 150 keV the proportion of characteristic radiation amounts to between 10 and 28% of the energy flux. Above 150 keV the proportion of characteristic radiation diminishes and at 300 keV becomes negligible in comparison to the x-ray bremsstrahlung.

Thus the choice of the target material (and hence the atomic number) determines for a given electron energy the *intensity of radiation (quantity)* and the *radiation energy (quality)* of the characteristic radiation. In tungsten the energy values of the characteristic radiation lie between 57 and 69 keV, in tin between 25 and 29 keV, and in lead between 72 and 88 keV.

The energy flux of the bremsstrahlung continuum is determined by the size of the field of the braking nucleus and thus by the atomic number of the atom. The higher the nuclear charge of the target atoms, the more efficient the generation of x-ray bremsstrahlung. Thus, for example, the energy flux of bremsstrahlung, given the same voltage and current, is larger in an x-ray tube with a tungsten target (atomic number $Z = 74$) than in an x-ray tube with a tin target ($Z = 50$). In any case tin is ruled out because of its relatively low melting point of 232 °C as opposed to tungsten with the highest melting point of all metals, 3370 °C. A high melting point, along with good thermal conductivity and a high heat capacity, is a primary requirement of the target material because of the predominant production of heat in the generation of x-rays. For this reason neither platinum ($Z=78$) nor lead ($Z=82$), for example, come into consideration.

It can be derived mathematically that for an optimum choice of material in the case of a fixed anode for long-time operation, the value

$$Z\vartheta_{max}\lambda$$

and for a rotating anode

$$Z\vartheta_{max}\sqrt{\lambda\varrho c}$$

must be as high as possible.

Z	Atomic number	λ	Thermal conductivity
ϑ_{max}	Maximum permissible temperature	ϱ	Density
c	Specific heat		

In Table 3.1 these values are listed for suitable materials. The value of ϑ_{max} is based on a vapor pressure of $1.33 \cdot 10^{-2}$ Pa.

As a rule, the maximum permissible focal spot temperature is 20 to 30% below the melting point of the target material.

Table 3.1
List of possible anode materials and order of their suitability for fixed anodes and rotating anodes

Element	Atomic number Z	Permissible temperature ϑ_{max} at 1.33×10^{-2} Pa in °C	Thermal conductivity λ W/cm K	Fixed anodes		Rotating anodes		
				$Z\vartheta_{max}\lambda$	Order of suitability	$\sqrt{\lambda\varrho c}$	$Z\vartheta_{max} \times \sqrt{\lambda\varrho c}$	Order of suitability
Cu	29	1032	3.98	119113	8	3.68	110135	10
Mo	42	2167	1.38	125599	7	1.88	171106	8
Ag	47	832	4.18	163450	4	3.18	124350	9
Ta	73	2587	0.55	103868	9	1.13	213402	6
W	74	2757	1.3	265223	1	1.81	369273	1
Re	75	2557	0.71	136160	6	1.38	264650	4
Os	76	2280	0.87	150754	5	1.77	306706	3
Ir	77	2220	1.46	249572	3	2.06	352136	2
Pt	78	1742	0.71	96472	10	1.41	191585	7
Au	79	(1063)	3.14	263687	2	2.81	235975	5
U	92	(1132)	0.25	26036	11	0.75	78108	11

From Table 3.1 tungsten emerges as an outstanding anode material for both short and long load times. This is on account of its high atomic number, its high melting point and – compared to other materials with a high melting point – its good thermal properties.

Because of the high thermal conductivity and heat capacity of copper, a higher specific performance can be obtained by embedding a tungsten disk of an optimized thickness in copper [3.4].

3.1.4 Intensity (energy flux density) of x-radiation

The energy flux density of x-radiation may be defined as the number of photons per unit of area and time multiplied by their energy. The energy flux density is given in units of $J/m^2\,s = W/m^2$. It changes with the voltage and the current

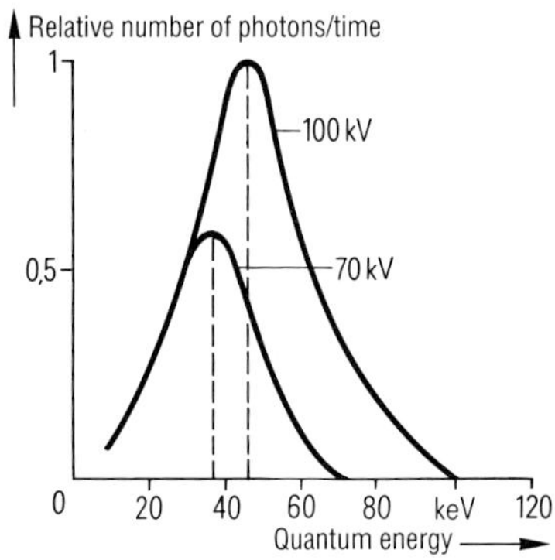

a) Influence of voltage

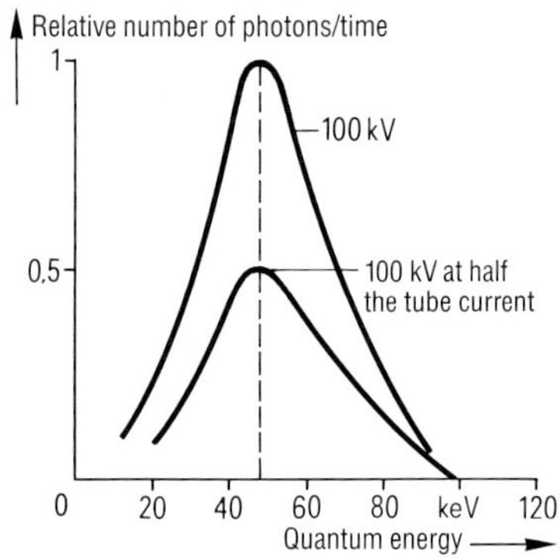

b) Influence of current

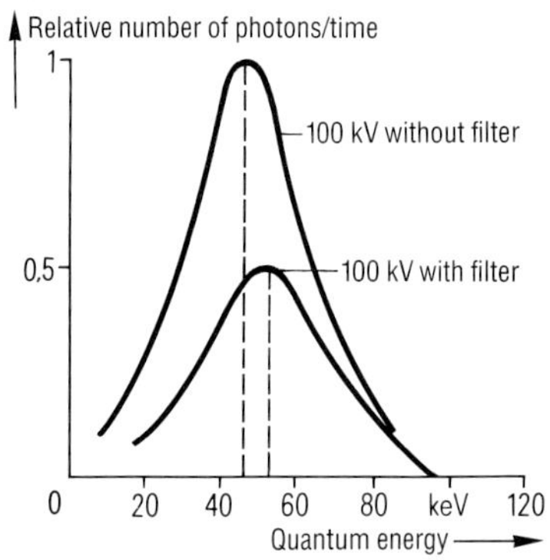

c) Influence of filtration

Fig. 3.7
The influence of voltage (a), current (b) and filtration (c) on the spectrum of a diagnostic tube (2-pulse generator). The maximum value of the 100 kV spectrum has been set equal to 1

as well as by being affected by the target material and the filtration (inherent filtration in the target).

The value of the peak voltage determines the maximum energy (quality) of the x-rays generated. At the same time, by raising the voltage, the quantity of radiation is increased (Fig. 3.7). The energy flux density is proportional to U^2.

Furthermore, the number of x-ray quanta is proportional to the number of electrons that hit the target. The larger the current in the tube (mA), the greater the energy flux. The quality of the x-radiation is not influenced by a change of current.

The energy flux density ψ of the radiation generated is proportional to the atomic number of the target material, the current in the tube and the square of the tube voltage:

$$\psi \sim ZIU^2. \tag{3.6}$$

The quadratic dependence upon voltage only holds exactly for unfiltered radiation. The filtration which occurs as a result of the glass envelope and any additional filters, including the patient, causes a hardening of the radiation. In this way the intensity is reduced at all wavelengths. However, the long-wavelength energy range is absorbed more strongly. Thus, besides the reduction in energy flux density, there is also a shift in the spectrum towards higher energies. The maximum energy is not affected by this. If the radiation is measured at the photographic plane, exponents for U are found between 2 and 5 depending on the thickness of the irradiated object. A change in voltage thus has a much stronger effect on the energy flux density than a change in the tube current.

Two concepts have been introduced in radiology to characterize x-radiation:

The half-value thickness (HVT) is the thickness of the additional filter which has to be placed in the ray path to reduce the dose rate (energy flux density) by half. Up to 150 kV, aluminum filters are used, and above this, copper filters. The homogeneity coefficient is the ratio of the 1st HVT to the 2nd HVT. Here the 2nd HVT is the thickness of the additional filter which is necessary to reduce again by half the dose remaining after the 1st HVT has been placed in the path of the radiation.

The 2nd HVT is greater than the 1st HVT because hardening of the x-radiation occurs due to the 1st HVT; the homogeneity coefficient after the 2nd HVT is, however, improved (Fig. 3.7).

3.1.5 Efficiency of bremsstrahlung generation

By the efficiency of bremsstrahlung generation is meant the ratio of the energy flux of the bremsstrahlung to the energy flux of the incident electron beam.

Following equation (3.6) the energy flux density of the bremsstrahlung is proportional to the acceleration of the electron through the voltage U. The acceleration is in turn proportional to the acting force, that is to the attractive force of the nuclear charge (eZ) on the electron. Thus the radiation intensity for each passage through an atom is proportional to the square of the nuclear charge number (atomic number) Z. The total radiation intensity of an electron along its entire trajectory is the product of this with the number of atoms traversed. In a target with a low Z value, an electron of energy eU will travel through more atoms than in a target with a high Z value. Thus the number of atoms which an electron of a given energy traverses can, with sufficient accuracy, be taken to be inversely proportional to the atomic number of the braking material. The energy flux of the bremsstrahlung is therefore not proportional to Z^2 but is proportional to Z.

The efficiency of bremsstrahlung generation is thus found to be

$$\eta = kUZ. \tag{3.7}$$

Here k is a constant which has been established experimentally to be $1.1 \cdot 10^{-9}$. U is stated in volts, and Z denotes the atomic number of the target material.

For tungsten ($Z=74$) a tube voltage of 100 kV leads to an efficiency of 0.8%. The equation does not hold for very high operating voltages.

Since only a very small part of the total anode radiation field leaves the tube as useful radiation (useful radiation beam), the radiological yield is reduced once more to about a tenth of its previous size.

3.2 Interaction of x-rays and gamma rays with matter

Compared to light, x-rays and gamma rays are very short electromagnetic waves. However, the energy of their quanta is very high. Thus they can easily pass through matter. These quanta do, however, interact with the atoms of matter. Thus the primary beam loses a portion of its quanta. The number of penetrating quanta depends on the type of matter, its density and thickness, and on the energy of the quanta. In x-ray technology, if the radiation is captured after its emergence from the object under examination, e.g. by a luminescent screen, a photographic image of the interior of the object can be made.

In order to explain the interactions which the quanta undergo on passing through matter, there follows a discussion of the effects which occur, the quantitative description of the effects by means of coefficients, the interactions with real objects, and the most important effects allowing the detection of x-rays and gamma quanta.

3.2.1 Effects occurring when x-rays and gamma rays penetrate matter

The number of quanta $\mathrm{d}N$ interacting with the matter in a thin layer of thickness $\mathrm{d}x$ is proportional to the number of incident quanta N, the thickness of the layer $\mathrm{d}x$, and the total linear attenuation coefficient μ (a constant of the material depending on energy):

$$\mathrm{d}N = -\mu N \,\mathrm{d}x \tag{3.8}$$

(the minus sign is because the number of emerging quanta decreases).

After dividing by N and integrating over N and x between the limits N_0 and N, and 0 and d respectively

$$\int_{N_0}^{N} \frac{\mathrm{d}N}{N} = -\mu \int_{0}^{d} \mathrm{d}x \tag{3.9}$$

the *law of attenuation* is obtained

$$N = N_0\, e^{-\mu d}. \tag{3.10}$$

The law of attenuation states that the number N of quanta penetrating the material is proportional to the number of incident quanta N_0 and decreases exponentially with the linear attenuation coefficient μ and the thickness d of the material.

These observations hold for a particular energy $h\nu$ of the incident quanta. In the case of a spectrum $N_0(h\nu)$ one must integrate over $(h\nu)$.

The decrease in the number of quanta on passing through material can be explained by three effects: the photoelectric effect, scattering and pair production. These are described below.

The photoelectric effect

The x-ray or gamma quantum hits an electron of the inner atomic shell and transfers all its energy to this electron in the process. If the energy transferred is greater than the binding energy of the electron, the latter abandons its atom and travels through the material as a so-called free photoelectron. Its energy is then smaller than that of the colliding x-ray quantum by an amount precisely equal to the binding energy.

The vacancy created is filled by an electron from the outer atomic shells, while at the same time the energy released is emitted in the form of an electromagnetic quantum. In some of these processes the energy released may also be transferred directly to an electron in the more outlying shells. This electron is called an Auger electron and is emitted.

In Sect. 3.2.3 the photoelectric process in a single atom is examined more closely. In particular, the dependence of the absorption on the energy of the quantum and on the atomic number of the atom is explained, and the angular distribution of the photoelectrons and the energy transfer to the photoelectron described.

Scattering

The x-ray or gamma quantum can also interact with the electrons of the atomic shell without its energy being absorbed. It then leaves the atom again with a change of direction. If in the process it retains all its energy, this is called *coherent scattering* or *Rayleigh scattering*. If it loses part of its energy to the scattering electron, the effect is called *incoherent scattering* or *Compton scattering*.

In Sect. 3.2.4 the effects of scattering off free and bound electrons are explored in more detail and the quantitative relationships explained.

Pair production

If the energy of the quantum is greater than 1022 MeV, then, through interaction with the Coulomb field of the nucleus, the quantum may form an electron-positron pair. The two charged particles then fly apart, predominantly in the forward direction. This effect will not, however, be discussed further here, since it does not occur in the range of diagnostic beam energies and therefore cannot be considered for any applications. An exception is the opposite effect, the combination of a positron with an electron, with the emission of two 511 keV gamma quanta. This effect is exploited in nuclear medicine by means of the so-called positron camera.

3.2.2 Phenomenological description of the effects

Attenuation coefficients

The linear *attenuation coefficient* μ, which has already been mentioned to describe the intensity of the processes, is a quantitative measure for the sum of all attenuating processes. Special, specific coefficients are defined for the various processes, individually indicating to what extent the number of quanta arriving in a layer $\mathrm{d}x$ is reduced by the process in question, or, alternatively, how many quanta interact with the electrons or nuclei of this layer in a certain process. Thus following Fig. 3.8 the total linear attenuation coefficient μ is divided up initially into a linear *photoelectric absorption coefficient* τ, a linear *scattering coefficient* σ, and a linear *pair production coefficient* χ.

In the case of the scattering coefficient one distinguishes between the linear *coherent scattering coefficient* σ_R and the linear *incoherent scattering coefficient* σ_c. The latter coefficient must then be subdivided further if one wishes to characterize e.g. how in the Compton process the absorbed energy is distributed between the mean kinetic energy of the Compton electron η_σ and the mean energy of the scattered quantum σ_S (Fig. 3.8). Similarly the linear photoelectric absorption coefficient τ is subdivided into the coefficients η_τ and τ_{fl}, where η_τ is a measure of the mean transfer of energy to the photoelectrons and Auger electrons. τ_{fl} is a measure of the energy transfer to the fluorescence quanta. If one adds up the attenuation coefficients of those processes which lead to electron kinetic energies, this defines the energy transfer coefficient η.

The linear attenuation coefficients may also take the density of the interacting material into account and then they are called mass attenuation coefficients or mass absorption coefficients μ/ϱ. Since these coefficients in turn refer to a certain density ϱ in terms of mass/volume of an element and are in general not dependent on the instantaneous density ϱ_m of the material in question,

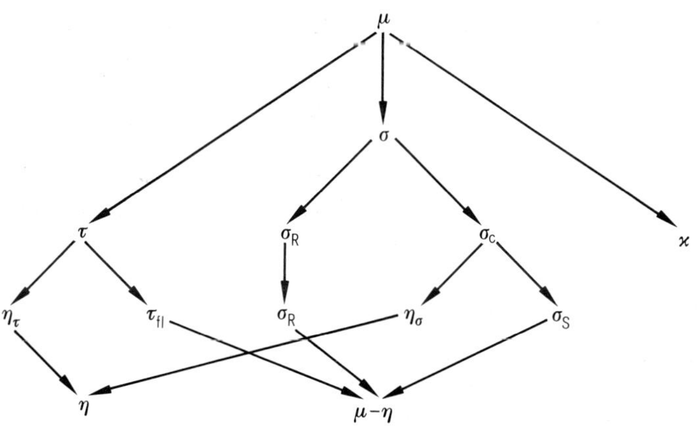

μ Total linear attenuation coefficient
τ Photoelectric absorption coefficient
σ Scattering coefficient
χ Pair production coefficient
σ_R Coefficient for coherent scattering
σ_c Coefficient for incoherent scattering, Compton coefficient
η_τ Kinetic energy transfer coefficient for photoelectric absorption
τ_{fl} Coefficient for energy transfer to fluorescence quanta in photoelectric absorption
η_σ Kinetic energy transfer coefficient in the Compton process
σ_S Transfer coefficient for the energy of the scattered quanta in the Compton process
η Energy transfer coefficient

Fig. 3.8 Linear attenuation coefficient

the linear attenuation coefficients μ may be calculated from the mass attenuation coefficients μ/ϱ and the instantaneous ϱ_m density of the material to be

$$\mu = \frac{\mu}{\varrho}\,\varrho_m.$$

If one wishes to calculate the effect on a real object of thickness d by integration over the "infinitesimally" thin layers of thickness dx – as in the integration in equation (3.9) – one should remember that neither multiple nor secondary processes are covered in this way (see Sect. 3.2.5).

Cross sections

Attenuation is often expressed in terms of the effect of an individual atom or even an individual electron by specifying the cross sections per atom or electron. Since the interactions essentially involve the electrons – with the exception of pair production, which is not considered here (see Sect. 3.2.1) – the cross section per electron would appear to be the measure which makes the most physical sense.

Thus, for the example of photoelectric absorption, we will now proceed to derive a relationship between the *mass absorption coefficient* τ/ϱ and the cross section for the absorption per electron σ_τ^e:

To begin with, one has for the *cross section per atom* σ_τ^a:

$$\sigma_\tau^a = Z\sigma_\tau^e \tag{3.11}$$

with atomic number Z and cross section per electron σ_τ^e.

Since the density ϱ is equal to the product of the number n_a of atoms per unit volume and the mass m of the atom, one has with m equal to the mass number A divided by the Loschmidt number or Avogadro's constant L

$$\varrho = n_a \frac{A}{L}. \tag{3.12}$$

Now, analogously to equation (3.8), one has for the quanta absorbed in a layer of thickness dx, on the one hand

$$dN = -\tau N\,dx, \tag{3.13}$$

where N is the number of incident quanta per unit area (1 m^2). In this layer of thickness dx, however, there are $n_a \cdot 1\,dx$ atoms, which each contribute to absorption with the mean cross section σ_τ^a. Thus one also has $\mathrm{d}N = -\sigma_\tau^a n_a \,\mathrm{d}x N$. If this is equated with equation (3.13), then it follows that $\tau = n_a \sigma_\tau^a$.

Equations (3.11) and (3.12) therefore imply the relationship

$$\tau = \varrho \frac{L}{A} Z \sigma_\tau^e$$

or

$$\frac{\tau}{\varrho} = L \frac{Z}{A} \sigma_\tau^e. \tag{3.14}$$

Z/A (except for hydrogen) is approximately equal to 0.5 (for more exact values of LZ/A see Table 3.2). Thus LZ/A = number of electrons/mass is practically independent of the atomic number Z. Z-dependence of the mass attenuation, absorption or scattering coefficients thus virtually only occurs as a result of the Z-dependence of the corresponding cross sections per electron.

However, in this approach one should realize that the various interaction processes are independent of neither the number of electrons per atom nor of the position of the electrons in the atom. The cross sections per electron are therefore merely an average over the electrons in an atom. Above all, they are not independent of Z. These problems will be examined later in more depth.

Table 3.2 Values of various materials

Material	ϱ Density g/cm^3	Z Effective nuclear charge	$\frac{LZ}{A}$ Number of electrons per g
Hydrogen	0.0000899	1	$6.00 \cdot 10^{23}$
Carbon	2.25	6	$3.01 \cdot 10^{23}$
Oxygen	0.001429	8	$3.01 \cdot 10^{23}$
Aluminum	2.7	13	$2.90 \cdot 10^{23}$
Copper	8.9	29	$2.75 \cdot 10^{23}$
Lead	11.34	82	$2.38 \cdot 10^{23}$
Air	0.001293	7.64	$3.01 \cdot 10^{23}$
Water	1.00	7.42	$3.34 \cdot 10^{23}$
Muscle	1.00	7.42	$3.36 \cdot 10^{23}$
Fatty tissue	0.91	5.92	$3.48 \cdot 10^{23}$
Bone	1.85	13.8	$3.00 \cdot 10^{23}$

3.2.3 The photoelectric effect, quantitative approach

Some aspects of the photoelectric effect will now be explained in more detail, without, however, describing its very complicated derivation.

Ionization, x-ray-induced fluorescence, Auger electrons

If an x-ray or gamma quantum is completely absorbed by a bound electron, then the electron leaves the atom with an energy E equal to the difference in energy between the colliding x-ray quantum and the binding energy of the electron (Fig. 3.9). If the electron comes from the outer shells which have low binding energy, then as a free photoelectron it takes over virtually all the energy of the quantum. If – particularly in the case of atoms with a high atomic number Z – the electron comes from the K or L shells, which have high binding energy, then its kinetic energy is considerably reduced compared to that of the colliding quantum. The resulting vacancy in the relevant electron shell is filled again. This can be by means of an electron from the more outlying shells or, in the case of a solid, by means of electrons from the bands. The vacancies which are subsequently created are also filled successively in the same way.

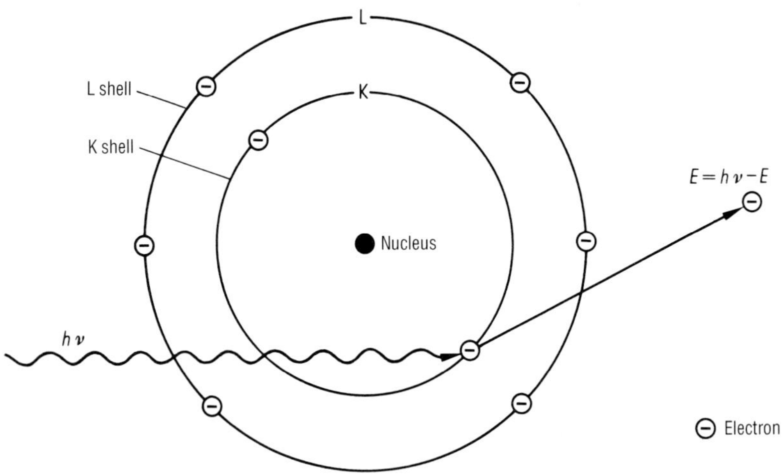

Fig. 3.9
The photoelectric effect:
A quantum with energy $h\nu$ collides with an atom with a nucleus and electron shells. An electron which is hit is emitted. It possesses the energy of the colliding quantum, minus its binding energy

Table 3.3
Some x-ray fluorescence lines of xenon (these are created by electron transitions between certain angular momentum states)

Transition	Name of line	Energy keV	Relative intensity
$L_{III} \to K$	$K_{\alpha 1}$	29.8	100
$L_{II} \to K$	$K_{\alpha 2}$	29.5	52
$M_{III} \to K$	$K_{\beta 1}$	33.6	20.2
$N_{II}/N_{III} \to K$	$K_{\beta 2}$	34.4	3.6

The discrete energies which are liberated in the process are emitted in the form of quanta. The discrete quantum spectrum ranges from very low energy values in the case of replacement by neighboring electrons from the outer shells, up to maximally the difference between the energy of a photoelectron and the energy of a K-electron. This energy naturally becomes higher with increasing Z, as is the case with the maximum energies of the individual series, the edges, which are identical to it. Here a series means the discrete energy values of all fluorescent quanta which result from electron transitions into *one* particular electron orbit.

As a result of the electron transitions, fluorescent x-radiation is created. This is a distinguishing characteristic of the atom in question and is therefore called characteristic radiation. It is indicated by the characteristic lines peculiar to the atom, e.g. $K_{\alpha 1}$, $K_{\alpha 2}$, $K_{\beta 1}$, $K_{\beta 2}$. In Table 3.3, as an example, some x-ray fluorescence lines of xenon are reproduced with their relative intensities.

However, the fluorescence lines are also superimposed on the bremsstrahlung spectra as a consequence of the inherent absorption of quanta from the bremsstrahlung spectrum in the anode material of the tube. As has already been mentioned in 3.2.1, the energy liberated in the atom may also directly release an electron from the same atom. Such a creation of so-called Auger electrons is not accompanied by any radiation. This process is therefore also called radiation-free transition or internal conversion. The probability of this process occurring is nearly 1 in the case of elements with a low atomic number Z and nearly 0 in the case of elements with a high atomic number (see [3.5]).

Dependence of the absorption on energy and atomic number

If the mass attenuation coefficient for photoelectric absorption τ/ϱ is plotted as a function of the energy $h\nu$ using log–log graph scales, there results the well-known steep decrease of this quantity with increasing energy $h\nu$ of the x-ray or gamma quanta. The graph is interrupted by peaks where the mass absorption coefficient increases by about a factor of 5. The corresponding energy

$h\nu$ is equal to the binding energy of a shell electron, e.g. a K-electron. If the energy of a quantum just exceeds the relevant binding energy, then its interaction and thus the effective cross section of the electron in question with the γ-quantum is particularly large. This is because absorption increases substantially more strongly than would correspond to the increased number of absorbing electrons. At the K absorption limit or K-edge of xenon, for instance, the number of absorbing electrons only increases by 2, from 52 to 54, but τ/ϱ increases by more than a factor of 5.

The dependence of τ/ϱ on $h\nu$ may be roughly described by an exponential law, where the exponent is equal to -2.7. For a precise description of the energy dependence it must be taken into account that this exponent changes with energy. Fig. 3.10 shows as an example the mass attenuation coefficient for photoelectric absorption in xenon.

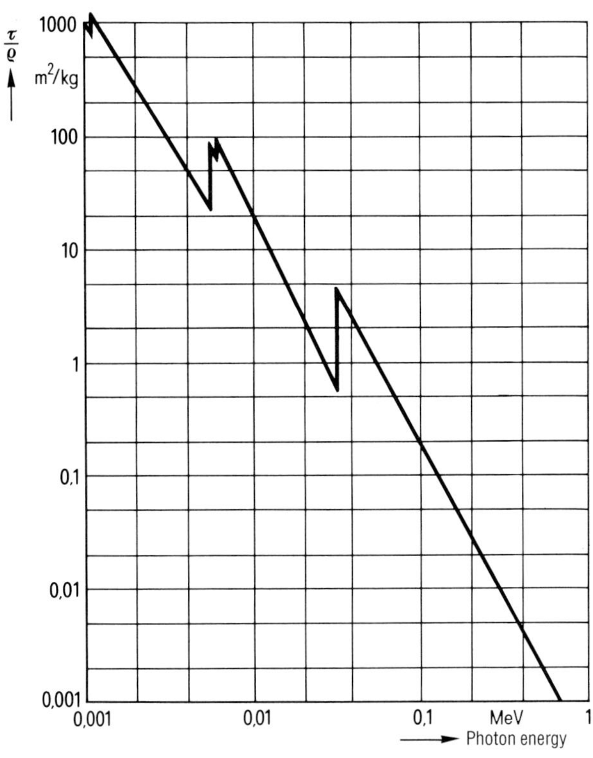

Fig. 3.10
Mass attenuation coefficient τ/ϱ for the photoelectric absorption process in xenon, as a function of photon energy

Similarly marked differences are obtained for the Z-dependence of τ/ϱ. Here, too, an exponential law holds with an exponent of about 3.

Angular distribution of the photoelectrons

According to the classical picture, the electrons of the atom are accelerated by the field strength of the electric vector of the incident wave. Since the electric vector is always perpendicular to the direction of incidence, one would expect the photoelectrons to be propelled outwards at an angle of exactly 90° to the direction of the incident x-rays. However, the x-ray quantum has a momentum, which it transfers to the atom and to the photoelectron. Bearing in mind the law of conservation of momentum, this gives rise to the butterfly-shaped figures shown in Fig. 3.11. The more energetic the incident quanta, of course, the more the photoelectron is, on average, catapulted out in the forward direction because of conservation of momentum. This can be seen clearly from the polar diagram of the photoelectrons.

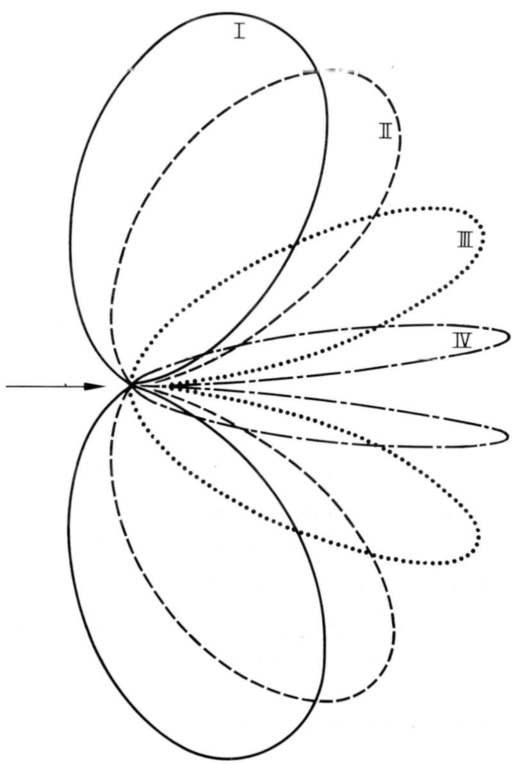

I 20 KeV
II 100 KeV
III 500 KeV
IV 1500 KeV

Fig. 3.11
Directional distribution of the photoelectrons as a function of the energy of the incident x-ray quanta

Energy transfer to the photoelectrons

If $\bar{E}_k$ is the average energy of the photoelectrons and Auger electrons which have been generated, then the energy transfer coefficient is without exception always given by:

$$\eta_\tau = \tau \frac{\bar{E}_k}{h\nu}.$$

The difference between τ and η_τ essentially gives the amount of energy from characteristic radiation (a small amount of bremsstrahlung is also contained in η_τ, around 2%).

3.2.4 Scattering processes

Classical scattering at free electrons

If a wave of frequency ν comes to interact with an electron, then one expects the electron as an oscillating dipole with frequency ν to itself transmit a wave of frequency ν. Thomson has calculated the cross section $\sigma_R^e/_{th}$ for this process; the following formula is obtained for the corresponding differential cross section of an electron:

$$\left.\frac{d\sigma_R^e}{d\Omega}\right|_{th} = \frac{e^4}{2m_0^2 c^4}(1+\cos^2\Phi). \tag{3.15}$$

If one integrates over the solid angle $d\Omega$, then one gets for the total classical scattering cross section per electron in m^2

$$\sigma_R^e|_{th} = 0.665 \cdot 10^{-28}, \tag{3.16}$$

i.e., the cross section for classical scattering is independent of the wavelength of the incident quantum. Since, as explained previously, the number of electrons per gram is almost independent of Z (equation 3.14), one would expect scattering to be independent of the energy and atomic number over the entire periodic system. However, this is not the case. The scattering of x-ray quanta depends both on Z and on the energy. This also holds for coherent scattering, i.e. for the scattering of x-ray quanta without a change in the wavelength, and in fact the coherent scattering cross section decreases very rapidly with energy. Only for very low energies ($h\nu$ tending towards 0) does the coherent scattering cross section for hydrogen for instance, agree with the Thomson value. Even

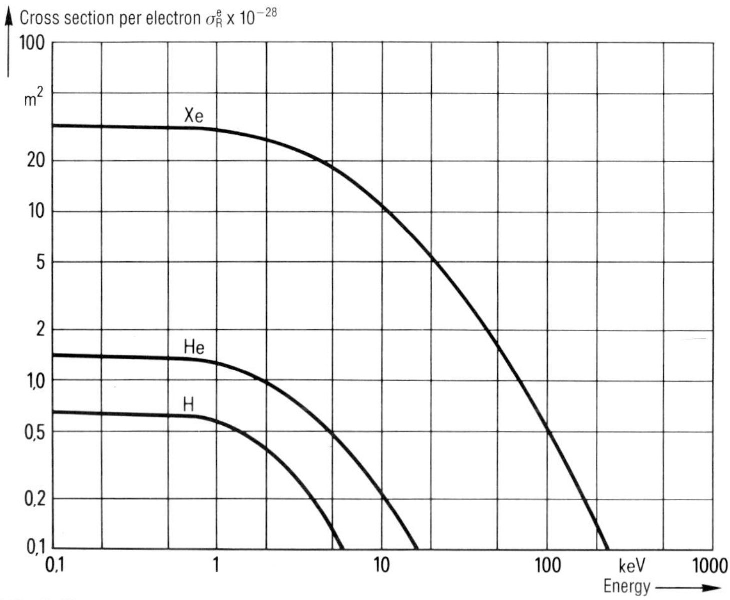

Fig. 3.12
Coherent scattering at bound electrons in various substances as a function of the energy

for helium it is already larger by about a factor of 3. Fig. 3.12 shows the cross sections σ_R^e for three elements. The reason for these deviations will be dealt with in the section entitled "Scattering, bound electrons".

Compton effect

The Compton effect provides clear evidence of the corpuscular nature of x-ray quanta. It is a description, together with the laws of conservation of energy and momentum, of the interaction of high-energy quanta with the quasi free electrons of the atoms. Since in the case of atoms with low Z the binding energy of the electrons is very small compared to the energy of the incident quanta, one may treat these electrons as quasi free. Extensive calculations are available for this case. Using conservation of energy and momentum, one can calculate for instance the energy E' of the recoil electron as a function of the energy $h\nu$ of the colliding quantum and the angle Φ through which the quantum is deflected from its original direction (Fig. 3.13), as well as the energy $h\nu'$ of the scattered quantum or the angle Θ of the recoil electron.

$$h\nu = 1h\nu' + E \qquad \text{(energy conservation)}$$

$$\frac{h\nu}{c} = \frac{h\nu'}{c}\cos\Phi + \sqrt{2mE'}\cos\Theta \qquad \text{(momentum conservation)}$$

$$0 = \frac{h\nu'}{c}\sin\Phi + \sqrt{2mE'}\sin\Theta.$$

Defining

$$\alpha = \frac{h\cdot\nu}{m_0 c^2} \quad \text{one deduces:}$$

$$E' = h\nu\cdot\frac{\alpha(1-\cos\Phi)}{1+\alpha(1-\cos\Phi)} \tag{3.17}$$

$$h\nu' = h\nu\cdot\frac{1}{1+\alpha(1-\cos\Phi)}. \tag{3.18}$$

Equation (3.17) shows that the energy transfer to the recoil electron is small when $h\nu$ is small and rises with increasing energy. The maximum transfer of energy occurs when $\Phi = 180°$, i.e. $\cos\Phi = -1$. This is shown in Fig. 3.14. If

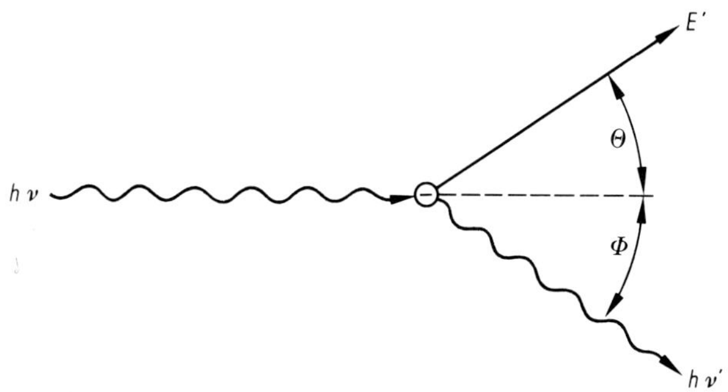

	Energy	Scattering angle	Mass	Momentum
Primary x-ray quantum	$h\nu$	–	–	$\frac{h\nu}{c}$
Scattered x-ray quantum	$h\nu'$	Φ	–	$\frac{h\nu'}{c}$
Recoil electron	E'	Θ	m	$\sqrt{2m_0 E'}$

Fig. 3.13
In the Compton process, an electron that is hit by a primary x-ray quantum is accelerated at an angle Θ and acquires a kinetic energy E'. The scattered x-ray quantum continues on its way with residual energy $h\nu'$ at an angle Φ

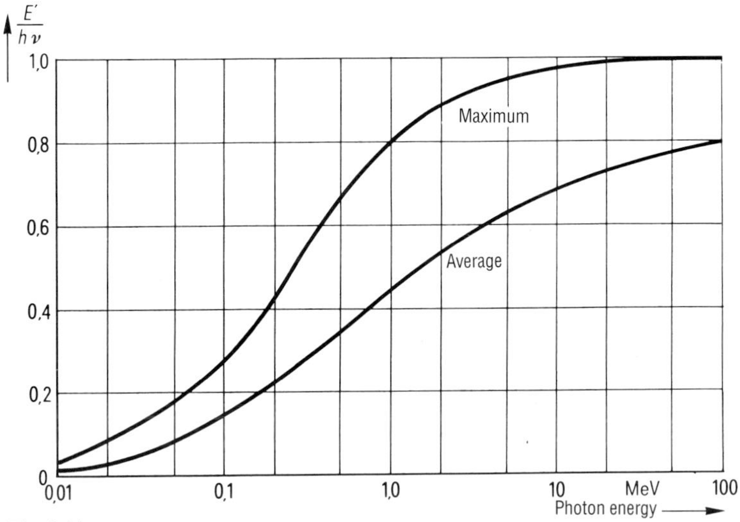

Fig. 3.14
Average and maximum energy transferred to the Compton (recoil) electron

one proceeds to calculate from equation (3.17) for $h\nu'$ the difference between the two wavelengths, one obtains

$$\lambda' - \lambda = \frac{h}{m_0 c}(1 - \cos \Phi). \tag{3.19}$$

This formula states that, leaving aside the dependence on the scattering angle, the wavelength increase is independent of the energy of the incident quantum. The universal constant $\frac{h}{m_0 c}$ is called the Compton wavelength. It has a value of 0.0024 nm.

Incoherent scattering off free electrons

Cross sections, free electrons

The cross section per electron and per solid angle $d\,\Omega$ in the case of incoherent scattering off free electrons is described by the Klein-Nishina formula:

$$\left.\frac{d\,\sigma_c^e}{d\,\Omega}\right|_{KN} = \frac{e^4}{2m_0^2 c^4}(1+\cos^2\Phi)\left\{\frac{1}{1+\alpha(1-\cos\Phi)}\right\}^2 \times\left\{1+\frac{\alpha^2(1-\cos\Phi)^2}{[1+\alpha(1-\cos\Phi)](1+\cos^2\Phi)}\right\}. \tag{3.20}$$

When $h\nu$ or α tends towards zero, one obtains – as should be the case – the Thomson equation (3.15) from the Klein-Nishina formula.

The curve of this differential cross section is depicted in Fig. 3.15. Integration over $d\,\Omega$ gives the linear scattering cross section for the electron.

The cross section per electron for the energy transfer to the electrons $\sigma^{e}_{c,\bar{k}}|_{KN}$ can be obtained for incoherent scattering by multiplying equation (3.20) by $E/h\nu$, using equation (3.17), and integrating over $d\,\Omega$. The result can be seen in Fig. 3.16.

For the ratio of the average transferred energy of the Compton electrons to the energy $h\nu$ of the primary quantum, one obtains, following Sect. 3.2.6.4, the curve labelled 'average' in Fig. 3.14 as the quotient of $\left.\frac{\sigma^{e}_{c,\bar{k}}}{\sigma^{e}_{c}}\right|_{KN}$. Here again, as was mentioned in the section before last, one sees that in the range of diagnostic interest the energy transfer is relatively small, averaging, for instance, only about 10% in the case of a 50 keV photon.

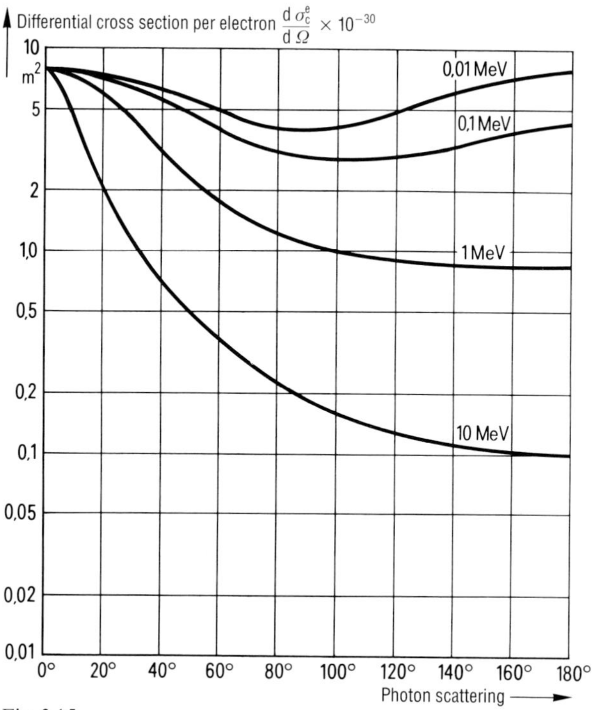

Fig. 3.15
Differential cross section $\left.\frac{d\sigma^{e}_{c}}{d\Omega}\right|_{KN}$, for an electron, according to the Klein-Nishina formula

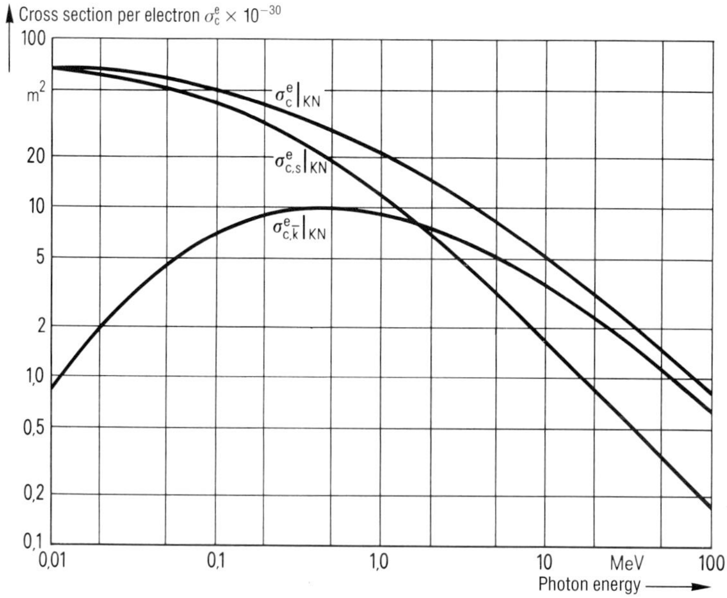

Fig. 3.16
Various cross sections per electron in the Compton process

Scattering at bound electrons

If the Compton electron is to leave the atom, it must be able to muster an amount of energy at least equal to its ionization energy. Thus the energy of the scattered quantum can never be equal to the energy of the incident quantum, as equation (3.18) would allow for the angle $\Phi=0$. If the energy of the incident quantum or the energy transfer in the primary collision is small, then there is a certain probability that the electron – because of its bond to the atomic nucleus – will oscillate instead of leaving the atom. However, the other electrons of the atom are also excited by the wave. Every electron emits a spherical wave. The coherently scattered wave comes about by vectorial addition of the amplitudes. Thus we are dealing with quite different processes than those which form the basis of not only the classical, but also the quantum-mechanical calculation of the "collision with a free electron". This is the reason why coherent scattering for increasing Z and low photon energies is significantly greater than is calculated according to the Thomson formula, and why the Compton process occurs much more rarely than calculated (Fig. 3.17).

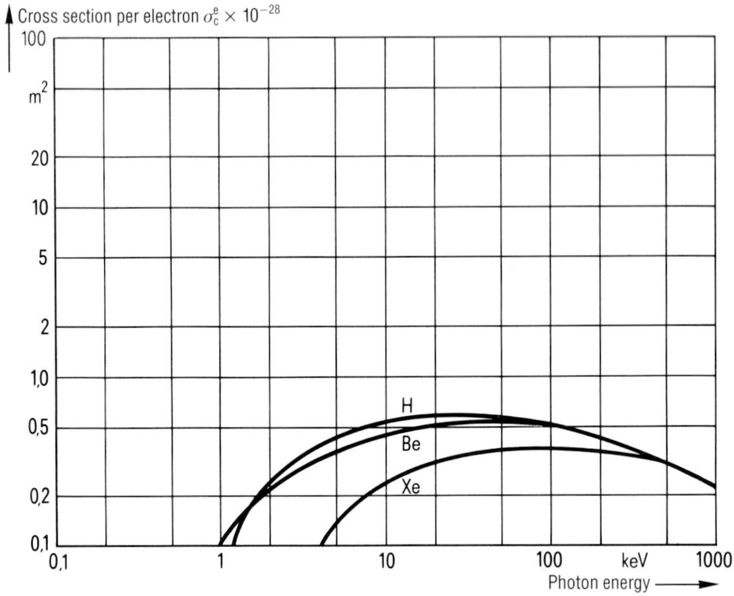

Fig. 3.17
Compton scattering at bound electrons

The relationship between the Thomson formula and coherent scattering leads to a factor $F^2(x, Z)$ where $F(x, Z)$ is the atomic form factor, and where

$$x = \frac{\sin \frac{\Phi}{2}}{\lambda}. \tag{3.21}$$

Combining the Klein-Nishina formula with the actual Compton scattering gives the incoherent scattering function $S(x, Z)$. Both functions are tabulated e.g. in Hubbel et al. [3.6].

General treatments of the interaction of x-rays and gamma rays with matter may be found in [3.5 to 3.9].

3.2.5 Interactions with real objects

Up to now our basic approach has been to discuss only interactions with individual atoms or the limiting case of infinitesimally thin layers.

If one wishes to quantitatively evaluate the effect of a real object, for instance, scattering in a real layer of thickness d, then an integration over $\mathrm{d}x$ – as carried out in equation 3.8 – is only possible if the expected contribution of multiple and secondary processes is small enough relative to the precision required. If this is not the case, more accurate calculations are necessary.

Scattering and energy absorption

If one wants to have accurate knowledge about the radiation which emerges behind a real object in terms of the number, direction and energy of the quanta, or about the energy absorption in the object under consideration, then one must follow the interactions of the relevant quanta and electrons in detail. To do this, one has to take into account multiple scatterings of the primary quanta and the fluorescence quanta associated with the photoelectric effect. In addition, when calculating the energy absorption, the secondary processes of the photoelectrons, Compton electrons and Auger electrons must also be taken into consideration. In a solid, the kinetic energy of these electrons is almost exclusively used for the creation of electron-hole pairs, whilst in gases and liquids it is used for the ionization and excitation of atoms or molecules, as the case may be.

Photoelectrons, Compton electrons and Auger electrons also cause other effects which, however, form a very small part of the energy transfer so that they can usually be ignored: bremsstrahlung, the formation of free valence electrons through the breaking up of chemical bonds, the creation of crystal defects, and the creation of photons, i.e. these electrons cause vibration of the molecular or lattice components.

Calculations of single and multiple scattering in an object (phantom) are carried out, e.g. with the help of the Monte-Carlo method in [3.10], as are calculations of the energy absorption in real receptor layers.

X-ray detectors

If one wants to detect x-ray or gamma quanta, one has to exploit the effects of their interaction with matter, as the quanta themselves move in empty space without changing their energy, so that for instance their path is not observable. Since photoelectrons, Compton electrons and Auger electrons generally possess a lot of energy, they are used to detect high-energy quanta. In actual fact these electrons are not made use of directly, their resulting products being used instead. In particular there are the following conversion mechanisms:

Chemical energy

Film: Fast electrons activate a grain of silver, which is then developed like ordinary photographic film.

Charge converters

Semiconductor detectors, high-pressure xenon gas detectors in computer tomographs, xeroradiography:

The electron-hole pairs or electron-ion pairs created by the fast electrons are separated by an external field and the current pulse is used to make a measurement. In xeroradiography a surface charge relief is produced.

Luminescence

Fluorescent screens for cassette recording and image intensifiers, Anger cameras, detectors in computer tomographs.

The fast electrons knock electrons in the crystal out of the valence band into the conduction band; the rule of thumb is that one needs on average three times the energy of the band gap for each pair production (electron/hole). The electrons can then either recombine directly with their hole (crystal luminescence), or they can diffuse to the bottom edge of the conduction band and return from there via the electron traps back to the valence band. Of course, some of the electrons may also recombine without emitting radiation, e.g. where there are defects in the crystal.

4 X-ray computed tomography

4.1 Principles of computed tomography

4.1.1 Introduction

Computed tomography is a special x-ray tomography method which is fundamentally different from the classical x-ray tomography method based on the blurring principle [4.1], in the way the image is formed. It is not absolutely essential to use a computer in order to carry out the method, so that the name computed tomography is actually misleading. However, the use of a computer to produce the images has proved to be extremely useful.

The method produces axial transverse tomograms, i.e. images of body layers which are essentially perpendicular to the longitudinal axis of the body. Although layers with corresponding orientation can be obtained using the classical photographic axial transverse tomography method [4.2, 4.3], these images usually have poor contrast. A large number of attemps have therefore been made to generate x-ray transaxial tomograms with better quality ([4.4], [4.5], [4.6]). In 1963 and 1964, A.M. Cormack was the first to describe an x-ray tomography method completely corresponding to computed tomography which made it possible to produce an image of a layer from a large number of lateral sections determined by x-ray techniques. It was subsequently discovered that the mathematical solution of this problem had already been given by Radon [4.9] in 1917. The first clinical application of computed tomography then followed in 1972 by Hounsfield [4.10] and Ambrose [4.11].

Classical x-ray techniques always produce a photographic recording of the two-dimensional shadow image of the three-dimensional object area projected by the radiation cone into the image plane. In images produced in this way, structures are necessarily superimposed from different object depths. Here, classical survey exposures or spot exposures can only be distinguished from classical tomograms by the fact that in the former the structures from different object depths have equally sharp images apart from small differences due to the radiation geometry whereas in the latter, with the exception of the structures in the layer concerned, the structures have more or less blurred images.

Computed tomography, however, avoids this superposition effect by only processing information on the layer, i.e. slice, of interest to the image. Thus, in the computer tomogram, an object detail exactly corresponds to an image detail and not to a large number of object elements lying behind each other in the

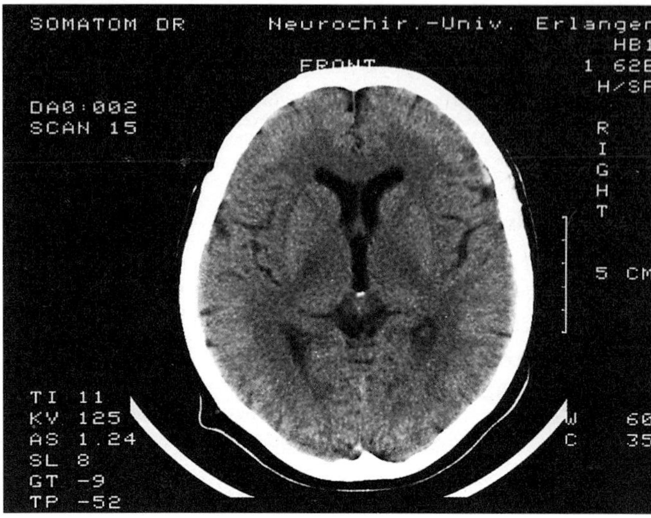

Fig. 4.1
Computer tomogram of a skull. The photograph shows a section at the height of the ventricles which can be easily distinguished from the cerebral matter without any contrast agent. White and gray cerebral matter can be distinguished in this image. Because of its high fat content, the white matter appears darker, i.e. with lower attenuation capacity than the gray matter

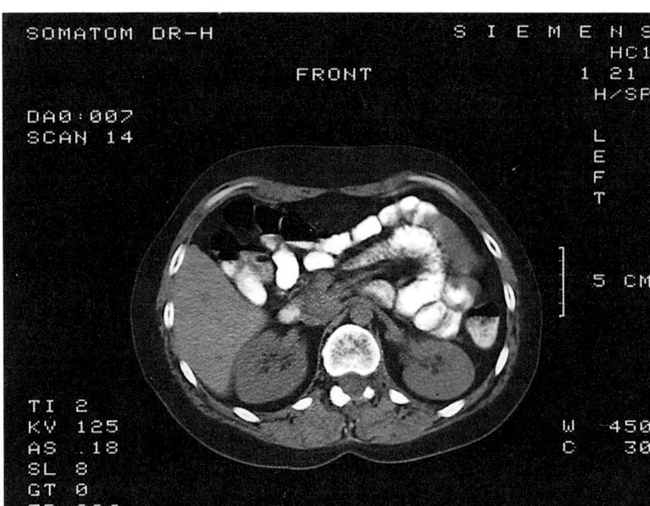

Fig. 4.2
Computer tomogram of an abdomen. The liver, kidneys, aorta, muscles and a large number of other details are clearly demarcated in this tomogram. Their different attenuation capacities can easily be seen

direction of radiation. Such an image which is free of superpositioning is called a substitution image. The capacity of computer tomographs to produce a substitution image instead of a superposition image is one of the main reasons for the high effectiveness of the method: computed tomography provides soft-tissue images with extremely high contrast, which cannot be achieved by classical methods. In addition, because of the special type of image generation, it produces images which can even be evaluated quantitatively.

As a result of these outstanding properties, computed tomography, only a few years after its introduction, has already established itself as an indispensable standard technique, at least in the field of neuroradiology (Fig. 4.1), but also in the radiological examination of other body areas (Fig. 4.2). Its scope of applications is constantly being widened.

In a large number of cases, the high-contrast soft-tissue images which can be obtained make it possible to image structures directly without using a contrast medium. For example, computed tomography enables the cerebral ventricles to be shown directly, so that the number of pneumoencephalograms has been considerably lowered through the introduction of this new technique. Frequently, an injection of contrast medium into the bloodstream can also be avoided. At least high-risk intraarterial contrast administration can be replaced by low-risk intravenous contrast administration. Here, the special advantage of the new imaging technique is not just in the reduction of the risk of a contrast agent accident, but in particular in the reproduction of the actual shape of the organs or lesions: conventional angiography often only produces indirect information, e.g. through vessel displacement. Although computed tomography does not make angiographic examination methods obsolete, it does provide in many cases a more rigorous indication for angiography.

The quantitative nature of the computer tomogram opens up completely new possibilities for image evaluation. However, we will not look at this any more closely here, since it will be treated in depth in section 8.2.

4.1.2 Basic principle

The most important components of a computer tomograph and their operation are shown in the form of a block diagram in Fig. 4.3. In order to generate an image of the body slice of interest, the attenuation of radiation by the object is determined for a large number of paths through the object slice by means of a measurement arrangement consisting of an x-ray tube and a radiation detector system. The simplest form of measurement system, shown in Fig. 4.3, uses an x-ray beam about the thickness of a pencil passing through the slice for measuring the attenuation. The attenuation is determined by first moving the measurement system perpendicular to this beam and parallel to the slice plane over the entire object cross-section. At the same time, the radiation intensi-

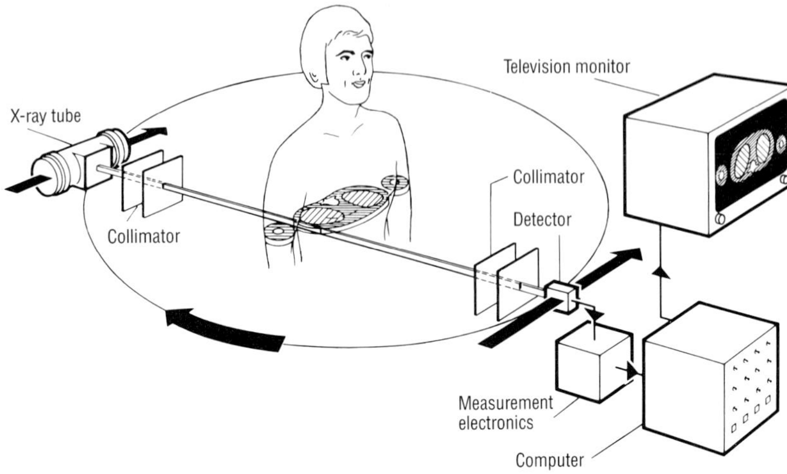

Fig. 4.3
Basic representation of a computer tomograph in the simplest design form. The measurement system, consisting of x-ray tube and radiation detector, is first moved linearly in the slice plane over the entire object cross section. The measurement system is then rotated about approximately 1° and then a new linear scanning movement performed, etc., until an angle of at least 180° has been traversed. Throughout the entire scanning process, the measurement signal obtained by an x-ray beam approximately the thickness of a pencil is recorded at fixed intervals and transferred to a computer. This computes a two-dimensional distribution of attenuation values corresponding to the object layer from the measurement values, which is finally displayed as a tomogram on a television monitor after conversion to video signals

ty at the detector is recorded at fixed predetermined intervals, so that an initial set of measurement values is obtained which corresponds to a lateral section of the slice and is called a projection. In contrast to classical x-ray technology, a large number of such projections is needed in computed tomography to generate an image. They are obtained by rotating the measurement system through a small angle of 1° about the system axis perpendicular to the slice plane after one projection is measured and then initiating another linear scanning process, etc., until the measurement system has traversed an angle of rotation of at least 180°. During the measurement process, the measurement values are coded in suitable form and transferred to a computer. With the present state of the art, every image requires a few hundred projections and every projection a few hundred measurement values, so that in total about 100000 to 1000000 measurement values are involved. The computer then calculates from all these measurement values a two-dimensional attenuation distribution corresponding to the object as an image of the slice, where object areas with high attenuation are assigned high numerical values and object areas with low attenuation are assigned low numerical values. Since the computer, just as it can only process a finite number of measurement values, can only calculate a finite number of attenuation values, the object slice must be thought of as divided into small volume elements ("voxels") with a square base, inside which the attenuation value is assumed to be constant (Fig. 4.4) and is then calculated by the computer. However, in practice the attenuation value of the object material will usually vary inside the individual layer elements, so that the calculated attenuation value is always obtained as an average over the volume element concerned. This should always be borne in mind, in particular in quantitative image evaluation.

At first, the slice image is only present in the computer in the form of a stored set of numbers and is thus not immediately accessible. The simplest way to make the image accessible to the eye is to print the attenuation values in an arrangement corresponding to the position of the volume elements assigned to them in the object layer. However, the visual evaluation of such an arrangement of numbers, also called a matrix, proves to be very laborious, especially because of the large number of matrix elements, which at present usually lies between 256 × 256 and 512 × 512. This image representation method is therefore only used in rare cases and then mostly only for parts of the image. Usually, the numerical matrix is converted into a black and white or color television image in which each image point ("pixel") corresponds to a matrix element and different gray or color tones are assigned to the different attenuation values.

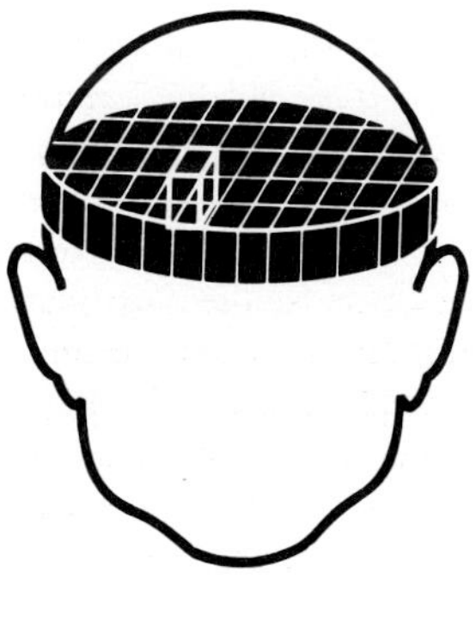

Fig. 4.4
Decomposition of the object slice into volume elements. The object layer is considered as made up of a large number of such small volume elements with a square base. The attenuation capacity of the object material is assumed to be constant inside these elements

4.1.3 Attenuation scale

For the attenuation of a monochromatic x-ray beam passing through a homogeneous material, we have

$$J = J_0 \, e^{-\mu x} \tag{4.1}$$

where

J is the radiation intensity behind the object
J_0 is the radiation intensity at the same point in the absence of the object
x is the object thickness
μ is the linear attenuation coefficient of the material for the radiation used.

The value of μ strongly depends on the radiation energy and is therefore only of limited use for characterizing the radiation attenuation capacity of an object in computed tomography, since it would only be possible to compare the results obtained with different equipment if all these different types of equipment were to use exactly the same radiation. This is why in computed tomography an

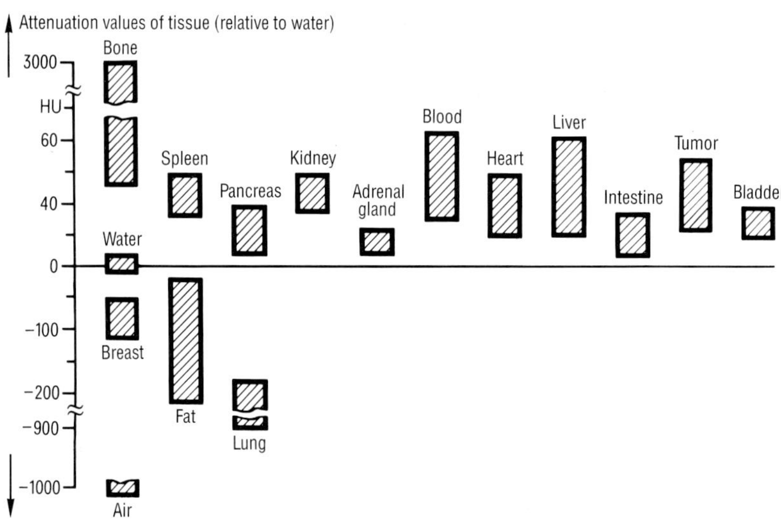

Fig. 4.5
Attenuation value ranges of different body substances and tissues. It can be seen that the attenuation value ranges corresponding to the individual substances frequently overlap. Therefore, it is not possible to unambiguously identify the substance from the attenuation value. This applies, in particular, to the different types of tumors

attenuation value is used which is the scaled relative deviation of the linear attenuation coefficient of the investigated object from the linear attenuation coefficient of a generally available reference material similar to the object. In practice, water is used as the reference material. The attenuation value is therefore given as

$$\mu_{rel}=k\,\frac{\mu_{object}-\mu_{H_2O}}{\mu_{H_2O}}. \tag{4.2}$$

As a rule, the factor k is chosen as 1000, so that in this scale water has the attenuation value 0 and air -1000, whereas very dense bone tissue lies around $+3000$ because its linear attenuation coefficient for the radiation energy values used in computed tomography is approximately four times that of water. The position of other tissue types on this scale is shown in Fig. 4.5.

4.1.4 Image generation

In order to construct a usable tomogram from the measured intensity profiles, a simple computational superposition of the individual intensity signals corresponding to the projection direction in the image matrix is inadequate (Fig. 4.6). Instead, the measured intensity J has to be converted to the quotient of the intensity J_0 (without attenuating medium) and J and then the logarithm of this quotient taken. In this way, values proportional to the linear attenuation coefficient of the object material are obtained before superposition. By taking the logarithms of both sides and rearranging, from the attenuation law – equation (4.1) – we obtain:

$$\mu=\frac{1}{x}\ln\frac{J_0}{J}. \tag{4.3}$$

However, even a superposition of the projections preprocessed in this manner still does not give us the required result. Such an image exhibits extensive blurring (Fig. 4.6a). In order to avoid such blurring, the preprocessed projections are convoluted with a filter function before superposition (Fig. 4.6b). Because of this preprocessing step, the entire image generation process described here, which is commonly used today in computed tomography, is called the convolution process. This convolution results in modified signals, which contain negative as well as positive components. If the filter function is suitably chosen, they have the properties that when the convoluted projections are superimposed, this extensive blurring is exactly cancelled out. One consequence of this convolution process and subsequent projection superposition is that every measurement value makes a contribution to every image point, even though with very different weighting. This is of special importance for the artifact behavior of computed tomography, which is completely different from classical x-ray techniques.

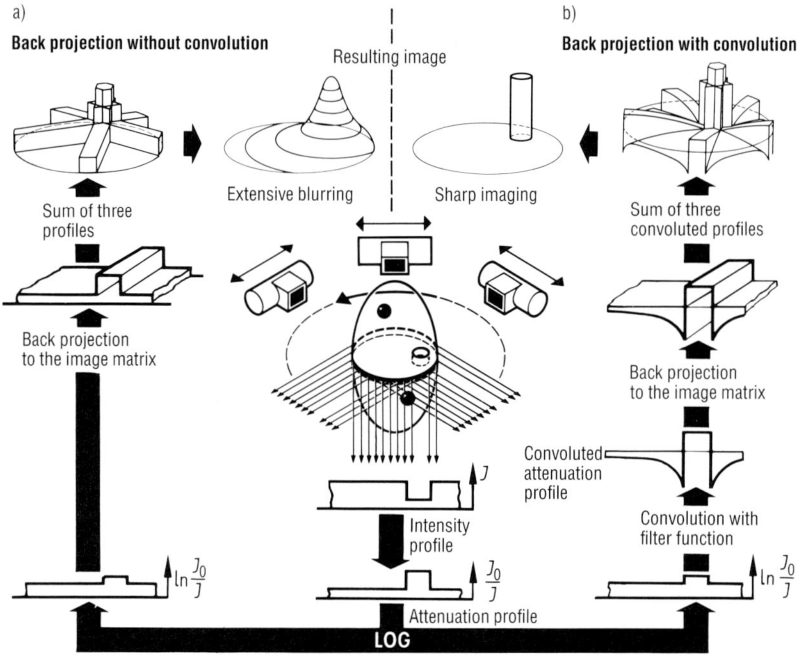

Fig. 4.6
Importance of convolution for image reconstruction in computed tomography. The intensity profiles J obtained by measurement are converted to attenuation profiles J_0/J, where J_0 is the intensity measured without the object in the radiation path. The attenuation profiles are then converted to logarithms, so that a quantity proportional to the attenuation coefficient is available for further processing. If, as shown in path a, the logarithmic attenuation profile is simply superimposed according to its projection direction, then there would be considerable blurring of the detail to be imaged. Therefore, in computed tomography, there is a specific alteration of the logarithmic attenuation profile, as shown in path b, by convolution with a suitable filter function. The convoluted profiles exhibit negative as well as positive components, whose contributions to the superposition image exactly cancel the extensive blurring when the filter function is correctly chosen

4.1.5 Types and properties of equipment

Since the introduction of computed tomography, considerable effort has been made to improve the effectiveness of the equipment, in particular to cut down the imaging time. This has led to the development of different scanning systems, which essentially differ in terms of the number and arrangement of the detectors. As the following comparison shows, each of the individual systems has certain advantages which are always offset by certain disadvantages.

The measurement system already mentioned, shown again in Fig. 4.7a with a single radiation beam of pencil thickness, is in fact the arrangement which is least commonly used for attenuation measurement: it only utilizes a vanishingly small fraction of the radiation generated in the x-ray tube. While the radiation released at the anode of the x-ray tube is emitted into all of the half space, i.e. a solid angle of $2\pi = 6.28$ radians, the radiation beam which is finally used for measurement only takes up a solid angle of approximately 10^{-4} radians. Since, on the one hand, the power of an x-ray tube is limited and, on the other hand, a certain amount of radiation (dose) is needed to produce a usable computer tomogram, and in addition the machine cannot be moved at unlimited speed, such a measurement system requires relatively long exposure times of the order of magnitude of a few minutes; it is therefore only suitable for the examination of stationary parts of the body or areas of the body which are easy to keep still, in particular for skull examinations.

The total examination time can be reduced by using a second detector directly following the first detector in the direction of the layer thickeness, otherwise keeping the same geometrical relationships, collimating the radiation beam correspondingly to both detectors and so processing the measurement data for two immediately adjacent slices at the same time. However, a real reduction in the exposure time for the same dose can only be achieved through increasing the number of measurement channels per layer by arranging several detectors next to each other in the scanning direction as is shown for example in Fig. 4.7b and collimating the beam at the x-ray tube to a fan shape. With such a measurement arrangement, utilizing the radiation generated in the x-ray tube in a much better way, it is possible to obtain the measurement data for a number of projections corresponding to the number of detectors at the same time, so that the system rotation angle between two linear scanning processes can be increased and thus the number of linear scanning processes and rotation steps decreased. Measurement times achieved with such equipment lie between 10 and 60 seconds, depending on the number of detectors per slice. However, there is a limit to any further reduction in the measurement time in these measurement systems for mechanical reasons, because of the alternating sequence of translational and rotational motions.

The shortest exposure times, of the order of a few seconds, can be obtained by using an x-ray fan covering the entire object cross-section in conjunction

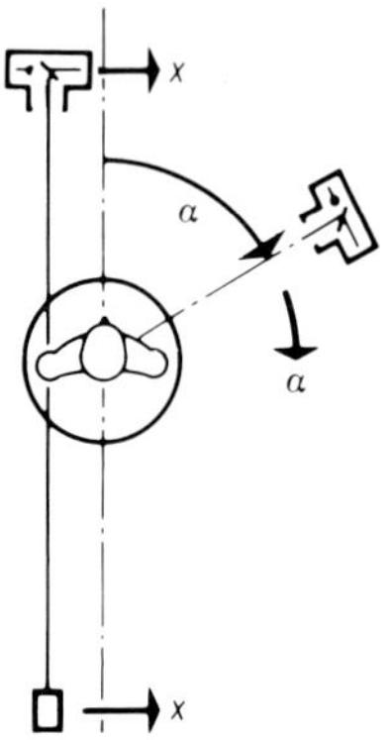

a) The parallel-beam system with only one measurement beam (see also Fig. 4.3), alternately moved in a translational and rotational manner, only poorly utilizes the radiation of the x-ray tube and requires a long measuring time

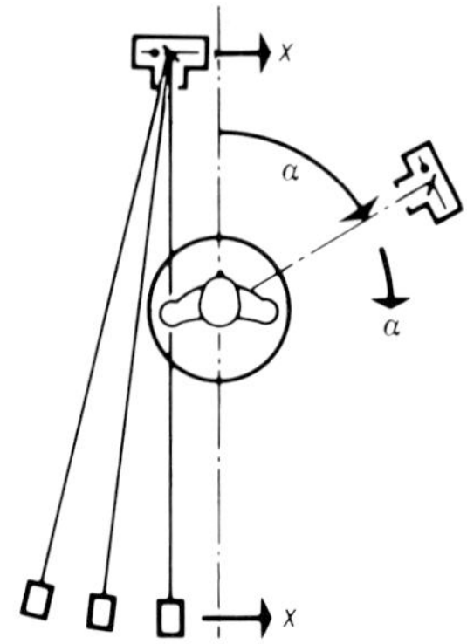

b) The parallel-beam system with several measurement beams makes better use of the generated radiation, reduces the number of movement steps and therefore cuts down the measurement time

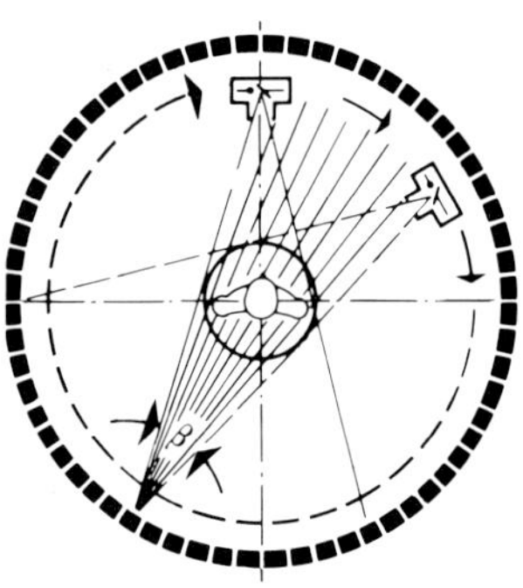

c) The ring-detector system has a fixed detector ring, operates with a fan-shaped x-ray beam simultaneously covering the entire patient cross section and therefore only requires a rotational movement of the x-ray tube

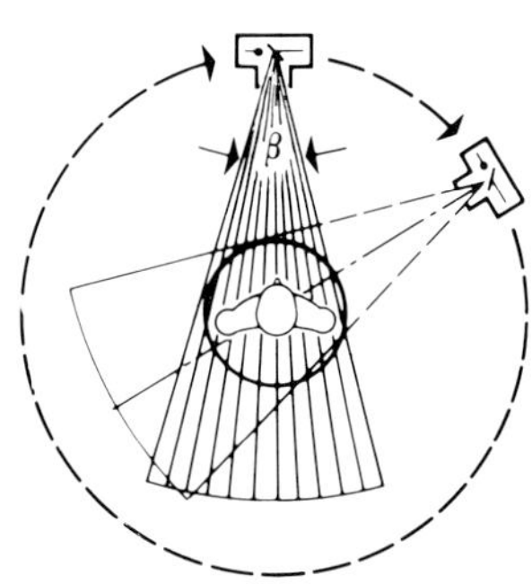

d) The fan-beam system has a multicellular detector system rotating about the patient together with the x-ray tube

Fig. 4.7
Scanning principles of different computed tomography systems

with a corresponding multi-cellular detector system. In this case, the radiation generated in the tube is optimally utilized and in addition it is only necessary for the system to execute purely rotational movements, which do not have to be in steps but can be performed continuously. Two different detector arrangements are possible, as shown in Figs. 4.7c and 4.7d: either a detector system which moves around the patient together with the tube or a stationary detector ring. In the case of the travelling detector system, the radiation is either switched on in pulses at fixed angular intervals or continuous radiation is used and the detectors are switched on and off. Only the second operating principle is common in equipment with a detector ring.

In contrast to translation-rotation systems, which always produce sets of measurement data for parallel projections and are therefore also called parallel beam scanners, in purely rotational systems primary sets of data are produced which correspond to central projections. Whereas in the case of a detector system moving together with the x-ray tube the projection center is always the tube focus (fan-beam scanner), in the case of a stationary detector ring, the individual detectors can also be interpreted as projection centers (ring-detector scanner), which is also usually the case in the corresponding equipment design.

It will be shown in Section 4.2 that a computer tomogram can be constructed directly from parallel projections as well as from central projections. However, since the amount of computation is greater in the latter case, in some types of equipment the sets of measurement data originally obtained as central projections are first rearranged to parallel projections before the actual reconstruction of the computer tomogram. In this case, though, it is no longer possible to process the measurement data in step with the data acquisition process, since all measurement data have to be collected first prior to complete rearrangement.

The reduction in scan time obtained by successively increasing the measurement beam in various scanning systems is offset by an increased level of scattered radiation at the detector entrance. Particularly with fan-beam equipment and ring detector equipment, which both operate with fan beams covering the entire cross section of the patient, it is necessary to reduce the amount of scattered radiation among the radiation which reaches the detector system. In fan-beam equipment, it is relatively easy to do this by installing an anti-scatter collimator focussed on the focal spot of the x-ray tube in front of the detector system. This collimator then rotates around the patient together with the measurement system (Fig. 4.8a). However, for ring detector equipment with the usual radiation geometry, as shown in Fig. 5.7c, it is not possible to have a fixed anti-scatter collimator in front of the detector system because this could only be focussed on the center of rotation and not on the focal spot (Fig. 4.8b). Instead, it would be necessary to provide a collimator with moving lamellae which would always have to be pointing at the focal spot. This is only possible by means of a complicated and very precisely operating mechanism. Since this is hardly feasible, the distance between patient and detector is chosen as large as possible, as in the well-known Groedel technique for classical radiography [4.12], in order to reduce the amount of scattered radiation in the signal which reaches the ring-detector equipment. However, in view of the equipment dimensions which are possible, the scattered radiation cannot be suppressed as drastically as by means of a collimator.

Apart from the various problems arising from scattered radiation, there are other important differences between the individual measurement arrangements in terms of image quality and image characteristics. These affect, for instance, the geometrical resolution and the image noise. In this respect, parallel-beam and ring-detector scanners behave in practically the same manner, because their scanning principles differ only slightly, whereas there are marked differences between these systems on the one hand and fan-beam scanners on the other hand.

For parallel-beam and ring-detector scanners, the linear distance or the angular distance of the individual measurement beams within a projection can be chosen independently of the width of the individual measurement beams in the scanning direction. On the other hand, for fan-beam scanners, the distance and the width of the individual measurement beams are fixed by the detector arrangement (Fig. 4.9). Since the measurement beam width b and the center-to-center distance a of the measurement beam components determine the spatial resolution d of the system according to the relationship

$$d=\sqrt{a^2+b^2} \tag{4.4}$$

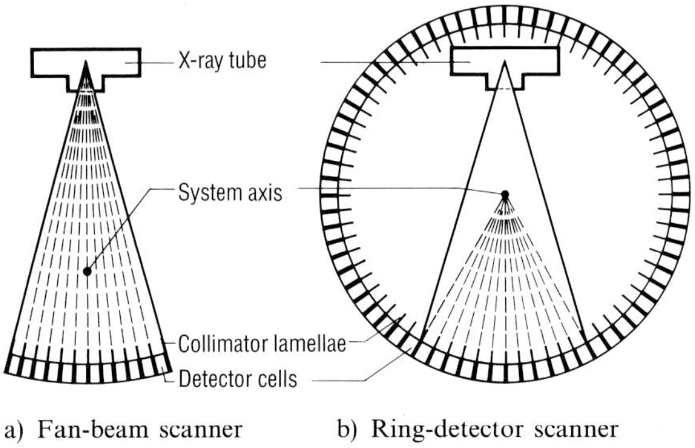

a) Fan-beam scanner b) Ring-detector scanner

Fig. 4.8
Possibilities for eliminating scattered radiation by a lamellar collimator connected to the detector system. For the fan-beam scanner (a) it is easily possible to insert a rigid anti-scatter collimator, focussed on the focal spot of the x-ray tube and attached to the detector system. For the ring-detector scanner in the usual arrangement (b), on the other hand, a rigid collimator could only be focussed on the center of rotation, so that shadows would be formed of the primary radiation towards the edge of the fan. In this case, the collimator lamellae would have to be moveable and would have to be kept pointed to the focal spot of the tube by a tracking mechanism

and the distance a fixes the noise-grain size in the reconstructed image. This means that, in contrast to fan-beam scanners, by means of a suitable choice of the distance a in parallel-beam and ring-detector scanners, the noise-grain size can to a large extent be selected independently of the spatial resolution. In another type of equipment, with fan-beam and flying focal spot, the focus is approximately fixed in space by periodic electron beam deflection for the duration of each readout cycle, whereas the fan-beams, due to the continuous detector movement A_D at the center of rotation, perform a swinging movement a about the focus (Fig. 4.9c). During this movement, n readouts can be made at the beam center distance a/n, as if the detector had an n times finer partitioning. This considerably increases the resolution, with the radiation beam width b remaining the same.

For parallel-beam, ring-detector and flying focal spot scanners, apart from the detector and focal spot width, the movement of the measurement beam influences the effective measurement beam width and thus also the geometrical resolution during a measurement interval. As shown in Fig. 4.10, this is not the case for conventional fan-beam scanners.

For a given image matrix, it is no longer possible to achieve any noticeable improvement in the image quality through increasing the number of measurement values in each projection and the number of projections above a certain

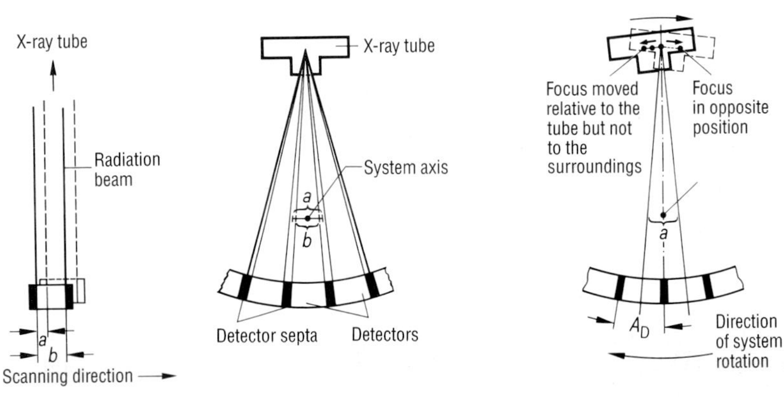

a) Parallel-beam scanner

b) Fan-beam scanner

c) Fan-beam scanner with flying focal spot

Fig. 4.9
Relationship between the measurement beam width and distance for different scanning systems. For parallel-beam systems (a), ring-detector systems and systems with flying focal spot (c), the center-to-center distance a of the individual measurement beams can be chosen independently of their width b by fixing the number of measurements. For fan-beam systems (b), the center-to-center distance a of the individual measurement beams is always greater than the measurement beam width b, because of gaps between the beam segments dictated by design

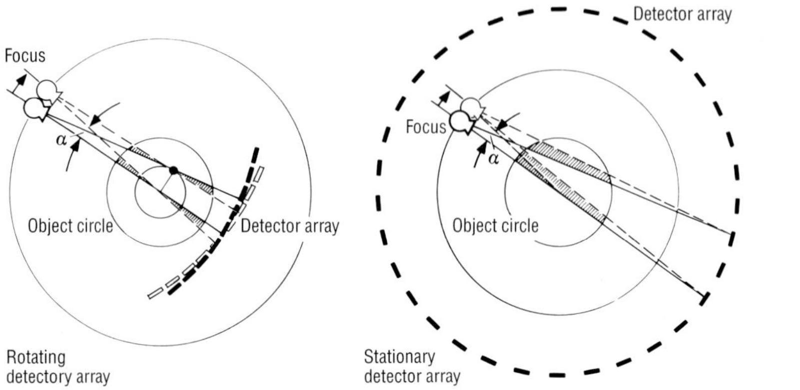

a) Fan-beam scanner b) Ring-detector scanner

Fig. 4.10
Effect of movement of the focal spot on the measurement beam width for different scanning systems. For conventional fan-beam systems (a) the focal spot and detector move together around the object, so that there is no blurring, i.e. broadening of the measurement beam, and thus no reduction in the geometrical resolution due to movement of the measurement system during the measurement process at the center of the image. However, in the ring-detector system (b), movement of the focus also produces such a blurring at the center of the image. The same applies to parallel-beam systems and flying focal spot systems

value. This results in a particular disadvantage of ring-detector scanners compared to fan-beam scanners in terms of the geometrical resolution: because of the high costs entailed, every effort is made to keep the number of detectors and measurement channels as small as possible to satisfy the specifications of image quality. Due to the equipment dimensions determined by the object sizes, this results in a relatively large detector distance for ring-detector systems compared with fan-beam systems having the same number of projections and thus a correspondingly large detector width, if the radiation in the detector plane is to be well utilized. However, the large detector width likewise leads to a relatively large measurement beam width and in turn to a correspondingly lower spatial resolution.

With some parallel-beam and ring-detector scanners, it is possible to reduce the detector width by additional collimation and thus increase the spatial resolution. However, in this case the radiation arriving in the detector plane is only partly utilized. This leads to higher image noise and thus also to a lower density resolution capacity for the same dose in the detector plane, which therefore indirectly means an increase in the radiation received by the patient.

The characteristics described above by no means cover all the differences between the various scanning systems. However, the comparison already makes it quite clear that every system has advantages and disadvantages, so that no single system can be regarded as optimal. The required image quality, costs and application determine which type of equipment is the best in each individual case.

4.1.6 Beam quality and measurement value corrections

Ideal measurement conditions would be present if it were possible to measure the radiation attenuation with monochromatic radiation, i.e. with radiation which only consists of quanta having the same energy (Fig. 4.11 a). In this case, practically only radioactive isotopes could be considered as a radiation source. However, there is no isotope which can emit a quantum energy suitable for computed tomography (60 – 80 keV) and which can be produced with sufficiently high specific activity to make sufficiently small sources available with adequate radiation intensity. Therefore, apart from special equipment for small object diameters, one is forced to use an x-ray tube as a radiation source for computer tomographs. However, the anode of an x-ray tube emits x-ray quanta with an energy varying from a few keV to a maximum energy of the order of 100 to 150 keV, depending on the voltage applied to the tube. A typical radiation spectrum of an x-ray tube for computed tomography is shown in Figs. 4.11 b and 4.11 c.

As they pass through the object, the various spectral components of the beam undergo very different attenuation, so that the attenuation law in the simple form of relationship (4.1) can only be applied to the individual energy components. In fact, for a homogeneous material, one measures

$$J = \int J_0(E)\, \mathrm{e}^{-\mu(E)x}\, \mathrm{d}E \tag{4.5}$$

and for an inhomogeneous material, one measures

$$J = \int J_0(E)\, \mathrm{e}^{-\int \mu(x,E)\mathrm{d}x}\, \mathrm{d}E, \tag{4.6}$$

where J_0 and μ depend on the quantum energy E and μ also depends on the position x along the measurement beam. No account has been taken here of the fact that the sensitivity of the detector system can also vary for the different spectral components.

The energy composition of the beam after passing through an object of given material, e.g. water, therefore depends on the object thickness (Fig. 4.11 b). In other words, the linear attenuation coefficient determined by (4.1) for the same material varies with the object thickness in such a way that it decreases with increasing object thickness. The lower energy soft radiation components are more strongly attenuated than the higher energy hard components, so that the mean energy of the radiation spectrum is shifted to higher energies after passing through an attenuating medium. This process is called hardening. A result of the hardening effect is that, for example, the measurement of a homogeneous object with elliptical cross-section gives a different attenuation coefficient in the direction of the minor semi-axis than in the direction of the major semi-axis. The results of the two measurements are therefore inconsistent and they must be brought into agreement by suitable measures before image reconstruction. A first step is to confine the spectral distribution by suitable prefiltering of the radiation. This removes the soft radiation components, which can only penetrate the object to a small extent and therefore only contribute to the radiation exposure of the patient without contributing to the signal intensity at the detector.

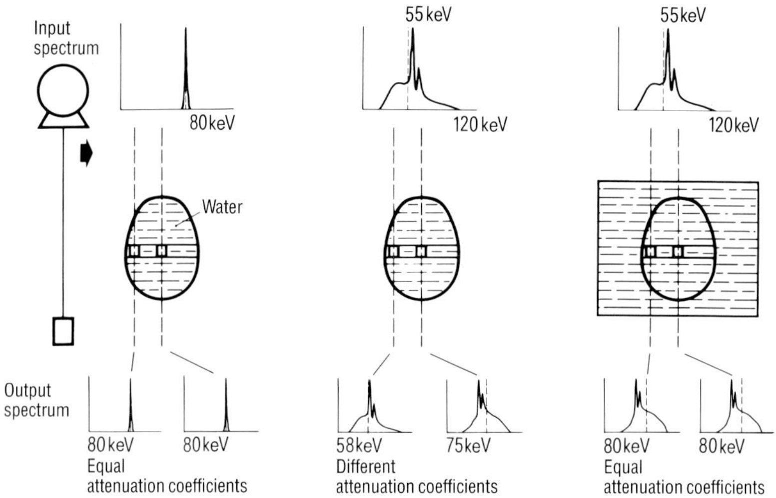

a) Monochromatic radiation

b) Radiation of an x-ray tube without compensation body

c) Radiation of an x-ray tube with compensation body

Fig. 4.11
Beam hardening and compensation body. Monochromatic radiation (a) would allow ideal measurement conditions. The measured radiation spectrum would be independent of the composition and thickness of the object. However, the radiation spectrum of an x-ray tube used in practice (b) covers a relatively large energy range. The soft spectral components are attenuated more strongly than the hard spectral components. This shifts the mean energy value of the spectrum to higher energy values when the radiation passes through the object: the radiation becomes harder. For one and the same material, we therefore have a different attenuation value for every material thickness without appropriate correction. By embedding the object in a compensation body (c) made of material similar to the object, effects of beam hardening, which are different for different object regions, can be reduced considerably

However, prefiltering is not sufficient to reduce the beam hardening effect to an insignificant level. Therefore, in the first computer tomographs, the object was embedded in a compensation medium of a material similar to the object (water and suitable plastics) to ensure that the path length of the radiation in the attenuating medium was the same in all directions, so that the signal changes at the detector were only caused by the small material and density differences in the object (Fig. 4.11 c). This type of correction was entirely sufficient and, in addition, ensured that the signal range at the detector was reduced to a minimum. It therefore contributed considerable advantages to the design of the detectors and associated measurement electronics. However, the compensation medium was a source of discomfort for the patient, caused problems in the examination of casualty patients and could only be offered at considerable costs for parts of the body with large variations in diameter (thorax and abdomen). This means of beam hardening correction was therefore very soon re-

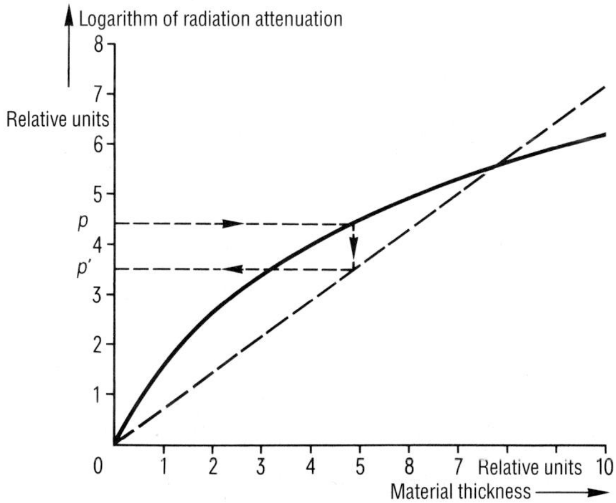

Fig. 4.12
Correction for beam hardening without compensation body. With the radiation quality chosen for the patient scans, the logarithm of the radiation attenuation is determined experimentally by measuring slices of different thickness of a material as similar as possible to the body. This generally gives a relationship such as shown by the solid curve. However, with no beam hardening effects, a straight line should be produced. We therefore choose a reference point on the measured curve and draw the dotted line through this point and the coordinate origin, which represents the required linear relationship between the material thickness and the logarithm of the attenuation. The corrected value p' corresponding to a measured value p of the logarithm of the attenuation is found by determining the material thickness associated with p on the measured curve and then reading off the value p' of the logarithm of the attenuation assigned to this material thickness from the straight line. In the computer, this correction process can be performed by accessing appropriate tables

placed by purely computational signal correction, although this considerably increased the costs of the measurement electronics because of the vastly greater signal range at the detector. In order to provide the basis for purely computational beam hardening corrections, the attenuations J_0/J are determined for different material thicknesses of a substance as similar to the body as possible, e.g. water (Fig. 4.12). The logarithms of these values would be linearly dependent of the layer thickness if there were no beam hardening. In practice, though, we do not obtain a straight line. We therefore choose a point on the curve, i.e. a specific material thickness, and draw a straight line between the coordinate origin and this point. The image reconstruction is then based on the corrected value of the layer thickness read from this straight line instead of the measured values lying on the curve. In the computer, this correction is carried out either by using look-up tables or by using a suitable approximation function.

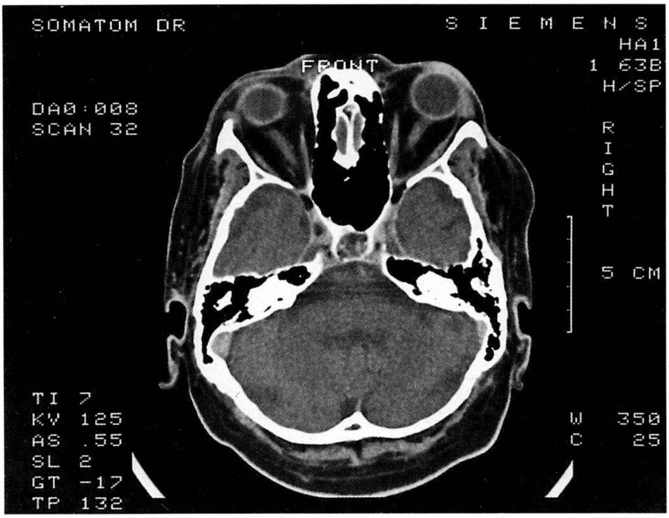

Fig. 4.13
Limits to the beam hardening correction. A beam hardening correction determined with, for example, material equivalent to soft tissue will only have an incomplete effect as soon as more extensive object structures occur in the slice under examination, for which the energy dependence of their attenuation capacity is different than that of soft tissue. This skull tomogram shows a typical artifact in the center of the image: a broad soft tissue band of apparently reduced attenuation capacity. This soft tissue area is reproduced with incorrect attenuation values since the extensive neighboring bone structures (petrous bones) have completely different beam hardening properties than the soft tissue

Of course, just as with the correction obtained using a compensation medium, this correction is only exact if the object consists entirely of materials which behave in completely the same way as the reference substance in terms of the energy dependence of its radiation attenuation capacity over the range in question. If, for example, water is taken as the reference substance, the correction for soft-tissue components will function very well, but may be inadequate if there is a large amount of bone in the slice. This is the cause of a typical artifact, shown in Fig. 4.13, observed in skull images showing the petrous bones: In a broad band between the petrous bones, the cerebral matter appears darker, i.e. less dense than in the rest of the image. In such a case, it is possible to make use of additional corrections which might possibly be carried out iteratively. These would ultimately produce a perfect reproduction of the morphology and attenuation values, but would also considerably increase the demands on computing resources.

Apart from the correction of the measurement values for the beam hardening effect described in detail above, there are several other corrections which have to be applied to the measurement values before the actual image reconstruction can start. These corrections concern, for example, the individual sensitivity, the offset, the spectral sensitivity distribution and the geometrical arrangement of the individual measurement channels. However, it would go well beyond the scope of this book to give an account of all the corrections which are necessary or conceivable. Further basic considerations on the principles of computed tomography can be found in references [4.13] to [4.19].

4.2 CT image reconstruction

As already explained in detail, x-ray computed tomography (CT) makes it possible to produce radiographical images of transaxial slices of the human body without disturbance due to shadows from adjacent layers. Moreover, in contrast to the classical x-ray image, the CT image is no longer a superposition image. What it reproduces is the local attenuation capacity, i.e. a physical property of the biological tissue, in the form of gray values.

Whereas in classical x-ray tomography, even though a sharp image is produced of one layer, the images of all the layers situated in the radiation paths are superimposed onto the desired layer image with a blurred appearance, in the CT procedure interference shadows arising from structures outside the layer concerned are excluded from the very start. The focal spot and the detector are always situated in the slice plane under investigation; the radiation beam only scans this slice (see Fig. 4.3). On the other hand, this means that every tissue structure in the slice itself produces an interference shadow. In other words, for a predefined position of focal spot and detector, the measured intensity distribution of the x-rays penetrating the object only provides information on the sum of all attenuations which the x-ray radiation has undergone in the object. The distribution of the attenuation capacity of the tissue along the scan beam cannot be taken from this single measurement value alone. A single projection is therefore not sufficient to determine the distribution of the attenuation capacity in the slice. As can be seen from the example of a parallel-beam scanner in Fig. 4.14, it is still not yet possible to identify tissue structures unambiguously when two mutually perpendicular parallel projections are taken after the manner of the well-known biplane technique in radiography. If, for instance, we replace the four symmetrically arranged rods (Fig. 4.14 left) by two rods of the same thickness with double the attenuation capacity (Fig. 4.14 right), a vertical and a horizontal projection give exactly the same measurement data in both cases: $P_V = P_V'$ and $P_H = P_H'$. Only another projection P_D or P_D' directed

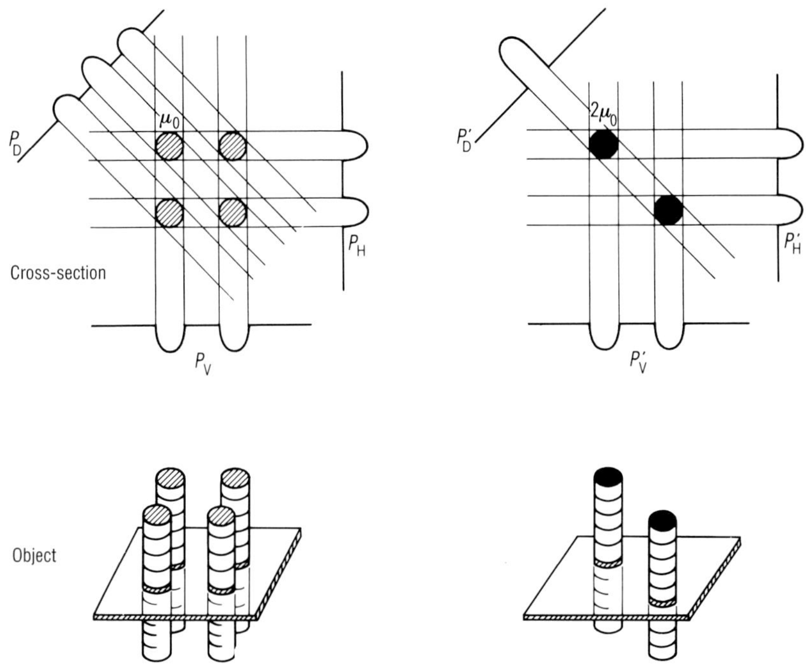

Fig. 4.14
Ambiguity of the scan data: the two rods to be imaged on the right have double the density of the four rods on the left, i.e. $P_H = P_H'$, $P_V = P_V'$. Only an additional diagonal projection P_D or P_D' makes it possible to distinguish between the two structures depicted here

along a diagonal makes it possible to distinguish the two object structures in this case. It is not difficult to imagine that even three projections are not sufficient for the unambiguous identification of more complicated structures. Even if many projections are used, there is always a certain residual uncertainty which increases with increasing fineness of the object structures.

However, objects with arbitrarily fine structure are never imaged in CT, because the effective width of the beam resulting from the detector width, the focus width and the movement of the measurement system – only allows a blurred representation of the object as imaged by the measurement system. In the language of communications theory, the measurement system carries out low-pass filtering and so simulates an object which only contains structures up to a certain level of fineness. Now, a finite number of projections is sufficient in order to unambiguously reconstruct this simulated, blurred image – now free of very fine structures. The question of determining this necessary number of projections will be considered below. The finite detector and focus widths in CT should not just be regarded as an evil, as a cause of the limitation in the resolution, but as a necessary condition for the unambiguous reconstruction of a CT image.

4.2.1 Principles of image reconstruction

The principles of image reconstruction in CT can be explained using the simplest design of a parallel-beam scanner. Fan-beam machines and ring-detector systems require more complicated algorithms, which however can be derived from the algorithms used with parallel-beam systems by a transformation of coordinates. Thus, restricting this discussion to the parallel-beam allows us to focus on the essential details.

This simple scanning principle is shown again in Fig. 4.15. The linear scanning movement takes place for the present in the η direction, characterized by the angle φ. The intensity J measured at the detector therefore depends, on the one hand, on the projection angle φ and, on the other hand, on the position η which the measurement system occupies at any point in time during the scanning movement and of course also on the intensity J_0 of the unattenuated radiation.

$$J = J(\varphi, \eta) = J_0 \, e^{-\int \mu \, d\xi}. \tag{4.7}$$

The path of the given scan beam through the object is taken as the integration path. The distribution of the attenuation coefficient μ in the slice under study can now be calculated from all the measured intensities $J(\varphi, \eta)$. The above integral equation is then solved for μ. However, it is more convenient to first transform equation (4.7) into a linear integral equation by referring the measured intensity $J(\varphi, \eta)$ to the intensity J_0, which is also known, and taking the logarithm:

$$p_\varphi(\eta) = \ln \frac{J_0}{J(\varphi, \eta)} = \int \mu \, d\xi. \tag{4.8}$$

In many CT systems, this logarithmic approach is already implemented as part of the scan data acquisition, so that the data $p_\varphi(\eta)$ (in digital form) is already transferred to the computer. The calculation of logarithms is therefore considered here as part of the measurement process and the function p_φ is regarded as a projection.

There are two different methods for solving the integral equation (4.8). In one method, it can be immediately written in discrete form, i.e. converted to a linear algebraic equation system which must then be solved. However, closed solution formulae can also be given for equation (4.8). In this case, the transformation to a discrete form is only carried out during the numerical evaluation of the solution formulas.

A minicomputer performs the actual image reconstruction. This computer usually has special arithmetic elements adapted to the requirements of the CT algorithms, permitting extremely fast processing.

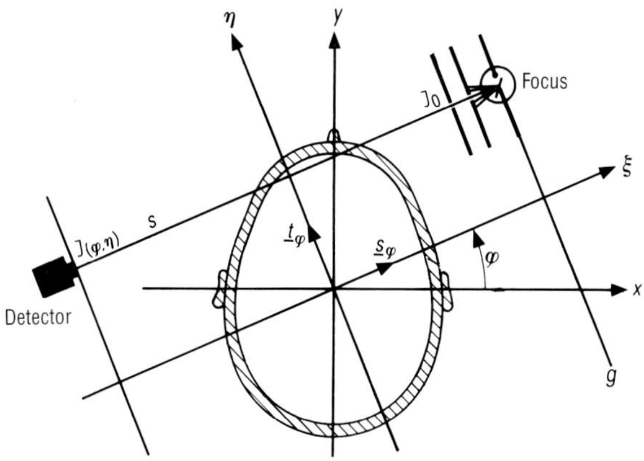

x, y Coordinates fixed in space
ξ, η Coordinates bound to the measurement system
φ Projection angle
$\underline{s}_\varphi, \underline{t}_\varphi$ Unit vectors
J Radiation intensity measured behind the object
J_0 Radiation intensity measured in front of the object

Fig. 4.15 Choice of coordinate systems

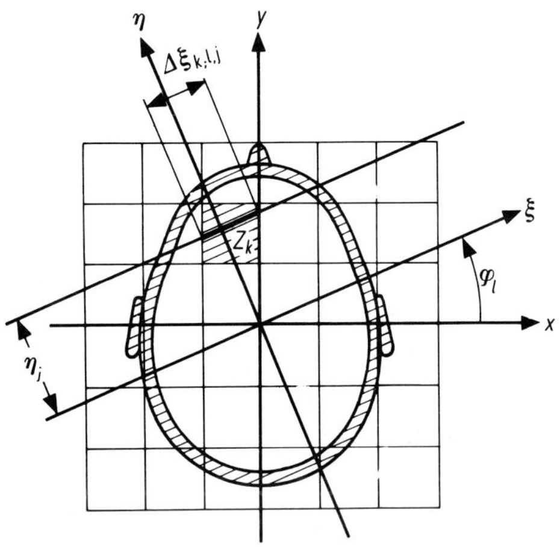

Fig. 4.16
Decomposition of the layer to be imaged into n square cells (pixels)

Z_k $(1 \leq k \leq n)$
$\Delta\xi_{k;l,j}$ Radiation path in the cell Z_k

Algebraic reconstruction methods

Historically, algebraic methods are the oldest reconstruction methods in computed tomography [4.20]. Even though there is hardly any likelihood today that they will again supplant the more modern integral transformation methods, they will be briefly described because they provide the simplest and most direct approach to understanding CT image reconstruction.

With these methods, the object is assumed to consist of small square cells (pixels) (Fig. 4.16). This finite number of pixels corresponds to an approximately equal number of measurement data; the linear scanning movements occur with a finite number of equally spaced angles φ_1 and for a predefined projection direction φ_1 the measured value is determined at a finite number of focus-detector positions η_j.

The measured value $p_{1,j}$, which refers to a scan beam passing through the object, is in this simple model the sum of the μ values of all the pixels encountered by the beam multiplied by the path length $\Delta\xi_{k;1,j}$ which the beam traverses in the cell:

$$P_{1,j} = \sum_k \mu_k \, \Delta\xi_{k;1,j}. \tag{4.9}$$

This extensive equation system consisting of up to a few hundred thousand variables can in practice only be solved iteratively for reasons of accuracy (rounding off errors!). Here, we will describe the best known iteration method for an extremely simple "object" consisting of four pixels with attenuation values 0.2, 0.3, 0.1 and 0.4 cm^{-1} (Fig. 4.17). (In the following, the unit cm^{-1} will be omitted in describing the attenuation values.)

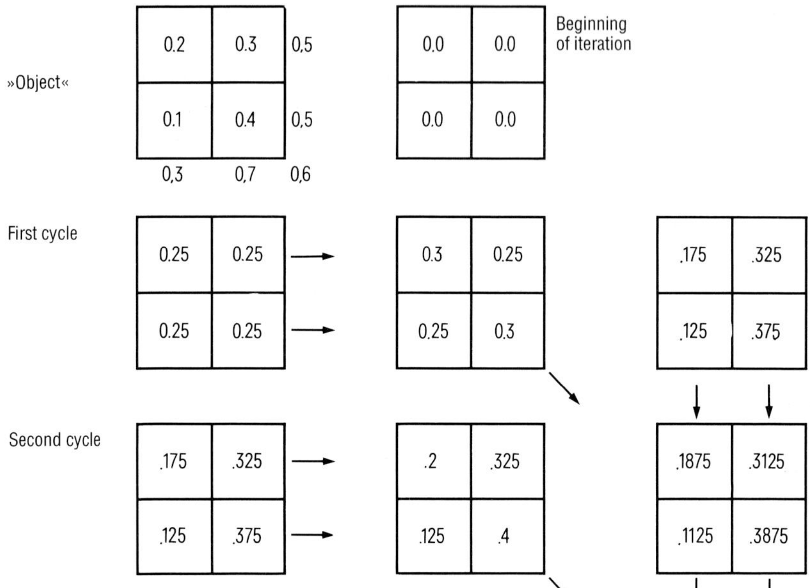

Fig. 4.17
Iterative image reconstruction using a simple example

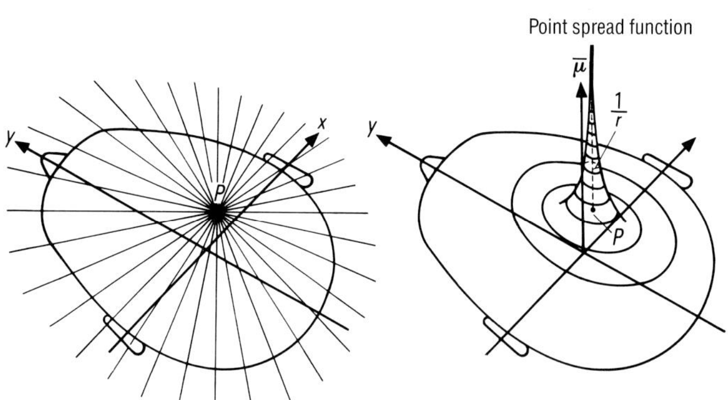

Fig. 4.18
Production of the point image in the form $1/r$ for simple back projection (r is the distance of a predefined point from the object point P)

Starting from the measurement values 0.5 and 0.5, i.e. the measured sums of the attenuation values, all attenuation values are initialized to 0.25 in the first cycle. However, this "image" only satisfies the two "horizontal measurements". The "diagonal measurement" is now satisfied by equally distributing the deviation of the measurement value 0.6 from the measurement value 0.5 which would be obtained if the object actually contained the attenuation values 0.25 and 0.25 along the diagonals, over the two diagonal elements. The two "vertical measurements" are then satisfied, completing an iteration cycle. At this point, the image matrix now no longer satisfies the "horizontal measurement", so that the correction loop has to be repeated until the "image" is finally stabilized.

Integral transformation methods (convolution methods)

Integral transformation methods ([4.21] to [4.25]) are based on solution formulas for equation (4.8) in which only the projections $p_\varphi(\eta)$ still have to be substituted by measurements. Several equivalent methods are available for the theoretical derivation of a solution formula. A particularly easy to visualize approach is the following (Fig. 4.18): we imagine an object which only consists of a single element and which attenuates the x-ray beam. During every linear scanning movement, only a single "measurement beam" is attenuated. Since, however, we now do not know which element on the beam line has caused this attenuation, it is uniformly distributed over the entire line passing through the element, which can be imagined as recorded onto a suitable two-dimensional storage device.

In practice, it is best to use a digital memory whose cell arrangement corresponds to the given division of the image into small pixels in a manner similar to that illustrated in Fig. 4.16.

Every direction, i.e. every angular setting of the scanning arrangement, is treated in the manner described above. The additive superposition of all scan lines then results in a spatial distribution which, as can be immediately seen, falls off from the attenuating object point as $1/r$, where r denotes the distance of a predefined observation point to the object point. By drawing circles of any arbitrary size about this point, there are then always the same number of straight lines uniformly distributed over the circumference of these circles, which increases in proportion to r. In the language of systems theory, we have defined here the point spread function of a linear, position-invariant imaging system, this imaging system consisting of the measurement of the integrals along any arbitrary straight lines and the back projection of the measured values onto the corresponding measurement lines. If, however, the object consists of many x-ray attenuating elements, or to be more exact, of a distribution of μ values, then this imaging system provides such a $1/r$ function for every object point weighted with the local attenuation coefficient. The superposition of all these functions leads to an approximation image $\bar{\mu}$, which in the language of mathematics is described as the convolution of the object function μ with the function $1/r$:

$$\bar{\mu} = \mu * \frac{1}{r}. \tag{4.10}$$

(A dimensional multiplicative constant has been omitted here.)

In graphic terms, this relationship states that every object point generates a point spread function of the form $1/r$, the center of which lies exactly at this object point and which must still be multiplied by the attenuation coefficient of the object at this position, that is weighted. Experience has shown that approximation images obtained by this simple principle are of practically no diagnostic value [4.26]. Neither fine structures nor small contrast differences can be identified in them. Nevertheless, if the blurring mechanism (described by the $1/r$ function) is known, they contain all the information on the irradiated slice!

Briefly stated, the convolution method attempts to reverse the known blurring process. We recall the generation of the image of an object point in the form $1/r$. This was produced by the superposition of all straight lines associated with the isolated object point, each line having a constant μ value. For a real object, when all the data of a projection are back-projected, the resulting image $\bar{\mu}_1$ has the appearance of Fig. 4.19. In order to arrive at the approximation image, $\bar{\mu}$, all these single-projection images have to be superimposed according to the projection direction. However, by modifying all back-projected values along the straight lines in such a way that a negative accompanying component

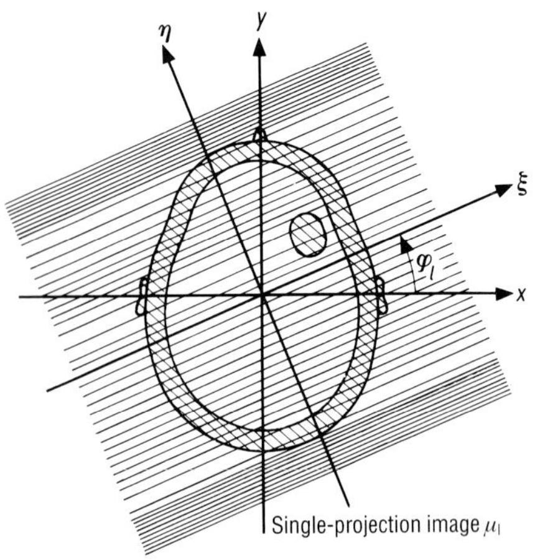

Fig. 4.19
Illustration of the single-projection image corresponding to projection 1

results to the right and left of every straight line as indicated in Fig. 4.20, top right, it is then possible to eliminate the $1/r$ blurring. The positive contributions still acting at any arbitrary distance from the object point along the straight line through the object point are then exactly compensated by the negative contributions of the projections directed oppositely to the projection in question. In the general case of a continuous object, this would be expressed mathematically as the convolution of the projections $p_\varphi(\eta)$ with the function shown in Fig. 4.32 (see page 136) (convolution kernel) and subsequent back projection of the convolution result to the storage device in the radiation direction.

This procedure will be explained using a simplified example (refer to appendix 4.2.3 for a more rigorous mathematical treatment). Fig. 4.20 gives a rough approximation of the convolution kernel by a simpler kernel which assumes only the values 1, $-{}^1/_2$ and 0. The three zones in which this kernel is not 0 each have the width of the x-ray scan beam. If two such single-projection images from mutually perpendicular directions are superimposed (Figs. 4.20a and b), a peak of height 2 is produced at the center; it is the "image" of the object point. However, two crossed bars of height 1 extend outwards from this peak to infinity. These bars again have two negative accompanying compo-

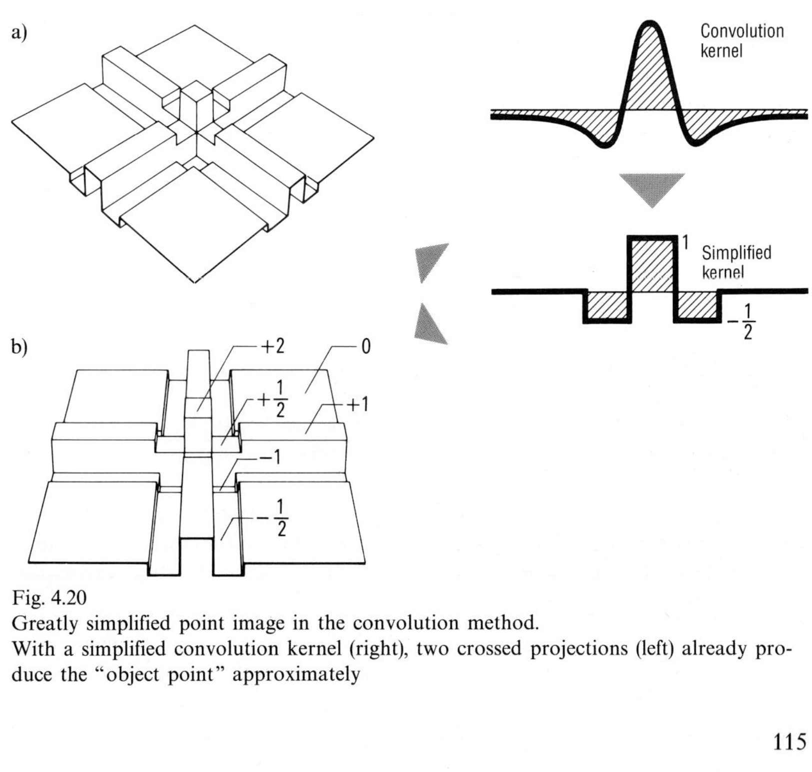

Fig. 4.20
Greatly simplified point image in the convolution method.
With a simplified convolution kernel (right), two crossed projections (left) already produce the "object point" approximately

nents with depth $-{}^{1}/_{2}$. The negative components are superimposed up to a depth -1 at their intersection points. However, the bars themselves are already partly compensated in the immediate vicinity of the "image point" by the negative components.

In practice, however, not just two crossed projections are used, but several hundred, which are turned to each other at small angular intervals $\Delta\varphi$. We imagine that we first superimpose a further pair of mutually perpendicular projections rotated by 45° (Fig. 4.20a). The result of this superposition is easy to visualize: at the center, the superposition of the four projections yields a peak of height 4. The height of the interfering bars is not increased by this, nor is the depth of their negative accompanying components. The signal-to-noise ratio is therefore improved. In addition, it can be seen that the immediate vicinity of the "image point" is made even more flat. The "holes" of depth -1 which were originally present have been partly filled by the incoming bars. If further such crossed projections are chosen, it can be seen that the central peak will become higher and higher. At the same time, a zone will extend around this peak whose μ values lie close to 0. The positive bars are exactly compensated by the negative accompanying components of neighboring projections.

However, it can also be seen that only a few projections are needed in order to obtain adequate sharpness in the reconstructed image. With an increasing number of projections, the central peak only becomes rounder but no longer narrower. At the same time, though, the ratio of the height of the central peak to the height or depth of the interference streaks becomes larger. The signal-to-noise ratio improves, i.e. the contrast resolution increases (Fig. 4.27 illustrates the effect of choosing too small a number of projections on the reconstructed CT image). On the other hand, the image sharpness is determined by the width of the bars and these in turn by the width of the scanning beam, i.e. primarily by the width of the detector or tube focus.

Critique of the various reconstruction principles

As already mentioned, the algebraic methods are hardly in use any more today. There are two main reasons for this: firstly, the image calculation is only possible after the acquisition of all scan data, so that the doctor has to wait for a longer time; secondly, the computing time is considerably longer than with the convolution method. However, since reconstruction methods are finding increasing application in such clinical areas as nuclear medicine and also ultrasound diagnostics, where the mathematical conditions for the convolution method are only satisfied inadequately, the flexible and versatile iteration techniques may well regain importance.

On the other hand, with the convolution method, every projection is immediately processed in the computer after its measurement, so that there is no waiting

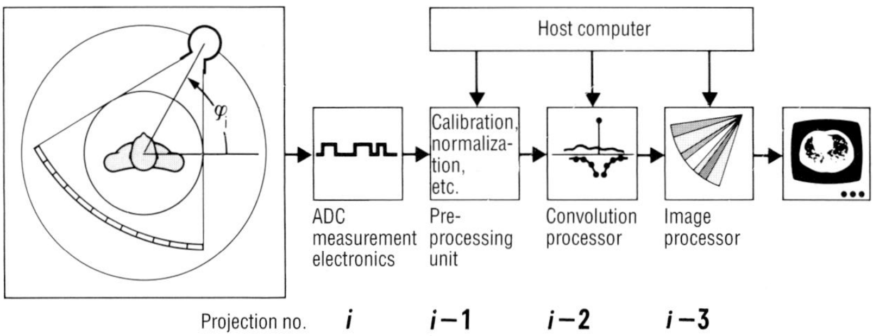

Fig. 4.21 Pipeline principle for reconstructing a CT image in real time

time for the doctor between the completion of the measurement and the appearance of the image on the screen.

In principle, all the above-mentioned considerations can be applied to the fan-beam system. However, the computer time required for image reconstruction increases unavoidably.

In order to reconstruct a CT image in real time, i.e. while the measurement data is being transferred to the computer, the so-called pipeline principle is used (Fig. 4.21). While projection No. i is undergoing analog-digital conversion and is being transferred to the computer, the immediately preceding measured projection is already undergoing the necessary preprocessing steps; its predecessor is convolved at the same time and its predecessor in turn already being back-projected. Of course, the processing speed for this operating principle is determined by the most critical time element in the chain, i.e. by the back projection. Therefore, special computers must be used, which have been especially designed for executing this operation. On the other hand, the pipeline principle cannot be applied to ring-detector systems with a stationary detector array. With this type of machine, we must first collect and rearrange all the measured values registered by a detector during the rotation of the tube before the convolution can take place.

Remarks on image reconstruction algorithms for the fan-beam principle

According to Jass [4.27], the convolution relationship (4.22) can be directly adapted to the fan-beam principle (Fig. 4.22). For this, the linear coordinate η must be replaced by the angular coordinate ψ and the filtering carried out using the function $\cos\psi\, p_\varphi(\psi)$. The position P at which the convolution product should be plotted must, however, already be included in the calculation of the convolution product; the distance from the image point P in question to

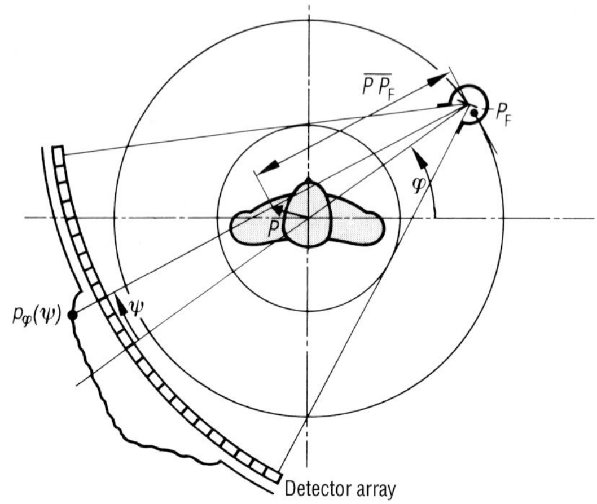

Fig. 4.22
Coordinate system of a fan-beam machine

φ Projection angle
ψ Angle within the fan
P Image point to be reconstructed
P_F Momentary focal spot
P_φ Projection

the momentary projection center P_F appears in the convolution integral. Under certain conditions, however, this distance can be eliminated from the convolution integral, so that the computational requirements are drastically reduced and resemble more the computational requirements of the convolution method for the parallel-beam scanner. This means that data processing can keep in step for fan-beam systems, with all the advantages for practical clinical operation. The Somatom fan-beam scanner, equipped with a special processor, functions according to this principle.

4.2.2 Image quality

The following are the principal criteria used for evaluating image quality in CT:

spatial resolution
contrast resolution (differentiation of fine differences in tissue density),
absence of all types of artifacts.

Apart from these, the following factors are of key importance in determining the image quality which can be attained in practice:

scan time and
required dose per image slice.

Since it seems hopeless to attempt to deal with all aspects of this comprehensive area, even in an approximate fashion, only characteristic differences between the CT image and the classical x-ray image will be indicated here.

Essentially, these differences arise from two sources. Firstly, the physical measurement process does not immediately yield the CT image. This can only be reconstructed with the help of the above-described mathematical transformation from all the measured data. The computing process destroys the local character of the measurement errors, unavoidable as in any measurement procedure, and distributes them over the entire image in a manner which is typical for the type of measurement error. The location at which an image distortion originates and the location of the distortion in the image are therefore no longer necessarily identical.

The second difference compared to classical radiography is discretization, i.e. the determination of the attenuation capacity of the tissue by only a finite number of measurement data. Only if certain rules are obeyed, of which the well-known Shannon sampling theorem [4.28] is the most important, is this procedure justified. The non-observance of these rules also produces image distortions unknown to classical radiography.

If we wish to understand the implications of the fact that the CT image is a computer-generated image derived from a few hundred thousand measured data, then we must keep in mind the two most important image reconstruction procedures. These are:

convolution, by means of which every projection is transformed so that negative projection values are also obtained, and
back projection, which imposes the convolved scan data in the direction of the scan beam onto the recording medium.

The different reaction of different scanner types to measured value disturbances

It is immediately understandable that disturbances in individual sample values of a single projection result in different image disturbances than uniform distortions of the measured data of a projection or even of all projections. This means that different CT scanning principles react to the same measured value disturbances with different image disturbances. For example, in a fan-beam scanner with a rotating detector array (see Fig. 4.7d), all data from a single projection are distorted in the same way as a result of fluctuations in the tube voltage, but different projections are distorted differently, whereas with a ring-detector scanner (see Fig. 4.7c) with stationary detectors, in which the data from one projection are collected during the movement of the x-ray tube, fluctuations in the measured data result in fluctuations within the projections. The following artifact examples relate to fan-beam scanners.

Typical CT image disturbances

The best way to understand image disturbances in computed tomography is to simulate their sources in a computer model. Synthetic scan data are generated which are distorted in a defined manner. In this way all other sources for measurement distortion, which are always present in reality, are eliminated. As in any measurement procedure, in computed tomography one has to distinguish between systematic and statistical measurement errors.

Systematic measurement errors

Distortion of a single measurement value

Let us consider the extreme case that one out of approximately 2×10^5 to 10^6 measured values is lost. This measured value disturbance is now also subjected to the convolution process for the affected projection, in the course of which accompanying components with opposite sign are produced to the right and left. The back projection thus generates a 3-line structure corresponding to Fig. 4.20, as shown in Fig. 4.23a.

Uniform distortion of a projection

We will again consider the extreme case in which an entire projection drops out. In this case, we do not have the reinforcing effect of the convolution operation on the distortion. We obtain the dark bars ascribed to objects of high density, as can be seen in Fig. 4.23b. It becomes clear that a serious disturbance in the measured data, namely the absence of an entire projection, which in this case involves 256 measurement values, results in a less pronounced image distortion than if a single measurement value drops out. In general, the following rule of thumb applies: disturbances in a single measured value within a projection are easier to recognize in the CT image than those which affect an entire projection in the same manner.

Statistical fluctuation phenomena

Here, we must first mention the so-called quantum noise, i.e. a physically unavoidable statistical fluctuation of the x-ray beam intensity, the effects of which can only be reduced by increasing the x-ray dose. In addition, however, statistical fluctuations are also involved to a certain extent in the electronics and the scanning mechanism.

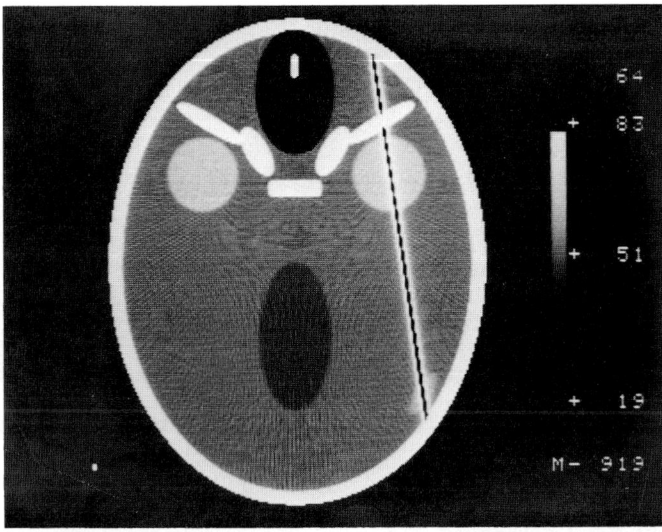

a) 3-line structure (white/black/white) when a single measured value is missing

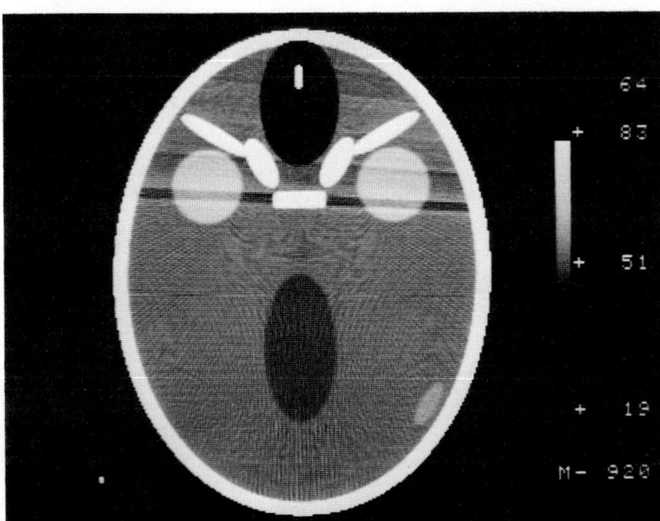

b) Interference structure when an entire projection is missing

Fig. 4.23
The simulated skull phantom shows a high-contrast structure ("bones", i.e. white), for example the "skull" and an "air inclusion" (black), as well as low-contrast structures, for example the "ventricle" and a small "hematoma" below the center of the image

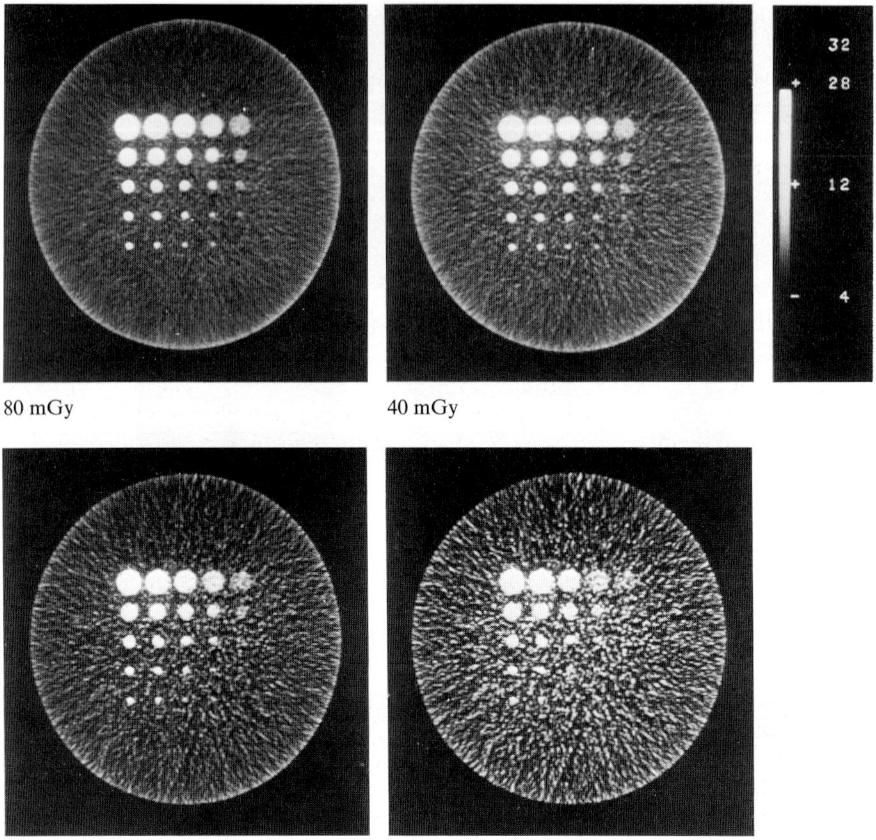

80 mGy 40 mGy

10 mGy 2,5 mGy

Fig. 4.24
"Button card": rods in the water bath. The density of the rods decreases from left to right. The preferential radial direction of the noise islands at the edge of the object should be noted. The dose per slice image is given in milliGrays (mGy)

Fig. 4.24 shows the so-called "button card", a simulated, water-equivalent plate, in which rods of variable diameter and variable density are embedded. The density decreases from left to right. With a decreasing x-ray dose per slice image, the noise disturbances are superimposed onto the object structures and make it difficult to identify them. A radial preferential direction of the noise islands to the edge of the object can be observed as an important characteristic of the CT image.

Basic remarks on the perceptibility of artifacts

It can be expected that statistical disturbances also make the recognition of systematic measurement errors more difficult. However, more exact investigations show that measurement errors associated with noise must reach an unacceptable level in many cases before they effectively mask systematic errors. Thus, in the case shown in Fig. 4.25, the fluctuation of the image noise is about the same as for the marked band or ring distortion structures immediately recognizable by the eye. The large "ventricle" below the center of the image differs from its environment by only half the noise fluctuation, σ, and the same applies to the "hematoma" which can still be recognized in the bottom right of the image.

Obviously, our visual perception system plays an important part in recognizing artifacts. The eye seems to look over the image for large simple structures and in this manner smooths over local statistical fluctuations in brightness.

Matching of the system parameters

The resolution capacity of a CT system is primarily determined by the scan beam width, i.e. by the effective widths of the focus and detector. If the beam width is predefined, the distances between the detectors, the angles between

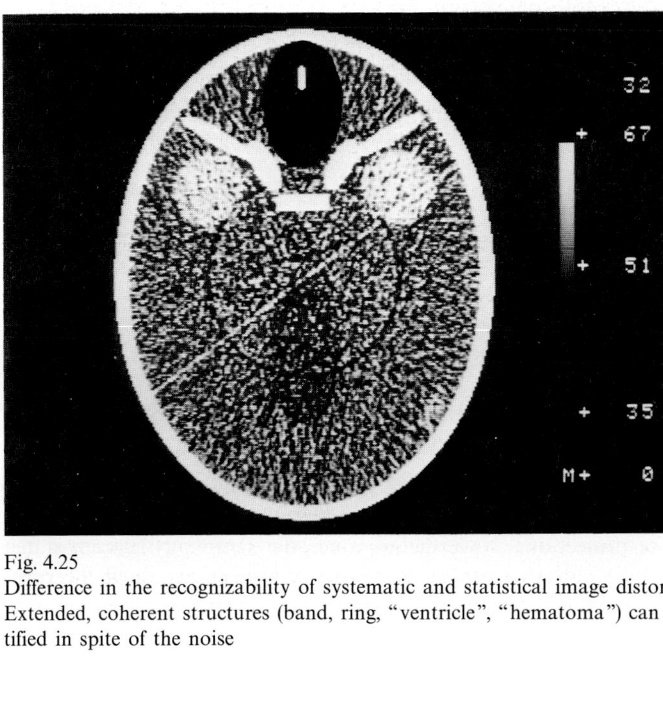

Fig. 4.25
Difference in the recognizability of systematic and statistical image distortions. Extended, coherent structures (band, ring, "ventricle", "hematoma") can be easily identified in spite of the noise

neighboring projection directions, the height of the slice to be measured and finally the fineness of the image matrix must be correctly matched to each other. The correct choice of these parameters is a complex optimization problem, which must take special account of the discrete nature of the data acquisition.

In order to be able to calculate an image from the measured data which is as true as possible to the object, it is necessary to fill up the measurement plane in all directions with measurement lines. Strictly speaking, this is not possible with a finite number of measurement lines. Fortunately, however, as was already emphasized earlier, the scan beam has a finite width, so that instead of the line integrals only integrals averaged over the finite-width measurement bands can be obtained. These can be approximately regarded as line integrals over an averaged, i.e. blurred, object function. The measurement system therefore produces a low-pass filtering of the object and thus suppresses fine structures. It is plausible that the remaining smoothed structures can be fully processed by scanning in finite steps, which is in fact essentially the statement of the Shannon sampling theorem [4.28]. Applied to functions of one variable (e.g. time), this states:

If point-like "samples" are taken from a frequency-band limited, i.e. low-pass filtered, function $g(t)$ at regular intervals ΔT, then the original function can be completely reconstructed from these "samples" alone, as long as the interval ΔT between neighboring samples is chosen sufficiently small. ΔT must be chosen so that at least two "samples" are still taken in each period from the highest frequency structures still contained in the function to be scanned.

The required number of projections and measured data per projection can be derived from this requirement for a given scanning beam width for every CT system. For example, for a parallel-beam machine in which the focus only traverses an angle of 180°, it can be estimated that the number of projections should be approximately $\pi/2$ times the number of measured values within a projection.

However, the situation is not so clear for fan-beam and ring-detector systems. During the scanning process, it can happen that – due to an exchange of roles between the focus and detector – scan beams are duplicated. The measured data are therefore not necessarily independent; their number is consequently not a direct measure for the fineness of scanning. This coincidence of the measurement beams can be avoided by mounting the detector array in a well defined position, slightly unsymmetrically to the center line of the focus-rotation center [4.29]. Fig. 4.26 shows the effectiveness of this simple trick.

Of course the requirement for a sufficiently fine scanning of the approximately band-limited projections must be balanced against the requirement for a sufficient number of projections. Nevertheless, since the sampling theorem states that, for restricted bands, increasing the number of projections above a certain limit does not bring any further benefit, it is part of the designer's job to exactly meet those hardware requirements which are necessary and at the same time

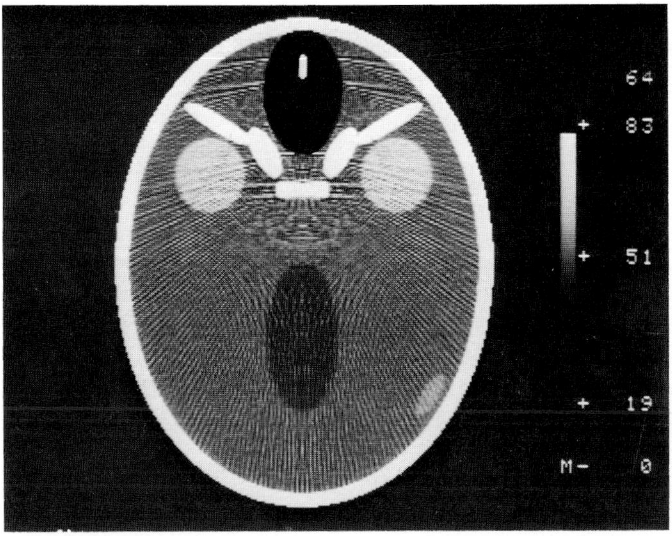

a) Centered detector array

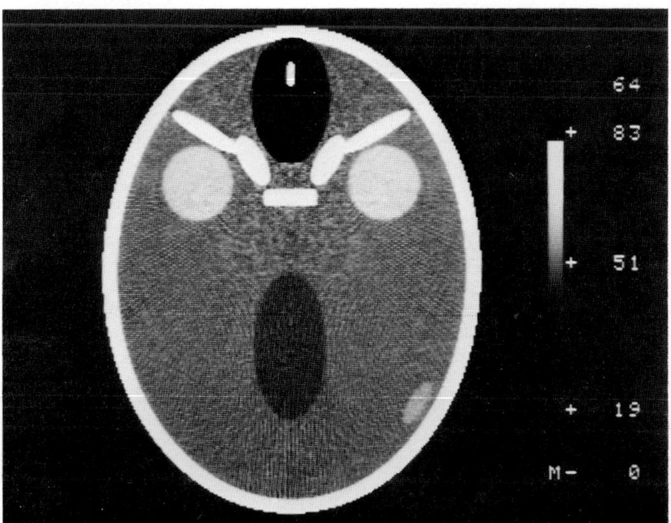

b) quarter shift offset of the detector array

Fig. 4.26
Reduction of artifacts by quarter shift offset of the detector array

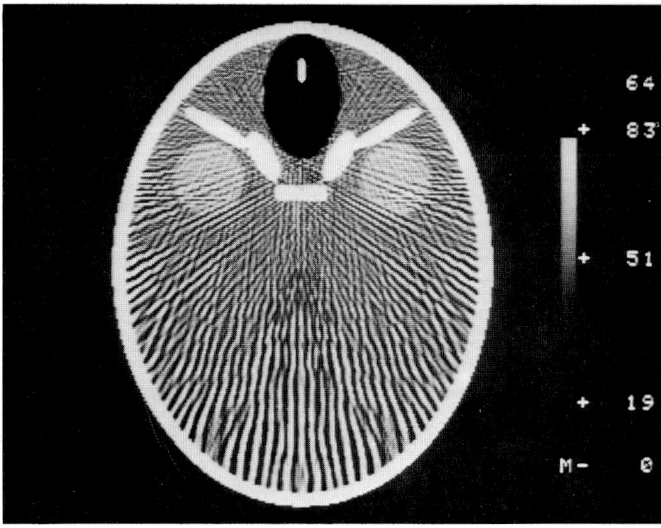

a) 180 projections

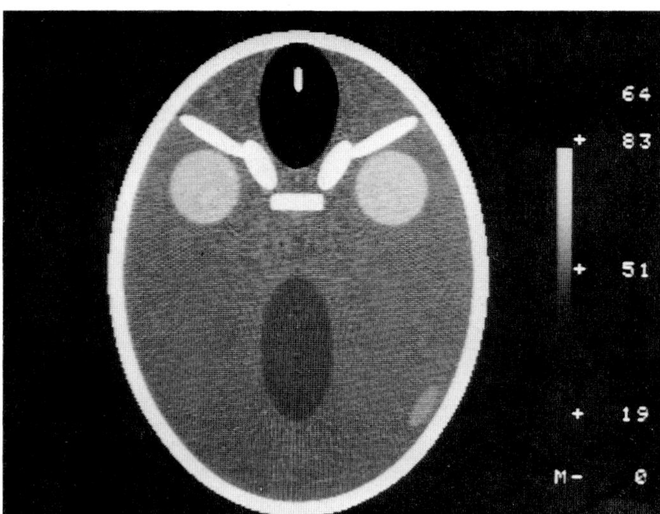

b) 720 projections

Fig. 4.27
Matching the number of projections to the scan beam width

just sufficient. Fig. 4.27a shows the case of faulty matching of the number of projections to the scanning beam width. For an effective scan beam width of approximately 1.5 mm, 180 projections are obviously still not sufficient, while according to Fig. 4.27b 720 projections are already clearly sufficient. The easily recognizable dark "ventricle" (fine contrast −5‰) in the bottom third of the image could not be made visible with 180 projections, just as with the clearly recognizable "hematoma" (fine contrast +5‰) with 720 projections at the bottom right. Thus, faulty matching of the number of projections to the scan beam width may make the recognition of large low-contrast structures very difficult.

The last example illustrates the problems of discretization, namely the fact that the CT image is obtained from individual data samples. If, in order to limit the computational requirements, the number of detectors is kept constant, but – in order to increase the spatial resolution – the focus and detectors are chosen to be very narrow, the artifacts of Fig. 4.28 will then result.

Such a measure would consequently not result in the desired improvement in detail sharpness, but in fact generate new image distortions. From classical

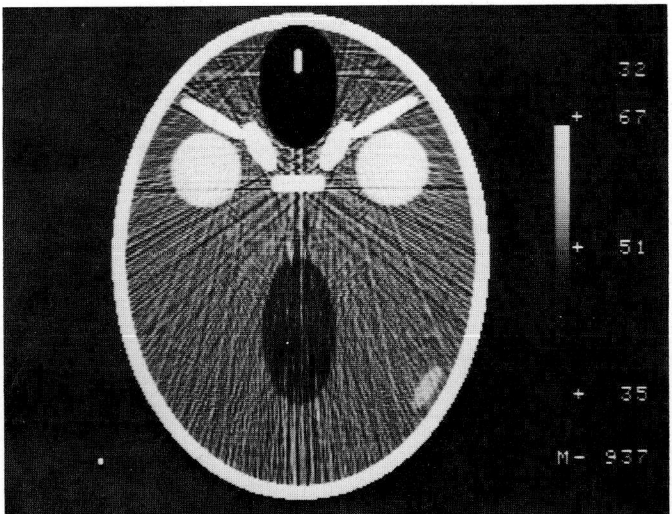

Fig. 4.28
Scanning with an "ideal", infinitely thin scanning beam but a finite number of measured data

radiography there is no parallel to such a phenomenon, arising specifically from the discretization of data. In radiography, one would expect that if the focus and detector are made smaller (for the latter we can consider using a film with sharper definition), an increase in spatial resolution without extensive distortion should result.

Discussion of a few frequently observed CT artifacts

Table 4.1 classifies the possible noise sources, dividing them into different groups with typical examples of each.

From the group of physically induced measurement errors, we consider here the beam hardening effect (see Sect. 4.1.6) and the non-linear partial volume effect, which nearly always occur together in an actual CT image and can therefore hardly be separated.

As already mentioned, an x-ray tube emits radiation of varying energy. However, since biological tissue absorbs soft x-rays more strongly than hard x-rays, when the scan beam penetrates the center of the body the x-rays emerging are harder than when the beam penetrates the body peripherally.

Table 4.1 Causes of CT artifacts

Physical causes
● Quantum noise ● x-ray scattering by the patient ● Beam hardening ● Non-linear partial volume effect
Patient-related effects
● Movement of the patient or of individual organs ● Overcharge of the data acquisition system due to metallic foreign objects
System-related causes
● Design insufficiencies Faulty matching of scan parameters Inadequacies in the image reconstruction algorithm ● System faults, such as Non-uniform scanning movement Fluctuations in the x-ray tube voltage Temperature drift in the measurement electronics

In the first case, this means that the detector sees a smaller attenuation capacity for the tissue. Modern CT systems are generally able to correct for this systematic error, in most cases adequately for diagnostic purposes.

However, this correction is based on the assumption, which is not strictly correct, that only varying tissue density is responsible for the differences in attenuation capacity of the tissue and not differences in atomic composition. Therefore, when bones are irradiated there are always residual errors which, for example, appear as dark bars between the petrous bones in cranial scans.

On the other hand, the non-linear partial volume effect arises as a consequence of the exponential, i.e. non-linear, attenuation of the radiation when high-contrast structures are only partially immersed in the slice to be imaged. This effect therefore always accompanies the beam hardening effect with bones. Rührnschopf and Kalender [4.30] succeeded in discovering the main differences between these effects by the skillful use of linear and non-linear combinations of the measured data from neighboring slices (Fig. 4.29). This eliminated soft-tissue structures which would hamper the interpretation. In this way, it was possible to show that the non-linear partial volume effect was the cause of the star-shaped artifact emerging from the protuberantia occipitalis in the fossa posterior. In principle, it is possible to largely eliminate the beam hardening effect with the help of intermittent spectral measurements [4.19], but the price for this is a considerable increase in expenditure.

On the other hand, correction methods based on the estimated bone distribution derived from the normal monospectral CT image have not gained acceptance,

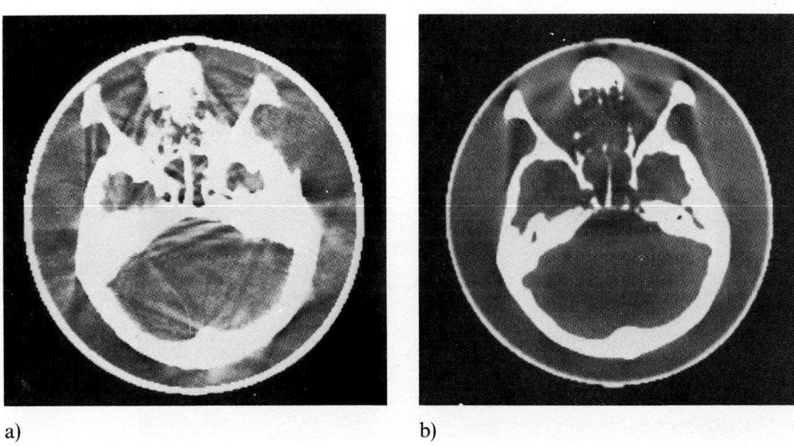

a) b)

Fig. 4.29
Isolated display of the non-linear partial volume effect (a) and the radiation hardening effect (b)

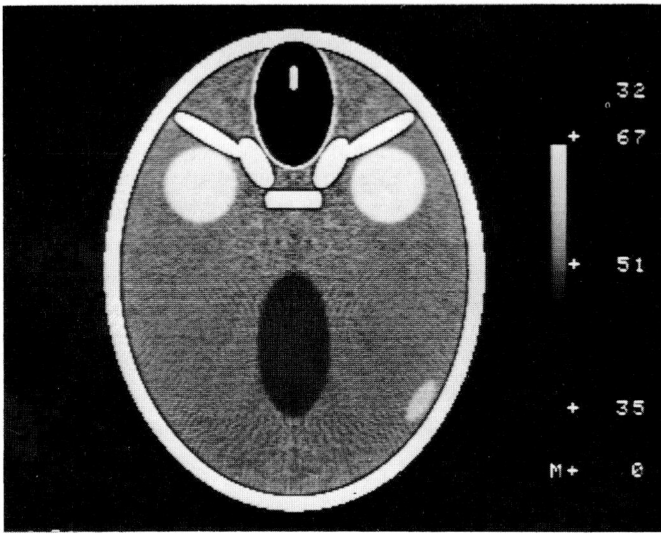

Fig. 4.30
Simulation of a high detail sharpness by modification of the convolution in order to emphasize the edges. The apparent "subarachnoidal space" should be noted

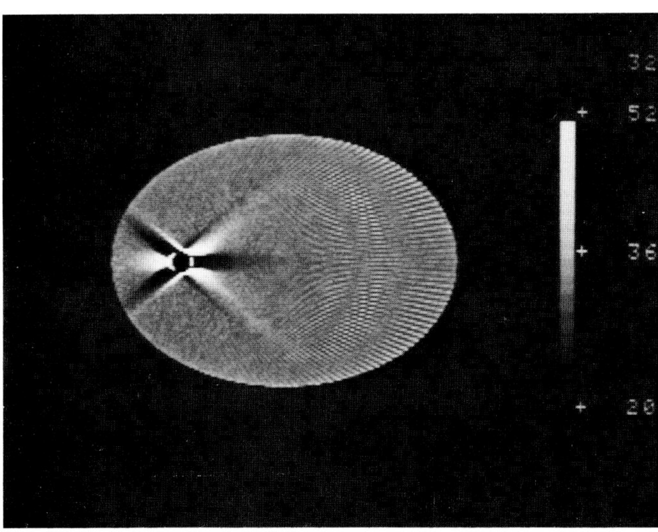

Fig. 4.31
Interference structure in the form of a cross produced by moving an "intestine" filled with contrast medium during the scan

one reason being that they require a very exact specification of the calcium content of the bone.

The non-linear partial volume effect can only be reduced by using thinner slices.

Fig. 4.30 shows an example from the group of system-related measurement errors. Here, the convolution method was modified in order to ensure edge enhancement, such as at the borders between bones and soft tissue. Many manufacturers provide the user with such means for specific alteration of the image character. Despite their undisputable usefulness in terms of diagnosis, the risk of an incorrect interpretation must be pointed out: the "subarachnoidal space" apparently shown in Fig. 4.30 is a pure artifact (compare with Fig. 4.27b).

As an example of a patient-related image distortion we show a motion artifact caused by peristalsis. If an "intestinal balloon" wetted with contrast agent is moved somewhat from its resting position during the scan time and then moved back, the image shows a typical distortion structure in the form of a cross (Fig. 4.31). Although such a structure is relatively easily recognized as a motion artifact in the CT image, the combination of several such artifacts can make it considerably more difficult to interpret the image.

4.2.3 Mathematical appendix: description of the convolution method

Filter equation

Equation (4.8) assigns a function $p_\varphi(\eta)$ of the variables φ and η to the distribution of the attenuation coefficients μ in the intersection plane. This function is called the Radon transform of μ. Already in 1917, Radon developed an integral transformation for recovering the function μ from the projections $p_\varphi(\eta)$ [4.21]. The relationships between the Radon transformation and the Fourier transformation [4.31] make it possible to represent the Radon inverse transformation in terms of the generally more commonly used Fourier transformation.

If one neglects higher-order physically caused effects, the CT measurement process represents a linear, position-invariant system in which the point spread function is derived as $1/r$. A real distribution of μ values provides the superposition of all point images weighted according to this distribution, i.e. the convolution product

$$\bar{\mu}(\underline{r}) = \iint \mu(\underline{r}') \frac{\gamma}{|\underline{r}-\underline{r}'|} \mathrm{d}^2 \underline{r}'. \tag{4.11}$$

This can be written in the more compact form

$$\bar{\mu} = \mu * \frac{\gamma}{r}, \tag{4.12}$$

where $\gamma = 1/\text{cm}$ is a constant which ensures that the physical dimensions are the same on both sides of the equation (4.12).

In order to obtain the distribution $\mu(r)$ from this relationship, we first make use of the two-dimensional Fourier transform $F_2\{\bar{\mu}\}$ and obtain, with the help of the convolution theorem,

$$F_2\{\bar{\mu}\}(\underline{v}) = F_2\{\mu\}(\underline{v}) \cdot \frac{\gamma}{v}, \tag{4.13}$$

with

$$F_2\left\{\frac{1}{r}\right\} = \frac{1}{v} \quad \text{and} \quad v = |\underline{v}|.$$

$\underline{v}$ denotes the two-dimensional frequency vector (see Sect. 2.2 for the meaning of the frequency vector).

We now obtain the required solution of equation (4.8) from equation (4.13), the so-called filter equation

$$\mu(\underline{r}) = \frac{1}{\gamma} F_2^{-1}\{v F_2\{\bar{\mu}\}\}(\underline{r}),$$

which, however, is best generalized to

$$\mu^*(\underline{r}) = \frac{1}{\gamma} F_2^{-1}\{H(v) F_2\{\bar{\mu}\}\}(\underline{r}). \tag{4.14}$$

Here, $H(v)$ represents a suitable filter function. If, for example, one knows that the measured spatial frequency spectrum has already fallen off to zero above a frequency limit v_0, $H(v)$ can be arbitrarily chosen for $v \geq v_0$.

The filter equation (4.14) provides the possibility for influencing the nature of the image in a controlled manner by a suitable choice of $H(v)$. For example, by raising the filter function for high spatial frequencies, the contour sharpness can be enhanced or images with low noise can be obtained with the help of suitable band-pass filters.

Nevertheless, one of the disadvantages of an image reconstruction algorithm based on equation (4.14) would be that at best the superposition image $\bar{\mu}$ could be reconstructed in the computer during the scan process, but the filtering could only be carried out after completion of the scan. Concurrent data processing would therefore be impossible.

One-dimensional form of the filter equation

We will show below how to simplify the filter equation to make it suitable as a basis for the real-time processing of scan data.

Let the unit vector which points in the direction of the linear scanning movement be denoted by $\underline{t}_\varphi$ (see Fig. 4.15). The unit vector $\underline{s}_\varphi$ perpendicular to it points in the direction of the scan beam. Then, the approximation image $\bar{\mu}$ introduced in equation (4.12) can be expressed in terms of the projections p_φ:

$$\bar{\mu}(\underline{r}) = \gamma \int_0^\pi p_\varphi(\underline{r} \cdot \underline{t}_\varphi)\, \mathrm{d}\varphi. \tag{4.15}$$

Equations (4.14) and (4.15) represent the relationship between the projections and the distribution μ. It can be shown that equation (4.15) also yields the point spread function γ/r.

Since the function $\gamma p_\varphi(\underline{r} \cdot \underline{t}_\varphi)$ only varies along one direction, namely along the scanning direction $\underline{t}_\varphi$, but not along the direction of the beam $\underline{s}_\varphi$, it can be regarded as a stripe image.

If we now wish to transform the filter equation with the help of equation (4.15) so that the superposition is only performed after the filtering, then we first calculate the Fourier integrals

$$F_2\{p_\varphi(\underline{r} \cdot \underline{t}_\varphi)\}(\underline{v}) = \iint p_\varphi(\underline{r} \cdot \underline{t}_\varphi)\, \mathrm{e}^{-j2\pi \underline{r} \cdot \underline{v}}\, \mathrm{d}^2 \underline{r},$$

by introducing the coordinate transformation

$$\xi = \underline{r} \cdot \underline{s}_\varphi, \qquad \eta = \underline{r} \cdot \underline{t}_\varphi, \qquad u = \underline{v} \cdot \underline{s}_\varphi, \qquad v = \underline{v} \cdot \underline{t}_\varphi \tag{4.16}$$

Since $\underline{r} \cdot \underline{v} = \xi \underline{u} + \eta v$ and $\mathrm{d}^2 \underline{r} = \mathrm{d}\xi\, \mathrm{d}\eta$, we obtain

$$\begin{aligned} F_2\{p_\varphi(\underline{r} \cdot \underline{t}_\varphi)\}(\underline{v}) &= \int_{-\infty}^{+\infty} p_\varphi(\eta)\, \mathrm{e}^{-j2\pi\eta v}\, \mathrm{d}\eta \int_{-\infty}^{+\infty} \mathrm{e}^{-j2\pi\xi u}\, \mathrm{d}\xi \\ &= F_1\{p_\varphi\}(v) \cdot \delta(u). \end{aligned} \tag{4.17}$$

Here $\delta(u)$ is the well-known Dirac function.

The two-dimensional spectrum of a stripe image $\gamma p_\varphi(\underline{r} \cdot \underline{t}_\varphi)$ is therefore concentrated on a straight line in the frequency plane. This line runs parallel to the scanning direction. If we now substitute equation (4.15) into the filter equation (4.16), taking into consideration equation (4.17), then after exchanging the order of integration and setting $\nu^2 = u^2 + v^2$, we obtain

$$\mu^*(\underline{r}) = \int_0^{\pi} F_2^{-1}\{H(\nu)\, F_2\{p_\varphi(\underline{r}\cdot\underline{t}_\varphi)\}\}\,\mathrm{d}\varphi$$

$$= \int_0^{\pi}\int_0^{\infty} H(|v|)\, F_1\{p_\varphi\}(v)\,\mathrm{e}^{j2\pi\eta v}\,\mathrm{d}v\,\mathrm{d}\varphi$$

$$= \int_0^{\pi} F_1^{-1}\{H(|v|)\, F_1\{p_\varphi\}(v)\}\,\mathrm{d}\varphi. \tag{4.18}$$

This relationship represents a version of the filter equation (4.14) which allows concurrent image reconstruction, because it now contains only computational operations which can be executed with the individual projections p_φ. Every projection can be filtered immediately after its measurement and back-projected. However, the filtering can also be performed directly on the measured values without having to proceed via the Fourier space. If we choose the one-dimensional convolution kernel $h(\eta)$ so that

$$H(|v|) = F_1\{h\}(v) \tag{4.19}$$

the convolution theorem along with equation (4.11) yields

$$\mu^*(\underline{r}) = \int_0^{\pi} (h * p_\varphi)(\underline{r}\cdot\underline{t}_\varphi)\,\mathrm{d}\varphi$$

$$= \int_0^{\pi}\left(\int_{-\infty}^{+\infty} h(\underline{r}\cdot\underline{t}_\varphi - \eta)\, p_\varphi(\eta)\,\mathrm{d}\eta\right)\mathrm{d}\varphi. \tag{4.20}$$

$\mu^*(\underline{r})$ now represents a superposition of one-dimensional convolution results.

Discretization of the filter equation

For digital data processing, φ can only assume M different, normally equidistant, positions φ_m:

$$\varphi_m = m\Delta\varphi \quad \text{with } \Delta\varphi = \frac{\pi}{M} \quad \text{and} \quad 1 \le m \le M.$$

The projections, too, are only known at N equidistant points $\eta_n = na$, where the measured projection values only represent approximation values for $p_\varphi(\eta_n)$, denoted by $\bar{p}_{\varphi,n}$; a is the sampling interval.

These approximation values must now either be filtered after discretization of equation (4.18), which can be facilitated by the fast Fourier transformation (FFT), or discretely convolved using equation (4.20) with a suitable numerical sequence h_k. If we consider the values $\bar{p}_{\varphi,n}$ as the scanning values of a continuous function $\bar{p}_\varphi(\eta)$, the question arises under what conditions the actual convolution integral to be calculated

$$g(\eta) = \int_{-\infty}^{+\infty} \bar{p}_\varphi(\eta')\, h(\eta - \eta')\, \mathrm{d}\eta' \tag{4.21}$$

may be replaced by discrete convolution expressions of the form

$$g_k = a \sum_{n=-\infty}^{+\infty} \bar{p}_{\varphi,n} \cdot h_{k-n} \tag{4.22}$$

(For formal reasons, the summation and integration limits are assumed to be infinite).

There is a simple answer to this question. If we assume that the functions $\bar{p}_\varphi(\eta)$ and $h(\eta)$ are frequency-band limited with a bandwidth $B \leq 1/(2a)$, then the following relationship applies exactly

$$a \sum_{n=-\infty}^{+\infty} \bar{p}_{\varphi,n} \cdot h_{k-n} = \int_{-\infty}^{+\infty} \bar{p}_\varphi(\eta') \cdot h(ak - \eta')\, \mathrm{d}\eta', \tag{4.23}$$

if the h_k are chosen as sampling values $h_k = h(ak)$ of the continuous kernel $h(\eta)$. This follows immediately from the representation which is valid for any functions $f(\eta)$ of bandwidth B:

$$f(\eta) = \sum_{k=-\infty}^{+\infty} f\left(\frac{k}{2B}\right) \cdot S_k(\eta), \tag{4.24}$$

where $S_k(\eta)$ is an abbreviated notation for

$$\frac{\sin 2\pi B(\eta - k/(2B))}{2\pi B(\eta - k/(2B))}$$

and from the easily verified relationship

$$\int_{-\infty}^{+\infty} S_k(\eta') \cdot S_n(\eta - \eta')\, \mathrm{d}\eta' = a \cdot S_{k+n}(\eta). \tag{4.25}$$

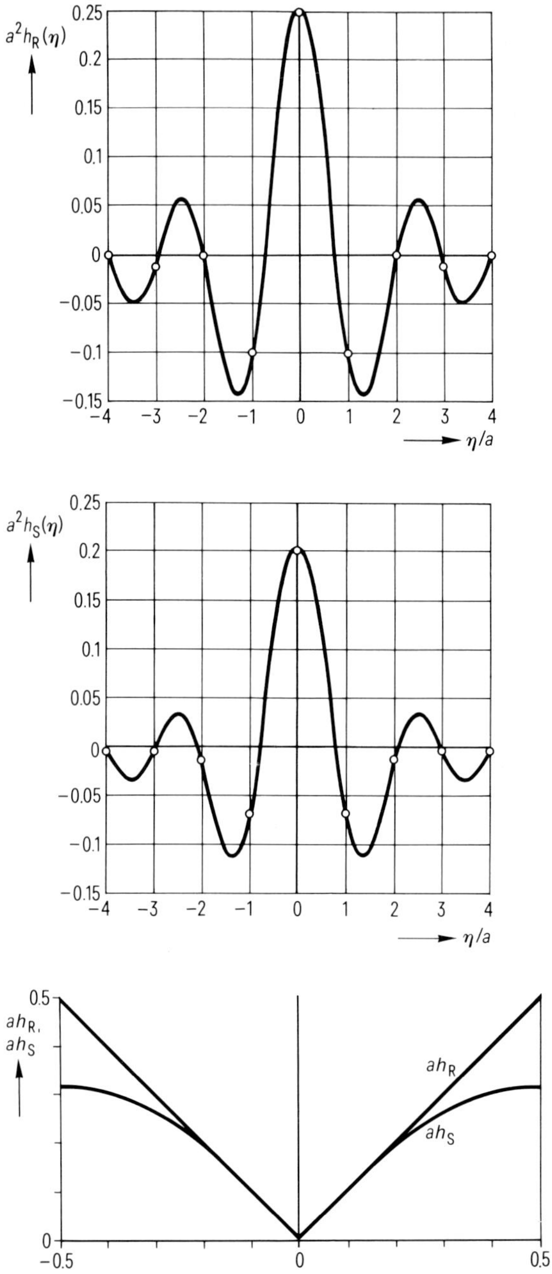

a) Ramachandran-Lakshminarayanan kernel

b) Shepp-Logan kernel. Solid lines represent $h(\eta)$ and circles h_k (cf. Table 4.2)

c) Representation of the filter functions corresponding to h_R and h_S

a sampling interval length

Fig. 4.32 Illustration of the two most common convolution kernels

The most common convolution kernels in x-ray computed tomography are the kernel $h_R(\eta)$ of Ramachandran and Lakshminarayanan [4.24] and the kernel $h_S(\eta)$ of Shepp and Logan [4.25].

The former, historically older, represents the implementation of the frequency filtering

$$H_R(v) = |v| \cdot \text{rect}(a v) \tag{4.26}$$

and the latter the implementation of the frequency filtering

$$H_S(v) = |v| \cdot \left| \frac{\sin \pi v a}{\pi v a} \right| \cdot \text{rect}(a v). \tag{4.27}$$

Here, rect(x) is the well-known rectangular function, which is 1 for $|x| \leq 1/2$ and 0 for $|x| > 1/2$. These kernels and their Fourier transforms, i.e. their associated frequency filters, are compared in Table 4.2. A graphical representation is shown in Fig. 4.32.

Table 4.2
Equivalent representations of the two most important convolution kernels

	Kernel of		
	Shepp and Logan	Ramachandran and Lakshminarayanan	
h_k	$-\frac{2}{\pi^2 a^2} \frac{1}{4k^2 - 1}$	$\frac{1}{4a^2}$	$k = 0$
		0	k even, $\neq 0$
		$-\frac{1}{\pi^2 a^2 k^2}$	k odd
$h(\eta)$	$-\frac{2}{\pi^2 a^2} \frac{1 - 2\frac{\eta}{a} \sin \pi \frac{\eta}{a}}{4\left(\frac{\eta}{a}\right)^2 - 1}$	$\frac{1}{2a^2} \left\{ \frac{\sin \pi \frac{\eta}{a}}{\pi \frac{\eta}{a}} + \frac{\cos \pi \frac{\eta}{a} - 1}{\left(\pi \frac{\eta}{a}\right)^2} \right\}$	
$H(\lvert v \rvert)$	$\lvert v \rvert \cdot \left\lvert \frac{\sin \pi v a}{\pi v a} \right\rvert \text{rect}(a v)$	$\lvert v \rvert \, \text{rect}(a v)$	

5 Magnetic resonance imaging

5.1 Basic principles

In common with all other imaging processes in medical diagnostics, magnetic resonance tomography makes use of the interaction of anatomical structures within the human body with a radiation field. This interaction, however, should not be so weak that no radiation re-emerges from the object to be measured, nor so strong that the biological tissue is damaged. In the case of electromagnetic waves, the shortwave region (<0.05 nm) has been used in medical diagnostics ever since the discovery of x-rays in 1895; the longwave region (>0.3 nm) has only come to be employed since 1973, in the field of magnetic resonance tomography. The limits placed on spatial resolution (image sharpness) by the wavelength are circumvented by superimposing two fields. With the aid of a radiofrequency field in the MHz range and a locally variable static magnetic field, the sharp resonance absorption of magnetic nuclei in biological tissue is used in order to obtain the spatial distribution of the nuclear magnetization.

In particular, hydrogen atoms, which occur naturally in large numbers, allow medically meaningful images to be formed with a spatial resolution comparable to that of x-ray computed tomography and which show previously unseen contrasts between tissues. In addition, it is even possible to detect magnetic nuclei, such as ^{13}C, ^{19}F, ^{23}Na, ^{31}P, in spite of their low concentration in biological tissue; nevertheless, the value of the information thus gained does not approach that obtained through proton resonance.

Below we briefly describe the basic physical principles underlying magnetic resonance (MR) and the various methods of obtaining spatial resolution, as well as discussing some aspects of proton magnetization images and spectroscopy. A detailed description and discussion can be found in the relevant literature.

5.1.1 Macroscopic magnetization

All atomic nuclei with an odd number of protons or neutrons – i.e. roughly two-thirds of all stable atomic nuclei – possess an intrinsic angular momentum $\hbar\vec{I}$ or a (dimensionless) spin $\vec{I}$. This is always coupled with a magnetic dipole moment, which is proportional to the angular momentum:

$$\vec{\mu}=\gamma\hbar\vec{I}. \tag{5.1}$$

$\hbar$ Planck's constant ($h/2\pi=1.055\cdot 10^{-34}\,\mathrm{Ws^2}$)

γ Gyromagnetic ratio
(for the proton, for example, $\gamma/2\pi=42.577$ MHz/T)

In an externally applied magnetic field of flux density $\vec{B}$, this dipole moment has the potential energy

$$\boldsymbol{H}=-\vec{\boldsymbol{\mu}}\vec{B}. \tag{5.2}$$

It is known from quantum mechanics that particles cannot continuously change their angular momentum and their energy, but that these can only assume discrete values. These values emerge as expectation and eigenvalues of operators which replace the classical physical quantities. In this sense equations (5.1) and (5.2) are to be understood as operator equations.

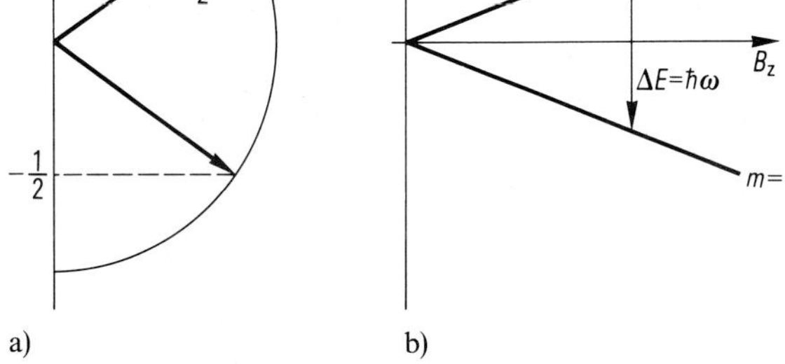

Fig. 5.1
(a) Possible orientations of a nuclear spin $I=1/2$ in a magnetic field (the magnitude of the spin vector is $\sqrt{I(I+1)}$), and (b) energies of a nuclear spin $I=1/2$ as a function of the magnetic field. For a quantum transition the difference in energy has to be added or removed in the form of light quanta of energy $\hbar\omega$

The magnitude of the nuclear spin (spin quantum number I) is the eigenvalue of the operator $\boldsymbol{I}^2$

$$\langle \boldsymbol{I}^2 \rangle = I(I+1) \tag{5.3}$$

(e.g. for the proton $I=1/2$ and for ^{23}Na $I=3/2$) and the component parallel to the magnetic field m is the eigenvalue of the operator $\boldsymbol{I}_z$

$$\langle \boldsymbol{I}_z \rangle = m(-I \leq m \leq I). \tag{5.4}$$

In a magnetic field B_z a nucleus with the quantum number I may therefore assume $2I+1$ discrete energy states (Fig. 5.1 a):

$$\langle \boldsymbol{H} \rangle = E_m = -\gamma \hbar B_z m. \tag{5.5}$$

A change in such a level always entails the absorption or emission of a photon (Fig. 5.1 b):

$$\hbar\omega = E_{m-1} - E_m = \gamma \hbar B_z. \tag{5.6}$$

Such processes were observed as hyperfine structure very early in optical spectroscopy of fluorescent gases and correctly interpreted by Pauli [5.4] in 1924.

In matter, atomic nuclei do not occur singly but only as an ensemble; for example 1 mm^3 of water contains $6.7 \cdot 10^{19}$ protons. In an external magnetic field, occupation of the energy states described by equation (5.5) proceeds in accordance with Boltzmann statistics:

$$N_{m-1}/N_m = e^{-\gamma \hbar B_z / kT}. \tag{5.7}$$

k is the Boltzmann constant ($k = 1.38 \cdot 10^{-23}$ Ws/K).

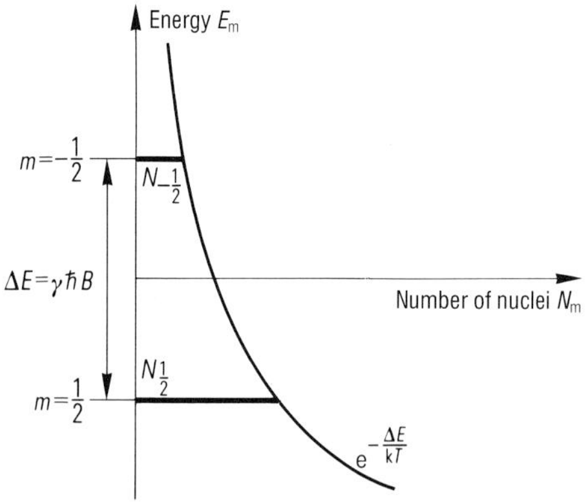

Fig. 5.2
Occupation of the energy states of a spin ensemble for $I=1/2$ according to the Boltzmann distribution

A surplus of nuclear magnetic moments aligned parallel to the magnetic field (for the same reason that the air pressure in the Earth's gravitational field decreases with increasing height) therefore results. Usually the magnetic interaction energy $\gamma\hbar B_z$ is much smaller than the thermal energy kT (for protons in a magnetic field of flux density 1 T (Tesla), the magnetic energy at room temperature is approximately a factor $8\cdot 10^5$ smaller than the thermal energy). The exponential function in equation (5.7) can therefore be linearized. This leads to a macroscopic angular momentum with an associated magnetic moment, given by equation (5.1).

$$m_N = NI(I+1)\,\gamma^2\hbar^2 B_z/3kT. \tag{5.8}$$

N is the number of nuclear spins

Instead of the macroscopic magnetic moment, the ratio of magnetic moment to sample volume, i.e. the nuclear magnetization, $M = \mathrm{d}m_N/\mathrm{d}v$, is often specified.

5.1.2 The Bloch equations

The phenomenon of nuclear magnetic resonance can be treated both in the framework of classical mechanics and in that of quantum mechanics. Since the mathematical formalism is simpler in classical mechanics, this will be the description chosen here, although an occasional recourse to the microscopic picture (as sketched in Section 5.1.1) will be unavoidable. The juxtaposition of the two representations – the quantum mechanical, in which according to Fig. 5.1 a spin can only assume discrete angles with respect to the external magnetic field, and the classical, in which – as will be shown in the following exposition – the macroscopic magnetization of equation (5.8) precesses around an external field with an arbitrary angle – occasionally leads to difficulties in comprehension. Thus, the reader should bear in mind the Bohr correspondence principle, which says that in the case of large quantum numbers (in this case, of many particles), the results of quantum mechanics become indistinguishable from the classical results.

In the case of thermal equilibrium, the magnetic moment (from equation (5.8)) of a probe with nuclear spins aligns itself parallel to the external magnetic field. If this equilibrium is disturbed, for example by suddenly changing the direction of the external magnetic field, then a torque $\vec{m}\times\vec{B}$ acts on the magnetic moment of the sample. Following the law of conservation of angular momentum, this torque causes a change in time of the angular momentum $1/\gamma\,\mathrm{d}\vec{m}/\mathrm{d}t$ of the probe, where

$$\frac{1}{\gamma}\,\mathrm{d}\vec{m}/\mathrm{d}t = \vec{\omega}_\mathrm{L}\,m/\gamma = \vec{m}\times\vec{B}. \tag{5.9}$$

This results in the precession of the nuclear magnetization around the direction of the magnetic field with the Larmor frequency

$$\omega_L = \gamma B_z \tag{5.10}$$

analogously to the precession of an obliquely oriented top around the normal (Fig. 5.3). This precession (nuclear magnetic resonance) can be detected easily by measuring the induced alternating voltage in a coil surrounding the sample. It is the classical analog of the quantum transition expressed by equation (5.6).

For hydrogen nuclei, which are the most frequently occurring in nature, one obtains at 1 T a resonance frequency of 42.577 MHz. Table 1 shows resonance frequencies of other nuclei found in biological tissue and their relative sensitivity to detection at the same measuring frequency, taking into account their natural abundances.

Experience shows that after a finite period of time the thermal equilibrium which had previously been disturbed is reestablished. This process is described following Bloch (5.5) by phenomenologically adding relaxation terms to equation (5.9). It is assumed here that the components of the nuclear magnetization parallel and perpendicular to the magnetic field tend to their respective equilibrium states (M_0 and 0 respectively) at a rate proportional to the respective deviation from equilibrium:

$$\begin{aligned} \mathrm{d}M_z/\mathrm{d}t &= \gamma(\vec{M} \times \vec{B})_z + (M_0 - M_z)/T_1, \\ \mathrm{d}M_{x,y}/\mathrm{d}t &= \gamma(\vec{M} \times \vec{B})_{x,y} - M_{x,y}/T_2. \end{aligned} \tag{5.11}$$

M_0 denotes the equilibrium magnetic moment according to equation (5.8), T_1 the time constant (longitudinal relaxation time) with which the magnetization along the direction of the basic field is restored, and T_2 the time constant with which the transverse component decays (transverse relaxation time). The longitudinal relaxation is associated with the emission of energy to the surroundings (the crystal lattice in which the atomic nuclei are embedded) – thus it

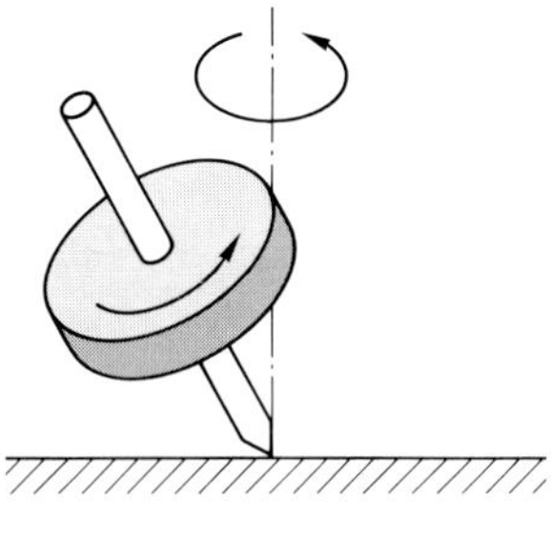

Fig. 5.3
Precession of a top
in a gravitational field

Table 5.1
MR detection capabilities for various elements in biological tissue. The final column gives the relative edge length of the cube which would result in a constant signal

Element Isotope	MR frequency in MHz (at 1T)	Average detection sensitivity in tissue at constant frequency	Resolution
^{1}H	42.58	100	1
^{2}H	6.53	0.006	25
^{13}C	10.71	0.025	16
^{14}N	3.08	0.31	7
^{17}O	5.77	0.049	13
^{19}F	40.06	0.006	25
^{23}Na	11.26	0.1	10
^{31}P	17.24	0.14	9
^{35}CI	4.17	0.0084	23
^{39}K	1.99	0.011	21

is often referred to as spin-lattice relaxation (the probe therefore heats up; this effect is hardly measurable, however). The disappearance of the transverse magnetization is due to the mutual interaction of the nuclear spins, and is thus often referred to as spin-spin relaxation. Since in the case of transverse relaxation the longitudinal component of the magnetic moment, which determines the energy of the spin ensemble (equation 5.2), remains the same, the spin system does not lose any energy in the process and only the relationship of the phases of the individual spins to one another is lost. T_1 is an energy effect and T_2 an entropy effect.

5.1.3 Relaxation

The relaxation times express the mobility of the molecules in which the nuclei under consideration are located. Each nucleus is surrounded by other magnetic moments which are in constant thermal motion (Brownian molecular motion) and produce a continuously changing magnetic perturbation field. Spectral components which correspond to the precession frequency of the nuclear magnetization induce the longitudinal relaxation; the transverse relaxation, on the other hand, is determined by the frequency of collisions between the molecules as a whole.

The time behavior of the molecular motion is described quantitatively by the autocorrelation function $K(t)$. This is a measure of how long a molecule can 'remember' colliding with another molecule. If on the average two collisions are separated by the correlation time τ_c, then given stochastic molecular motion one can assume an exponential decay for the autocorrelation function:

$$K(t) = K(0)\,\mathrm{e}^{-\frac{|t|}{\tau_c}}. \tag{5.12}$$

In between two collisions the magnetic field b with components b_x, b_y, b_z, which acts from the nucleus (or possibly from the electron spin) of the one molecule on the nucleus of the other molecule, changes statistically by an amount $\pm b$. According to equation (5.10) the nucleus precesses with an additional phase $\delta\varphi = \pm\gamma b_z \tau_c$ around the z-component of this perturbation field. After n collisions, the result is therefore an average squared dephasing angle

$$\langle\varphi^2\rangle = n\,\delta\varphi^2 = n\gamma^2 b_z^2 \tau_c^2. \tag{5.13}$$

(for the average dephasing angle, of course, $\langle\varphi\rangle = 0$).

The time needed to dephase by one angular unit is the transverse relaxation time,

$$T_2 = \frac{n\tau_c}{\langle\varphi^2\rangle} = \frac{1}{\gamma^2 b_z^2 \tau_c}. \tag{5.14}$$

The reciprocal of the longitudinal relaxation time $1/T_1$ is a measure of the probability of transitions between two neighboring energy levels which a magnetic nucleus may assume in an external magnetic field following equation (5.5). This transition probability is proportional to the square of the average transition energy of the nuclear magnetic moment $\vec{\mu}$ with the stochastically fluctuating perturbation field $\vec{b}$ of the neighboring molecules

$$|\langle m+1|\vec{\mu}\vec{b}|m\rangle|^2 = \hbar^2\gamma^2(b_x^2 + b_y^2)\,\boldsymbol{I}(\boldsymbol{I}+1) \tag{5.15}$$

and to the probability $J(\omega)$ that the perturbation field has precisely the resonance frequency ω. The latter is given by the Fourier transform of the autocorrelation function, expressed in equation (5.12)

$$J(\omega) = \int K(t)\,\mathrm{e}^{i\omega t}\,\mathrm{d}t = \frac{2K(0)\,\tau_c}{1+\omega^2\tau_c^2}. \tag{5.16}$$

The reciprocal of the longitudinal relaxation time $1/T_1$ then follows by taking the product of equations (5.15) and (5.16), taking into account the normalization of $K(0)$, to give

$$1/T_1 = \frac{\gamma^2(b_x^2 + b_y^2)\,\tau_c}{1+\omega^2\tau_c^2}\,\boldsymbol{I}(\boldsymbol{I}+1). \tag{5.17}$$

Although the arguments for the derivation of T_1 and T_2 are only plausibility arguments, the results are essentially correct. For liquids, the correlation time is given by the ratio of viscosity to temperature. Biological tissue behaves in a similar manner to a viscous liquid.

Fig. 5.4 shows the relaxation time functions T_1 and T_2 measured by Bloembergen [5.6] for glycerine as a function of the ratio of viscosity to temperature. For T_2 there is a monotonic decrease according to equation 5.14 and for T_1 also a decrease according to equation 5.17, provided that the collision frequency is higher than the Larmor frequency ($\omega\tau_c \ll 1$, rapid molecular motion) and an increase when it is lower than the Larmor frequency ($\omega\tau_c \ll 1$). If $\tau_c \approx T_2$, i.e. $\tau_c \geq 1/\gamma b_z$, the transverse relaxation is no longer influenced by collisions; T_2 is then independent of the autocorrelation time.

For nuclei with a nuclear spin $I > 1/2$, the electrostatic interaction of the nuclear quadrupole moment with the electric field gradient, formed at the site of the nucleus because of the molecular structure, leads to additional relaxation. The short relaxation times of such nuclei often make the experimental observation of nuclear resonance more difficult.

Table 5.2 gives the order of magnitude for the relaxation times of protons in biological tissue [5.7]. The frequency dependence of T_1 may be described approximately by

$$T_1 \sim \omega^{0,3}. \tag{5.18}$$

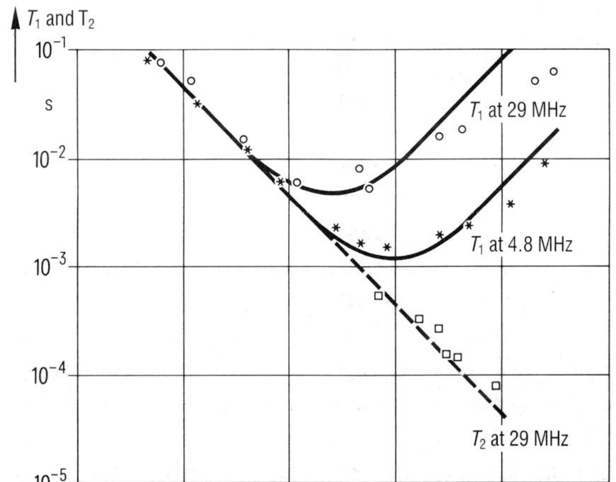

Fig. 5.4
Relaxation times T_1 and T_2 for the magnetic resonance of protons in glycerine as a function of the ratio of viscosity η to temperature θ [5.6]. η/θ is proportional to the autocorrelation time, τ_c

Table 5.2 Typical relaxation times T_1 (at 1 T) and T_2 [5.7].

Tissue	T_1 in s	T_2 in ms	Tissue	T_1 in s	T_2 in ms
Muscle	0.73 ± 0.13	47 ± 13	Spleen	0.68 ± 0.19	62 ± 27
Heart	0.75 ± 0.12	57 ± 16	Fat	0.24 ± 0.07	84 ± 36
Liver	0.42 ± 0.09	43 ± 14	Gray matter	0.81 ± 0.14	101 ± 13
Kidney	0.59 ± 0.16	58 ± 24	White matter	0.68 ± 0.12	92 ± 22

The transverse relaxation is independent of the Larmor frequency, in agreement with equation (5.14), but often several time constants are observed simultaneously.

It is the great range of values which the relaxation times assume in biological tissue which makes them so useful in medical diagnostics. When the spatial distribution is displayed, large contrasts are produced and diseased areas can be localized at once as a result of conspicuous differences in relaxation times. It is hoped that, in the future, T_1 and T_2 can be used to differentiate between tissues. Furthermore, functional studies can be carried out by adding paramagnetic contrast substances in order to shorten the relaxation times.

5.1.4 The magnetic resonance experiment

In the case of pulsed magnetic resonance, the equilibrium of the magnetization for a sample in a magnetic field is disturbed by a radio frequency (RF) pulse which matches the frequency of the Larmor precession. The linearly polarized radio-frequency field in the coil surrounding the sample can be thought of as the sum of two oppositely rotating circularly polarized fields, one of which has the same direction of rotation as the Larmor precession. Thus, in a reference frame which rotates at the nuclear precession frequency (rotating frame), a constant magnetic flux density B_1 acts, which in accordance with equation (5.9) causes the magnetization to precess about the axis of the B_1 field. In the laboratory system, the magnetization describes a combined precession movement around the basic static magnetic field B_z and the co-rotating field vector of the radio-frequency field B_1, which corresponds to a spiral path on the surface of a sphere (Fig. 5.5). The contrarotating radio-frequency field acts in the rotating reference frame as a perturbation having twice the Larmor frequency, with an effect which averages out.

Under the assumption that for the duration t of the radio-frequency pulse relaxation effects do not yet play a role, then the angle α which arises due to the influence of this pulse between the magnetization and the static magnetic field is

$$\alpha = \gamma B_1 t. \tag{5.19}$$

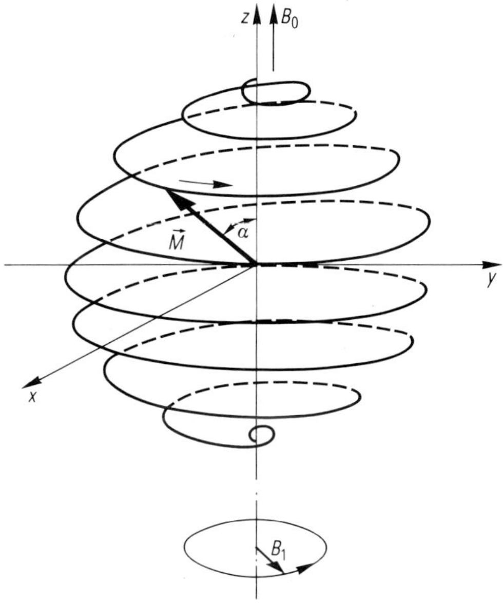

Fig. 5.5
Motion of the nuclear magnetization vector $\vec{M}$ under the influence of the static magnetic field B_0 and the circularly-polarized high frequency field B_1 with the Larmor frequency γB_0. The initial position of $\vec{M}$ is parallel to B_0; after time t, M is oriented an angle $\alpha = \gamma B_1 t$ to the direction of the static field

If the radio frequency pulse is switched off after the magnetization has reached a position perpendicular to the constant magnetic field ($\alpha = 90°$, hence a 90° pulse), it precesses with the maximum possible angle about the static field. Solving the Bloch equation (5.11) for the precessing transverse magnetization gives

$$M_{xy}(t) = M_0\, e^{\left(-i\gamma B_z t - \frac{t}{T_2}\right)} \tag{5.20}$$

and for the longitudinal magnetization

$$M_z(t) = M_0 (1 - e^{-\frac{t}{T_1}}). \tag{5.21}$$

The precessing transverse magnetization can be detected easily via the signal induced in the radio-frequency coil (free induction decay, FID). The complex Fourier transform of this signal gives the magnetic resonance line – the dependence of the transverse magnetization on the frequency (Fig. 5.6). The real part of the Fourier transform describes the so-called absorption line

$$M_x(\omega) = \frac{M_0}{\pi} \frac{T_2}{1 + (\omega - \omega_0)^2 T_2^2}, \tag{5.22}$$

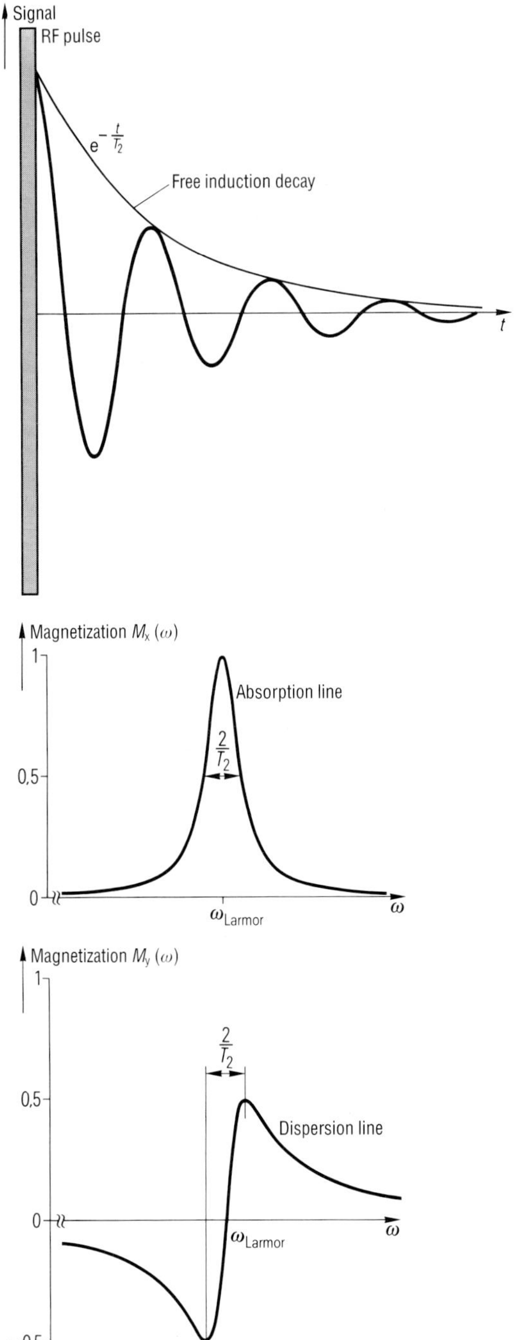

Fig. 5.6
(a) Induction signal following a 90° pulse about the y-axis of the rotating frame:

In order to be able to evaluate the phase of the transverse magnetization as well as its absolute value, the induction signal is mixed with an alternating voltage signal of similar frequency, giving a signal with the difference frequency (phase-sensitive demodulation)

(b) Absorption signal:

The real part of the Fourier transform of the time signal in (a) represents the frequency dependence of the x-component of the precessing magnetization vector

(c) Dispersion signal:

The imaginary part of the Fourier transform of the time signal in (a) represents the frequency dependence of the y-component of the precessing magnetization vector and the imaginary part the dispersion line

$$M_y(\omega)=\frac{M_0}{\pi}\frac{T_2^2(\omega-\omega_0)}{1+(\omega-\omega_0)^2 T_2^2}. \tag{5.23}$$

The half-width of the absorption and the distance between the inflection points of the dispersion line are given by the transverse relaxation time T_2:

$$\Delta\omega=2/T_2. \tag{5.24}$$

Protons in distilled water exhibit a line width of less than 1 Hz. Absorption and dispersion may also be measured directly by recording the effective resistance and inductivity of the coil surrounding the sample as a function of the frequency or of the field strength of the static magnetic field, e.g. by means of a bridge (continuous wave, CW). Because of the relatively long time required for taking measurements in comparison with the pulse method, continuous wave methods have, however, declined in importance.

The measurement of the transverse relaxation time T_2 through the duration of the free induction decay or through the line width only functions with very homogeneous magnetic fields. In practice the magnetic field usually varies from place to place, resulting in differing precession frequencies for the magnetization. Because of destructive interference, one therefore observes a shortened free induction decay (FID) or a (inhomogeneous) broadening of the line width. The form of the resulting resonance line essentially depends on the nature of the field distribution for the magnetic field ΔB_z; giving the effective transverse relaxation time

$$1/T_2^*=1/T_2+\gamma\Delta B_z \tag{5.25}$$

only describes the influence of field inhomogeneities in a general way since, of course, normally the signal decay is no longer exponential.

5.1.5 Pulse method for determining T_2

The destructive interference of precessing nuclei in inhomogeneous magnetic fields is reversible: if, after the free induction signal has decayed, a second radio-frequency pulse is applied which flips the component of magnetization perpendicular to the B_1 direction (in the rotating frame) by 180° (180° pulse, Fig. 5.7) the previously diverging magnetization converges again [5.8]. The Hahn spin-echo is observed with a reduced amplitude because of the transverse relaxation which has occurred in the meantime (Fig. 5.8).

Transverse relaxation is, however, not the only mechanism which determines the amplitude of the spin-echo. In the case of liquids in particular, molecules

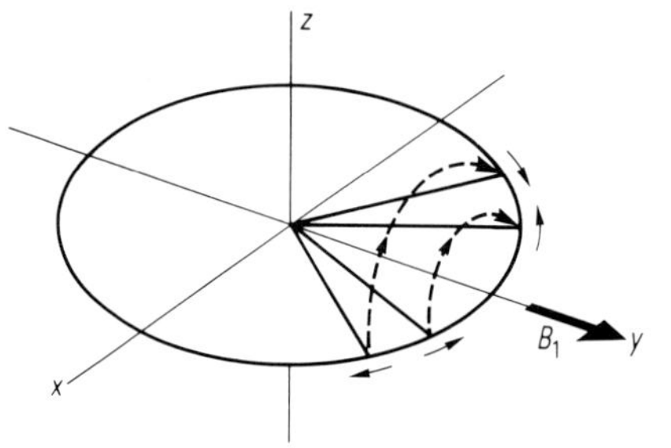

Fig. 5.7
A 180° pulse inverts the precession of two spins in relation to each other. View in the rotating frame

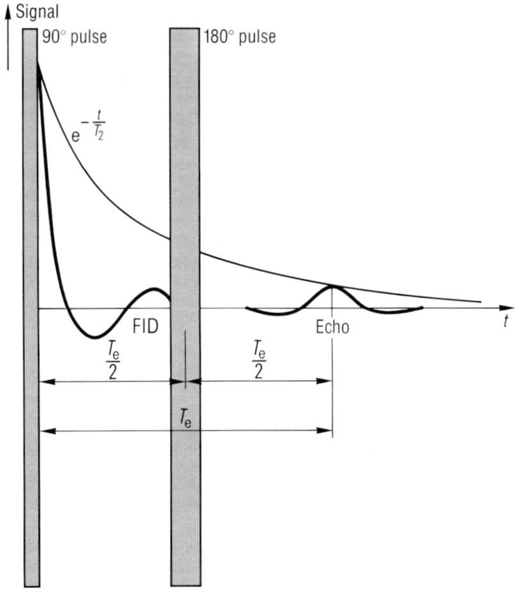

Fig. 5.8
The free induction decay signal (FID) which rapidly decays following a 90° pulse as a result of field inhomogeneities can be induced to occur again by means of a 180° pulse (with a reduced amplitude due to the transverse relaxation)

diffuse (according to the self-diffusion coefficient D) during the echo time T_e between the 90° pulse and observation of the echo from one position in the inhomogeneous static magnetic field to another; in accordance with the field difference (expressed by the magnetic field gradient G), the nuclei precess there with a different Larmor frequency and thus no longer contribute fully to the echo amplitude. This is given by the expression

$$M(T_e) = M_0\, e^{-\frac{T_e}{T_2} - \frac{D\gamma^2 G^2 T_e^3}{12}}\,. \tag{5.26}$$

To determine T_2 and the self-diffusion coefficient D, the spin echo experiment is repeated with various echo times T_e and the ratio of logarithm of echo amplitude to echo time T_e plotted as a function of the echo time T_e^2. A straight line is obtained, which at $T_e = 0$ assumes the value $1/T_2$ and has a slope equal to the product $D \cdot G^2$ of the self-diffusion coefficient and field gradient squared.

A method of determining T_2 over a very much shorter measuring period was described by Carr and Purcell [5.9]: after applying a 90° pulse, a series of 180° pulses is made to follow after a time gap $T_e/2$. The 180° pulses are separated from each other by a time gap T_e (Fig. 5.9). Spin echoes then appear between the 180° pulses, the amplitude of the kth spin echo being given by

$$M(k) = M_0\, e^{-k\frac{T_e}{T_2} - \frac{D\gamma^2 G^2 T_e^3 k}{12}}\,. \tag{5.27}$$

If the echo time T_e is chosen to be very short, then the influence of diffusion in the Carr-Purcell sequence can be kept small.

In practice the exact 180° condition on the refocussing pulses required for the Carr-Purcell experiment cannot be met; the unavoidable inhomogeneity of the radio-frequency coil surrounding the sample already prevents this. In

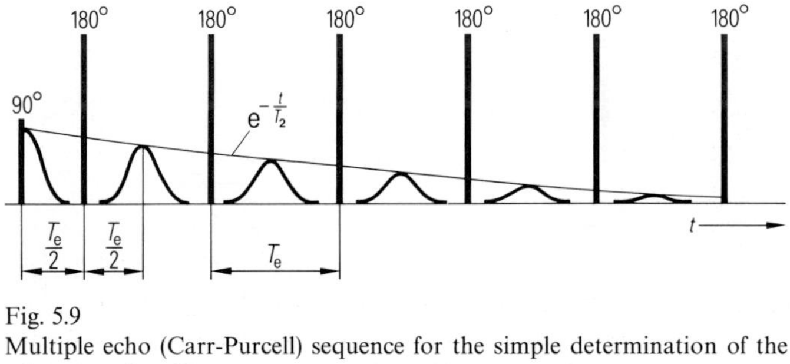

Fig. 5.9
Multiple echo (Carr-Purcell) sequence for the simple determination of the transverse relaxation time T_2

order to avoid cumulative deviations from equation (5.27) resulting from this, one can either alternate the phase of every second 180° pulse by 180° (Carr modification), or one can shift the phase of all the 180° pulses by 90° with respect to the 90° pulse (Gill-Meiboom modification [5.10]). All even echoes then show the correct amplitude, whereas the odd echoes are somewhat reduced, but not cumulatively.

5.1.6 Pulse method for determining T_1

The amplitude of a spin echo produced by a 180° radio-frequency pulse is determined through T_2; an RF pulse sequence consisting of three 90° pulses (Fig. 5.10) also generates a spin echo, the stimulated echo [5.8], the amplitude of which is characterized by T_1. After the second 90° pulse, the primary echo, characterized by T_2, appears, but with (compared to a 180° echo) half the amplitude. The other half of the signal is transformed into longitudinal magnetization and undergoes longitudinal relaxation during the time gap t between the second and third RF pulses. The third RF pulse transforms this longitudinal magnetization back into transverse magnetization. After a time $T_e/2$ following the third RF pulse, the stimulated echo appears with amplitude

$$M(t+T_e) = 1/2\, M_0\, e^{-\frac{t}{T_1}-\frac{T_e}{T_2}-\frac{1}{8}D\gamma^2 G^2 (2/3\, T_e^3 - 2\, T_e^2\, t)}\,. \tag{5.28}$$

By systematically altering the time interval t between the second and third RF pulse it is then possible to determine T_1; however, as mentioned before, a priori the stimulated echo can only give a signal corresponding to half the total magnetization.

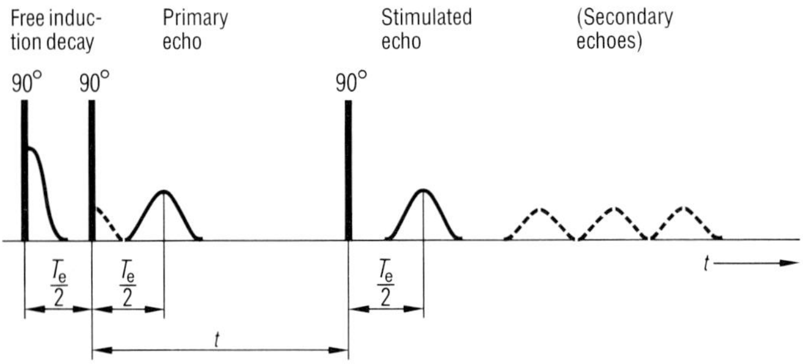

Fig. 5.10
Sequence of three 90° pulses for generating the stimulated echo. If there is a deviation from the 90° condition extra secondary echoes appear

If the 90° condition is not met exactly, three further (secondary) echoes appear, which can be explained as normal (i.e. determined by T_2) echoes and which are generated by the third RF pulse and the free induction decay after the first and second RF pulses, as well as by the first echo.

Another method of determining the longitudinal relaxation time consists in first inverting the magnetization by means of a 180° pulse and then probing the longitudinal magnetization resulting after time t

$$M_z(t) = M_0(1 - 2\,\mathrm{e}^{-\frac{t}{T_1}}) \tag{5.29}$$

by means of the free induction decay (FID) produced by a 90° pulse (Fig. 5.11, inversion recovery). By repeating this sequence with various inversion times t, T_1 can be calculated. If, in particular, we look for the value t_0 at which $M_z(t)$ passes through zero, we find

$$T_1 = t_0/\ln 2. \tag{5.30}$$

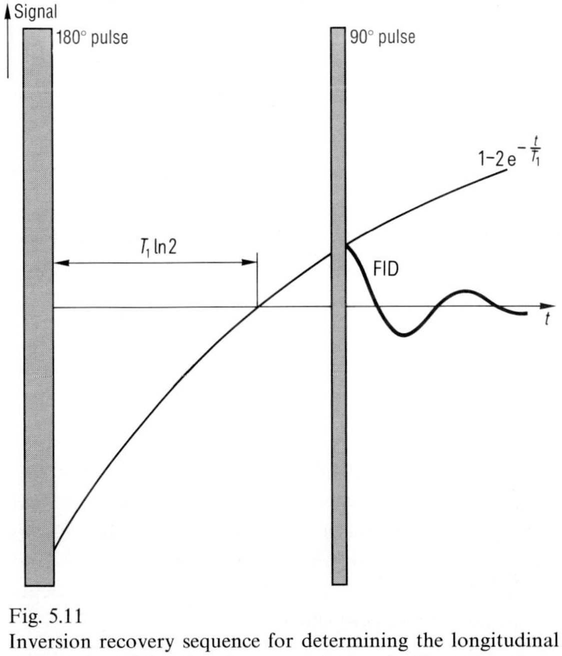

Fig. 5.11
Inversion recovery sequence for determining the longitudinal relaxation time T_1. By means of a 180° pulse, the magnetization is directed antiparallel to the constant magnetic field; (tending to decay back to the equilibrium state with the time constant T_1). The instantaneous value of the longitudinal component can be measured by flipping it by means of a 90° pulse into the transverse plane and evaluating the nuclear induction signal

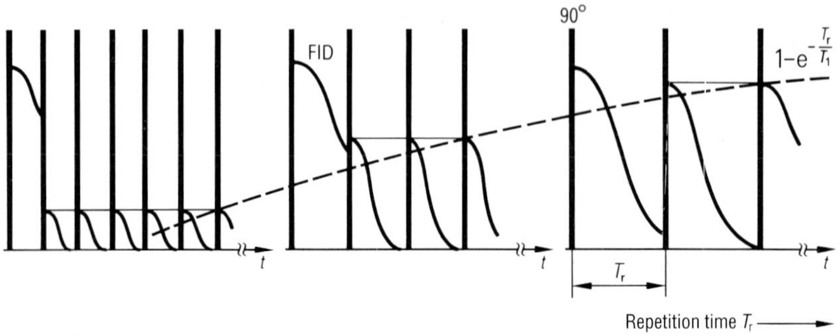

Fig. 5.12
Saturation recovery sequence for determining the longitudinal relaxation time T_1. The amplitude of the free induction decays for several 90° pulses following each other with the repetition time T_r depends exponentially on the ratio T_r/T_1. The magnetization settles into equilibrium after the second 90° pulse

Another method of determining T_1 involves generating free induction decays by means of 90° pulses which are repeated with repetition time T_r (Fig. 5.12). The initial amplitude of these FIDs is then given by

$$M(T_r) = M_0 (1 - e^{-\frac{T_r}{T_1}}). \tag{5.31}$$

For short repetition times the signal vanishes, i.e. the spin system 'saturates' (saturation recovery). To calculate T_1, the magnetic resonance signal is recorded as a function of the repetition time.

5.1.7 Magnetic resonance spectroscopy

It has already been mentioned that the gyromagnetic ratio is a fixed constant for each nuclear species. In experiments where the atomic nuclei under investigation are embedded in different molecules, however, for the same magnetic field slightly different resonance frequencies are observed. This is caused by the molecular electrons responsible for the chemical bonds. These screen the external magnetic field, with the result that the atomic nucleus 'sees' different fields depending on the nature of the bond (chemical shift).

$$B_k = B_0 - \delta_k B_0. \tag{5.32}$$

In a molecular complex there are often several resonance lines, which may be attributed to individual groups of molecules. In quantitative terms the chemical shift δ_k is usually given in ppm (parts per million) relative to a reference line.

Besides the chemical shift, one also often observes a fine splitting of the magnetic resonance lines (Fig. 5.13). This is caused by the magnetic interaction (spin-spin coupling) between the nuclei, which does not act through space but again indirectly via the electrons of the chemical bonds. Such spectra are analyzed by using the energy function (Hamiltonian operator) with interaction energy J_{kl} between the different spins $\vec{I}_k$

$$\boldsymbol{H} = -\sum_{k} B_z(1-\delta_k)\,\boldsymbol{I}_{zk} + \sum_{k,l} J_{kl}\,\vec{\boldsymbol{I}}_k\,\vec{\boldsymbol{I}}_l, \tag{5.33}$$

whose eigenvalues and eigenfunctions are constrained to describe the measured spectrum in accordance with the molecular model adopted. In physical chemistry, elucidation of the molecular structure is often made possible in this way. In medicine it is hoped to be able to detect typical metabolites noninvasively in-vivo via their spectra.

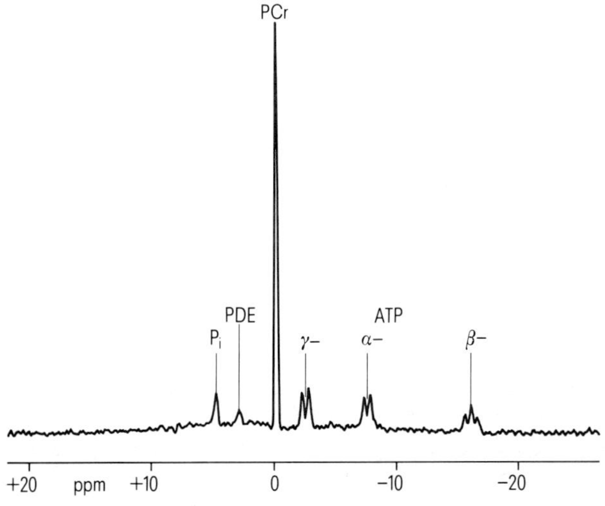

Fig. 5.13
^{31}P-spectrum of a human thigh muscle recorded with a surface coil at 2 T. On the basis of their different chemical shifts, the metabolites adenosine triphosphate (ATP), phosphocreatine (PCr), inorganic phosphate (P_i) and phosphodiester (PDE) can be distinguished. The three ATP lines correspond to the three locations of the phosphorous atom in the molecule; the lines are split further because of the interaction of the nuclei with other nearby nuclei

5.1.8 Signal-to-noise ratio

Nuclear magnetic resonance in-vivo is only meaningful if the parameters of interest, such as number of nuclei, relaxation times, diffusion constant, chemical shift, spin-spin coupling, etc., can be measured in a way which permits spatial resolution, i.e. in a small subvolume V (Voxel) of the patient to be examined (Fig. 5.14). Before going into the various methods of spatial resolution, however, the fundamental limit which restricts such measurements will be defined.

This limit has its origin in the fact that the thermal motion of the electrons in the coil for detecting the magnetic resonance and the Brownian molecular motion in the object to be measured (the human body) produce a noise voltage [5.11], which competes with the magnetic resonance signal. Following Nyquist, this is given by:

$$U_N = \sqrt{(2/\pi)\, k\, T_N\, R \Delta\omega}. \tag{5.34}$$

T_N is the noise temperature
R is the resistance of the detection coil and
$\Delta\omega$ is the detection bandwidth (angular frequency).

The product $T_N\, R$ can be resolved into a coil part and a sample part

$$R T_N = R_{coil}\, T_{coil} + R_{sample}\, T_{sample}. \tag{5.35}$$

The resistance R_{sample} imparted to the measuring coil because of the sample may be calculated from the dissipated power converted in the sample

$$P_{sample} = 1/2 \int_{sample} \sigma E^2 \, dv. \tag{5.36}$$

where

σ is the electrical conductivity and
E is the electric field strength.

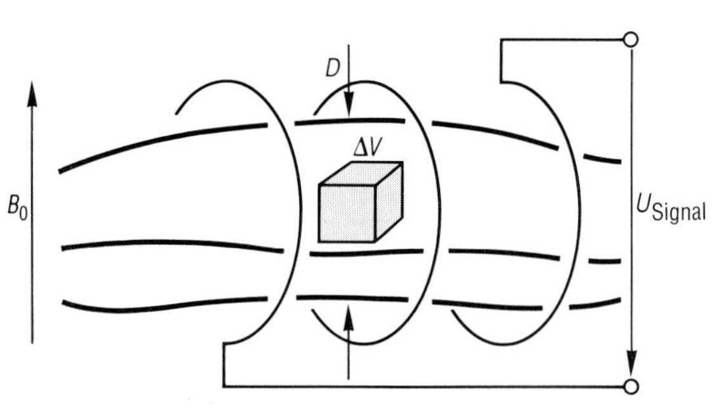

Fig. 5.14
Detection element ΔV inside a patient, surrounded by a radio-frequency coil

From Maxwell's equations we obtain for a homogeneous radio-frequency magnetic field with angular frequency ω and amplitude B_1

$$E = 1/2\,\omega B_1 r_\perp, \tag{5.37}$$

where

$r_\perp$ is the radius perpendicular to the B_1-field,

with the result that the power converted in the sample is

$$P_{\text{sample}} = 1/8\,\omega^2 \sigma B_1^2 \int\limits_{\text{sample}} r_\perp^2\,\mathrm{d}v. \tag{5.38}$$

This is proportional to the "moment of inertia"

$$\Theta = \int\limits_{\text{sample}} r_\perp^2\,\mathrm{d}v, \tag{5.39}$$

and thus depends on the shape of the sample and its orientation. For a cylindrical sample of length l and diameter D, with the RF field oriented perpendicularly to the axis,

$$\Theta = \frac{\pi}{64}\left(D^4 l + \frac{4}{3} D^2 l^3\right)$$

and, with the RF field oriented parallel to the axis,

$$\Theta = \frac{\pi}{32} D^4 l.$$

From the dissipated power it is then possible to calculate the sample resistance, according to the ratio of dissipated power to effective value of the current squared, giving

$$R_{\text{sample}} = 1/\sigma \omega^2 B_i^2\,\Theta, \tag{5.40}$$

where B_i denotes the field per unit of current, i.e. a geometrical factor for the RF coil. For the center of a cylindrical coil

$$B_i = \frac{\mu_0}{2n\sqrt{a^2 + l^2/4}}. \tag{5.41}$$

μ_0 Permeability in a vacuum $= 1.256 \cdot 10^{-6}$ Vs/Am
n Number of turns
l Length of coil
a Radius of coil.

The pure coil resistance R_{coil} can also be expressed by the quality factor of the coil

$$Q_0 = \frac{\omega \cdot (\text{energy stored in the coil})}{\text{power dissipated in the coil}} \tag{5.42}$$

and is therefore found to be

$$R_{coil} = \frac{\omega B_i^2 \, V_{sample}}{2 \mu_0 \, \eta \, Q_0}. \tag{5.43}$$

Here V_{sample} represents the useful volume in the coil taken up by the sample, while for the 'field distribution factor' or 'filling factor'

$$\eta = B_i^2 \, V_{sample} / \int B_i^2 \, \mathrm{d}v. \tag{5.44}$$

The noise voltage given by equation (5.34) is to be compared with the voltage induced in the coil by the precessing magnetization (equation 5.8)

$$U_{Signal} = M B_i \, \omega \Delta V \tag{5.45}$$

following a 90° pulse.

The signal-to-noise ratio is then seen to be independent of the geometrical factor of the coil and is given by

$$S/R = \sqrt{\frac{\pi}{18 k^3}} \, I(I+1) \, \hbar^2 \gamma \frac{N_v \, \omega}{T_{sample} \sqrt{\dfrac{V_{sample} \, T_{coil}}{2 \mu_0 \, \eta \, Q_0 \, \omega} + \dfrac{1}{4} \sigma \Theta T_{sample}}} \frac{\Delta V}{\sqrt{\Delta \omega}}. \tag{5.46}$$

where

N_V is the spin density.

For small samples and a low coil quality factor Q_0, the signal-to-noise ratio is proportional to the measuring frequency $f^{3/2}$; for a high coil quality factor and a low coil temperature, it is directly proportional to the measuring frequency. For a fixed sample volume V_{sample}, the quality of the magnetic resonance coil is determined only by the product of the field distribution factor (filling factor) and the unloaded quality factor ηQ_0. In magnetic resonance tomography the latter is usually so large that the noise induced by the patient predominates over the coil noise, with the result that (for constant detection bandwidth) the signal-to-noise ratio may be regarded as proportional to the static magnetic field strength[1].

[1] Increasing the signal-to-noise ratio by restricting the detection band width is only possible to a limited extent; in order for there to be no loss of information, it is necessary that $\Delta\omega > 1/T_2$. Of course the S/R can also be increased by multiple (n) measurements (S/R $\sim \sqrt{n}$), but this is at the expense of increased measuring time. The number of measurements for a given measuring time T_M is limited by T_1 ($n \sim T_M/T_1$). The relaxation times T_1 and T_2 of the sample and the measuring time T_M can be taken into account in equation (5.46) by replacing $1/\sqrt{\Delta\omega}$ by $\sqrt{T_2 \cdot T_M / T_1}$. These physical dependences are the reason why the number of protons that can be detected by means of a magnetic resonance experiment is limited. At room temperature $5 \cdot 10^{18}$ protons in a liter of physiological saline solution in a magnetic field of 1 T give roughly S/R ≈ 1 ($n = 1$). For comparison: 1 mm^3 of water alone contains $6.7 \cdot 10^{19}$ hydrogen nuclei.

5.2 Methods of spatial resolution

5.2.1 Classification of imaging procedures

To localize the magnetization, magnetic field gradients are superimposed onto the homogeneous static magnetic field during the excitation and measurement of the magnetic resonance signal, with the result that the frequency of the magnetic resonance signal becomes a function of position. Various strategies have been developed for the effective measurement of the spatial distribution of the nuclear magnetization [5.12].

If one imagines the object to be measured as being divided into N^3 volume elements (voxels), then in the simplest case each voxel can be measured in turn; the measuring time for the whole object is thus proportional to N^3. If it is possible to simultaneously register an entire row consisting of N voxels, then in order to obtain the contribution of an individual voxel it is necessary to measure the row N times under different conditions. The measuring time for the whole object thus remains the same, but the signal-to-noise ratio is improved by a factor of $\sqrt{N}$ in comparison to the point-by-point measurement. This is due to each volume being measured N times, although under different measuring conditions, thus reducing the noise by averaging. Extending this principle to the scanning of surfaces and volumes (Fig. 5.15) leads, given the same measuring time, to a further improvement in the signal-to-noise ratio by a factor of $\sqrt{N}$ in each case.

In spite of the above considerations, scanning by volume is not always the most advantageous procedure; this is because the relaxation times T_1 and T_2 of the object being examined place constraints on the times within which a measurement can be repeated. Within the transverse relaxation time T_2 typically N measuring points can be scanned; after each excitation of the total object volume, it is then necessary, before being able to measure a further N points, to wait a time of the order of the longitudinal relaxation time T_1, during which the excited nuclear spin system returns to its original state. In order to scan the entire volume one must therefore figure with measuring times of $N^2 T_1$; thus for a 64^3 matrix and typical measurement repetition times of 0.5 s, this would amount to 34 min.

For planar scanning, the measuring time is only of the order of NT_1, i.e. in the above example around 30 s, so that in the interest of improving the spatial resolution the scan matrix may be enlarged to $N=256$. The measurement of further layers (or 'slices') in the object is also possible without a significant increase in the measuring time, since other slices which have not previously been excited can be measured in the relaxation pauses.

Often, it is not actually interesting to study the spatial distribution of the magnetization at all, but rather to conduct as precise a determination as possible of a particular magnetic resonance parameter – for example the spectral splitting – at a particular location.

Limiting the object to be measured to a partial volume can be done in various ways: by employing a measuring coil which only receives signals from the subregion of interest. These so-called surface coils are popular, because of their improved signal-to-noise ratios compared with whole-body coils (equation 5.46): in this way the 'moment of inertia' (equation 5.39) can be significantly reduced; on the other hand, the inhomogeneity of the radio-frequency field is a disadvantage.

Limiting the resonance volume by shaping the main static magnetic field [5.13, 5.14] has not proved acceptable, since this 'field focus" is technically difficult to vary with the necessary flexibility in regard to its position and range. This is where the strength of 'selective excitation' lies.

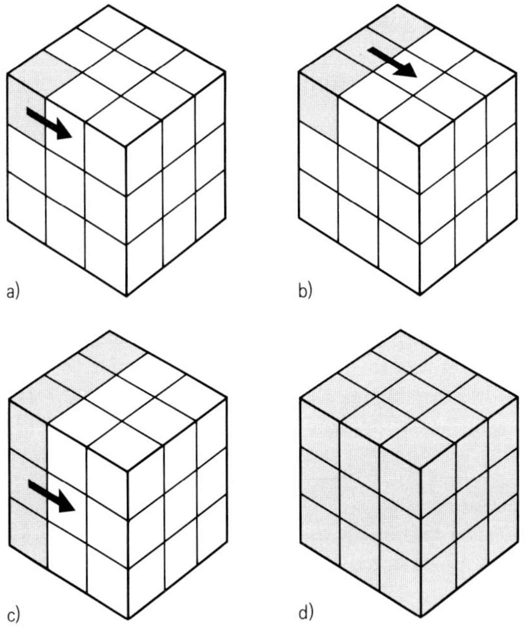

Fig. 5.15
Point (a), line (b), surface (c) and volume (d) scanning of an object in a three-dimensional scan matrix

5.2.2 Selective excitation

It has already been mentioned in Section 5.1.5 that the actual magnetic resonance signal is preceded by the excitation caused by a radio-frequency pulse, the frequency of which coincides with the Larmor frequency. If during a 90° pulse a magnetic field gradient G_z is superimposed onto the object to be measured in addition to the homogeneous main static magnetic field B_0 (Fig. 5.16), then the resonance frequency varies according to

$$\omega_{\text{Larmor}} = \gamma(B_0 + G_z z) \tag{5.47}$$

along the object, and only those nuclei in the slice with position

$$z = (\omega_{\text{Larmor}} - \gamma B_0)/\gamma G_z \tag{5.48}$$

are excited. Thus, only these nuclei yield a magnetic resonance signal, while all the others remain unaffected. In a similar way the magnetization in a slice can be inverted by means of gradient-superimposed (selective) 180° pulses.

The case of a selective 90° pulse will be examined in the following in greater detail. For small angles of rotation about the axis of the RF-field $\gamma B_1\,\mathrm{d}t$ the Bloch equations can be linearized, giving (5.9) for the response of the spin system to an amplitude-modulated RF pulse of frequency ω_{Larmor}

$$\mathrm{d}M_\perp = \gamma M_0\, B_1(t)\, \mathrm{e}^{(-i\omega t)}\,\mathrm{d}t, \tag{5.49}$$

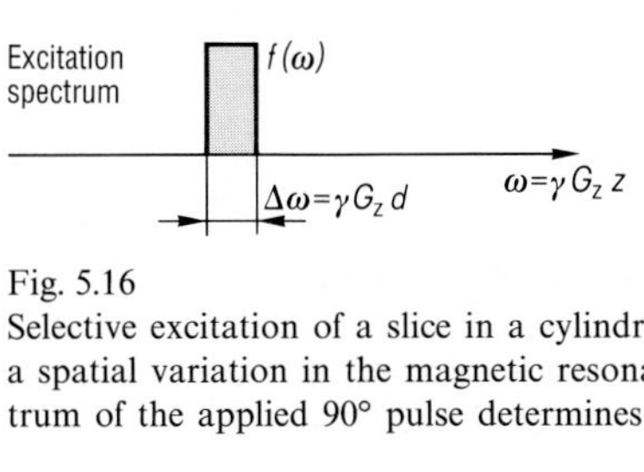

Fig. 5.16
Selective excitation of a slice in a cylindrical object. A gradient along the object allows a spatial variation in the magnetic resonance frequency, with the result that the spectrum of the applied 90° pulse determines position and thickness of the slice

i.e. to a first approximation, the spatial dependence of the transverse magnetization (in the frame rotating with γB_0) is given by the Fourier transform of the selective radio-frequency pulse

$$M_{\perp}(z)=\gamma M_0 \int_0^{t_{\max}} B_1(t)\,\mathrm{e}^{-i\gamma G_z z t}\,\mathrm{d}t. \tag{5.50}$$

Here, the x and y components of the transverse magnetization have been combined in the complex quantity $M_{\perp}=M_x+iM_y$.

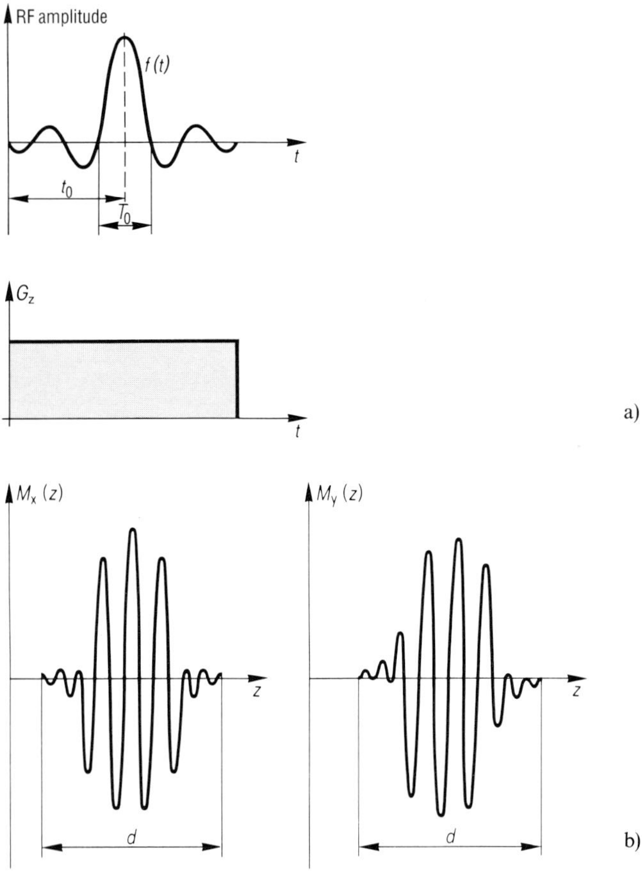

Fig. 5.17
(a) To excite a rectangular slice, the radio frequency of the 90° pulse is modulated with a sinc ($\sin x/x$) function
(b) x and y magnetization (in the rotating frame) as a function of the slice thickness following selective excitation; the magnetization rotates in a spiral fashion

In order to achieve as rectangular a distribution of the transverse magnetization as possible over the thickness of the slice, it is necessary to impose a time dependence on the exciting RF pulse, corresponding to the sin x/x (sinc) function (Fig. 5.17a):

$$B_1(t) = B_1(t_0)\frac{\sin\left(\frac{1}{2}\gamma G_z d(t-t_0)\right)}{\frac{1}{2}\gamma G_z d(t-t_0)}. \quad 0 \le t \le 2t_0 \tag{5.51}$$

where

d is the slice thickness desired and
t_0 is the half-length of the pulse.

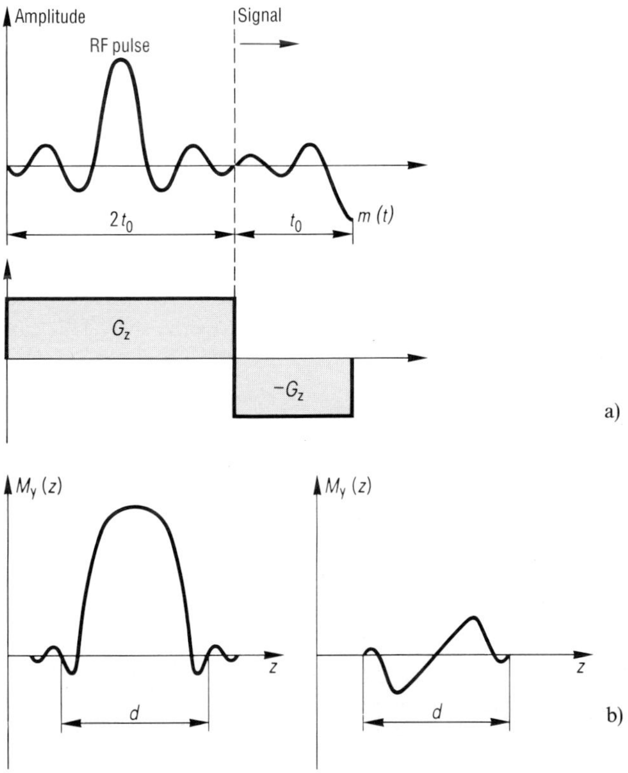

Fig. 5.18
(a) In order to realign the transverse magnetization, which rotates immediately after the selective 90° pulse, an interval with a reversed-polarity field gradient is added on after the RF pulse.
(b) x and y magnetization as a function of slice thickness for selective excitation with refocussing. The remaining oscillation is an expression of the non-linearity of the Bloch equations. It can be improved by means of modified RF modulations

In accordance with equation (5.50), it follows for the transverse magnetization that

$$M_{\perp} = M_0 \operatorname{rect}\left(|z| - \frac{d}{2}\right) e^{i\gamma G_z z t_0} \tag{5.52a}$$

(rect = rectangular function)

an oscillating function (Fig. 5.17 b) with width

$$d = 4/\gamma G_z T. \tag{5.52b}$$

where

T is the distance between the two innermost zeroes of the sin function.

Although the 'selective RF pulse' has flipped each 'spin' into the transverse plane along the slice, this is only in its own co-rotating frame. After termination of the RF pulse the magnetization is therefore rotated. Reversing the polarity of the field gradient during a period t_0 (Fig. 5.18 a) following the RF pulse [5.15] aligns (refocusses) all spins so that they are parallel again (Fig. 5.18 b). Instead of the reversed gradient it is also possible to use a 180° pulse and a gradient with the same polarity.

Linearization of the Bloch equations is a good approximation up to angles of rotation of 30°, but larger angles, such as 90° or 180°, require numerical solutions. Thus, for a sinc-shaped 90° pulse with subsequent refocussing there still remains a small oscillation of the magnetization across the slice. This can be avoided by means of modified RF pulse shapes.

5.2.3 Imaging procedures

In order to measure the spatial distribution of the precessing transverse magnetization following a selective slice excitation, a magnetic field gradient G is superimposed onto the main static magnetic field in the slice. As a result, the Larmor frequency is constant in strips perpendicular to the direction of the gradient – the amplitude of the magnetic resonance signal as a function of the frequency corresponds in each case to the sum of all the 'spins' in this strip, i.e. it represents the projection of the magnetization onto the field gradient [5.16].

Following Fig. 5.19 one obtains for the projection

$$P(r, \varphi) = \int M_{\perp}(x, y)\, \mathrm{d}l. \tag{5.53}$$

What is actually measured experimentally is the time signal; for a frame rotating with γB_0

$$m_{\perp}(t, \varphi) = \int P(r, \varphi)\, e^{-i\gamma G r t} \mathrm{d}r. \tag{5.54a}$$

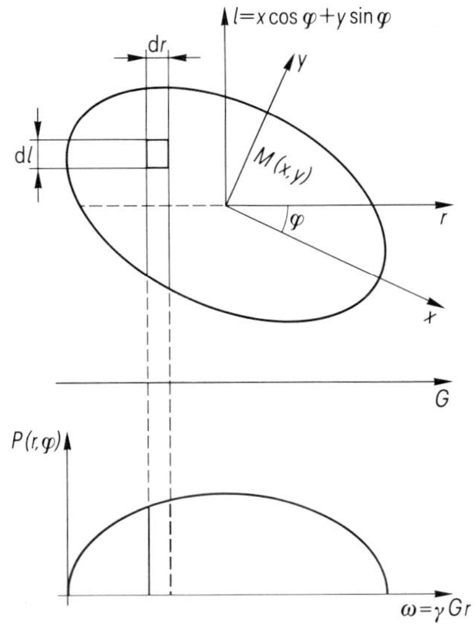

Fig. 5.19
The magnetic resonance signal as a function of the frequency for an object in a linear magnetic field gradient G represents the projection of the transverse magnetization onto the direction of the gradient

Introducing a 'normalized time'

$$k=\gamma G t \tag{5.55}$$

the measured signal

$$m_{\perp}(k, \varphi)=\int P(r, \varphi)\, \mathrm{e}^{-ikr} \mathrm{d} r \tag{5.54b}$$

and the projection

$$P(r, \varphi)=\int m_{\perp}(k, \varphi)\, \mathrm{e}^{ikr} \mathrm{d} k \tag{5.54c}$$

are seen to be Fourier transforms of each other. Inserting equation (5.53) into equation (5.54) it then follows that a set of measured signals $m_{\perp}(q, \varphi)$ in successively rotated gradients is the two-dimensional Fourier transform of the magnetization

$$m_{\perp}(k, \varphi)=\int M_{\perp}(x, y)\, \mathrm{e}^{-i(k_x x+k_y y)} \mathrm{d} x\, \mathrm{d} y. \tag{5.56}$$

The space defined by the Fourier inverse of the space in which the object to be measured is located is thus scanned by means of a grid in polar coordinates. However, the pictorial representation of the magnetization takes place in Cartesian coordinates. Instead of a re-interpolation of the measured data onto a Cartesian grid and a two-dimensional Fourier transform, it is also possi-

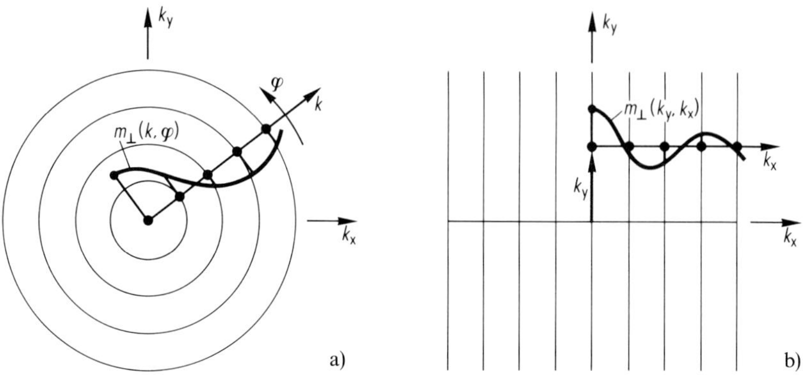

Fig. 5.20
Scanning of the Fourier space by means of (a) polar and (b) Cartesian coordinates

ble to calculate the projection from the measured signal by means of a one-dimensional Fourier transform and then reconstruct the image through filtered back projection.

Unlike x-ray computed tomography, which only permits the construction of images from successively rotated projections, magnetic resonance tomography offers another possibility. Instead of employing a grid in polar coordinates, one can scan the Fourier space with a grid in Cartesian coordinates (Fig. 5.20). This then allows a direct reconstruction of the image by means of the two-dimensional 'Fast Fourier Transform (FFT)' [5.17] within a few seconds.

After excitation of a slice in the object through a selective RF pulse, the magnetization is dephased for a certain length of time t_y in the gradient G_y and then read out within a time t_x in the projection gradient G_x (Fig. 5.21 a). After a certain waiting period, during which thermal equilibrium is reestablished, this sequence is repeated with different values for the gradient G_y or coding time t_y [5.18]. The precessing transverse magnetization in the rotating coordinate frame as a function of the dephasing gradient strength or time and the readout time is then given by

$$m_\perp(G_y\,t_y, t_x) = \iint M_\perp(x,y)\,e^{-(i\gamma(G_y y t_y + G_x x t_x))}\,dx\,dy. \tag{5.57}$$

A two-dimensional Fourier transform applied to this signal directly yields the desired spatial distribution of the transverse magnetization.

5.2.4 Pulse sequences and contrast

In practice, a sequence modified from that shown in Fig. 5.21 a is used (Fig. 5.21 b), which measures a spin echo signal. The reason is that, on the one hand, inhomogeneities in the main static magnetic field are compensated

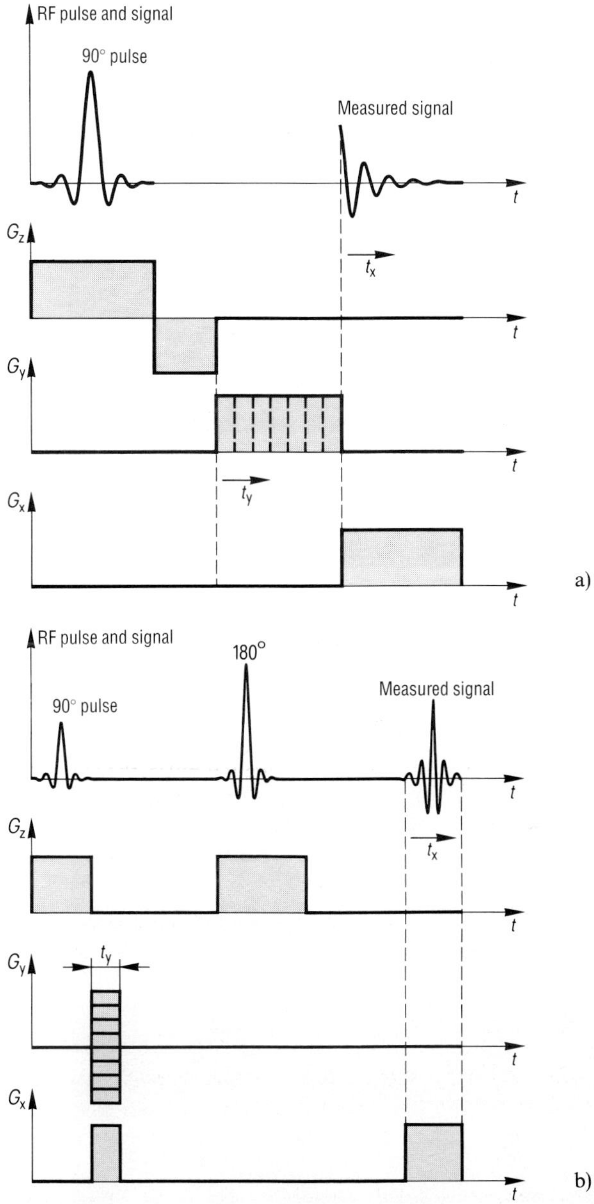

Fig. 5.21
(a) Sequence for measuring a slice by scanning the Fourier space in Cartesian coordinates. After a selective excitation in the gradient G_z, the magnetization is first coded with G_y and then read out in G_x.
(b) Sequence for measuring a slice with a spin-echo sequence

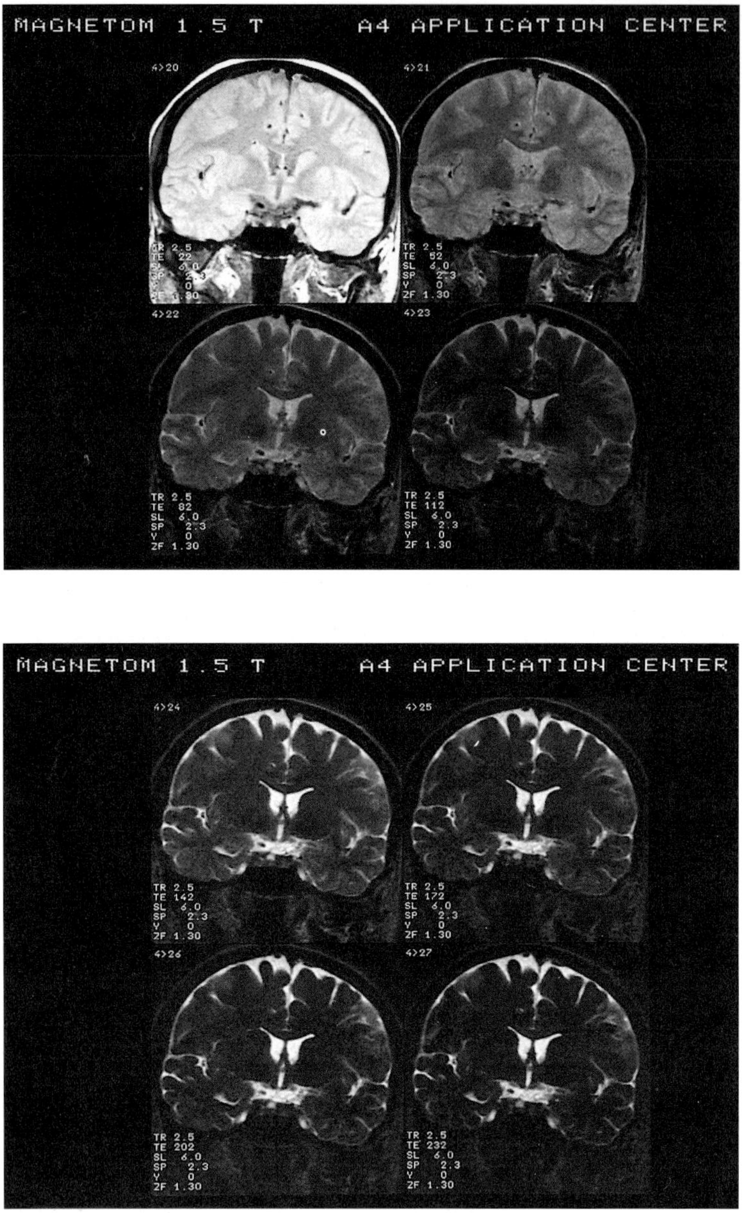

Fig. 5.22
Multiple echo image of a normal volunteer: the echo time increases by 30 ms from image to image. Areas with long transverse relaxation times remain bright

for, at least in the direction of the coding gradient and, on the other hand, that by reading out the spin echo a whole line of the Fourier space is scanned, and not just half a line as before. The total scan time is thus halved.

According to the sampling theorem, the size of an image element (pixel) is determined by the duration of the maximum scanning period

$$\Delta x, y = \pi/\gamma G_{x,y}\, t_{x,y\ max}; \tag{5.58 a}$$

and the size of the scan matrix then follows from the maximum object diameter D according to

$$N_{x,y} = D/\Delta x, y. \tag{5.58 b}$$

In practice $N_{x,y}$ is rounded up to a power of two, in order to be able to employ the fast Fourier transform (FFT) algorithm.

As already mentioned, the use of a selective 180° pulse permits the measurement of additional slices in the breaks between repetitions without prolonging the measuring time. The repeated application of 180° pulses in a sequence allows several images to be constructed with varying T_2 weighting for a single slice, from which the transverse relaxation times can then also be calculated locally. Fig. 5.22 shows an example of such a multiple-echo series.

The local transverse magnetization in a spin-echo sequence may be influenced externally through the echo time T_e and the time interval T_r with which the sequence is repeated. For a single echo sequence

$$M_\perp(x, y) = N_v \left(1 - 2\,e^{-\left(T_r - \frac{T_e}{2}\right)\frac{1}{T_1}} + e^{-\frac{T_r}{T_1}}\right) e^{-\frac{T_e}{T_2}}. \tag{5.59 a}$$

where

N_v is the local spin density.

For the case $T_r \gg T_e$ this relation may be simplified to

$$M_\perp(x, y) = N_v\, e^{-\frac{T_e}{T_2}} \left(1 - e^{-\frac{T_r}{T_1}}\right). \tag{5.59 b}$$

The contrast resulting in the image of the magnetization is given by the difference in signals $M_1 - M_2$ between two regions of unequal magnetization. By choosing the pulse parameters T_r and T_e it can be enhanced, inverted, or even made to vanish. The head scan images in Figs. 5.23 a and 5.23 b are instructive; here white matter yields a stronger signal than gray matter for short repetition times, whereas for long repetition times and long echo times the situation is

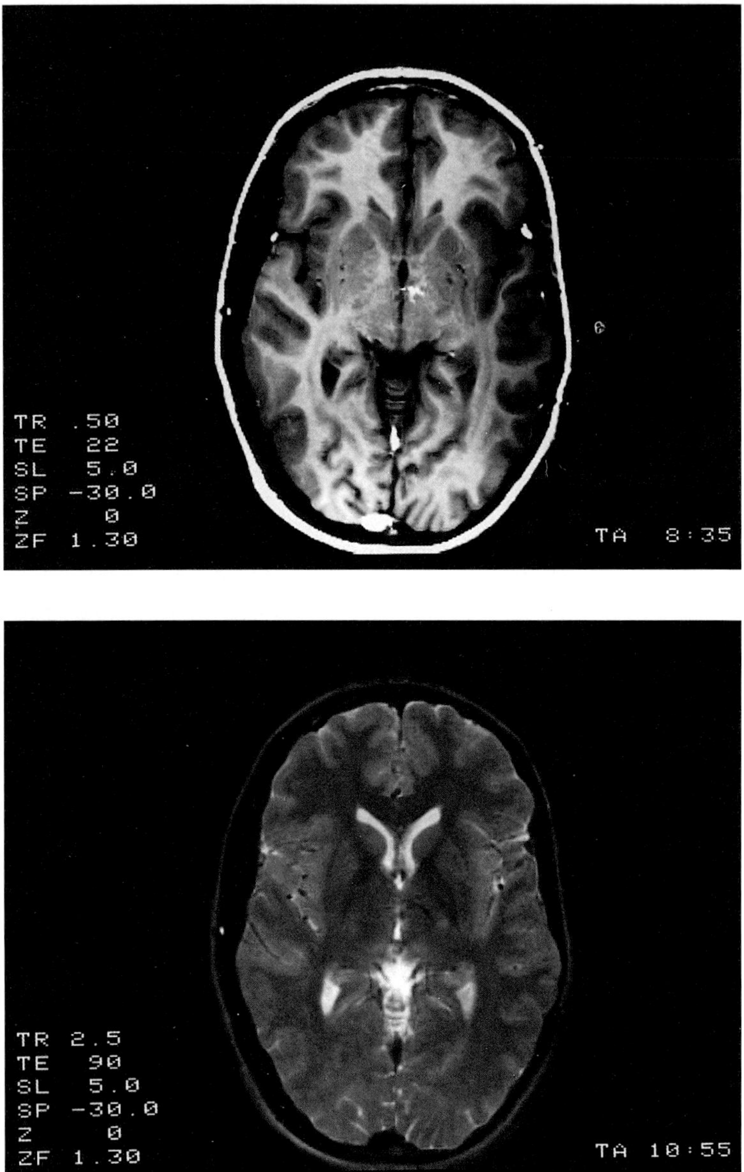

a)

b)

Fig. 5.23
(a) Head scan taken with a repetition time of 500 ms and an echo time of 22 ms. The white matter appears brighter than the gray matter.
(b) The same slice as in (a), but with a repetition time of 2.5 s and an echo time of 90 ms. The white matter now appears darker than the gray matter

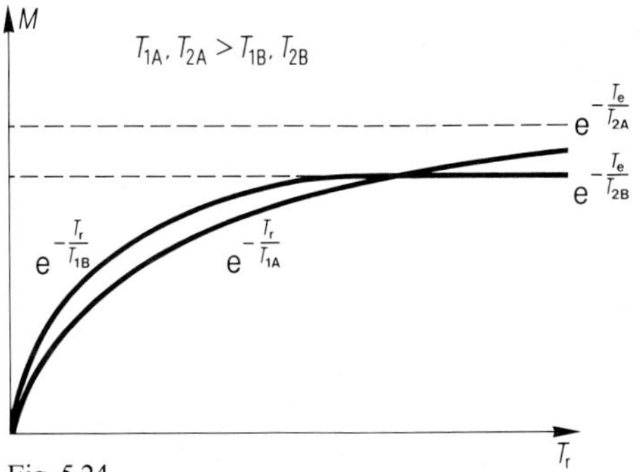

Fig. 5.24
Dependence of the transverse magnetization on the repetition time for tissue with larger and smaller T_1 and T_2 values, respectively

reversed; Fig. 5.24 illustrates this graphically. In addition two images taken with different repetition times and the same echo time also make it possible to determine quantitatively the distribution of the longitudinal relaxation times T_1.

5.2.5 Flow in the magnetic resonance image

It has already been mentioned in Sect. 5.1.5 that the magnetic resonance signal is not only characterized by the relaxation times, but also by the diffusion of the nuclei under observation. However, in biological tissue the diffusion constant is so small that it does not lead to any effect in a normal spin-echo image – in order to determine the diffusion constant, additional strong gradients are required before and after the 180° pulse. On the other hand, the nature of the image is significantly influenced by flowing nuclei, i.e. by blood flow.

Here, it is necessary to make a fundamental distinction between two cases: flow perpendicular to the excited slice and flow within the excited slice. In the first case it is observed that the magnetic resonance signal increases initially at low velocities and then decreases strongly at high velocities (Fig. 5.25). The initial increase in signal, which is often described as a paradoxical enhancement, can be explained by the fact that in the repetition pauses, nuclear spins which no longer carry any magnetization from the previous excitation, i.e. which are unsaturated, flow into the slice under examination. At high velocities, on the other hand, some of the excited spins flow out of the slice being measured between the 90° and 180° pulse and therefore no longer contribute to the magnetic resonance signal.

Formally, this may be described by introducing effective relaxation times T_1' and T_2' [5.19], which are shortened compared to the original relaxation as a result of flow terms

$$1/T_1' = 1/T_1 + v/d, \qquad (5.60\,\text{a})$$

$$1/T_2' = 1/T_2 + v/d, \qquad (5.60\,\text{b})$$

where

v is the velocity of flow perpendicular to the slice and
d is the thickness of the slice.

If we examine vessels containing flowing matter within a slice by means of a multiple echo sequence, then in all odd-echo images we observe a signal intensity which decreases with the flow velocity; the signal intensity remains the same, however, in the even echoes (at least for laminar flow).

This is due to the fact that if transverse magnetization flows along a field gradient G, then in the time $T_e/2$ between the 90° and 180° pulses a phase shift builds up relative to static magnetization,

$$\varphi = \int_0^{T_e/2} \gamma G v \,\mathrm{d}t = \gamma G v \, T_e^2/8 \qquad (5.61)$$

which is inverted by the 180° pulse and assumes the value $\gamma G_v \, T_e^2/4$ in the

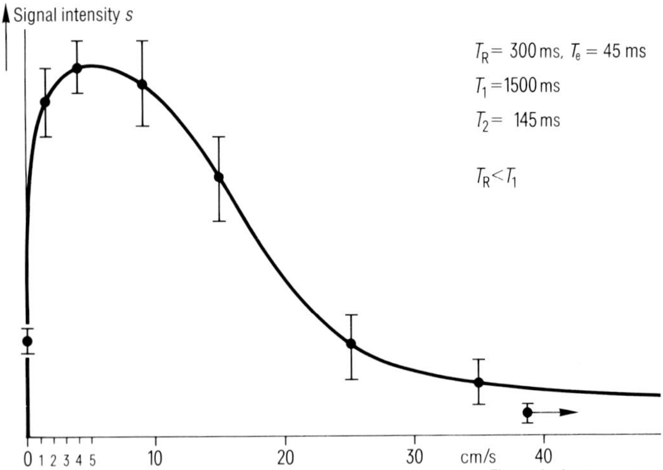

Fig. 5.25
Dependence of the signal intensity of matter flowing perpendicular to the slice on the flow velocity

echo (Fig. 5.26). This phase is reduced to zero again in the second and all subsequent even echoes.

In magnetic resonance tomography, the phase shift due to flow is produced (in the odd echoes) by the gradient used for imaging. The distribution of phases, which is linked to the distribution of flow in the vessels, is then (as a consequence of the vectorially averaged magnetization over the slice, which is represented in the image) the cause of reduced signal intensity. Fig. 5.27 gives an example of this. Thus, in principle, magnetic resonance imaging offers the possibility of noninvasive angiography for large vessels.

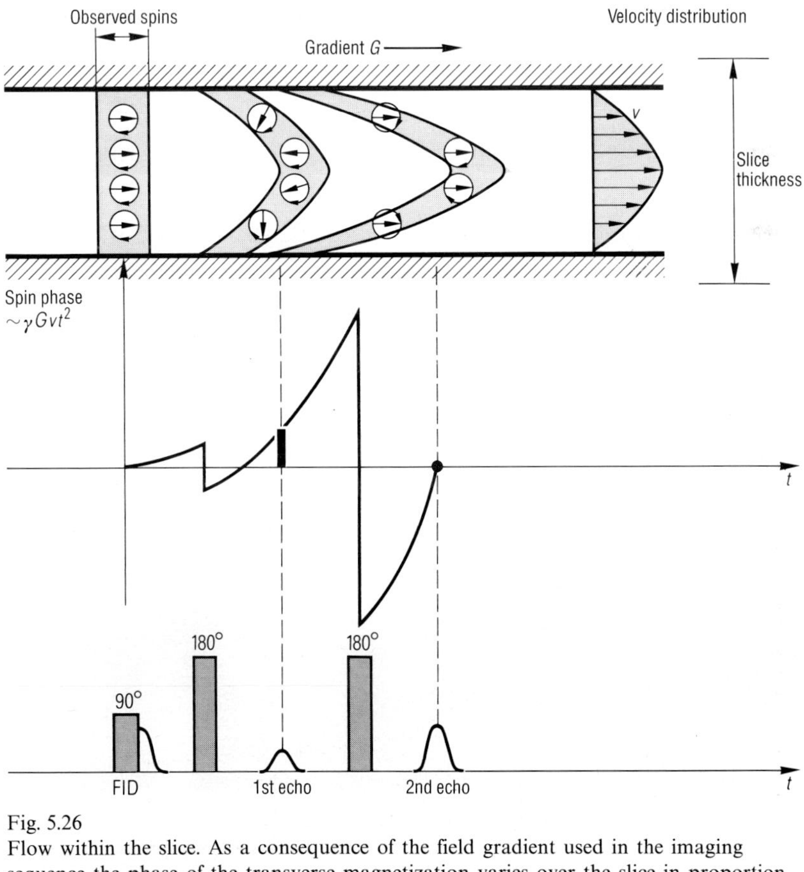

Fig. 5.26
Flow within the slice. As a consequence of the field gradient used in the imaging sequence the phase of the transverse magnetization varies over the slice in proportion to the velocity, so that in the first echo a reduced average signal results; in the second echo the phase shift has been compensated

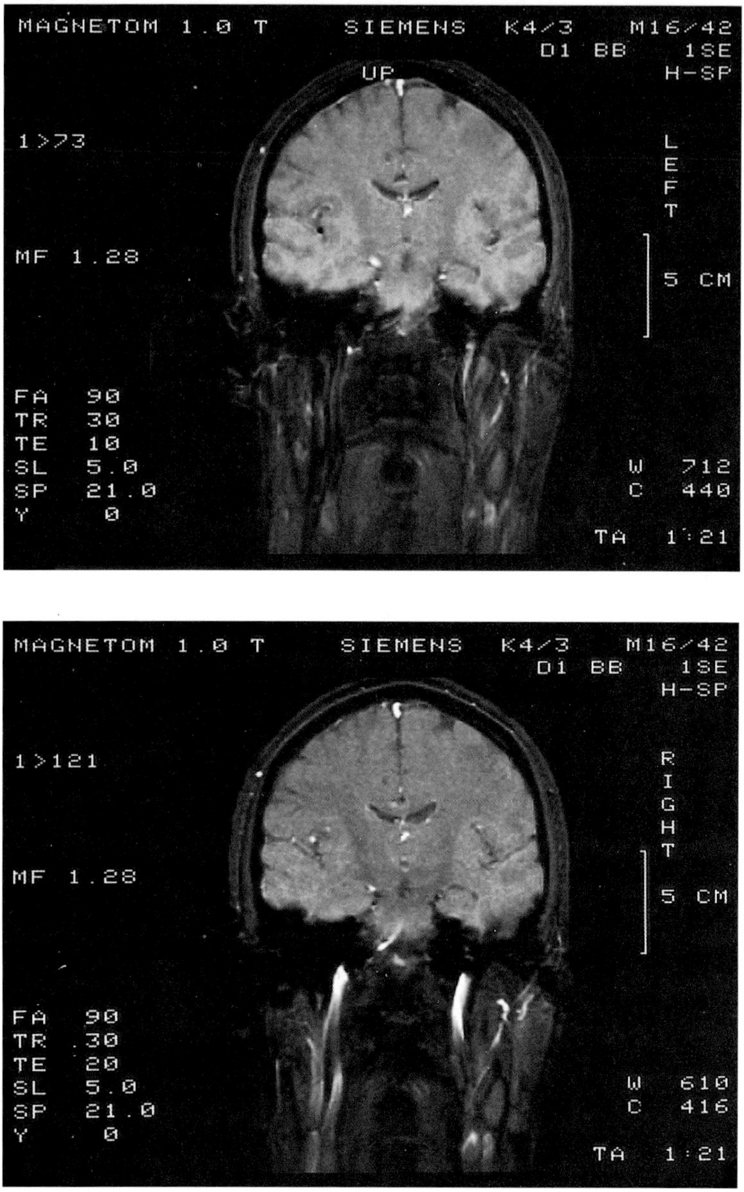

a)

b)

Fig. 5.27
(a) Magnetic resonance tomogram from the first echo obtained from the area of the carotid arteries in a normal volunteer; the flow in the vessels appears dark.
(b) The corresponding image from the second echo, in which the carotid arteries appear bright; only where turbulent flow occurs is the signal intensity diminished

5.2.6 Spatially resolved spectroscopy

For the magnetization measurement described up to now, spatial resolution was obtained by relating the MR frequency to the position with the aid of magnetic field gradients. However, if one is interested in the spatial distribution of chemical shifts and spectral splitting, it is of course not permissible for an additional magnetic field to be acting during signal acquisition. Various procedures have been developed for spatially resolved spectroscopy, in which this requirement is fulfilled. Essentially they may be reduced to two principles, those pre-coding the magnetic resonance signal and those employing a volume-selective excitation.

Fig. 5.28 shows a pulse sequence for the first case, designated as 'chemical shift imaging' (CSI). Following a (generally non-selective) 90° pulse, a combination of magnetic field gradients G_x, G_y, G_z are switched on for a specified length of time and then the magnetic resonance signal is read out in the absence of any gradients. This signal is then given by

$$m_\perp(G_x t_x, G_y t_y, G_z t_z, t) = \int M_\perp(x, y, z, \omega)\, e^{-i\gamma(G_x x t_x + G_y y t_y + G_z z t_z + \omega t)} \mathrm{d}x\, \mathrm{d}y\, \mathrm{d}z\, \mathrm{d}\omega. \tag{5.62}$$

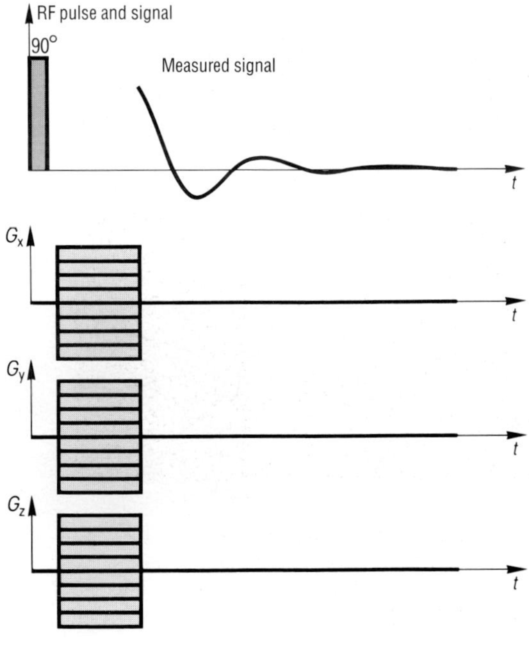

Fig. 5.28
Principle of the sequence for spectroscopic imaging: the magnetic resonance signal is coded by a combination of the three gradients G_x, G_y, G_z and then read out in the absence of a gradient

This sequence is repeated as often as necessary with other gradient combinations until the desired spatial resolution results in accordance with equations 5.58a and b. A four-dimensional Fourier transform of this set of signals then yields the desired spatial distribution of the resonance lines.

If a sample with a uniform resonance frequency is used, e.g. water, the procedure described yields the spatial distribution of the static magnetic field [5.20]. However, even a spatial resolution as coarse as that given by 16^3 image elements and a typical repetition time of 1 s would require a measuring period of over one hour. Instead of the non-selective RF excitation pulse, therefore, one generally uses a selective pulse and only determines the distribution of the resonance frequencies in a single slice. The pictorial representation of the data can be given in the form of a summed image, which shows the magnetization of all the spectral lines as a gray shade value; with this image it is possible to call up the desired spectrum of the labelled pixels by means of a cursor from the image evaluation console. A pictorial representation of the magnetization of a frequency component can, however, also be given; this would correspond, e.g. to the distribution of a chemical compound.

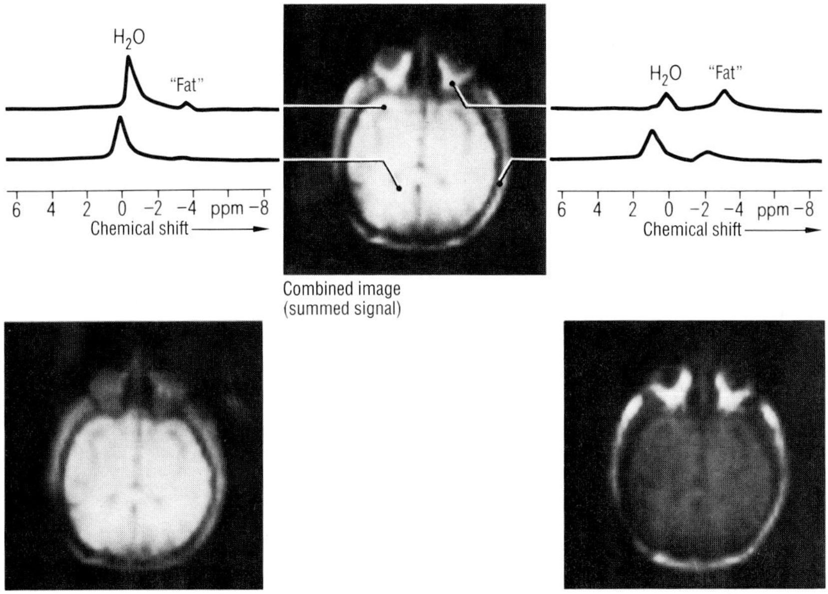

Fig. 5.29
Example (showing the human head) of spectroscopic imaging by means of protons. A 32 × 32 matrix was used in conjunction with selective excitation

For the magnetic resonance of hydrogen nuclei in the human body, however, nearly always only those two components which are due to lipids and to water are observed in the spectrum (Fig. 5.29). Given this information, lengthy measurements to gather data for a multidimensional Fourier transform are of course pointless.

A procedure has been described by Dixon [5.2] in which one specifically measures the fat and water distribution and where only twice the measuring time needed for a single image is required. In addition to the image obtained by the standard spin-echo sequence, a second image is constructed in which the 180° pulse is shifted relative to the half-way point between the 90° pulse and the middle of the measurement period. In this extra time interval, phase shifts build up between the spins (Fig. 5.30), which may be ascribed to different chemi-

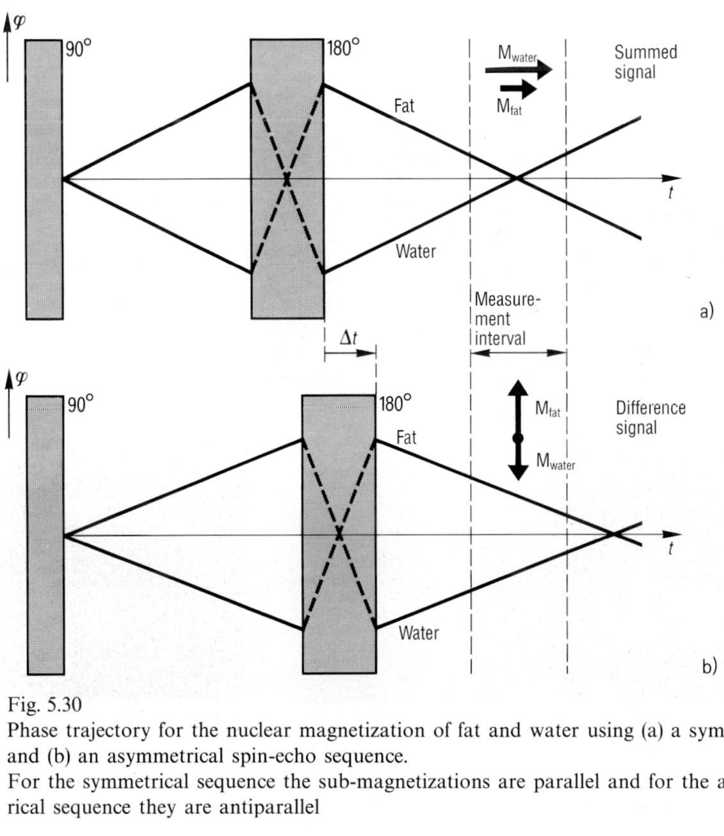

Fig. 5.30
Phase trajectory for the nuclear magnetization of fat and water using (a) a symmetrical and (b) an asymmetrical spin-echo sequence.
For the symmetrical sequence the sub-magnetizations are parallel and for the asymmetrical sequence they are antiparallel

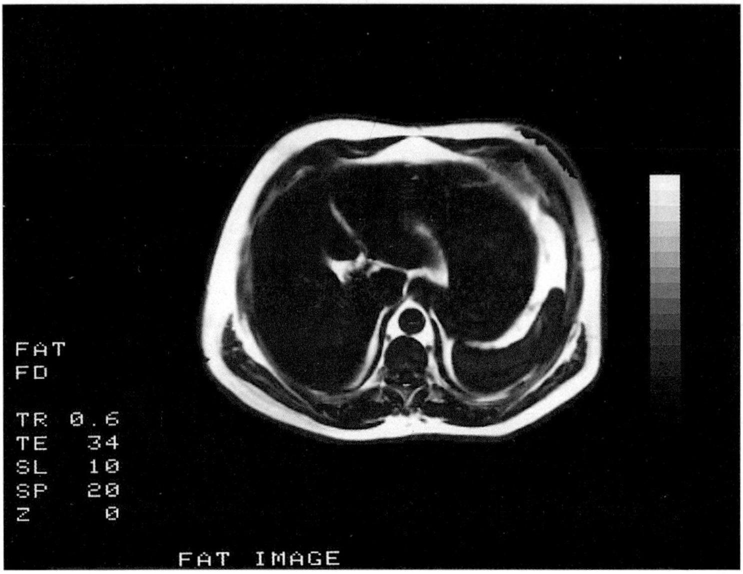

a)

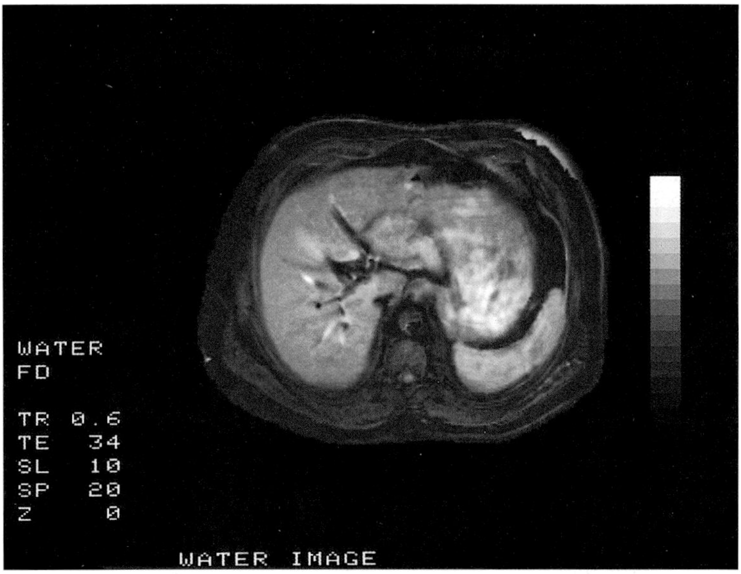

b)

Fig. 5.31
Calculated pure fat image (a) and pure water image (b) obtained using the Dixon sequence. To correct field inhomogeneities, a circular water phantom was employed, the contour of which can still be recognized in the images

cal shifts (but may also be due to static field inhomogeneities). If, in particular, a time shift of the echo is performed,

$$\Delta t = \frac{\pi}{\gamma \delta B_0}, \tag{5.63}$$

where

δ is the difference in the chemical shifts between fat and water

then at the time of signal readout, the magnetization of the lipids is antiparallel to that of the water. This means that by addition and subtraction of the image generated with the 'symmetric' echo, a pure fat and a pure water image may be calculated (Fig. 5.31).

It has already been mentioned that, for an asymmetrical 180° pulse, effects arise which are not only due to different chemical shifts but also to field inhomogeneities. For the condition given by equation (5.63), this means that the difference vector for the magnetizations of fat and water is locally rotated with respect to the sum vector, i.e. the pure fat and the pure water image can only be calculated if this angle is known. To obtain this angle, it is necessary to carry out a calibration measurement with a homogeneous phantom. The comparison of the 'image in phase' with the image 'out of phase' yields the distribution of the phases caused by field inhomogeneities.

Metabolites, e.g. lactate, occur in tissue only in a concentration 10000 times smaller than that of lipids or water. Detecting them by means of proton resonance therefore functions only if the strong water and fat signals are not excited or suppressed in the process. For this purpose, special pulse sequences [5.22] have been developed in analytical spectroscopy. In order to be able to use them selectively with regard to position, we can by way of example ensure by means of so-called selective saturation pulses that the magnetization is oriented only along the static magnetic field in the subvolume of interest and is otherwise distributed as randomly as possible in space (Fig. 5.32a); then the application of an arbitrary non-selective sequence only yields information from the previously selected subvolume.

One method of selective saturation consists in first rotating the whole magnetization into the transverse plane by means of a non-selective 90° pulse, and then, with a selective RF pulse in a magnetic gradient, rotating all the spins from one slice back again. The spins outside the slice remain in the transverse plane and dephase in the field gradient and then no longer yield a signal. Immediately repeating this sequence in the two other orthogonal gradients first selects a strip from the slice and then, from this, a cube (Fig. 5.32b).

As mentioned in Table 5.1, the detectability of heavy nuclei is about 1000 times smaller than that of protons. Field strengths substantially larger than 1 T are required in order to be able to resolve the spectral splitting. Detection is consequently limited to relatively large volumes. Imaging with such nuclei requires very long measuring times and even then only gives very coarse spatial resolution and a poor signal-to-noise ratio. The best solution is to make use of surface coils, frequently in conjunction with an additional localization procedure.

Apart from the methods of selective excitation or selective saturation already briefly described, one procedure seems especially well suited to achieving additional localization. This procedure, 'rotating frame spectroscopy', does not require magnetic field gradients and only utilizes the radio-frequency field gradient of a surface coil [5.23, 5.24]. The problems associated with the rapid switching of magnetic fields, e.g. of eddy current compensation, are avoided by this method; the measurement can start immediately after the RF pulse without losing any signal due to transverse relaxation.

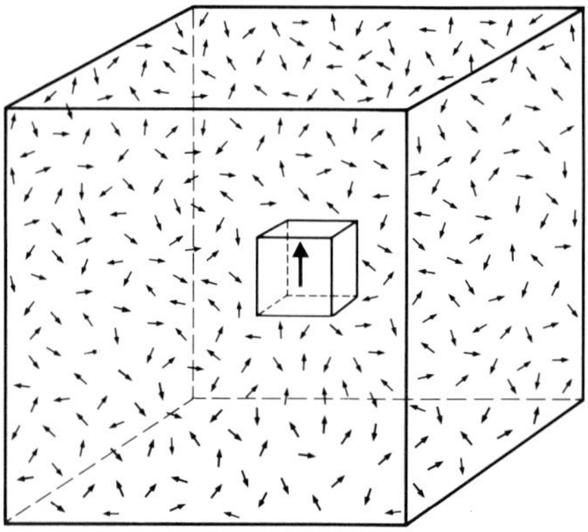

a)

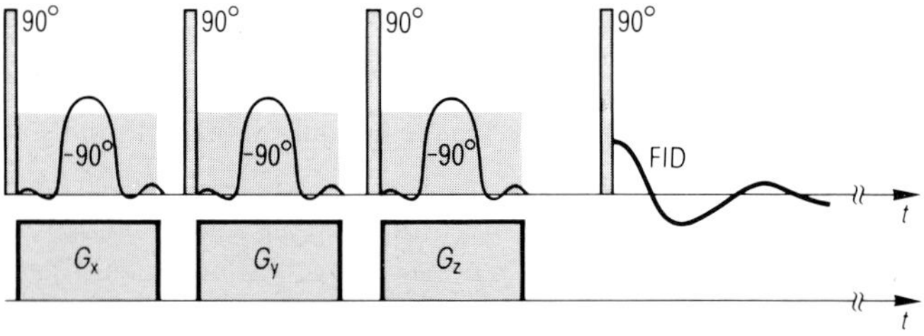

b)

Fig. 5.32
(a) With selective saturation, the magnetization is dephased outside the subvolume ΔV of interest.
(b) Principle of the selective saturation sequence: With a non-selective 90° pulse, transverse magnetization is generated. In each case this dephases in the magnetic field gradient, while selective 90° pulses restore the equilibrium magnetization in the desired volume element. A final non-selective 90° pulse then reads out the magnetic resonance signal from this volume element only

If we transmit an RF pulse through a surface coil, nuclear spins in its vicinity are rotated away from the equilibrium orientation by a larger angle than distant ones. This is demonstrated in Fig. 5.33, in which the transverse magnetization of a phantom is depicted following excitation by means of a surface coil. For the shells with no signal

$$\sin \alpha = \gamma B_1(r)\, t = n\, 180° \; (n = 0 \ldots n_{max}), \tag{5.64}$$

where

B_1 is the RF field strength at position r and
t is the duration of the RF pulse.

With rotating frame spectroscopy, we detect nuclear magnetic resonance spectra on these shells: If r denotes the position of constant field strength $B_1(r)$ (given by the geometry of the surface coil), then the transverse component of the magnetic moment following an RF pulse is given by

$$m_\perp(\alpha, t) = \int m_\perp(r, \omega) \sin(\alpha(r))\, e^{-i\omega t} \mathrm{d}r\, \mathrm{d}\omega. \tag{5.65}$$

By varying the field strength or the length of the RF pulse successively, the two-dimensional Fourier transform of this set of signals described by equation (5.65) then gives the spectra on the shells characterized by equation (5.64).

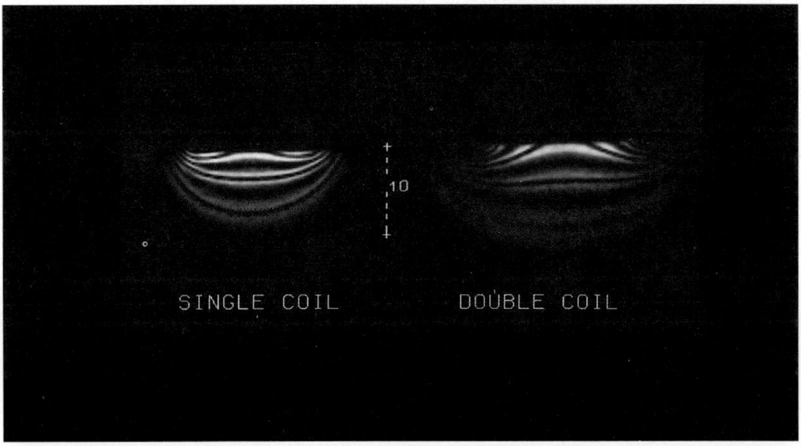

Fig. 5.33
(left) Distribution of the transverse magnetization beneath a single surface coil which has been subjected to a radio frequency pulse.
(right) Distribution of the detected transverse magnetization beneath a concentric double coil in which the outer coil was used for transmitting and the inner coil for receiving

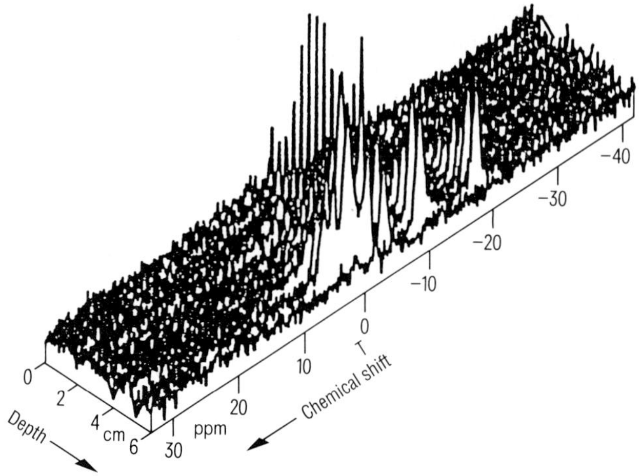

Fig. 5.34
Rotating frame spectrum of the human liver. The surface spectrum corresponds to a muscle spectrum, whereas the more deeply lying spectrum indicates the presence of sugar phosphates and phosphodiester, but no longer any phosphocreatine

When using single coils placed over the body, even the 'deepest' spectrum still contains information from the surface, because of the curvature of the shells. If concentric double coils are used, with the outer coil transmitting and the inner coil receiving, then the latter essentially cuts out parallel planes from the excited shells (Fig. 5.33b). An in-vivo phosphorus spectrum of the human liver, obtained by using a double coil and rotating frame spectroscopy, is shown in Fig. 5.34.

6 Ultrasonic techniques

The principal methods used in ultrasonic diagnostics are based on the reflection principle, i.e. acoustic energy is sent into the body and the reflected energy received and evaluated at the point of transmission. Besides this, there are also transmission techniques – as yet only of secondary importance – which evaluate transmission waves.

The preferred form of presentation of the data gathered is the optical image. Ultrasonic images are determined by different physical parameters than those which play a key role in the other methods discussed in this book. Hence different medically relevant information can be expected, with the result that the procedures can complement each other. The strength of ultrasonics is shown in soft tissue diagnostics. Internal organs – even ones which are moving – may be depicted without being subjected to the dangers of radiation and without contrast agents.

Ultrasonics can be regarded as an extension of the over 200-year-old technique of percussion (Auenbrugger, 1761) [6.1]. The techniques of sonar (Langevin, 1918) [6.2] and of non-destructive materials testing based on reflection (Firestone, 1942) [6.3] then entered the scene and prompted the first experiments with reflection techniques on biological tissue (Ludwig and Struthers, 1949) [6.4], which led to the present-day A-Scopes (Wild, 1950; Leksell, 1955) [6.5, 6.6]. Transmission techniques also originated in materials testing (Sokolov, 1929) [6.7], and in medicine were first applied to the brain (Dussik, 1942) [6.8].

Echo sectional imaging methods were first employed to produce images of mammary tumors using a frequency of 15 MHz (Reid and Wild, Howry and Bliss, 1952) [6.9, 6.10]. For books about ultrasound, see the bibliography [6.11, 6.12, 6.13, 6.83].

6.1 Basic physical principles

6.1.1 Ultrasonic field parameters and derived concepts

Sound is bound to a material medium. The nature of the material influences the acoustic process. Thus, in soft body tissues, as in liquids, practically the only waves which occur are longitudinal. The form of this type of wave which is easiest to describe is found in the special case of plane waves. Since it is bound to matter, this process can, to a first approximation, be well illustrated using a solid model.

In Fig. 6.1, as a model of the (loss-free) material medium, molecules and binding forces are represented in the form of balls suspended between springs. The hallmark of a longitudinal wave is that the balls move to and fro exclusively in the direction of the vertical springs, i.e. in the direction of the sound propagation, about a resting position fixed in space. The shaded planes connect all those balls together which are in the same state of motion, and thus e.g. have the same velocity. For a plane wave, they should be thought of as infinitely extended planes.

The way the process of motion arises can be illustrated more precisely if a single vertical chain of molecules from the previous model is viewed at different moments in time, and these configurations juxtaposed as shown in Fig. 6.2:

Suppose the excitation starts with the displacement of the uppermost molecule on the left (1st row, 2nd column). Because of the springs (omitted in this figure), the displacement is transmitted to the second molecule lying below (2nd row, 3rd column). The inertia of this molecule causes a time delay in the transmission of the excitation. The process continues until the vibrational state of the final column has been reached, as shown in Fig. 6.1.

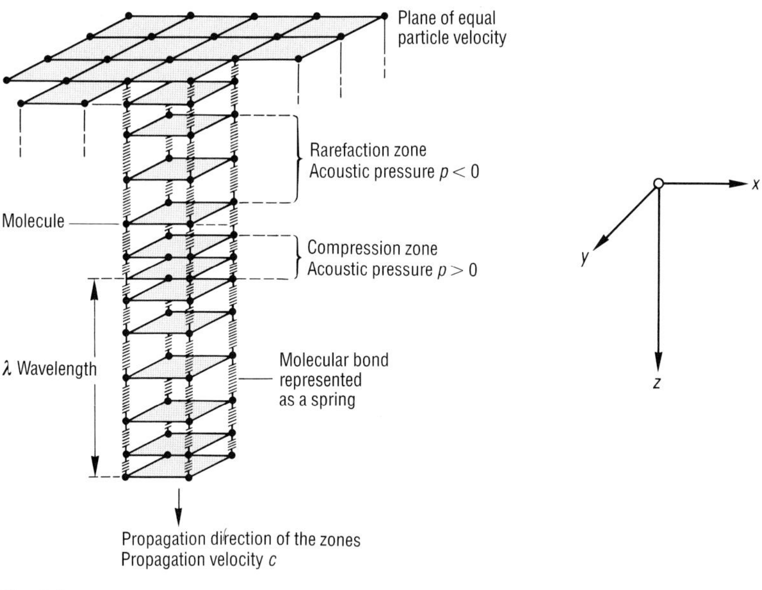

Fig. 6.1
Plane, longitudinal sound wave in a crystal-lattice type model (three-dimensional)

Thus it becomes clear that:

● The ultrasonic beam does not come about due to migration of molecules, but instead the molecules oscillate around their equilibrium position at the excitation frequency. Resonances of the spring-mass systems do not occur because the kinetic energy of each molecule can be transferred to the neighboring molecule, whereby a spatially propagating wave is formed and perfect damping occurs. The displacement of the particles from their rest position is called *elongation* ξ, and the velocity of the motion of the particles to and fro is called the *sound particle velocity* v (in m/s)

$$v = \frac{d\xi}{dt}. \tag{6.1}$$

● A high molecular density corresponds to an increase in pressure, and a low molecular density to a decrease in pressure relative to the sound-free state. These pressure changes, i.e. the pressure difference from the normal pressure, are referred to as *acoustic pressure* p:

$$1\ \text{Pa} = 1\ \text{N/m}^2 = 10\ \mu\text{bar}.$$

● Similar states of pressure, sound velocity, elongation, etc., (compression or rarefaction zones, oscillation nodes and bulges – in short, the excitation) propagate with a velocity specific to the material, the *propagation velocity* c. The stiffer the springs and the smaller the molecular masses, the greater the propaga-

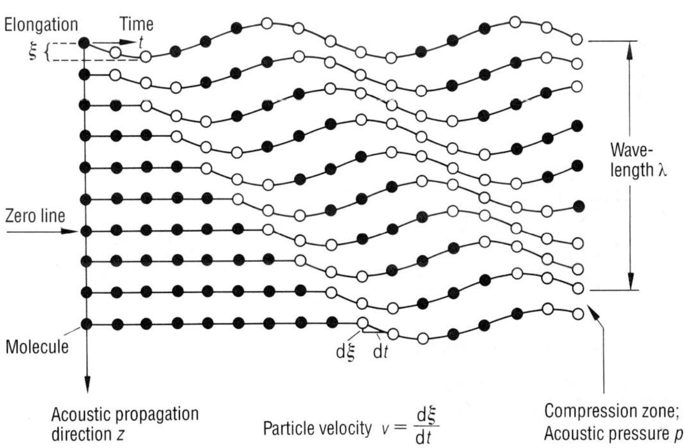

Fig. 6.2
Excitation of an ultrasound longitudinal wave in a one-dimensional model

tion velocity (in m/s). From the wave equations which will be given later, it can be shown that

$$c=\sqrt{\frac{E}{\varrho_-}}. \tag{6.2}$$

E Modulus of elasticity
ϱ_- Density at rest

▻ The smallest distance between excitation states of the same type (e.g. of maximum compression) is called the *wavelength* λ. The greater the propagation velocity c and the smaller the frequency f, the greater the wavelength (in m).

$$\lambda=\frac{c}{f}. \tag{6.3}$$

▻ In the case of a variable excitation frequency, the maximum acoustic pressure (degree of compression), for example, remains constant, if the excitation has a constant maximum particle velocity (not elongation). Hence the wave motion is best described by the two parameters particle velocity v and acoustic pressure p.

▻ The acoustic pressure p increases (see Fig. 6.2) with the magnitude of the imposed particle velocity v. In addition, it is dependent upon the properties of the medium. At the intensities usual in diagnostics, there is a linear relationship. The material-specific constant of proportionality is known as acoustic impedance (or wave resistance) Z (measured in kg/m^2 s).

$$p=Zv. \tag{6.4}$$

Pressure and velocity oscillate in the plane wave with the same relative phase. On the other hand, for the case of spherical waves, there is a phase shift between p and v. Intuitively, one can see that for a given sound velocity and a material with propagation velocity c, the stiffer the springs, the greater the acoustic pressure p which occurs. It can be shown from the wave equations to be given later on that the proportionality constant between impedance Z and modulus of elasticity E assumes the form:

$$Z=\frac{E}{c}. \tag{6.5}$$

From this follows, using equation (6.2):

$$Z=\varrho_-\,c=\sqrt{\varrho_-\,E}. \tag{6.6}$$

The designation wave resistance is analogous to electrical resistance. As impedance rises, it increasingly 'inhibits' the build-up of velocity (current) for a given acoustic pressure (voltage). Thus, for a particular value of the particle velocity, the greater the impedance, the greater the acoustic pressure that has to be generated.

▻ Linked to the motion (velocity) of the molecules is the transport of energy. The upper left-hand particle in Fig. 6.2 (1st row, 2nd column) exerts a pressure p on the molecule lying below (2nd row, 2nd column) accelerating it. The (potential) energy expended in the first time interval (column 1 to column 2) per unit of area ψ is $\mathrm{d}\psi = p\,\mathrm{d}\xi$. The power density

$$J = \frac{\mathrm{d}\psi}{\mathrm{d}t} = p\frac{\mathrm{d}\xi}{\mathrm{d}t} = pv$$

is transferred in the form of kinetic energy to the 2nd molecule, i.e. is transported. The acoustic intensity (power density) J in W/cm^2, i.e. the instantaneous power passing through a unit area, is thus

$$J = pv. \tag{6.7}$$

The analogy with instantaneous power in the case of an electrical resistance (current times voltage) thus also holds true here. For a constant velocity (current), e.g. the maximum velocity, the greater the resistance which has to be overcome, the more acoustic pressure (voltage), as well as power, which have to be brought to bear. The maximum values or amplitudes of v and p in water for a sinusoidal excitation of arbitrary frequency may be taken from Fig. 6.3.

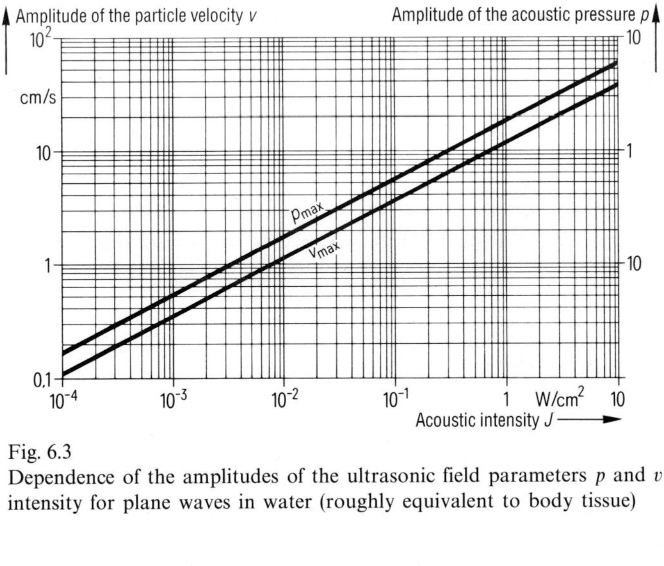

Fig. 6.3
Dependence of the amplitudes of the ultrasonic field parameters p and v on the intensity for plane waves in water (roughly equivalent to body tissue)

For an arbitrary impedance Z the following formulas hold:

$$\frac{p_{max}}{\mu\,\text{bar}} = \sqrt{200 \cdot 10^5 \frac{Z}{\text{g/cm}^2\,\text{s}} \cdot \frac{J}{\text{W/cm}^2}}, \tag{6.8}$$

$$\frac{v_{max}}{\text{cm/s}} = \sqrt{10^7 \frac{\dfrac{J}{\text{W/cm}^2}}{\dfrac{Z}{\text{g/cm}^2\,\text{s}}}}. \tag{6.9}$$

The amplitude of the elongation follows from

$$\xi_{max} = \frac{1}{2\pi f} v_{max}. \tag{6.10}$$

Ultrasound is used to denote sound waves with frequencies above the audible range, i.e. greater than about 16 kHz. Typical values for diagnostic instruments are:

Frequency range 1 to 10 MHz (usually 2 to 5 MHz).

Wavelength λ 1.5 to 0.15 mm in soft tissue, averaged over time at a fixed position,

Acoustic intensity $J < 100$ mW/cm^2, usually 1 to 10 mW/cm^2 (pulsed sound),

Acoustic pressure $p < 0.57$ bar,

Particle velocity $v < 3.5$ cm/s,

Elongation $\xi < 2 \cdot 10^{-6}$ mm (at 3 MHz)

Particle acceleration $< 7 \cdot 10^4 g$ (at 3 MHz), where g is the acceleration due to gravity.

The instantaneous values of the power density may lie up to a factor of 10000 and those of the field parameters (p, v, etc.) up to a factor of 100 above the stated averages.

Table 6.1 gives typical values for various media. The values may be taken to be virtually independent of the frequency, i.e. dispersion does not play a significant role [6.15, 6.42, 6.65].

Table 6.1
Typical values for the propagation velocity c, density ϱ and impedance Z

Substance	c m/s	ϱ g/cm^3	$Z=\varrho c$ g/cm^2 s
Fat	1470	0.97	$1.42 \cdot 10^5$
Bone marrow	1700	0.97	$1.65 \cdot 10^5$
Muscle	1568	1.04	$1.63 \cdot 10^5$
Brain tissue	1530	1.02	$1.56 \cdot 10^5$
Bone (compact)	3600	1.7	$6.12 \cdot 10^5$
Bone (porous)			(2.2 to $2.9 \cdot 10^5$)
Water (20 °C)	1492	0.9982	$1.489 \cdot 10^5$
Air (NN)	331	0.0013	$0.00043 \cdot 10^5$

6.1.2 Wave equations and the plane wave

The intuitively derived equations above follow from an infinitesimal calculation which will be given here for the ball and chain model (Fig. 6.4) for the simple case of a plane wave.

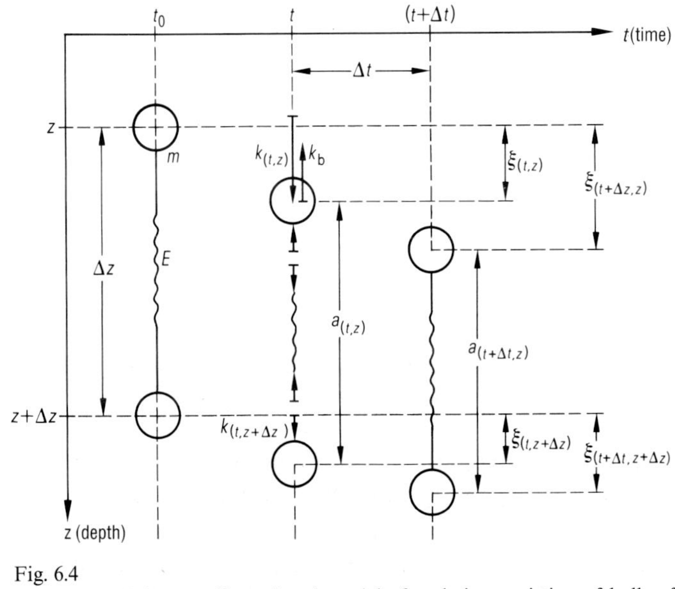

Fig. 6.4
Excitation of the one-dimensional model of a chain consisting of balls of mass m and massless springs of elastic modulus E

▻ According to Newton's second law of mechanics (force equals mass times acceleration), one has for the acceleration $\frac{\partial^2 \xi}{\partial t^2}$ of the mass m by the spring forces $K_{(z)}$ and $K_{(z+\Delta z)}$

$$K_{(t,z)} - K_{(t,z+\Delta z)} = m \frac{\partial^2 \xi}{\partial t^2}.$$

This holds strictly in Lagrangian coordinates, i.e. if $\xi_{(z)}$, $K_{(z)}$ are always assigned to the same ball at $(z+\xi)$ and their values are plotted at z. In Eulerian coordinates – i.e. if $\xi_{(z)}$, $K_{(z)}$ are assigned to the (oscillating) mass particle which is at position z, and their values are plotted at z – a 'convective' term also comes into play. This leads to a slight non-linearity, which expresses itself e.g. in the ultrasonic radiation pressure.

To relate these values to the macroscopic variables (pressure p, density ϱ) let the volume element $\Delta V = \Delta F \Delta z$ be assigned to a ball-spring pair, where ΔF represents a square with edge length equal to the lateral distance between the balls. It then follows that

$$\frac{K_{(t,z)} - K_{(t,z+\Delta z)}}{\Delta z \, \Delta F} = \frac{m}{\Delta z \, \Delta F} \cdot \left. \frac{\partial^2 \xi}{\partial t^2} \right|_t .$$

With $\frac{K}{\Delta F} = p$ and $\frac{m}{\Delta z \Delta F} = \varrho$ – this becomes in the limit $\Delta z \to 0$.

$$\left. \frac{\partial p}{\partial z} \right|_t = -\varrho \left. \frac{\partial^2 \xi}{\partial t^2} \right|_t$$ (*Equation of motion* according to Newton's second law of mechanics) (6.11)

▻ The relative change in the volume element $\frac{\Delta(\Delta V)}{(\Delta V)}$ between the positions of two molecules in the model with regard to the period of time Δt is then given by

$$\frac{\Delta(\Delta V)}{(\Delta V)\Delta t} = \frac{\Delta F \, a_{(z,t+\Delta t)} - \Delta F \, a_{(z,t)}}{\Delta F \, \Delta z \, \Delta t}$$

$$= \frac{\Delta z - \xi_{(z,t+\Delta t)} + \xi_{(z+\Delta z,t+\Delta t)} - (\Delta z - \xi_{(z,t)} + \xi_{(z+\Delta z,t)})}{\Delta z \, \Delta t}$$

$$= \frac{-\frac{\xi_{(z,t+\Delta t)} - \xi_{(z,t)}}{\Delta t} + \frac{\xi_{(z+\Delta z,t+\Delta t)} - \xi_{(z+\Delta z,t)}}{\Delta t}}{\Delta z}$$

$$= \frac{\frac{\xi_{(z+\Delta z,t+\Delta t)} - \xi_{(z,t+\Delta t)}}{\Delta z} - \frac{\xi_{(z+\Delta z,t)} - \xi_{(z,t)}}{\Delta z}}{\Delta t} .$$

In the limit as $\Delta z \to 0$ and $\Delta t \to 0$, this becomes

$$\frac{1}{\Delta V} \cdot \frac{\partial \Delta V}{\partial t} = \frac{\partial}{\partial z} \cdot \frac{\partial \xi}{\partial t} = \frac{\partial}{\partial t} \cdot \frac{\partial \xi}{\partial z}.$$

By formally differentiating the equation $\varrho - = \frac{m}{\Delta V}$ one obtains $\frac{\partial \Delta V}{\Delta V} = -\frac{\partial \varrho}{\varrho_-}$ and hence the *continuity equation*

$$\frac{\partial v}{\partial z} = \frac{\partial}{\partial t} \cdot \frac{\partial \xi}{\partial x} = -\frac{1}{\varrho_-} \cdot \frac{\partial \varrho}{\partial t}. \tag{6.12}$$

▻ According to Hooke's Law (the relative change of length is proportional to the tension) one has

$$\frac{K_{(z+\Delta z,t)}}{E\,\Delta F} = \frac{\xi_{(z,t)} - \xi_{(z+\Delta z,t)}}{\Delta z} = \frac{-a_{(z,t)} + \Delta z}{\Delta z},$$

$$\frac{K_{(z,t)}}{E\,\Delta F} = \frac{\xi_{(z-\Delta z,t)} - \xi_{(z,t)}}{\Delta z} = \frac{-a_{(z+\Delta z,t)} + \Delta z}{\Delta z},$$

$$\frac{K_{(z+\Delta z,t)} - K_{(z,t)}}{E\,\Delta F\,\Delta z} = -\frac{a_{(z,t)} - a_{(z-\Delta z,t)}}{\Delta z^2} = -\frac{\Delta F\,a_{(z,t)} - \Delta F\,a_{(z-\Delta z,t)}}{\Delta F\,\Delta z^2}.$$

In the limit $\Delta z \to 0$ this becomes, using $\frac{\partial \Delta V}{\Delta V} = -\frac{\partial \varrho}{\varrho_-}$,

$$\frac{1}{E} \cdot \frac{\partial p}{\partial z} = -\frac{1}{\Delta V} \cdot \frac{\partial \Delta V}{\partial z}$$

or the *equations of state* according to Hooke's Law

$$\frac{1}{E} \cdot \frac{\partial p}{\partial z} = \frac{1}{\varrho_-} \cdot \frac{\partial \varrho}{\partial z} \tag{6.13}$$

expressed in a different form

$$p_\sim = \frac{E}{\varrho_-}\varrho_\sim.$$

$p_\sim$ Variable pressure
$\varrho_\sim$ Variable density

By partial differentiation and mutual substitution, using the abbreviation introduced in equation (6.2), the *wave equations* for the case of a plane then follow:

$$\frac{\partial^2 p}{\partial z^2}=\frac{1}{c^2}\cdot\frac{\partial^2 p}{\partial t^2} \quad \text{or} \quad \frac{\partial^2 v}{\partial z^2}=\frac{1}{c^2}\cdot\frac{\partial^2 v}{\partial t^2}. \tag{6.14}$$

The simplest form of electromagnetic oscillations may be described by a relation which is formally identical to this (the differences lie in the vectorial nature of the electromagnetic variables as opposed to *p*, which is a scalar). Hence in some simple cases similar relations hold, so that one occasionally speaks of 'acoustic optics'. Furthermore, the law of linear superposition holds, and in particular also Huygen's principle.

In the special case of a sinusoidal excitation, the solution to the wave equation is the wave field represented in Fig. 6.2/

$$p=\hat{p}\cos\left(\omega t-\frac{\omega}{c}z\right), \tag{6.15}$$

$$v=\frac{\hat{p}}{Z}\cos\left(\omega t-\frac{\omega}{c}z\right), \tag{6.16}$$

$$\xi=\frac{\hat{p}}{Z\omega}\sin\left(\omega t-\frac{\omega}{c}z\right). \tag{6.17}$$

$\hat{p}$ Peak value of pressure
z Propagation coordinate

6.1.3 Physical effects

The ultrasonic wave may be reflected, refracted, diffracted, scattered or absorbed. These phenomena are the subject of this section.

Reflection

If a plane sound wave penetrates along the normal from a first medium with impedance Z_1 into a directly adjoining second medium with impedance Z_2, then a sudden change in the velocity and the pressure has to occur in the transmitted wave, in order for the conditions $Z_1=p_1/v_1$ and $Z_2=p_2/v_2$ to be simultaneously fulfilled. Such a disturbance of the wave field causes the reflection of a part of the incident wave (acoustic intensity J_i). Incident and reflected waves are superimposed additively (hence e.g. the doubling of amplitude in a standing wave).

The reflection process is illustrated by the ball model in Fig. 6.5:

At their two ends, the springs, assumed massless, in the *boundary layer* can only absorb forces which are equal in magnitude. This corresponds to the boundary condition $p_1 = p_2 = p$, i.e. equal acoustic pressure on both sides in the immediate vicinity of the boundary layer. If one demands equal energy density in front of and behind the boundary layer, this implies that $J = p v_1 = p v_2$, or $v_1 = v_2$. This contradicts the condition $Z_1 \neq Z_2$.

The assumption $J_i = J_r + J_t$; $p_1 = p_i + p_r$; $p_2 = p_t$ resolves the contradiction, i.e. for the superposition of incident and reflected waves, the continuity condition holds for p and v in the boundary layer; the values of the incident wave, however, jump to those of the transmitted wave. This leads to the *reflection coefficient* R for plane boundary surfaces perpendicular to the direction of the acoustic waves,

$$R = \sqrt{\frac{J_r}{J_i}} = \frac{p_r}{p_i} = \frac{Z_2 - Z_1}{Z_2 + Z_1} \tag{6.18}$$

J_r, p_r Acoustic intensity and pressure of the reflected wave

J_i, p_i Acoustic intensity and pressure of the incident wave

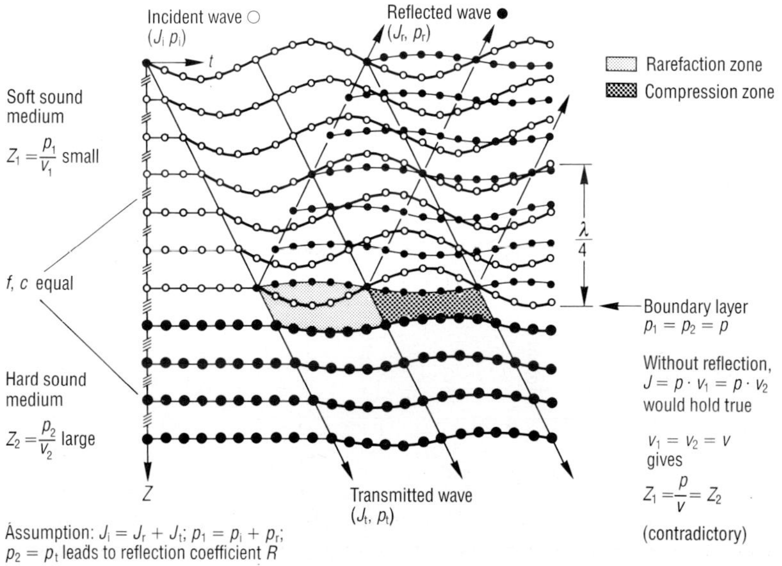

Fig. 6.5
Sound reflection and sound transmission at boundary layers between media with different acoustic impedances

and to the *transmission coefficient* τ

$$\tau=\sqrt{\frac{J_t}{J_i}}=\sqrt{1-R^2}=\sqrt{\frac{4Z_1 Z_2}{(Z_1+Z_2)^2}}, \tag{6.19}$$

$$\frac{p_t}{p_i}=\tau\sqrt{\frac{Z_2}{Z_1}}=1+R=\frac{2Z_2}{Z_1+Z_2}. \tag{6.20}$$

J_t, p_t Acoustic intensity and pressure of the transmitted wave

For $R>0$, it follows from equation (6.20) that $p_t>p_i$. The excess of p_t over p_i may also be interpreted as the cause of a reflected wave.

Between soft biological tissues, there are small energy reflection coefficients of a few thousandths up to several percent (Table 6.2) [6.18, 6.20, 6.22]. The attenuation due to reflection thus remains relatively small in soft tissues; the tissue-air boundary, on the other hand, results in virtually *total reflection*. Hence air-filled organs and tissues lying behind these cannot be examined with ultrasound. For the same reason, the air (even thin layers) must be excluded from the contact zone between the transducer and the surface of the skin by means of a coupling gel or oil. For a more detailed discussion of the permeability of thin layers, see [6.17]. Bones embedded in soft tissue also lead to strong reflections [6.21].

Table 6.2
Typical values for the magnitude of the reflection coefficient R between different tissues (from Erikson, Fry, Jones [6.18])

Water	Fat	Muscle	Skin	Brain tissue	Liver	Blood	Cranial bone	Plexiglas (perspex)
Water	0.047	0.02	0.029	0.007	0.035	0.007	0.57	0.35
Fat		0.067	0.076	0.054	0.049	0.047	0.61	0.39
Muscle			0.009	0.013	0.015	0.02	0.56	0.33
Skin				0.022	0.0061	0.029	0.56	0.32
Brain tissue					0.028	0.00	0.57	0.34
Liver						0.028	0.55	0.32
Blood							0.57	0.35
Cranial bone								0.29

If a plane wave is incident obliquely on a smooth, infinitely extended boundary, then the following law familiar from optics applies:

$$\alpha_1 = \alpha_3. \tag{6.21}$$

α_1 Angle of incidence with respect to normal
α_3 Angle of reflection

In this context, a boundary may be described as smooth if its surface roughness (e.g. the effective value of the roughness depth) is small compared to the wavelength.

Figure 6.6 shows how this law can be applied to the case of an ultrasonic beam, i.e. an ultrasonic field bounded perpendicularly to the direction of propagation. If the ultrasonic field within the beam can be taken, to a first approximation, to be planar (far field), then the following equations hold:

$$\frac{J_r}{J_i} = \left(\frac{Z_2 \cos\alpha_1 - Z_1 \cos\alpha_2}{Z_2 \cos\alpha_1 + Z_1 \cos\alpha_2}\right)^2, \tag{6.22}$$

$$\frac{J_t}{J_i} = \frac{4 Z_1 Z_2 \cos\alpha_1 \cos_2}{(Z_2 \cos\alpha_1 + Z_1 \cos\alpha_2)^2}. \tag{6.23}$$

Refraction

Figure 6.6 also illustrates the phenomenon of refraction. As in optics,

$$\frac{\sin\alpha_1}{\sin\alpha_2} = \frac{c_1}{c_2}. \tag{6.24}$$

α_1, α_2 Refraction angles with respect to normal

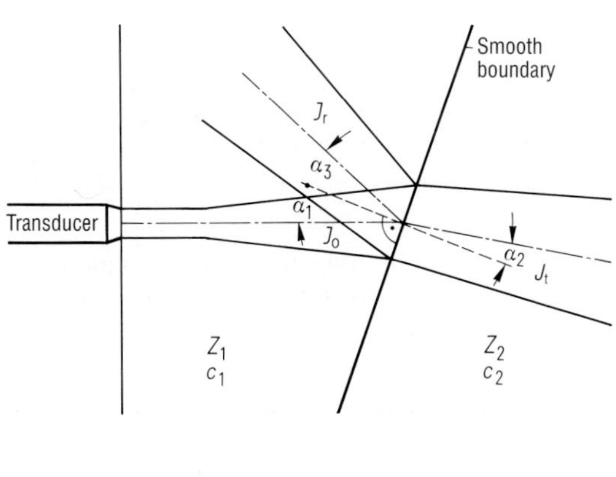

Fig. 6.6
Behavior of an ultrasonic beam at a smooth plane boundary

Accordingly, it is possible, for example, to construct lenses and thus to focus ultrasound waves [6.14, 6.23, 6.24].

Because of the small variations in the propagation velocity in soft biological tissue, the deviations from propagation along a straight line remain relatively slight in this case. This no longer holds true for the passage of sound waves through bone ($c = 3360$ m/s) [6.21].

Diffraction

If, for example, a disk which is impenetrable to sound is placed in a plane wave, there will be a shadow zone behind the disk. Although the ultrasonic intensity in this zone is less than that in the incident field, it is not zero. The incomplete screening is caused by diffraction around the edges of the disk. The explanation can be found by reference to Huygen's principle in the same way as in optics. The main role of diffraction is in connection with the generation of acoustic beams (see Section 6.1.4).

Scattering

If an ultrasonic wave passes through a medium containing areas (e.g. corpuscles) which are small compared to the wavelength and which differ from the surrounding medium in regard to their impedance, a 'nondirectional reflection' (spherical waves) results, which is referred to as scattering. It is usually described by means of a *scattering cross section* σ. This is the surface area with which it is necessary to multiply the intensity J of the incident beam in order to obtain the total scattered power P_a:

$$P_a = \sigma J. \qquad (6.25)$$

P_a Intensity of scattered sound
σ Scattering cross section

The scattering cross sections for individual particles (e.g. air bubbles) or collections of particles (e.g. blood) can be taken from the literature [6.15, 6.25 to 6.27]. Instead of σ, the scattering coefficient may also be given; this is the scattering cross section relative to the scattering volume. The differential backscattering coefficient, which describes the backscattering coefficient relative to the solid angle [6.26, 6.78], may also be found in the literature.

The transition between pure reflection and scattering occurs when sound penetrates through a plane *rough boundary*. The echoes of an incident acoustic beam are found in the region of a cone about the reflection axis for smooth boundaries (Fig. 6.7). The width of the cone depends on the wavelength, the roughness depth (standard deviation), and the correlation function of the roughness [6.28, 6.66, 6.68, 6.69]. To a first approximation, the smaller the wavelength and the larger the effective roughness depth, the wider the cone. Figure 6.8 shows an example for an average roughness depth of 100 μm [6.61].

Owing to the effect described above, non-normally acoustically irradiated boundaries, i.e. boundaries which lie obliquely to the acoustic beam, as well as curved boundaries, can also be detected by conventional ultrasonic echo techniques (see section 11).

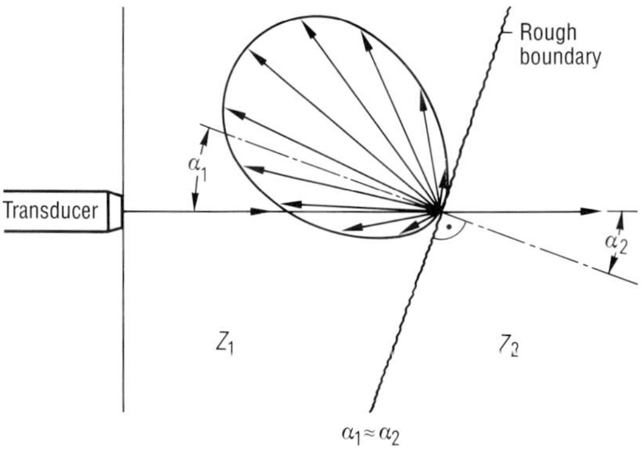

Fig. 6.7 Scattering from rough plane boundaries

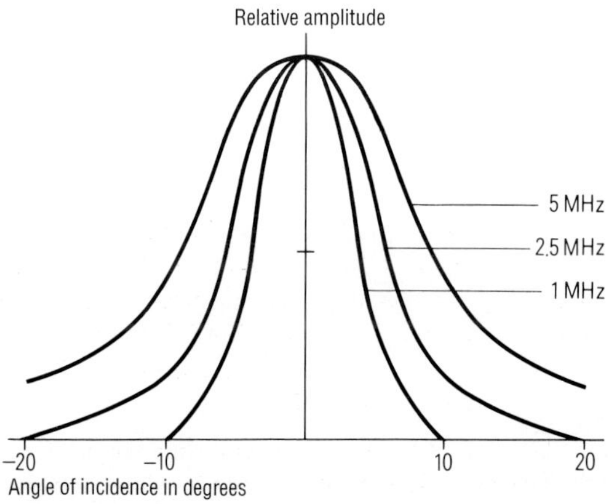

Fig. 6.8
Angular dependence of backscattering from a boundary with an average roughness depth of 100 μm (about 30 μm effective) from Kresse [6.61]

Absorption

The intensity of an acoustic beam may decrease along the direction of propagation for various reasons: The acoustic beam can, for example, spread out and become distributed over a progressively increasing area (rarefraction, geometrical damping, see section 6.1.4). Attenuation can also occur through reflection and scattering. In biological tissue at normal diagnostic frequencies (1 to 10 MHz), the strongest effect, however, (e.g. 82% [6.79]; figures quoted in the literature vary), stems from absorption. By this is meant a transformation of energy from acoustic energy into heat through 'internal friction' in the medium. The decrease of the ultrasonic intensity with increasing path length z obeys the exponential law (see Fig. 6.9)

$$\frac{J_z}{J_0} = e^{-2\beta z} \tag{6.26}$$

J_z Ultrasonic intensity at depth z
J_0 Initial value of ultrasonic intensity ($z=0$)
β Absorption coefficient in N_p/cm

The factor 2 in the exponent is omitted when the ratio of the ultrasonic field parameters p or v is required. In an echo system, the outward-and-return path length should be taken as the distance travelled. Instead of the absorption coefficient β, a measure of the attenuation α is often given:

$$\begin{aligned} \alpha &= 10 \lg \frac{J_0}{J_z} = 20 \beta z \lg e \\ &= 8.68 \beta z. \end{aligned} \tag{6.27}$$

α Absorption attenuation in dB.

Biological tissue possesses the peculiarity that the *absorption coefficient* increases almost linearly with the frequency over a wide frequency range (0.2 to 100 MHz) (in other substances it usually increases quadratically) [6.15, 6.42, 6.65, 6.70].

$$\beta = \frac{\beta_0}{f_0} f, \tag{6.28}$$

β_0 Absorption coefficient at frequency f_0.

Thus, the relative absorption attenuation is usually given as:

$$\frac{\alpha}{zf} = 8.68 \frac{\beta_0}{f_0} \quad \text{in} \quad \frac{\text{dB}}{\text{cm MHz}}. \tag{6.29}$$

Figure 6.10 shows typical values for the most important body tissues [6.62].

At diagnostic frequencies, bone tissue exhibits substantially higher attenuation values than soft tissue. Water, on the other hand, has a negligibly small absorption effect.

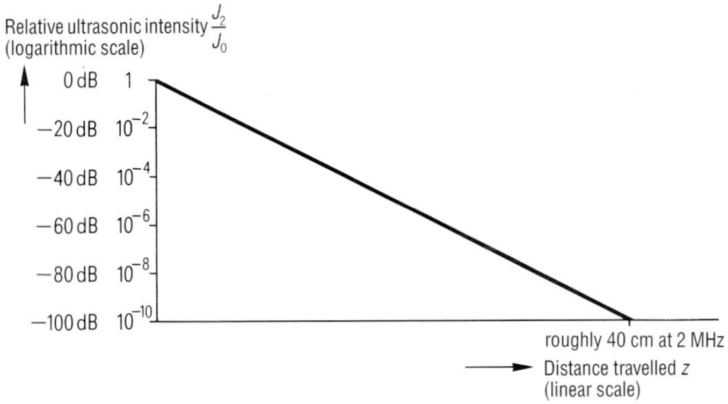

Fig. 6.9
Absorption-caused decrease of the ultrasonic intensity as a function of the distance travelled

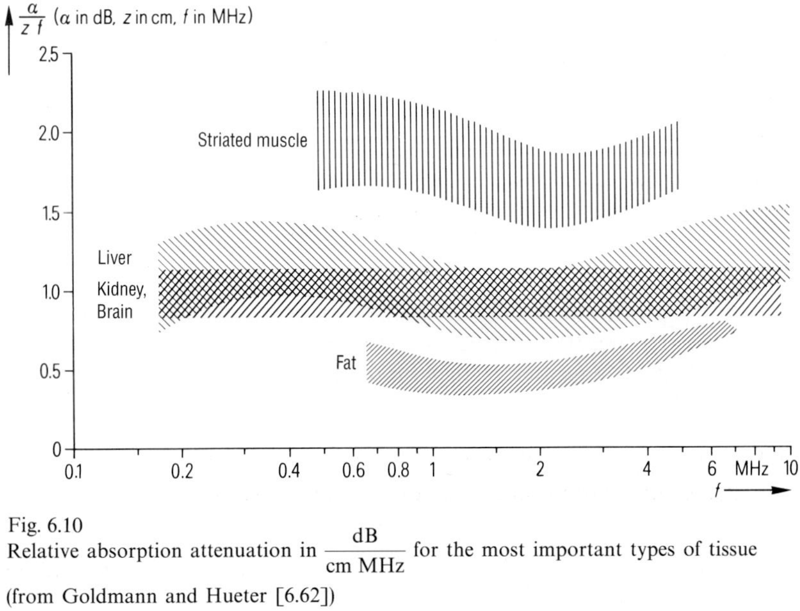

Fig. 6.10
Relative absorption attenuation in $\frac{\text{dB}}{\text{cm MHz}}$ for the most important types of tissue (from Goldmann and Hueter [6.62])

If the decrease in amplitude in tissue of average attenuation α/zf for a certain distance travelled z is plotted as a function of the frequency, then it can be seen that absorption attenuation follows the behavior of a strong low-frequency bandpass filter, i.e. the higher frequencies are attenuated more strongly than the lower ones. Accordingly, pulse spectra or pulse shapes can become noticeably changed. In the case of a distance travelled of 40 cm (corresponding to 20 cm of image depth in an echo system) the principal frequency of a typical pulse falls to about half its value. This has consequences for the spatial resolution (see section 6.3.2).

6.1.4 Acoustic beam and transducer

In medical ultrasound diagnoses, the acoustic beams used are as narrow as possible. The intensity of such an ultrasonic field should fall off as fast as possible from a given value towards the edge (x and y direction), i.e. perpendicular to the direction of propagation. This property should remain unchanged along the propagation coordinate z.

The acoustic field of a vibrating piston (plane transducer) [6.29] fulfils this condition to a first approximation. One can think of this field as the result of a screen with a hole in the plane wave. The ultrasonic field passing through the hole is noticeably affected by diffraction effects. These effects are known mainly from optics. There, however, they are not so much in evidence, because the ratio of the wavelength to the standard hole diameters is significantly smaller.

The diffraction effects lead to a strong local inhomogeneity of the amplitudes of the field in the immediate vicinity of the hole (or of the transducer surface). This part is known as the *near field* (or the Fresnel zone) as opposed to the adjoining *far field* (or the Fraunhofer zone, boundary at $z = a^2/\lambda$).

Figure 6.11 shows the dependence of the acoustic pressure on the central axis on the distance from the plane of the screen. In the near field, of length a^2/λ ($2a$ is the hole diameter), there are a/λ maxima. The amplitude decreases in the far field in inverse proportion to the distance z.

Figure 6.12 shows the loci (contour lines) of all points in the xz plane in which the acoustic pressures (in particular the acoustic pressure extrema) are smaller by a ratio, given as a parameter, than on the central axis at the same distance z. The near field has roughly the diameter of the aperture and displays inhomogeneity of pressure. In the far field a linear rarefaction of intensity can be seen (see Section 6.1.3 Absorption) as the distance increases, which corresponds to a diameter enlargement of the sound beam.

By analogy with antenna theory, a different representation of the far field is often chosen. The relative acoustic pressures are plotted on a circle intersecting the central axis, of radius z above the center of the transducer, as a function of the angle subtended with the central axis. Hence one also speaks of lobes (*sound beams*) if the directional characteristic is meant.

The half-angle subtended follows from

$$\tan \Theta_{3\,\mathrm{dB}} = 0.26\,\frac{\lambda}{a},$$

$$\tan \Theta_{6\,\mathrm{dB}} = 0.35\,\frac{\lambda}{a},$$

$$\tan \Theta_{10\,\mathrm{dB}} = 0.40\,\frac{\lambda}{a},$$

$$\tan \Theta_{\infty\,\mathrm{dB}} = 0.61\,\frac{\lambda}{a}. \tag{6.30}$$

$\Theta_{\mathrm{n\,dB}}$ Angle between central axis and locus for n dB (see Fig. 6.12).

Between the near and far field there is a constricted zone, also called the *natural focus*. This is located at the focal distance z_f and has the focal diameter d_f.

The following equations may be used in its calculation:

$$z_{\mathrm{f}\,3\,\mathrm{dB}} = 0.75\,\frac{a^2}{\lambda}, \qquad d_{\mathrm{f}\,3\,\mathrm{dB}} \approx a,$$

$$z_{\mathrm{f}\,6\,\mathrm{dB}} = 0.9\,\frac{a^2}{\lambda}, \qquad d_{f\,6\,\mathrm{dB}} \approx 1.6\,a. \tag{6.31}$$

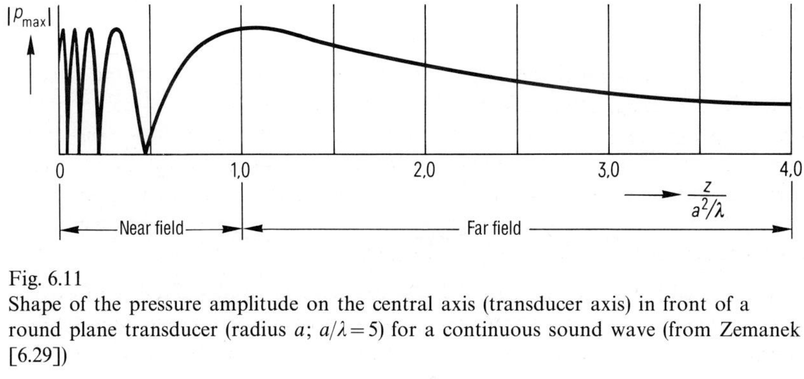

Fig. 6.11
Shape of the pressure amplitude on the central axis (transducer axis) in front of a round plane transducer (radius a; $a/\lambda = 5$) for a continuous sound wave (from Zemanek [6.29])

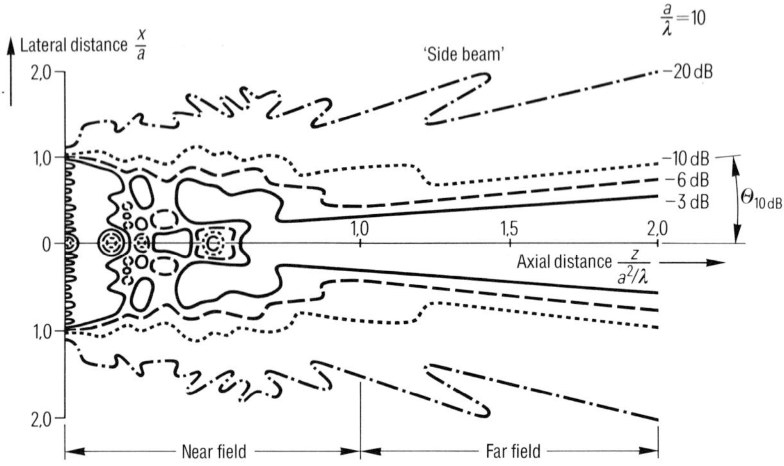

Fig. 6.12
Pressure amplitude contour lines for a plane round transducer (radius a; $a/\lambda=10$ corresponding to $a=7.5$ mm, 2 MHz) for a continuous sound wave (from Zemanek [6.29])

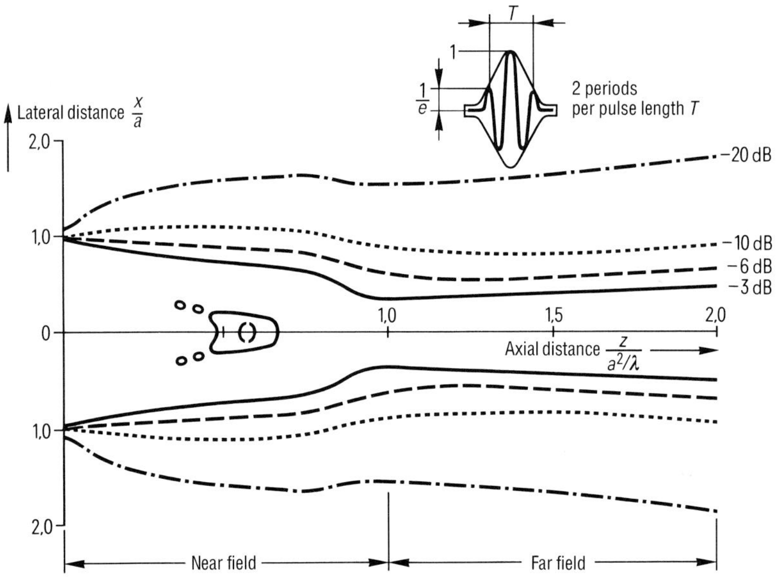

Fig. 6.13
Pressure amplitude contour lines for a plane round transducer (radius a; $a/\lambda=10$ corresponding to $a=7.5$ mm, 2 MHz) for a pulse with Gaussian envelope (from Weyns [6.30])

The majority of ultrasound diagnostic instruments use pulsed sound and not continuous sound. A pulse usually contains three or four periods and accordingly only has a short spatial length (e.g. 3 mm in the z direction). The ultrasonic field contour lines for this case indicate the lateral boundaries of the moving sound-filled area and its change in shape along the z axis.

In particular, the interference structures of the near field and the 'side lobes' depend on the pulse length (more precisely, the number of periods per pulse) [6.30]: compare Figs. 6.12 and 6.13. The shorter the pulses, the broader the frequency band of the pulse spectrum (a large bandwidth is roughly 50% of the average frequency). Hence the result is a superposition of many fields of the type shown in Fig. 6.12 for various frequencies and a 'smearing out' of the extreme values.

For generating and receiving ultrasound, practically only the inverse or the direct *piezoelectric effect* is used in diagnostics. To this end, piezoceramic transducer plates are employed. For these, the reciprocity theorem applies (Rayleigh, Helmholtz, Carson), i.e. the same transducer can convert electrical energy into mechanical energy and vice versa. Hence the aforementioned contour line diagrams can also be viewed as a reception sensitivity curve.

The transducer may be described over a broad frequency range by a transmission line model [6.31]. Over the region of thickness resonance, there are equivalent circuit diagrams in the form of an electrical triple gate [6.32]. The ratio of converted to absorbed energy in the static case (frequency zero) is given by the coupling factor K. For the dynamic case, more precisely in the region of the fundamental resonance of the transducer plate, this ratio is given by the factor $8/\pi^2 K_T^2$ for a transducer acoustically matched on both sides and no electric load (e.g., no imposed current). The thickness coupling factor K_T for good transducers is about 0.5.

Figure 6.14 shows the typical *design of an ultrasound transducer* [6.33, 6.34].

It is the job of the *backing*, in the case of transmission, to absorb ultrasonic power radiated in the backward direction and, in the case of receiving, to absorb ultrasonic power passing through the piezodisk. The withdrawal of energy thus achieved leads to the suppression of the intrinsic resonances of the piezodisk, i.e. to increased broadness of bandwidth and hence to improved pulse transmission behavior or to suppression of reflections, as the case may be. For this purpose, the impedance is chosen to be as close as possible to that of the piezoceramic material (backwards matching).

The *transformation or matching layer* serves the purpose of acoustic matching forwards to the body tissue, i.e. of bridging the large gap between the impedance of the backing (e.g. $30 \cdot 10^6$ kg/m^2 s) and that of tissue ($1.5 \cdot 10^6$ kg/m^2 s). Without matching, there would be an incomplete energy conversion due to reflections [6.35, 6.15].

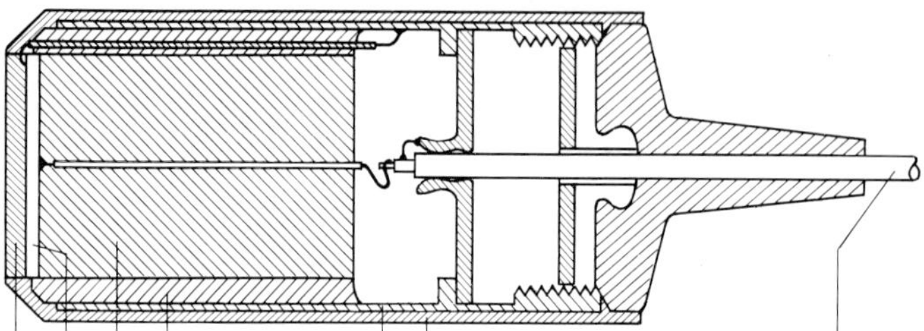

Fig. 6.14
Typical design of an ultrasound transducer for A scan or Compound Scan

Good energy conversion achieves damping by radiating the energy and thus leads to the desired short pulse shapes. In addition, fewer strong multiple reflections arise in this way between the transducer surface and the outer body layers.

The matching layers are usually made of a plastic material with an impedance lying between that of the insulating block and that of tissue (as close to the geometric mean as possible) and with a thickness of an odd multiple of $\lambda/4$.

Focussing transducers [6.15, 6.36] contain curved radiating surfaces (e.g. spherical calottes). Occasionally lenses are also used (e.g. made of plexiglas) [6.14, 6.23, 6.24]. These, however, cause the pulse shapes to deteriorate if the impedance matching cannot be achieved.

For further details concerning the physical background, see also [6.11 to 6.19].

6.2 Technical procedures

An introduction to the systems theory of pulse echo techniques may be found in [6.81] and to the systems theory of Doppler methods in [6.80]. Established technical imaging procedures are treated in Chapter 11, 'Sonography'. In this section new approaches will be described.

6.2.1 The Doppler methods

In Doppler methods [6.15 and 6.16a] (areas of application: vascular diagnostics, fetal heart rate; see Fig. 6.15), an acoustic beam which is not necessarily pulse-shaped, such as a continuous beam, is directed at the area to be examined. The sound which is scattered from the heart wall or from moving blood corpuscles and received again is shifted in its frequency in accordance with the *Doppler effect*, e.g. when the corpuscles approach the transducer, the frequency is slightly increased. For the frequency difference Δf relating to a blood corpuscle of velocity v_d,

$$\Delta f = 2 f_0 \frac{v_d}{c} \cos \varphi \tag{6.32}$$

f_0 Transmission frequency
φ Angle of incidence between beam axis and direction of flow.

In accordance with the *velocity distribution* in the area of flow probed by the ultrasound signal, a *noise signal* results from the superposition of the signals of all the blood corpuscles. The difference is generated by demodulation.

The frequency range of the noise for normal transmission frequencies (1 to 10 MHz) and for physiological velocities of movement lies in the audible range. In the case of blood flow detectors operating qualitatively, it is made audible by means of a loudspeaker and/or the spectrum of the electrical signal is analyzed [6.37, 6.38, 6.46, 6.71, 6.72].

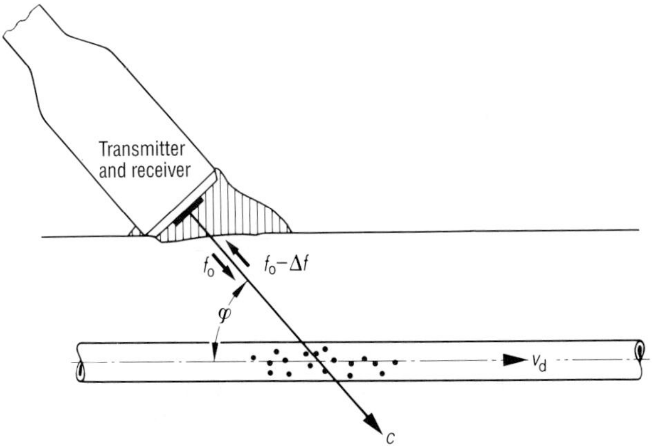

Fig. 6.15 Doppler effect used to detect blood flow velocity

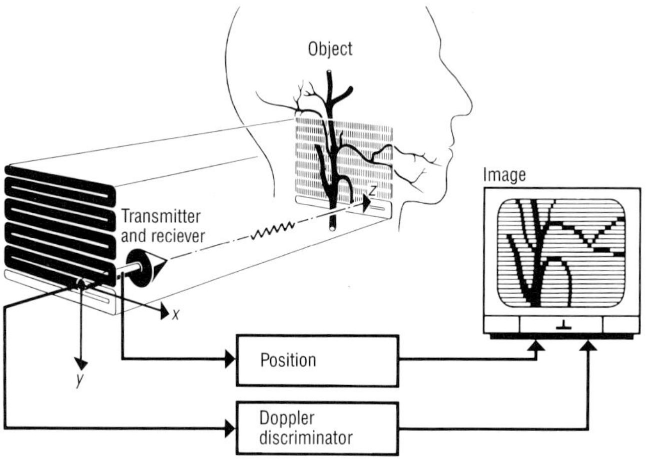

Fig. 6.16 Principle of angiography using ultrasound

On the basis of the above principle, imaging systems can also be designed which specifically reproduce the physiological quantity 'blood flow' [6.39 to 6.41, 6.43, 6.44]. One can, for example, probe an area of the skin with as narrow as possible a beam either mechanically (systematically zigzagging to and fro) (Fig. 6.16) or by hand. The coordinates of the scanning movement can then be transferred to a cathode ray tube and a dot produced on the screen whenever Doppler signals are received from inside the body.

In this way, using a continuous wave device, a three-dimensional section of the body is scanned. When using pulsed Doppler devices, the scanning can be confined to a plane. The most common form of this technique nowadays is to use part of a B-scope; in this method, the B-scan slice is scanned using pulsed Doppler methods and the Doppler image superimposed in color onto the B-image (color flow imaging). Such imaging procedures may also be described as ultrasonic angiography. They achieve the same spatial resolution as standard ultrasonic methods, a few centimeters penetration depth and do not rely on any contrast media.

More information concerning conventional technical procedures can be found in [6.45 to 6.47].

6.2.2 Other methods

Apart from the methods based on reflection discussed in Chapter 11, 'Sonography', there are various other procedures which are not as yet widely in use.

The most important of these employ transducers placed opposite each other for transmission and reception, i.e. based on *transmission*:

Acoustical holography [6.48]

Ultrasonic camera [6.49 to 6.51]

Ultrasonic computer-aided tomography [6.52 to 6.55]

These methods have the advantage that different physical sound parameters determine the image (e.g. the damping) and hence also allow obtaining different information. A disadvantage common to all these methods is that it is only possible to send ultrasound through the human body at a few places, because in most cases air cavities or bones, for example, prevent or disrupt the passage of ultrasound.

6.3 Limitations of the methods (image quality criteria)

All the devices which function according to the principles described above and in chapter 11 are limited in their performance. The limitations can be either of a fundamental nature or else specific to the particular device. Here only the fundamental limits set on the methods by physics or medicine will be indicated, as opposed to those imposed on the instruments because of technical considerations. The limitations of the methods and instruments determine the 'image quality'. This concept involves a number of aspects, the most important of which (in relation to the echo system) will be discussed below (see also [6.56]).

6.3.1 Penetration depth, signal dynamics

All the procedures mentioned are limited with respect to signal strength (size of amplitude). On the one hand, to avoid tissue damage (section 6.4) the body may only be subjected to a limited average ultrasonic intensity, which means that for medical reasons the achievable signal strength has an upper limit (e.g. 0.25 W for a strong echo, acoustically). On the other hand, arbitrarily small signals cannot be received and processed, because the thermal noise (in the acoustical and electrical transmission path) caused by the Brownian molecular motion is unavoidable and sets a physical lower limit (e.g. $2.5 \cdot 10^{-11}$ W of equivalent acoustic noise). The maximum possible amplitude or power ratio between the strongest signals and the noise is of the order of 100 dB for echo systems, irrespective of the particular device.

Since the effective amplitudes are determined above all by the damping in the tissue, Fig. 6.9 may also be regarded as the graphical representation of the maximum signal-to-noise ratio or the dynamic range of the signal.

In order to cite a maximum *penetration depth* $\hat{z}$ or the image depth for imaging systems, it is therefore necessary to specify a signal-to-noise ratio corresponding

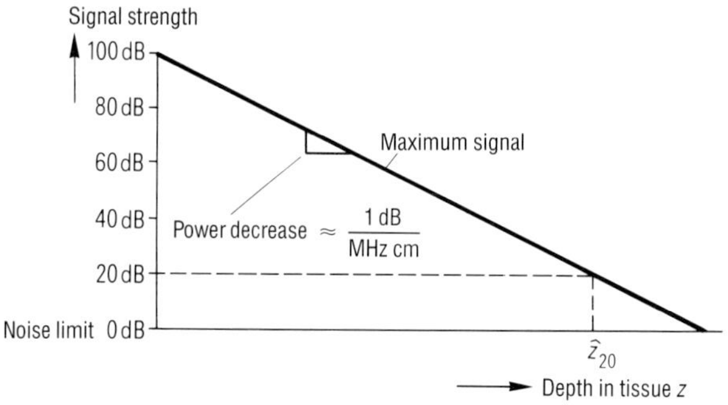

Fig. 6.17 Interrelationship of signal dynamic range and penetration depth $\hat{z}$

to the example of z_{20} for a 20 dB dynamic range of the signal in Fig. 6.17. In regard to the signal strength, this could be based on 'maximally occurring values', which should also be given (acoustic standard reflector). Apart from this (because of the frequency dependence of the absorption, section 6.1.3) the penetration depth depends on the proportion of low frequencies in the pulse spectrum technically evaluated by the apparatus (thus in the final analysis, also on the pulse shape). If this proportion is increased, a greater penetration depth can be achieved at the expense of a deterioration in the spatial resolution (see section 6.3.2). Accordingly, the maximum achievable spatial resolution at the greatest image depth should also be given.

In the design of instruments, one always has to find a compromise between the required maximum path length (e.g. the penetration depth in the echo system) and the spatial resolution or ultrasonic frequency, assuming some average value for the attenuation due to absorption (e.g. 1 dB/MHz cm). One would like to choose the ultrasonic frequency to be as high as possible, because the attainable spatial resolution increases with increasing frequency, i.e. with decreasing wavelength. On the other hand, this causes a drop in the penetration depth.

6.3.2 Spatial resolution

In ultrasonic technology, spatial resolution is taken to mean the capacity of an imaging system to reproduce two echoing point-like reflectors close together in the imaging plane as separate image points. Points which lie just outside the imaging plane are, however, also registered because the slice thickness of the scan is not infinitesimally thin. From the imaging of a spherical or cylindrical surface it can be shown that the above definition, which is the usual one, is thus too strict without modification. In the limiting region of small contours, the spatial resolution also depends to a considerable extent on the slice thickness of the scan, i.e. on the transverse dimension of the ultrasonic beam in the direction perpendicular to the scanning plane (y-direction) [6.57]. This aspect will not, however, be elaborated further here.

The physical limitation with respect to spatial resolution is due to the nature of ultrasound. In echo methods, for example, a point-like reflector – because of the geometrical shape of the ultrasonic field – is reproduced as an oval shaped illuminated area with its major axis perpendicular to the direction of the sound, instead of as a dot of infinitesimally small diameter. The brightness decreases towards the edges. The stronger the echo, the greater the area.

Elongation in the direction of the sound (minor axis) occurs primarily because the ultrasonic pulses and the echo signals received cannot be made arbitrarily short. The higher the frequency selected, the shorter they may be. An ideal pulse (with steep edges) of duration Δt would result in a minor axis of $c/2\Delta t$ on a screen which reproduces the original size (1:1 scale). Two reflectors then have to be further apart than this distance in order to be reproduced separately. Because of inevitable frequency band limitations, the pulses, however, have sloping – and not steep – edges (see Fig. 6.13 and $f_1(z)$ in Fig. 6.18) – hence the decrease in brightness towards the edge – and the question arises of how to describe the length of these pulses in an appropriate way.

Elongation perpendicular to the direction of the sound (major axis) is determined by the width of the ultrasonic beam in the scanning direction. The higher the ultrasonic frequency, the smaller this may be (in addition, focussing measures are possible). The reflector produces echoes as long as it is located in the ultrasonic field in front of the transducer. Thus, it also produces echoes when, after a sideways shift (scan), it no longer lies centrally in front of the transducer,

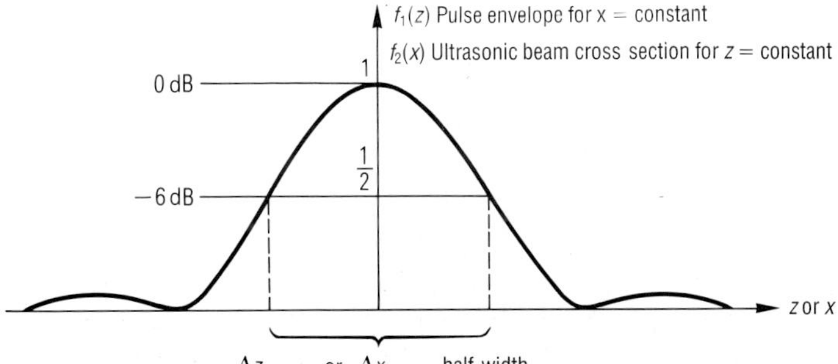

Fig. 6.18
Curves with sloping edges, pulse responses or point spread functions for the position coordinates x or z (measurement by means of reflection of a steel ball in a water or oil bath

but is only picked up by the edge of the ultrasonic field intended to generate the adjacent lines of the image. The decrease in the echo intensity in the direction of the scan (see $f_2(x)$) in Fig. 6.18 can be taken, for example, from the contour line representation (see section 6.1.4), if one doubles these parameters to take account of both transmission and reception (in the same transducer). Here too it is not possible to find a clearly recognizable lateral boundary, so that the beam width and the lateral resolution remain amplitude-dependent and thus lacking in sharpness.

In echo methods it is customary to give the *half-widths* $\Delta x_{-6\,\mathrm{dB}}$ and $\Delta z_{-6\,\mathrm{dB}}$ as an approximate measure of the *spatial resolution*. These are obtained from the curves with sloping edges $f_1(z)$ or $f_2(x)$ by measuring the distance between the points on the curve which have half the maximum value (−6 dB). Typical values are about 0.5 to 1 mm in the direction of depth and 2 to 6 mm in the scanning direction.

This measure corresponds roughly to the limiting value of the resolution which may be achieved under optimum conditions. This is shown in Fig. 6.19 using the example of a Gaussian curve for both $f_1(z)$ or $f_2(x)$.

Two adjacent points may individually yield the distribution functions $f_1(z)$ and $f_1'(z)$, and together the sum curves $b(z)$. The depth of the crevasse of the sum curve takes the value of 1 dB exactly when the points are contracted together to a distance d corresponding to a decrease in amplitude of −6.8 dB, i.e. roughly $\Delta x_{-6\,\mathrm{dB}}$ and $\Delta z_{-6\,\mathrm{dB}}$. A variation in light intensity of 1 dB can just barely be recognized under optimum conditions. This illustrates how spatial resolution and amplitude resolution are interrelated (see sections 1.4.3ff and 6.3.3).

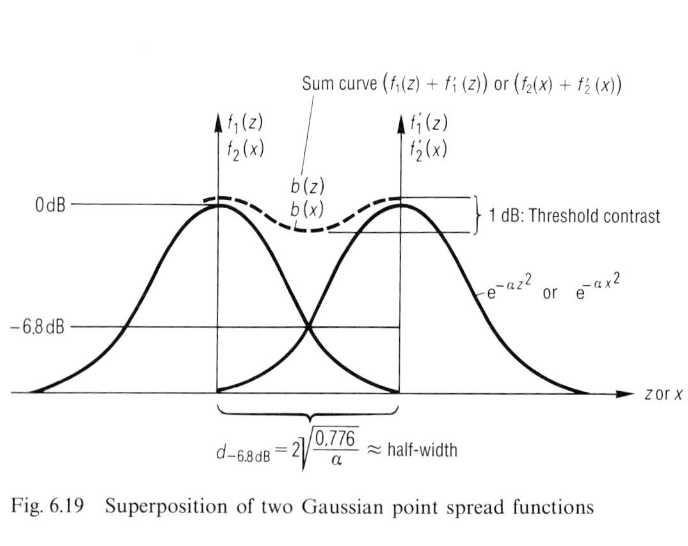

Fig. 6.19 Superposition of two Gaussian point spread functions

In x-ray technology, the *resolving power* is given in line pairs or periods per milimeter together with the corresponding reduction in amplitude strength. In sonography, taking the example of the above Gaussian functions of the form

$$f_1(z) = e^{-\alpha z^2}, \tag{6.33}$$

$$f_2(x) = e^{-\alpha x^2}, \tag{6.34}$$

following Fig. 6.19, the relation to the x-ray case is seen in the following way:

$f_1(x)$ and analogously $f_2(z)$ can be understood as the pulse response describing the system (pulse: jump in impedance in the point reflector), or alternatively as the point spread function. Because of the constant spectral density of a Dirac pulse (a short pulse in comparison with the spatial resolution), the Fourier transform of the pulse response describes the frequency dependence of the system [6.58]. The magnitude of the frequency dependence is called the *modulation transfer function* (MTF).

If, instead of a single pulse, a pulse sequence is applied in the shape of a rectangular point or line grid $a(x)$ (Fig. 6.20) to the system input, one obtains as the superposition of all the pulse responses the sum curve $b(x)$ with spectrum $B(\omega)$. This spectrum contains virtually only a stationary part and the fundamental frequency $2\pi/x_0$ if the gap between the pulses x_0 is of the same order of magnitude as the spatial resolution. The same components of the spectrum of $B(\omega)$ can be obtained (sequentially in time), if, instead of the point grid, sinusoidal inputs of frequencies $\omega = 0$ and $\omega_0 = 2\pi/x_0$ and amplitude A_0 are used (frequency characteristic point of view). If x_0 is exactly the distance

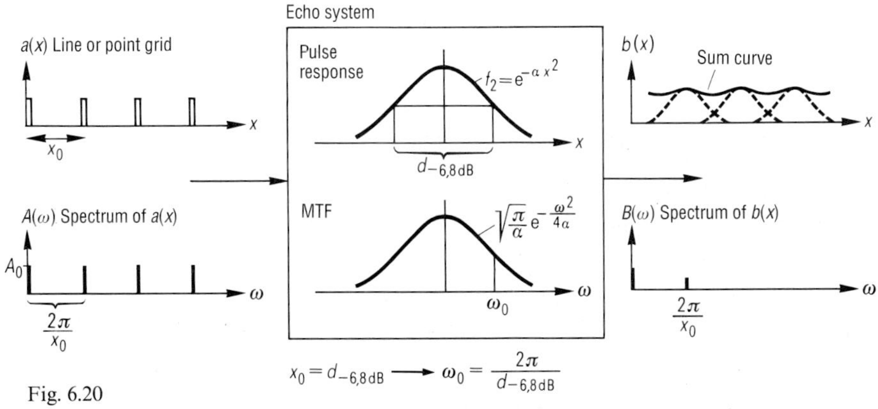

Fig. 6.20
Interrelation of line grid density $1/x_0$ and limit frequency ω_0 for the modulation transfer function (MTF)

at which 1 dB of variation results in the sum curve $b(x)$ (Fig. 6.19)

$$x_0 = d_{-6.8\,\mathrm{dB}} = 2\sqrt{\frac{0.776}{\alpha}}, \tag{6.35}$$

which then corresponds to the angular frequency

$$\omega_0 = \frac{2\pi}{x_0} = \frac{2\pi\sqrt{\alpha}}{2\sqrt{0.776}} \tag{6.36}$$

at which the modulation transfer function has fallen off by the factor

$$e^{\frac{-\omega_0^2}{4\alpha}} = e^{\frac{\pi^2}{4\cdot 0.776}} = 0.042 \mathrel{\hat{=}} -27.5\ \mathrm{dB} \tag{6.37}$$

Here too it can be seen that the half-widths yield an absolute upper limit because the drop in amplitude obtained virtually exhausts the range of brightness modulation which can be read from the screen by the eye (see section 6.3.3). Thus the spatial frequency $f_0 = \omega_0/2\pi$ can also be given as a measure of resolving power for a predetermined decrease in the transfer function (separately for the x and z functions).

The frequency dependence of the absorption (see section 6.13) enters into the MTF. Thus, the MTF as well as the spatial resolution is dependent upon the depth. If special measures are not taken, therefore (passband filter or frequency-dependent depth gain control [6.73]), the spatial resolution decreases with depth. The order of magnitude of this effect for maximum image depth is roughly a factor of 2.

6.3.3 Amplitude resolution

Up to now, when dealing with amplitudes, either ultrasonic pressures, particle velocities or, for example, the analogous voltages have been meant. The *interference signals* superimposed on these signals may be regarded as a limit on the accuracy with which an amplitude can be given, or on the amplitude resolution. Near the skin, the amplitude of a strong echo can be resolved with $10^{-3}\%$ accuracy, corresponding to a 100 dB signal-to-noise ratio and, at a large image depth for 20 dB signal strength, only with 10% accuracy.

In an ultrasonic image the above amplitudes are translated into brightness values. One could, for example, select a linear relationship with the photometric scales (for example, of light intensity in cd/m^2), i.e. of the light wavelength-dependent effect on the eye (γ correction). The upper limit of the light intensity could be set in such a way that flickering of the image remained tolerable. Then one would have to check whether the echo signal dynamics of e.g. 50 dB at average image depth could be perceived by the eye. This is definitely not the case (see section 1.4.3ff.) [6.74 to 6.76]. An eye that is adapted to the average light intensity of the screen, i.e. that has an optimum amplitude resolution, can take in a *brightness range* $L_{min}:L_{max}$ of about 1:30, i.e. about 30 dB. Echo amplitudes more than 30 dB below the maximum value of the light intensity are not seen. Furthermore, within this range, it is not possible to detect arbitrarily small differences. At most 35 different values (shades of gray) can be seen. The echo amplitudes which have been made visible are evaluated logarithmically by the human eye according to the Weber-Fechner Law, i.e. the distinguishable differences in light intensity are separated by constant logarithmic distances. The levels of brightness perceived by the eye can be described by the relation:

$$i = n \frac{1 + \lg \dfrac{L}{L_{max}}}{\lg \dfrac{L_{max}}{L_{min}}}. \tag{6.38}$$

i	Levels of brightness perceived by the eye	L_{max}	Maximum light intensity
L	Photometric light intensity	L_{min}	Minimum light intensity
		n	Maximum number of levels (35)

The signal dynamic range of about 30 dB is resolved to about 1 dB, corresponding to roughly 12% of the current value. The limit of spatial resolution depends on this value.

By selecting a different modulation characteristic, a higher signal dynamic range, for example, can then also be made visible between L_{min} and L_{max} (as for compression and windowing in CT). At the same time, however, the limiting values of the amplitude and spatial resolutions fall or, in the case of deviation from the logarithmic law, become dependent on the level.

The echo amplitude depends on the jump in impedance, on the damping by the path covered, on the geometric shape of the reflector (scattering, angle-dependent reflection), and on the shape of the ultrasonic field (contour lines and their distortion). Echo methods reach one of their limits, for example, when purely tangentially insonated boundary surfaces can no longer (e.g. as a contour) be picked up. The higher the signal dynamic range presented (compression), the less pronounced the effect [6.83].

6.3.4 Tissue inhomogeneity

The inhomogeneous spatial distribution of the acoustic impedances is the prerequisite for any ultrasonic echo image. Organs may, for example, be distinguished from each other in the impedance level or through the inhomogeneity of the spatial impedance distribution within the organ. The first of these leads to the *contour*, the second to the *structure* in the image. In this process, both the amplitude differences (see contrast) and the differences in the spatial distribution (echo density) are evaluated.

The differences of inhomogeneity in the impedance distribution among organs can be very pronounced (e.g. liver tissue/cyst) with the result that they are clearly visible in the image.

However, the opposite situation may also be encountered – almost identical echo structure of different neighboring regions (e.g. tumors in mammary tissue) – which makes detection impossible if there is no contour in the image.

In the case of two or more very large jumps in impedance after one another (e.g. boundary layers: from bones to soft tissue and from transducer to soft tissue) interfering multiple reflections may occur. These arise when a returning echo is reflected, propagates like a transmitted pulse back into the tissue and once again causes echoes there. In this way virtual image points are produced. Normally, this effect occurs in the region below the visibility threshold because of the small energy reflection coefficients involved and the damping caused by the tissue.

Besides the inhomogeneity with respect to the acoustic impedance, further inhomogeneities in other acoustic parameters are found in tissue. In particular, the spatially uneven distribution of the propagation velocity and the damping due to absorption sets a physical-medical limit. Even more so than for instance in sonar or radar technology, the propagation velocity and the damping due to absorption vary along the acoustic transmission path between the transducer and the target area to be imaged, with the result that the phases and amplitudes of signals which have followed different trajectories cannot be precisely determined in advance [6.59]. This places limitations on all ultrasonic systems.

In echo systems, for example, it is necessary to strive for as narrow an ultrasonic beam as possible (by means of focussing) in order to achieve a high lateral resolution. In accordance with Huygen's principle the ultrasonic beam can, with respect to amplitude and phase, be regarded as the linear superposition of many spherical waves which have all followed different paths from the transducer aperture to the same point in the object. The superposition is perturbed mainly because of the spatially differing propagation velocities, and the ultrasonic beam width may become enlarged or the beam become deflected [6.60, 6.77]. This perturbation effect becomes more evident, the narrower one attempts to make the ultrasonic beam at a given frequency. This is because the aperture which receives or transmits the signals must, among other things, be enlarged (focussing), which causes more inhomogeneous tissue to be acoustically irradiated. The phase distribution on the transducer surface becomes increasingly perturbed.

For the case of reflection techniques, the spatially inhomogeneous velocity distribution in the area under investigation also involves some uncertainty concerning the depth measurement, because primarily only times are measured and converted into depths using an expectation value for the velocity. Because of the finite spatial resolution in the direction of propagation, the effect of this when irradiating soft tissue is, however, only of secondary importance. When irradiating bones within soft tissue, on the other hand, noticeable errors occur, because the propagation velocity in bone is more than double that in soft tissue.

Similarly the inhomogeneity with respect to absorption leads to errors in echo systems because only an average expectation value for the damping can be preselected. Thus, the echo amplitudes of areas which are imaged through the accumulations of water or blood (cysts and hemotomas with low damping), bones or stones (high damping, possible ultrasonic shadow zones), may under certain circumstances be highly distorted. Areas behind accumulations of air (intestine, lung) cannot be imaged at all. 'Errors' of this kind are, however, sometimes used for diagnostic purposes.

6.3.5 Line density

It is necessary to distinguish between the line density (number of lines per scan width) of the acoustic scanning (line density D) and of the optical reproduction in the image. With the aid of storage memories, the optical line density can be made higher than the acoustic line density.

The acoustic lines quantize (chop) the point image function in the scanning direction. According to the sampling theorem, the line density has to be chosen sufficiently high so that the MTF in the x-direction is not significantly distorted. This condition is met by most instruments, which means that the finite line density does not make the spatial resolution noticeably worse.

Conversely, therefore, an optical line density above this value does not increase the spatial resolution (no gain in information); it does, however, contribute to an increase in contrast and to a more 'pleasant' appearance of the image.

6.3.6 Image frequency

For real-time instruments, the image frequency is of importance. Here too, one must distinguish between the repetition frequency of the spatial scanning movement (acoustic) and the number of the (optical) images offered per unit of time. Through temporary storage, the latter can be chosen to be higher than the acoustic repetition frequency.

To resolve movement (e.g. within the body), the acoustic repetition frequency f_A must be chosen to be high. It is dependent on the line density D, scanning width $\hat{x}$ and image depth $\hat{z}_0$ (penetration depth). For standard systems without parallel operation

$$f_1 = \frac{c/2}{D\hat{x}\hat{z}_0}. \tag{6.39}$$

By raising the optical image frequency relative to the acoustic image frequency, flickering of the image can be reduced.

6.3.7 Geometrical display accuracy

The image display accuracy in regard to area and angles depend, on the one hand, on a knowledge of the exact value of the propagation velocity and, on the other hand, on the precision of the transfer of the spatial scanning process to the line deflection electronics. From the physical point of view, the limitations described in 6.3.4 apply. The principal problems in precision are specific to the instrument.

6.4 Safety considerations

The advantage of ultrasonic diagnostics lies in the fact that the patient is not subjected to radiation and in its safety, as long as the applied ultrasonic intensity does not exceed a fixed maximum value. A clearly-defined *damage level* does not appear to exist. Hence, it is understandable that there are differing maximum admissible values quoted in the literature. Nyborg separates the safe region from the potential damage region in Fig. 6.21 by means of two straight lines corresponding to $J \cdot t < 50\ \mathrm{Ws\ cm^{-2}}$ and $100\ \mathrm{mW/cm^2}$ intensity, respectively. The Nyborg report, which was compiled on behalf of the Food and Drug Administration in the United States and the American Institute for Ultrasound in Medicine [6.67] is regarded as the reference point for current thinking on the matter, given that there are still no internationally or nationally binding regulations with respect to diagnostic ultrasonics. In West Germany, for example, this limit has the status of a recommendation.

At high ultrasonic intensities, two principal types of damage are conceivable:

a) *Mechanical damage*, due to violent movement (in particular, acceleration) of the particles.
b) *Thermal*, and consequently *chemical damage*, due to the conversion of ultrasonic energy into heat.

Investigations into potential damage are concerned with the effect on the skeletal support muscles, nerves, liver, eye, erythrocytes, DNA, etc. [6.63 to 6.64, 6.46, 6.83]. Both 'macroscopic' damage, such as the rupturing of blood vessels or breaking up of cells, and 'microscopic' damage, such as breaking of chromo-

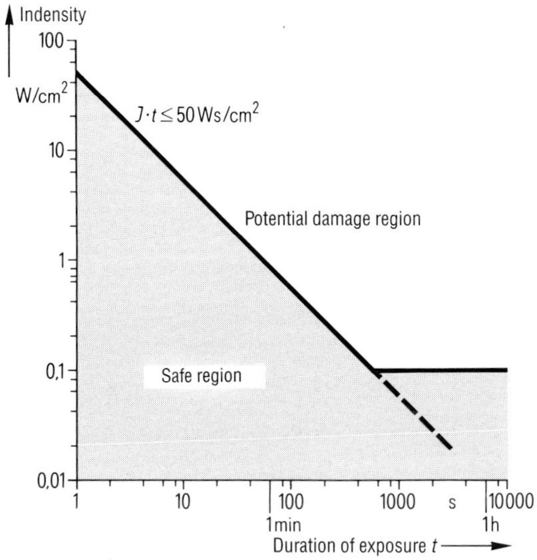

Fig. 6.21
Damage level for diagnostically applied ultrasound (from W.L. Nyborg, [6.67])

somes, are regarded as types of damage. The cell division ability (mitotic index) over several generations is also observed.

Potential damage depends on the intensity, the duration of exposure, the frequency, and the type of tissue. Only in the case of peak pulse powers over 1 kW/cm^2 of relatively long duration can degassing (pseudocavitation) and subsequent cavity formation (cavitation) occur, which can lead to mechanical damage. In diagnostic ultrasonics this power level is not reached, so that damage of the mechanical type does not occur. The main effect comes from the local increase in temperature.

Given the heat capacity of tissue, the time average of the ultrasonic intensity at a fixed position is a useful measure for the damage level. At normal ultrasonic intensities, the increase in temperature is very small [6.83].

Part 2 Technical solutions

7 X-ray diagnostics

Ever since the discovery of x rays by Wilhelm Conrad Roentgen in 1895, x-ray units for classical x-ray diagnostics have generally consisted of three basic components:

- the x-ray tube, which is supplied with power, switched and protected by the x-ray generator,
- the detector, which registers the radiation image after the x rays have passed through the patient, and
- the apparatus which takes care of the geometrical arrangement of tube, patient, and detector.

It was not until the advent of modern electronics in recent decades that there was any substantial progress in this area. The introduction of image intensifier television systems in the 1960s in particular, which made it possible to separate the locations of image viewing and image generation, created the conditions for adapting x-ray diagnostics to the specific demands of different specialities. Special equipment appeared – just to give a few examples – for gastrointestinal diagnostics, lung and skeletal diagnostics, urology, pediatrics, angiology, neurology, traumatology, and for taking x-rays in the operating room. The key factor in the specialization of x-ray diagnostics is to achieve the best direction of projection when arranging the tube and the detector with respect to the patient.

Further advances in electronics, with the possibility of digital image storage and processing, then led to the biggest breakthrough: digital subtraction angiography (DSA), i.e. the imaging of blood vessels in isolation.

In this section, the individual components of x-ray diagnostics will be dealt with first, such as x-ray tubes, intensifying screens, x-ray films, storage phosphor screens, x-ray generators, x-ray image intensifiers, x-ray television and digital image storage equipment. Afterwards x-ray systems, including invasive systems such as lithotripsy, will be described.

7.1 Image generation

7.1.1 The x-ray tube

As the source of radiation in the x-ray apparatus, the x-ray tube has a decisive influence on the image quality of the system. The following properties are of crucial importance:

▻ The hardness of the radiation, i.e. its penetration capacity, may be varied over a wide range by means of the magnitude of the voltage applied to the tube and thus may be optimally adapted to the object to be examined and to the method of examination.

▻ The radiation intensity (dose rate) may also be controlled over a wide range via the tube current.

▻ Finally, the focal spot size and the energy distribution in the focal spot are determining factors for the modulation transfer function (MTF) of the radiation source and thus contributing factors to the contrast and the resolving power.

The principle of the design of an x-ray tube can be taken from the example of the cross-section of the tube SR 70/7 used in dental x-ray units (Fig. 7.1): An evacuated envelope (1), which here simultaneously performs the task of high voltage insulation, contains the cathode assembly (2) and the anode (3) situated opposite one another. The electrons which are released and focussed in the cathode assembly are accelerated by the applied high voltage to 30

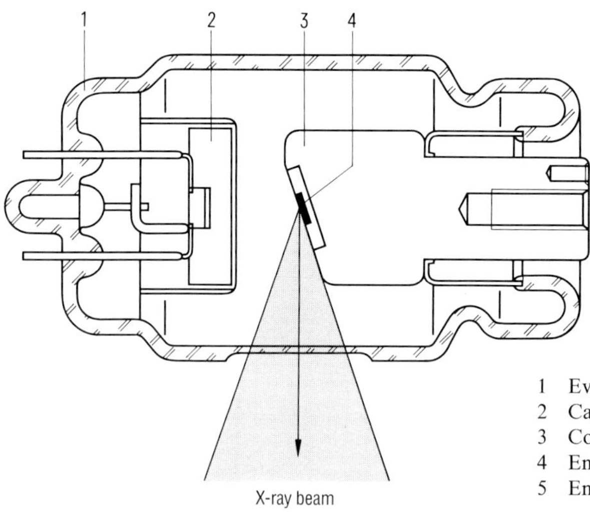

1 Evacuated glass envelope
2 Cathode
3 Copper anode
4 Embedded tungsten target
5 Emerging radiation

Fig. 7.1 Cross-section of the SR 70/7 stationary anode tube (HELIODENT) to 65% of the speed of light [7.1] (Fig. 7.2), and abruptly decelerated in the tungsten target (4) in the anode. In this process, as described in section 3.1, less than 1% of the electron energy is converted into x radiation; by far the largest part has to be dissipated as waste heat.

The individual assemblies in the x-ray tube will be treated in detail in the following sections.

Cathode assembly

In the vast majority of x-ray tubes used today, the cathode assembly consists of two parts: the electron source, usually a directly-heated helically-wound tungsten wire of 0.2 to 0.3 mm diameter, and an auxiliary electrode surrounding this (Wehnelt electrode). Other systems, for example multiple electrode systems with dispenser cathodes (electron guns), have up to now been confined to special applications because of their complex construction [7.2].

Electron emission

We begin with some basic remarks about the properties of a tungsten wire as an electron emitter. Apart from depending on the geometrical dimensions and the material constants, the number of electrons emitted from a metal depends in the first instance on the temperature. The emission current density

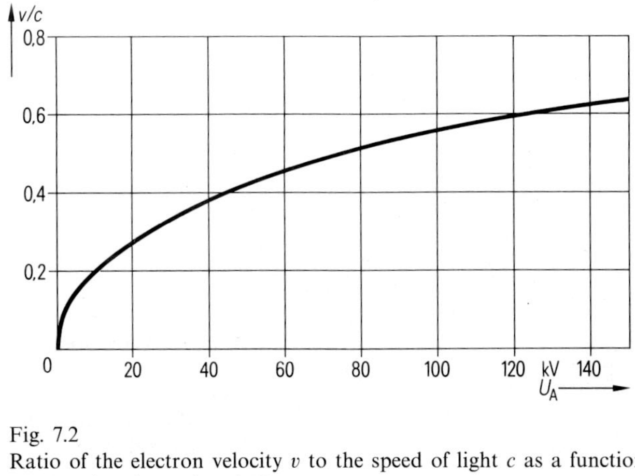

Fig. 7.2
Ratio of the electron velocity v to the speed of light c as a function of the anode voltage (acceleration voltage) U_A

j_e as a function of temperature is given by the Richardson equation

$$j_e = A_0\, T^2\, e^{-\frac{W}{kT}} \tag{7.1}$$

W Work function, for tungsten = 4.5 eV
k Boltzmann constant
T Temperature
A_0 Material constant, for tungsten $\approx 60 \dfrac{A}{\mathrm{cm}^2\,\mathrm{K}^2}$

and is depicted for tungsten in Fig. 7.3.

In order to obtain the currents of a few 100 mA up to 2 A required for x-ray images, emitter temperatures around 2700 K are needed. At such high temperatures a noticeable evaporation of the metal can be observed even for tungsten, which has a high melting point. This evaporation leads to the shortening of the life of the emitter, on the one hand via the deposition of metal on the inside of the glass envelope with consequent impairment of insulation, and, on the other hand, in a direct way due to the filament melting (Fig. 7.4). Because of this the filament is heated to the emission temperature only for the short exposure period. In order to keep the time until the emission temperature is reached below 1 s, the emitter is preheated to around 1500 K. At this temperature, there is so little metal evaporation that no negative effects on the useful life of the tube can be observed.

Anode current

The electrons, emerging with a low velocity from the emitter, form an electron cloud around it. They are accelerated towards the anode by the applied high voltage. Since the electron cloud partially screens the electric field generated, however, only a portion of the electrons are affected at low voltages. This then gives the characteristic curves depicted in Fig. 7.5 for the anode current.

For low voltages, the space charge law applies

$$I_A = \frac{4}{9}\varepsilon_0 \sqrt{2\frac{e}{m}} \cdot \frac{U_A^{3/2}}{d^2}, \tag{7.2}$$

I_A Anode current
ε_0 Permittivity of vacuum
e Electron charge
m Electron mass
U_A Anode potential
d Distance between cathode and anode

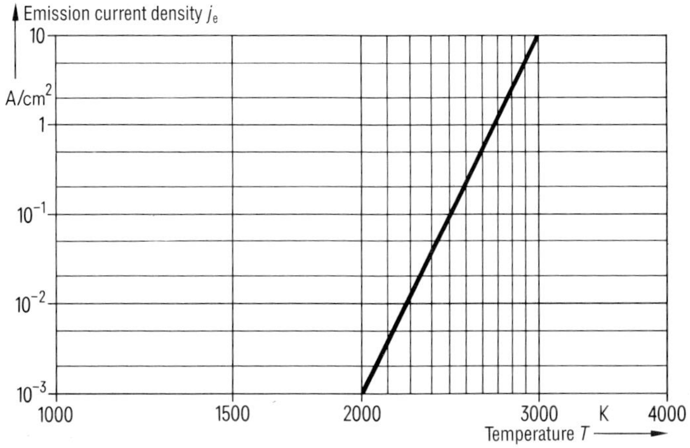

Fig. 7.3 Emission current density j_e as a function of the temperature T for tungsten

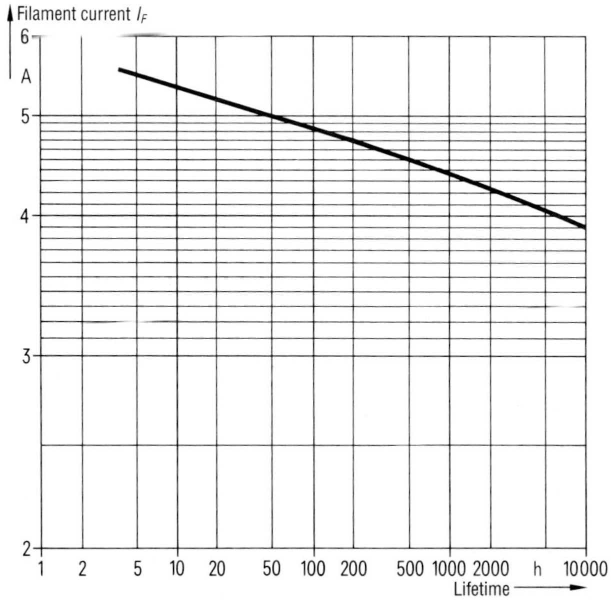

Fig. 7.4
Lifetime of a 0.2 mm diameter tungsten wire as a function of filament current. For radiography, filament currents are around 5 A, for fluoroscopy, filament currents are below 4 A.

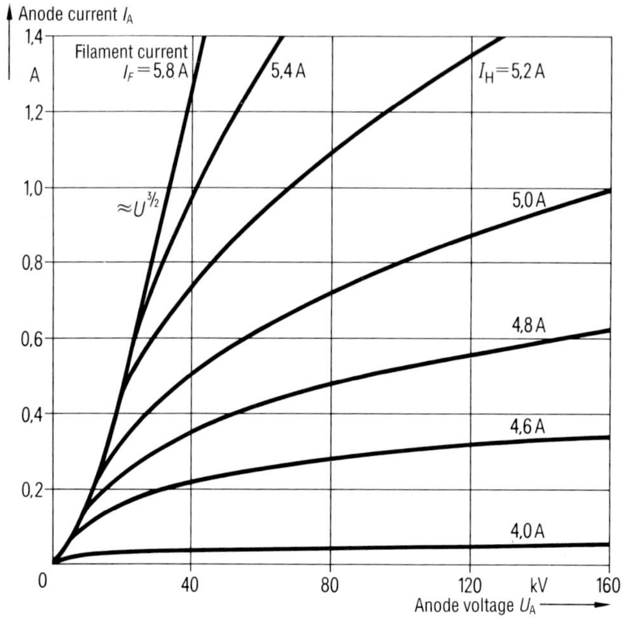

Fig. 7.5
Anode current I_A as a function of anode voltage U_A with the filament current I_F as a parameter

however, only as long as the electron density around the cathode is sufficiently high. For high anode potentials, all the electrons emitted are drawn off and one obtains the saturation current from emitter surface and current density according to the equation:

$$I_S = j_e \cdot A_E. \tag{7.3}$$

j_e Emission current density following equation (7.1)
A_E Emitter surface
I_S Saturation current

In this region, the current virtually only depends on the cathode temperature and consequently on the filament power: because of high field strengths in front of the emitter, the work function is reduced (Schottky effect). For x-ray tubes, this in fact still leads to a slight dependence of the saturation current on the anode potential, but may be ignored in the range $<5\%$. Further details may be found in the literature, e.g. in [7.1].

Focussing

If additional measures were not taken, the electrons emitted from the cathode and accelerated towards the anode would hit the anode in a widely smeared-out distribution, and would thus cause the x radiation to be created over a large area, which would lead to blurred images (Fig. 7.6a).

By means of an extra electrode of a suitable shape arranged around the cathode (Wehnelt electrode) and at the cathode potential, the path of the equipotential lines can be changed in such a way that the electrons are focussed at the

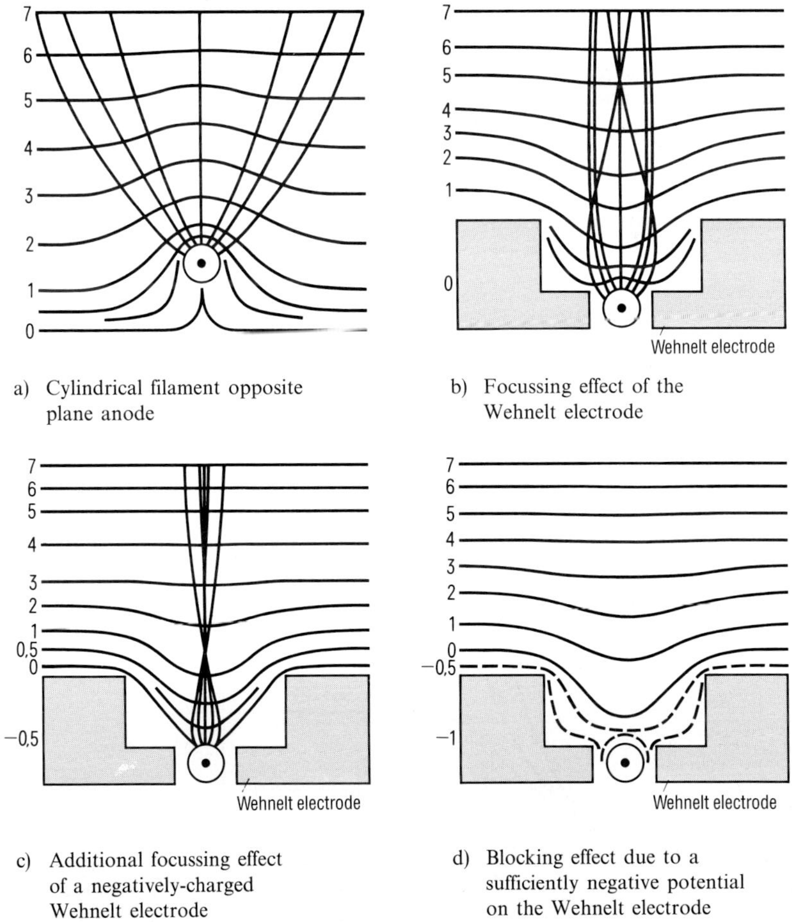

a) Cylindrical filament opposite plane anode

b) Focussing effect of the Wehnelt electrode

c) Additional focussing effect of a negatively-charged Wehnelt electrode

d) Blocking effect due to a sufficiently negative potential on the Wehnelt electrode

Fig. 7.6
Theoretical variation of the equipotential lines (relative potential values: 0 to 7) and electron trajectories

focal spot by the forces directed towards the central line joining cathode and anode (Fig. 7.6b). If the Wehnelt electrode is given an additional negative potential, this effect can be enhanced (Fig. 7.6c). It is, of course, a prerequisite that the geometry of the Wehnelt electrode, the emitter and the separation from the anode are optimally adapted to one another.

Furthermore, an electrode with a negative bias relative to the cathode provides an additional means of controlling the anode current, since, as can be seen from Figs. 7.6b and c, the field strength in front of the emitter is changed. In practice, however, this is only used in the case of x-ray tubes for switching on and off by means of a grid voltage (Fig. 7.6d) (grid pulsed operation) in the case of particularly short pulse times and fast pulse sequence frequencies.

A drawback of the Wehnelt electrode is that the effect of the anode potential on the emitter is reduced. The saturation value of the current is, therefore, only reached at higher anode potentials. At low anode potentials, especially for strongly focussed small focal spots, this arrangement operates in a part of the characteristic which is still essentially space-charge limited. This restricts the anode current. The attempt to achieve a greater anode current through increased heating of the emitter leads to the admissible temperatures being exceeded and thus to the emitter's destruction (Fig. 7.7).

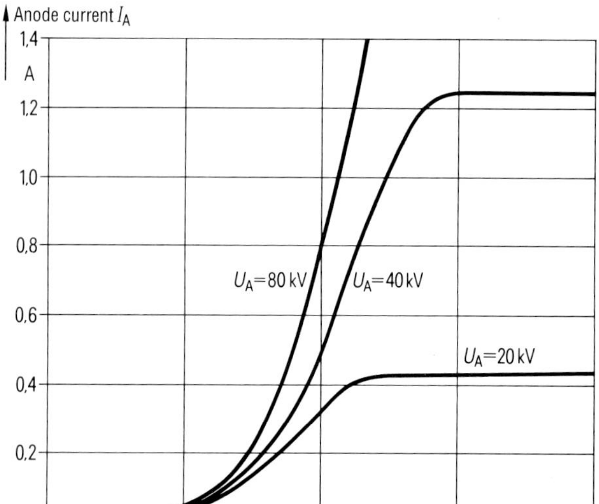

Fig. 7.7
Anode current I_A as a function of the filament current I_H with the anode voltage U_A as a parameter

Geometry of the focal spot

The area covered by the electrons and their distribution over the anode determine the size and structure of the focal spot, whose effective size is obtained from its projection in the imaging direction (Fig. 7.8).

It is thus immediately clear that for the various zones of a large-area image, differing focal spot sizes come into effect (Fig. 7.9).

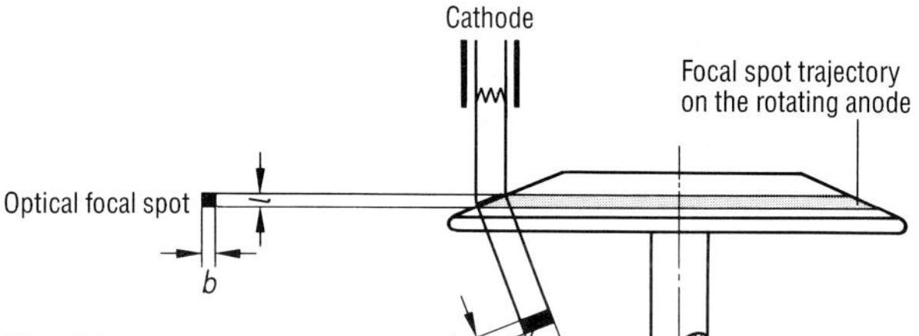

Fig. 7.8
Diagram of the relation between the electronic and the optical focal spot

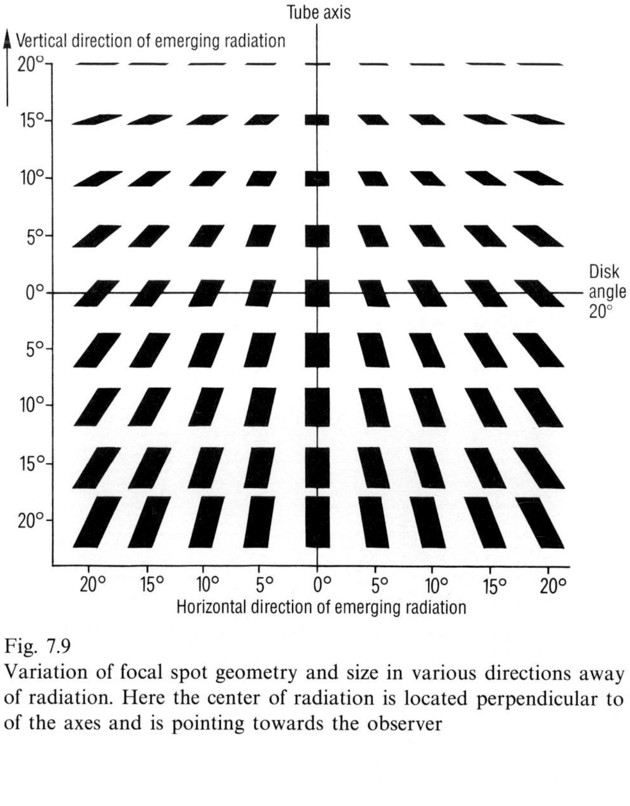

Fig. 7.9
Variation of focal spot geometry and size in various directions away from the center of radiation. Here the center of radiation is located perpendicular to the intersection of the axes and is pointing towards the observer

Usually the projection perpendicular to the tube axis is given as the focal spot size.

The focal spot size can be determined most easily with the aid of a pinhole image (Fig. 7.10). For more exact analyses of the focal spot with respect to its properties, however, narrow slits in the two major axes of the focal spot are used instead of the pinhole (Figs. 7.11 and 7.12). The images so obtained can be analyzed with a photometer so that one gets an image of the intensity distribution of the x rays in the focal spot. By means of a Fourier transform, the modulation transfer function, MTF, is obtained from this intensity distribution curve, being the fundamental measure of the imaging properties of the focal spot. It describes the contrast (in %) as a function of resolution (line pairs/mm).

As an example, Figs. 7.10 to 7.13 show the various quantities for the focal spot of an x-ray tube.

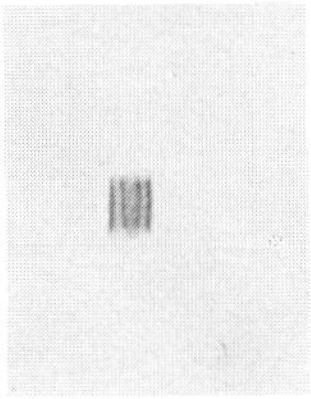

Fig. 7.10
Pinhole camera image of a 100 kW focal spot

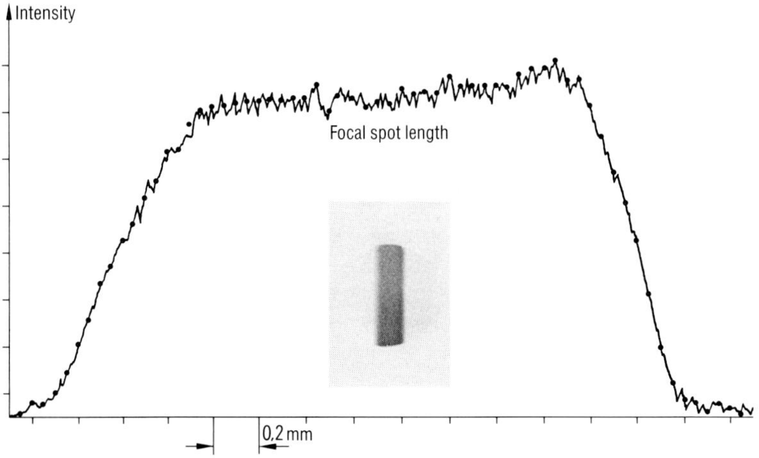

Fig. 7.11
Slot camera image of the length of the focal spot in Fig. 7.10 and photometric analysis

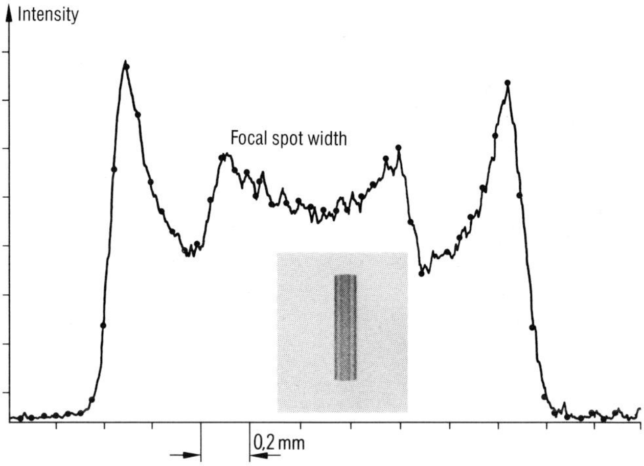

Fig. 7.12
Slot camera image of the width of the focal spot in Fig. 7.10 and photometric analysis

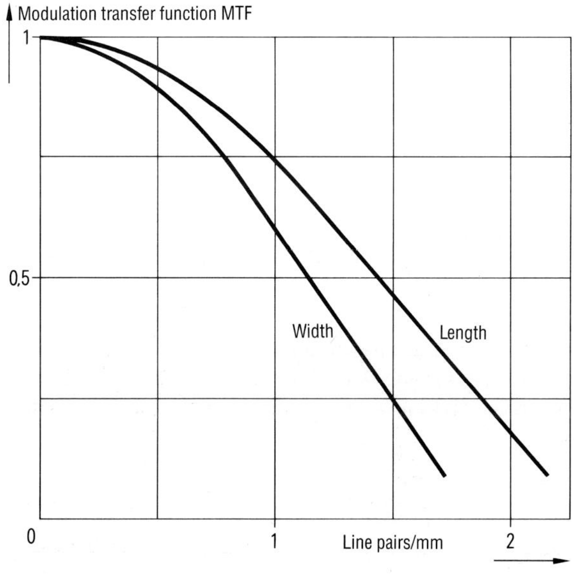

Fig. 7.13
Modulation transfer function calculated from the photometer curves of Figs. 7.11 and 7.12 for an imaging ratio of 1:1.3

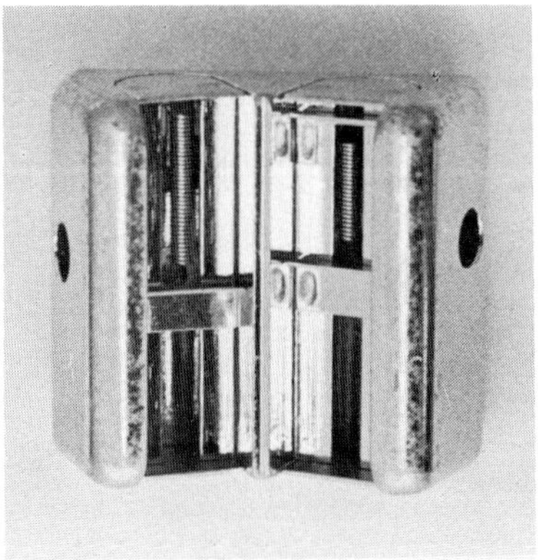

Fig. 7.14
Focusing head with two parallel emitters for focal spots of 0.6 and 1.2 mm projected one inside the other and for powers of 40 and 100 kW

Most x-ray tubes offer the possibility of working with two or more focal spots. The reason for this is that a simultaneous optimization of the size of the focal spot to achieve both high resolution and high power cannot be realized because of the limitations due to the properties of the anode material. Thus, in the case of two focal spots, which may be arranged one behind the other or next to each other, one will be designed for high resolution, and the other for high power. The construction of such cathodes for focal spots with 40/100 kW power and 0.6 and 1.2 mm focal size respectively, lying superimposed upon each other on the disk, is shown in Fig. 7.14.

Extrafocal radiation

A not inconsiderable proportion of the electrons which hit the anode leaves it again. Some of these electrons are scattered backwards elastically, i.e. without loss of energy, enter the opposing field between cathode and anode and fall back onto the anode, but outside the original focal spot. In this way extrafocal radiation is created outside the focal spot which in certain circumstances may also have a negative influence on the image quality if it is generated in the immediate vicinity of the focal spot and thus cannot be screened out. By arranging the tube assembly in an appropriate way, one aims to achieve electrical field distributions in the critical region of the anode which counteract this effect.

Anode assembly

In the following, the design characteristics of various kinds of anode are described; loading capacity is dealt with at the end of this section. From what was said in section 3.1.3, it follows that tungsten is the most suitable target material for use in x-ray diagnostics; only in the special case of mammography is molybdenum sometimes preferred. Because of the low efficiency of the conversion of the electrons' kinetic energy into x radiation, more than 99% of the energy introduced into the x-ray tube has to be carried off in the form of heat. The problems to be solved are those of the heat distribution in the anode and of the dissipation of the heat to the surroundings.

Stationary anodes

The tungsten target is embedded in a copper block. The heat is carried away by conduction via the stem to the surroundings. One method (which, however, is hardly ever used for diagnostic x-ray tubes) is to create additional convection by means of cooling boreholes in the anode block, through which water or oil is then pumped for cooling. The anode frequently has an electron capture hood with a beryllium window which lets through radiation easily, and this prevents the electrons which are reflected at the target from reaching the glass envelope and thus adversely affecting the disruptive strength of the tube. Because of the field-free space in front of the target, this design also largely stops the reflected electrons falling back and so reduces the undesirable extrafocal radiation. Stationary anode x-ray tubes are admittedly very reliable because of the simplicity of their construction, however, for many applications they are not suitable because of the power limit in the focal spot on the anode. The upper power limit is reached in particular for radiography by the temperature at the boundary between the tungsten target and the copper exceeding the melting point of copper. The maximum load for radiography is around 100 W/mm^2, and in continuous operation (fluoroscopy) it is 30 W/mm^2. Fig. 7.15 shows a cross-section of a typical stationary anode x-ray tube, the x-ray tube SRL 90/10/30.

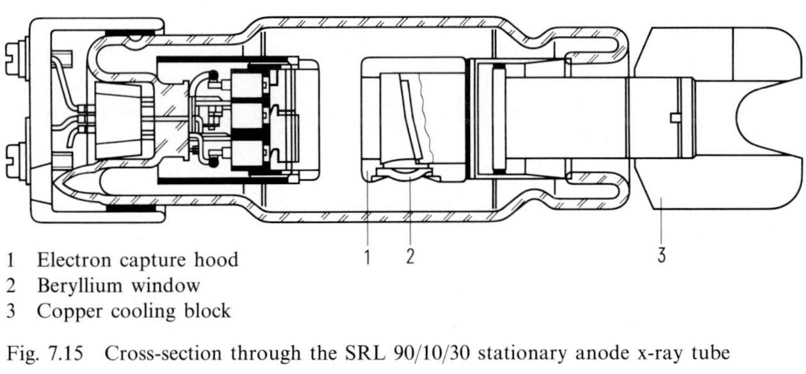

1 Electron capture hood
2 Beryllium window
3 Copper cooling block

Fig. 7.15 Cross-section through the SRL 90/10/30 stationary anode x-ray tube

Rotating anodes

The idea of letting the anode rotate in order to raise the rating occurred very early on. This first suggestion, which was made by Wood in 1897, was that the glass bulb should rotate as an anode around the cathode, which was also mounted so that it could rotate (Fig. 7.16). The actual technical realization of this idea, however, did not come about until 1929 with the advent of the rotating metal anode and the introduction in 1933 of the freely rotating anode disk made out of tungsten.

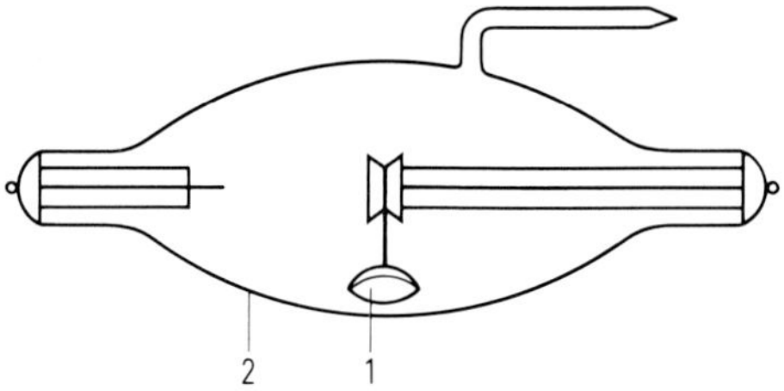

Fig. 7.16
The first idea for a 'rotating anode x-ray tube' by Wood in 1897. The cathode (1) is supported by bearings so as to be free to rotate inside the glass bulb (2), which functions here as the anode. It is held in position by gravity

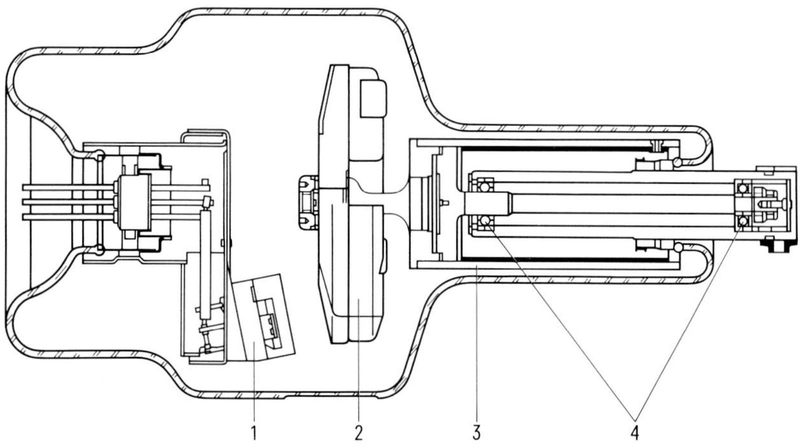

1 Dual focus cathode
2 Graphite-RTM compound anode
3 Rotor
4 Ball bearings

Fig. 7.17 Cross-section through a rotating anode x-ray tube

The construction of a modern rotating anode x-ray tube is shown in Fig. 7.17. It is powered with the aid of the rotor (3) made to act as a squirrel-cage rotor by means of the rotating field, which is generated by a stator outside the vacuum. The standard number of revolutions is around 3,000 r.p.m. and 9,000 r.p.m. respectively. For special applications with extremely high intensities in the focal spot, 17,000 r.p.m. are required. In these circumstances, operating in the vacuum and at high temperatures, the ball bearings have to satisfy exceptional demands.

The highest thermomechanical demands are placed on the anode disk. Originally it was made out of pure tungsten. Because of its restricted rating and lifetime, at the very least a rhenium-tungsten-molybdenum (RTM) compound anode (Fig. 7.18a) is used in x-ray tubes nowadays. By alloying a few parts of rhenium to tungsten, an improvement in the elastic properties and hence a substantially improved resistance to wear of the 1 to 2 mm thick covering layer are achieved (Fig. 7.18d). A disk base made of molybdenum gives an increased heat capacity compared to a tungsten anode with the same mass [7.11, 7.12].

The graphite RTM composite anode (Fig. 7.18b) represents a further advance in anode technology. This technology enabled the heat capacity and heat loss by radiation of the anode to be raised considerably. In modern high power x-ray tubes, as used for example in computed tomography, the CALOREX anode with a heat capacity of up to 2×10^6 Ws and a thermal dissipation power of up to 5 kW is exclusively used (7.18c).

Vacuum envelope

The vacuum inside an x-ray tube must meet the following requirements:

- It must be good enough to guarantee the insulation of the high voltage between the anode and the cathode.
- The electrons must be able to travel from cathode to anode without colliding with atoms of residual gas.
- The cathode surface must not be adulterated by the atoms of residual gas, in order to ensure the reproducibility and constancy of the emission currents.
- The vacuum must be maintained throughout the entire life of the x-ray tube.

Besides selecting suitable electrode materials readily susceptible to de-gassing, a prerequisite for generating and maintaining a vacuum of at least 10^{-5} mbar is an appropriate vacuum envelope. Apart from the technical requirements relating purely to maintaining a vacuum, the envelope should also fulfil the

Fig. 7.18
Comparison of the heat capacities of RTM and RTM-graphite anodes

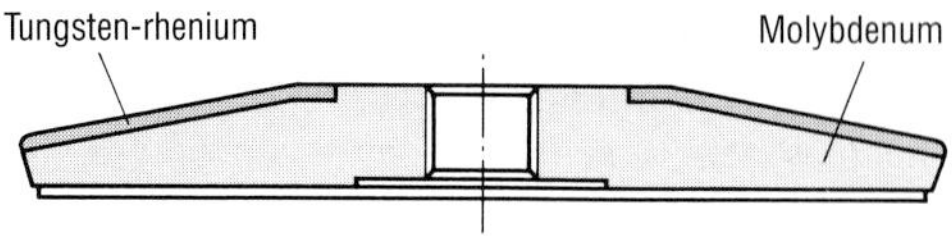

a) RTM anode for 250,000 Ws

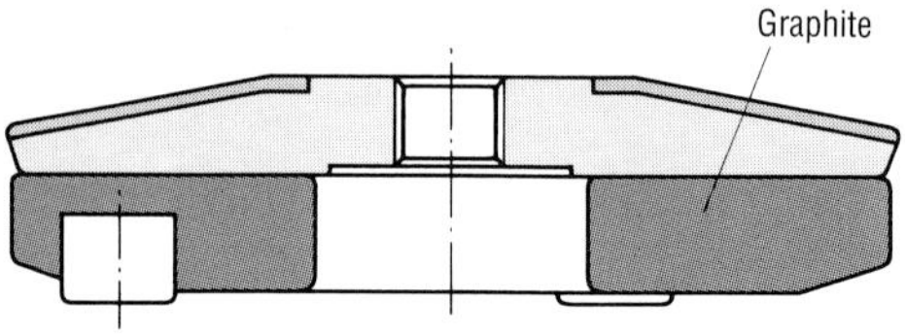

b) RTM-graphite anode for 400,000 Ws

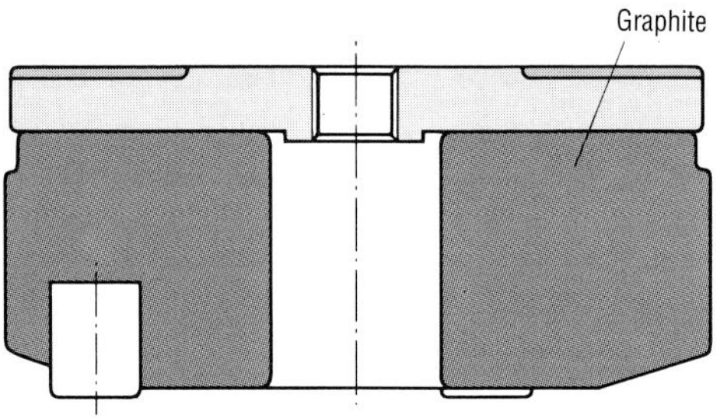

c) RTM-graphite anode for 1,000,000 Ws
(for computer tomographs)

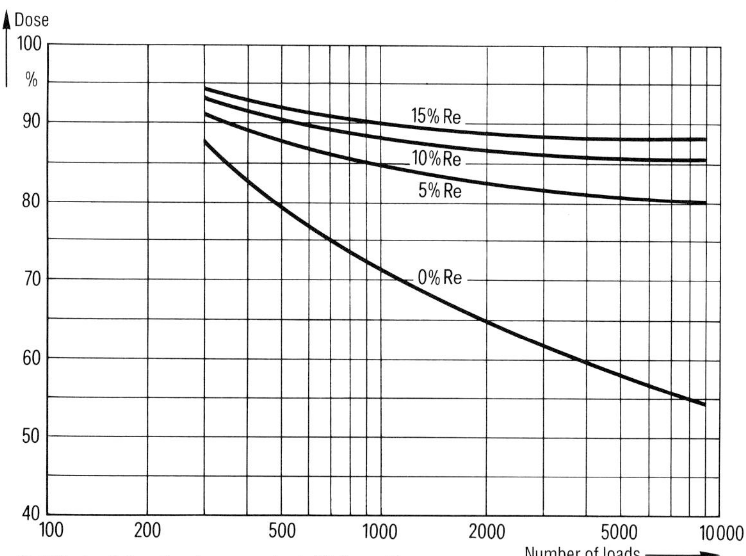

d) Effect of the rhenium content (Re) on the resistance to wear and tear of the tungsten anode covering layer following conditions:

- ▻ low x-radiation absorption,
- ▻ high temperature cycle resistance
- ▻ high insulation capacity, at least in those cases where it simultaneously takes care of the insulation of the cathode and anode,
- ▻ high permeability to radiated heat.

Glass satisfies all these requirements almost ideally, which is why up to this day glass has predominantly been used as the vacuum envelope for x-ray tubes (Fig. 7.17).

A drawback of the glass envelope construction is the deterioration of its insulating capacity due to vaporization from the anode and cathode, which is virtually unavoidable and which leads to metal deposits on the glass surface. One tries to overcome this disadvantage by using an appropriate design in which the central part of the tube is made of metal. Designs in which the entire vacuum envelope is made of metal and the insulation achieved using ceramic insulators in the anode and cathode assemblies aim to avoid the same problem. It is necessary to weigh up which design is preferable in each particular case, taking into account all the parameters pertaining to the operation of the tube.

X-ray tube assembly

In order to ensure the safe operation of the x-ray tube it is enclosed in a protective casing. Two kinds of design should be distinguished, the simple x-ray tube assembly (Fig. 7.19), which, apart from the tube, only houses the stator and a few control components, and the single-tank x-ray tube assembly. In the single-tank assembly, the tube is integrated with the high voltage generator. This kind of x-ray tube assembly was originally used almost exclusively for stationary anode x-ray tubes, but in the meantime has become very important for rotating anode tubes as well, because of the application of high frequency technology in generating high voltage.

The tube casing performs the following functions:

- ▻ high voltage insulation
- ▻ cooling
- ▻ protection against implosion
- ▻ protection against radiation.

The radiation protection in particular must be checked for each individual x-ray tube assembly by means of a suitable 4 π-measurement (Fig. 7.20).

The measurement is carried out as follows. The x-ray tube assembly is operated in the center of a C-arc of 2 m diameter which is fitted with ionization chambers.

By rotating the assembly, the entire volume is measured. Each time the chamber with the highest reading is electronically selected and recorded.

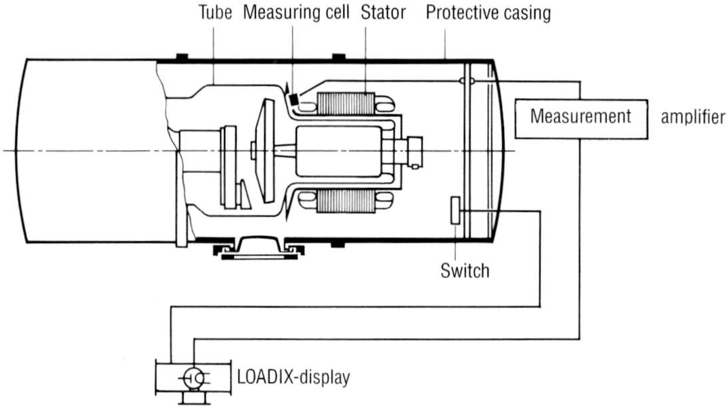

Fig. 7.19
The x-ray tube assembly consists of the protective casing and the built-in x-ray tube. The diagram also shows an instrument for monitoring the anode disk temperature (LOADIX)

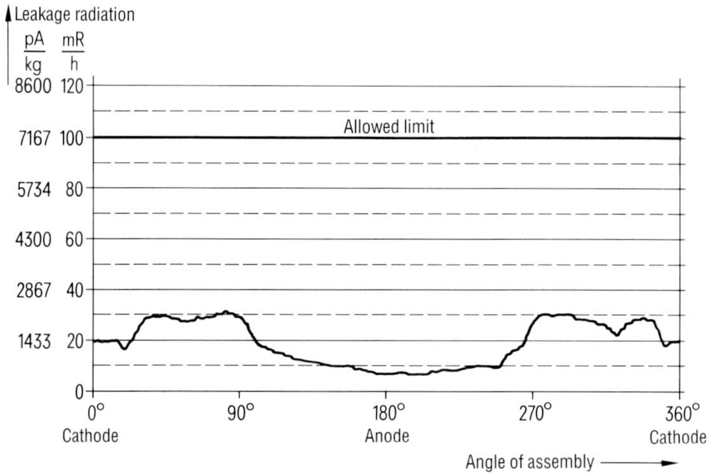

Fig. 7.20
Leakage radiation from a high power x-ray tube assembly. The measured values lie clearly below the allowed limits

Load capacity of x-ray tubes

The load capacity of x-ray tubes in operation is determined by the rapid rise in temperature in the focal spot. Fundamental work was done on this subject by Bouwers [7.3] and Osterkamp [7.4] for stationary anodes. The rise in temperature in this case for short load times (<0.05 s for standard focal spot dimensions) is given approximately by

$$\vartheta = \frac{2P}{A}\sqrt{\frac{t}{\pi \cdot \lambda \varrho c}} \tag{7.4}$$

P	Power input	λ	Thermal conductivity
A	Focal spot area	c	Specific heat
t	Load period	ϱ	Density

and for long load periods by

$$\vartheta = \frac{P \cdot R}{A \cdot \lambda}. \tag{7.5}$$

R Smallest dimension of the focal spot.

Once again it should be pointed out that in the case of a stationary anode tube a significantly lower value should be used for the maximum permissible focal spot temperature than that which follows from equation (7.5), since in this case the admissible temperature at the boundary between tungsten and copper would be exceeded. Furthermore, for very long load periods a further limit which is obtained from the thermal capacity of the anode and the thermal dissipation to the surrounding oil must often be taken into account.

With respect to rotating anodes, the focal spot temperature may be written following [7.5, 7.6, 7.7] as the sum of basic disk temperature θ_0, focal ring temperature θ_{v0} and temperature rise θ_R after several turns n of the rotating anode (Fig. 7.21):

$$\vartheta_{n0} = \vartheta_0 + \vartheta_{v0} + \vartheta_R.$$

Here the temperature rise may be calculated according to the equation (7.4) already given for the stationary anode, if for the load period one inserts the appropriate length of time a disk element with focal spot width 2δ stays in the electron beam. Given the mean focal track radius R and rotation frequency f, one then has:

$$\Delta t = \frac{\delta}{\pi \cdot R \cdot f} \tag{7.7}$$

or using equation (7.4)

$$\vartheta_R = \frac{2P}{A}\sqrt{\frac{\delta}{\pi^2 \cdot f \cdot R \cdot \lambda \cdot \varrho \cdot c}}. \tag{7.8}$$

The focal ring temperature is described by

$$\vartheta_{v0} = k\,\vartheta_R \sqrt{\frac{\delta}{\pi R}}\sqrt{n+1} \tag{7.9}$$

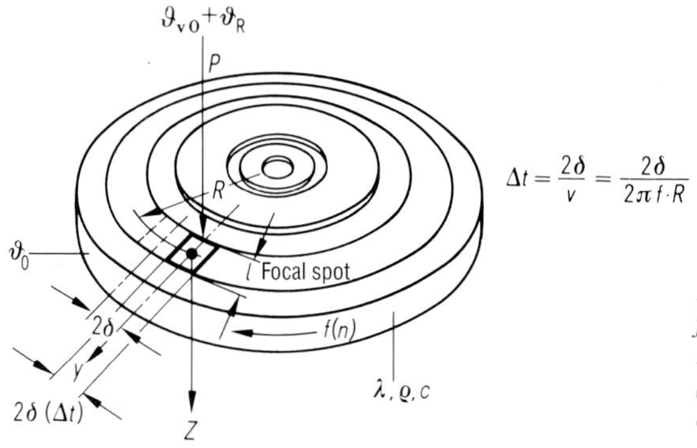

T time for one revolution
A Focal spot area ($2\delta l$)
f Rotation frequency
λ Thermal conductivity
ϱ Density
c Specific heat

Fig. 7.21 Geometrical relations at the rotating anode

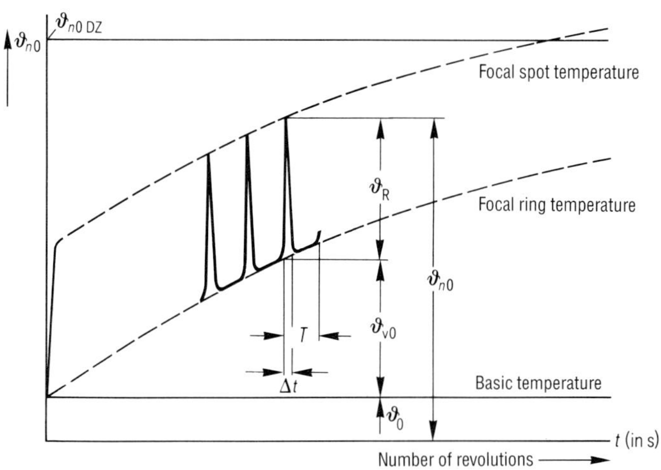

Fig. 7.22 Temperature increase in the focal spot on the rotating anode

Here k is a correction factor which takes into account the effects of the anode thickness, the thermal radiation at high temperatures and the heat diffusion in the radial direction. The result of these calculations is shown in Fig. 7.22.

From the calculations of the temperature distribution beneath the focal ring as a function of time and depth, which is given by

$$\vartheta_{z,t} = \frac{1}{2}\,\vartheta_R \sqrt{\frac{\Delta t}{t}}\, e^{-\frac{z^2 \varrho c}{4\lambda t}} \tag{7.10}$$

z Depth of anode

and is shown as an example in Figure 7.23, it follows that the temperature in the focal ring is virtually levelled out before each subsequent passage through the electron beam. It is, however, equally clear that very high temperature gradients occur, which, as already described, lead to the destruction of the anode surface. (Since in particular the mechanical stresses which arise in the direction of the circumference can lead to cracking of the disk, this is prevented by placing slits in the radial direction, Fig. 7.24).

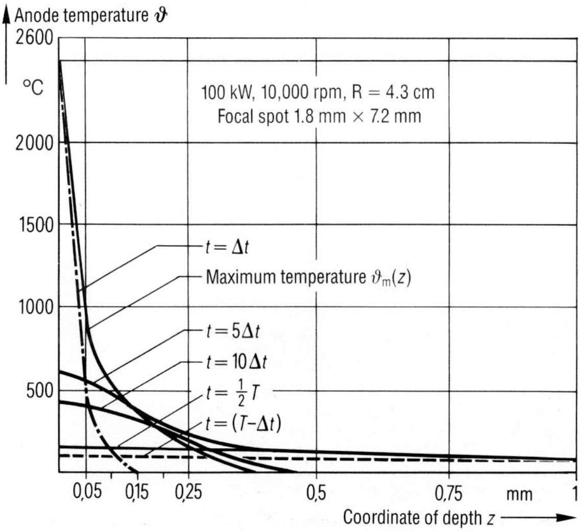

Fig. 7.23
Temperature of the anode beneath the focal ring after at most one revolution T

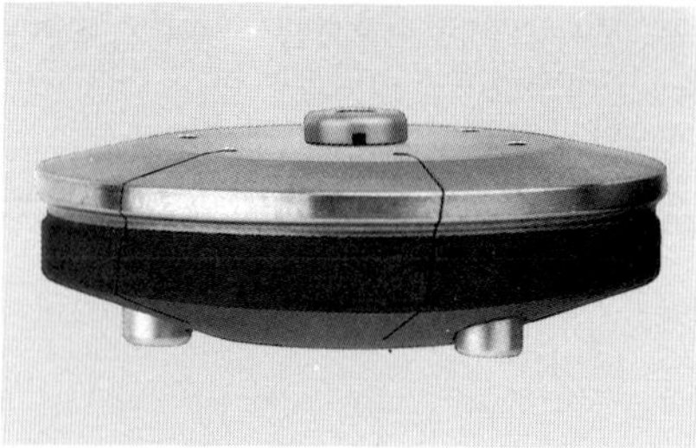

Fig. 7.24
Stress relieved CALOREX anode in which potential mechanical stresses are avoided by means of radial slits

An upper temperature limit ($\theta_{\mathrm{n_0\,z}}$) in the focal spot is reached when, as a consequence of the ionization of the evaporating metal, there is an arc discharge between cathode and anode. For reasons of safety during operation, a value for the admissible focal spot temperature is set which is lower by an amount

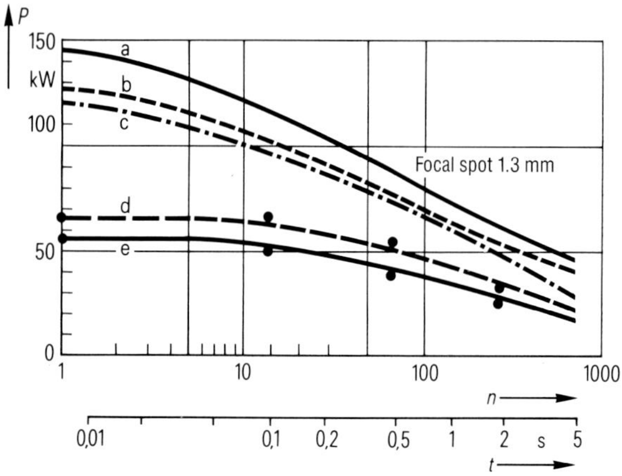

- a Metal-graphite anode (2 mm metal and 15 mm graphite and CALOREX anode design) at 150 Hz and 6 pulse operation
- b Graphite anode with 0.1 mm rhenium metal layer at 150 Hz and 6 pulse operation
- c RTM anode at 150 Hz and 6 pulse operation
- d RTM anode at 150 Hz, but 4 pulse operation
- e RTM anode at 50 Hz, but 6 pulse operation

Fig. 7.25
Rating curves of rotating anode x-ray tubes for constant focal spot temperature of 2500 °C and constant maximum temperature in the boundary layer between metal and graphite in compound anodes

$\Delta\theta_s$. Thus, by combining the equations (7.4 to 7.9) and solving for the power, one obtains

$$P = \frac{\pi(\vartheta_{n_0\,z} - \Delta\vartheta_s - \vartheta_0)\sqrt{\lambda\varrho c}\cdot l\cdot\sqrt{fR\delta}}{1 + k\sqrt{t\cdot f\cdot\dfrac{\delta}{\pi\cdot R}}}. \tag{7.11}$$

In any particular case a rating curve is valid only for an anode with a known basic temperature. The basic temperature of the anode depends on the preceding loads and interval periods.

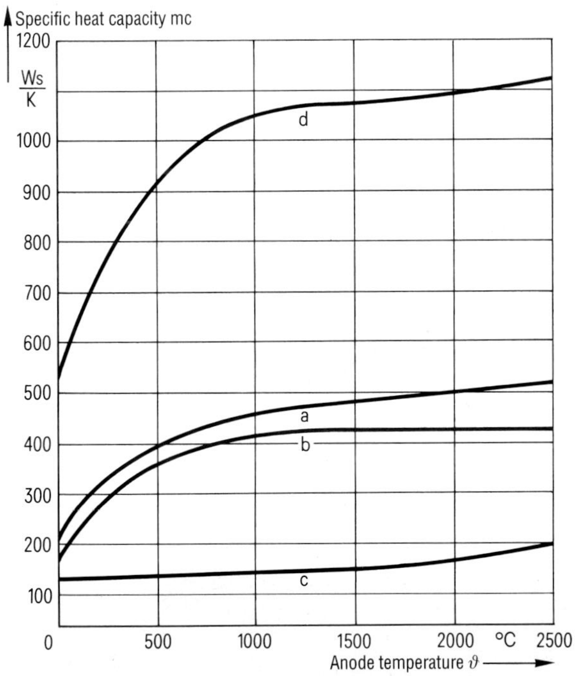

a Metal-graphite anode (2 mm metal and 15 mm graphite) and CALOREX anode design
b Graphite anode with 0.1 mm rhenium metal layer
c RTM anode
d RTM anode with 33 mm thick graphite disk as a CALOREX anode for the Opti 151 CT x-ray tube used in computed tomography

Fig. 7.26
Heat capacity as a function of the temperature for four different types of anode

From the heat capacity of the anode and the summed power, on the one hand (Fig. 7.26), and the cooling curve determined by the power radiated away

$$P = A_A \sigma_0 \varepsilon(T)(T_A^4 - T_0^4) \tag{7.12}$$

A_A Surface area of anode
σ_0 Constant of radiation
$\varepsilon(T)$ Specific emission capacity
T_A Anode temperature
T_0 Surrounding temperature

on the other hand, the basic temperature can be found in each case.

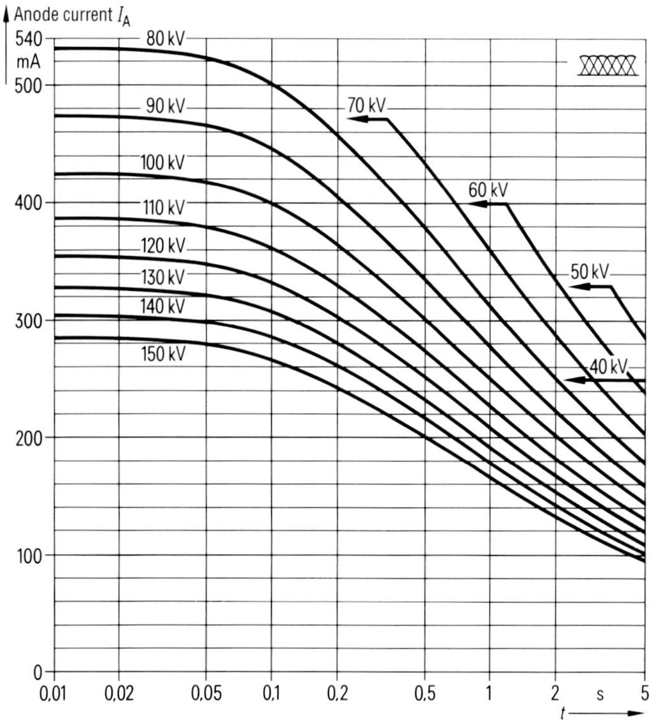

Fig. 7.27
Rating curves for a focal spot 0.6 mm, 40 kW, 150 Hz. The anode current as a function of the load period is valid for an anode preheated with 300 W with the anode voltage as a parameter. The sharp bends in the curves at low anode voltages are due to the limits on the emission of the cathode

For practical purposes, x-ray tube rating charts usually give the permitted anode currents as a function of the load period with the voltage as a parameter.

The sharp bends in the curves for low voltages are due to the limited emission capacity of the cathode. In these curves a basic thermal state (e.g. 300 W) is assumed. This is established by experience for normal operation of the x-ray tube. If the tube has previously had a higher load, the exposure power has to be reduced or a pause has to be made before the next exposure.

The thermal state can be monitored by means of direct measurement of the anode temperature, e.g. using the LOADIX system [7.8].

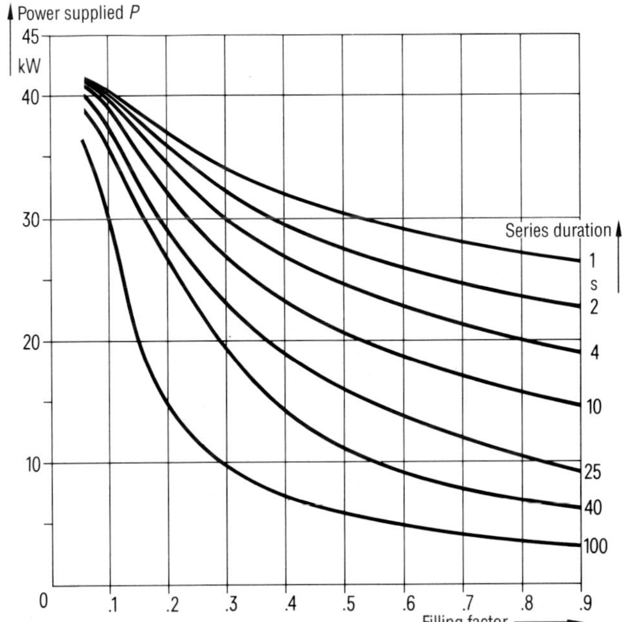

t_p (ms)								
1	100	200	300	400	500	600	700	800
2	50	100	150	200	250	300	350	400
4	25	50	75	100	125	150	175	200
6	16	33	50	67	83	100	117	133
10	10	20	30	40	50	60	70	80

Images/s →

Fig. 7.28
Serial rating curves for a focal spot 0.6 mm, 40 kW, 150 Hz, with the series duration as a parameter, as a function of the filling factor, which corresponds to the ratio of pulse length to pulse interval.

Modern x-ray installations offer an indirect, but very reliable method using a tube load calculator. This system, apart from monitoring the current thermal state of the anode, checks whether for the given exposure settings there is a danger of overloading.

In normal radiography, it is the permitted focal spot temperature limit which usually determines the power limit for the exposure. In serial exposure operation or in pulsed cineradiography, in which a large number of exposures is made quickly one after another over a long period, one has in addition a power limitation due to the permitted basic anode temperature. The permitted load values as a function of series duration, number of exposures per second and the duration of a single exposure can be taken from the relevant diagrams (Fig. 7.28). It also applies here that at the beginning of a series, the thermal reference power of the anode for which the diagram was determined must not be exceeded.

7.1.2 Scattered radiation and its reduction

7.1.2.1 Effect of scattered radiation on the x-ray image

The effects of x-radiation described in chapter 3 lead in radiography to the occurrence of scattered radiation in the object to be imaged, viz. the patient. Because of this, a 'veil' of scattered radiation is superimposed on the absorption image. The scattered radiation extends over the whole area of the image and, roughly speaking, this means that there is an additional homogeneous exposure (with a flat peak in the middle of the format). This additional exposure leads to a reduction in contrast in the radiograph depending on the intensity of the scattered radiation. The radiation contrast without scattered radiation, i.e. the primary radiation contrast C_0, is by definition

$$C_0 = \frac{J_u - J_l}{J_u + J_l}$$

J_u Higher value of intensity
J_l Lower value of intensity

For small differences in intensity, this gives approximately

$$C_0 \approx \frac{\Delta J_p}{2 J_p}$$

J_p Primary radiation intensity

The contrast with scattered radiation C_m is given by adding the intensity of the scattered radiation J_s to the intensity of the primary radiation J_p:

$$C_m = \frac{\Delta J_p}{2J_p + 2J_s} \tag{7.13}$$

From this it follows that

$$C_m = C_0 \cdot \frac{J_p}{J_p + J_s} = C_0 \cdot \frac{1}{1 + \frac{J_s}{J_p}} \tag{7.14}$$

If, for instance, the scattered radiation intensity is equal to the primary radiation intensity, then the primary contrast is reduced by half.

On closer inspection it turns out that the contrast of a detail depends on its distance from the image recording system (Fig. 7.29). The contrast of detail A which lies close to the film is greater than that of the more distant detail B, because in the latter case much more scattered radiation is able to fall into the shadow of the detail [e.g. 7.14].

Fig. 7.30 shows the considerable difference in image contrast between radiographs with substantially different proportions of scattered radiation. The scattered radiation in Fig. 7.30 b was reduced by a highly efficient scattered radiation grid.

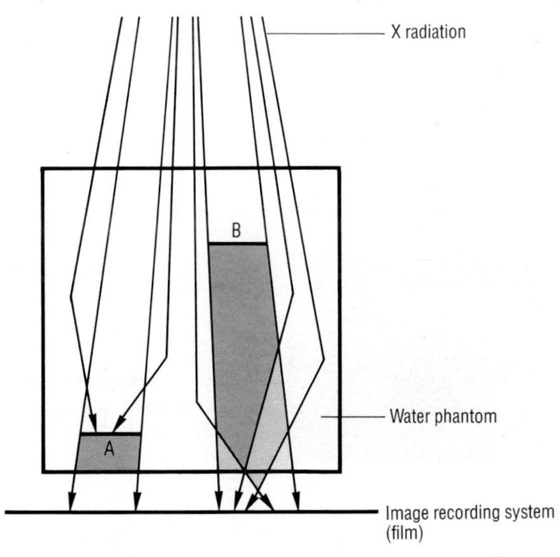

Fig. 7.29
Dependence of the contrast of a detail on its position in relation to the plane of the film

Fig. 7.30
Exposures of a pelvis phantom

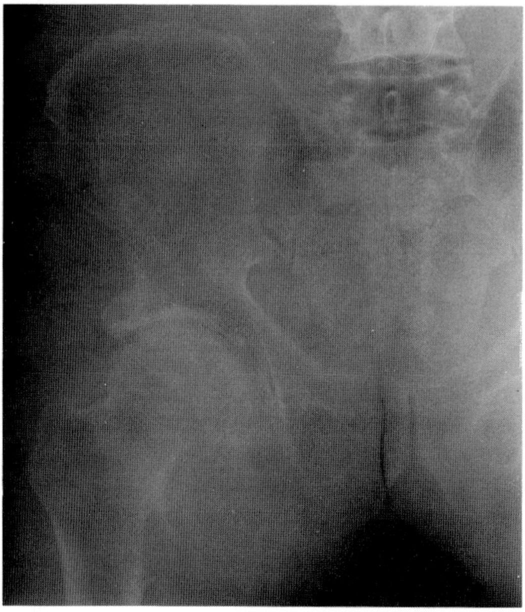

a) with a high proportion of scattered radiation and in consequence very blurred, 75 kV, without grid

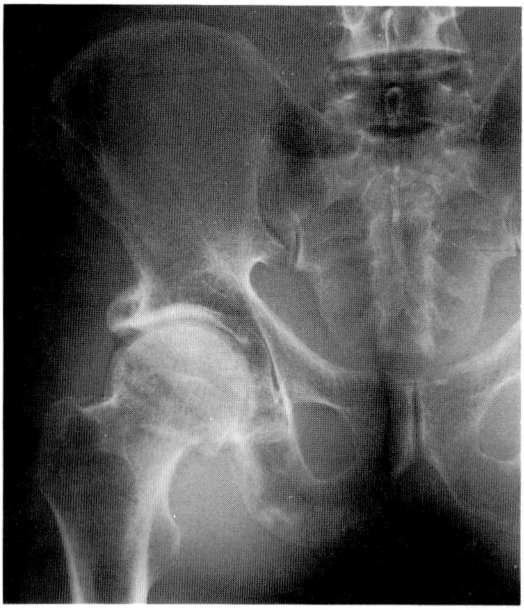

b) with a low proportion of scattered radiation, 75 kV, grid with grid ratio 12

7.1.2.2 Dependence of the percentage of scattered radiation on the beam parameters

The contrast-reducing effect of scattered radiation depends, as previously mentioned, on the ratio of scattered radiation to primary radiation. One frequently relates the percentage of scattered radiation P to the total radiation J_t:

$$P = \frac{J_s}{J_p + J_s} = \frac{J_s}{J_t} \tag{7.15}$$

How great is the percentage of scattered radiation? What does it depend on?

The view often put forward in the past that scattered radiation increases with tube voltage is not true in general. Fig. 7.31 shows that the percentage of

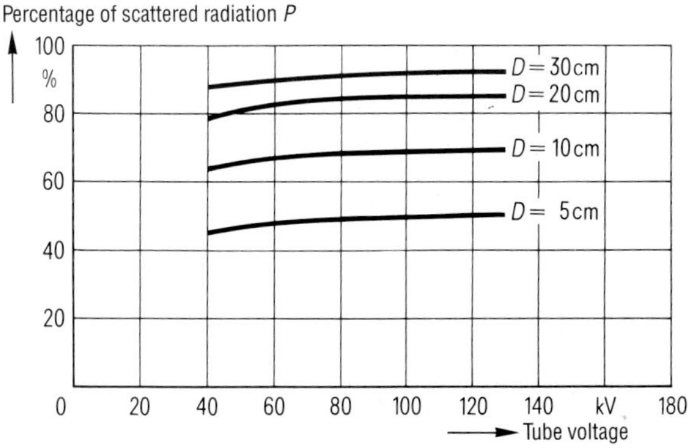

Fig. 7.31
Percentage P of scattered radiation in the total radiation J_t for various tube voltages and water phantom thicknesses D, field size 900 cm^2

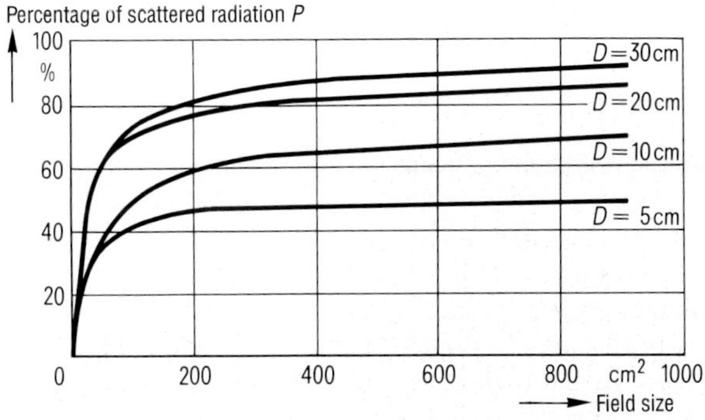

Fig. 7.32
Percentage P of scattered radiation in the total radiation j_t for a tube voltage of 100 kV, various field sizes and thicknesses of the water phantom (from [7.15])

Table 7.1
Scattered radiation proportions P and exposure lengthening factor V (using secondary radiation grids) for x-ray exposures of various parts of the body

Object	U_A	P	V(Pb 8/40)[1)]
Cranium p.-a.	70 kV	45%	2.6
Lung (average) p.-a.	120 kV	55%	2.6
Lung (thick) p.-a.	120 kV	65%	3
Bulbus p.-a.	80 kV	70%	4
Pelvis (average) p.-a.	80 kV	80%	5
Pelvis (thick) p.-a.	80 kV	85%	6
Pelvis from the side	80 kV	90 to 95%	7 to 8.5

[1)] The exposure lengthening factor V holds for a Pb 8/40 grid; for an explanation of V see 'Physical characteristics of grids' (page 257)

scattered radiation P is virtually constant in the voltage range important for diagnostics [7.15]. At most there is a slight increase in the percentage of scattered radiation with the tube voltage in the soft radiation range (20 to 40 keV).

It is easy to see that the percentage of scattered radiation must increase with the irradiated volume, i.e. with the size of the irradiated field and the thickness of the object. Fig. 7.32 illustrates the effect of the field size on the percentage of scattered radiation for water phantoms of varying thickness. It is noticeable that from a field size of 200 cm^2 onwards the scattered radiation virtually ceases to increase.

In Table 7.1, the percentages of scattered radiation are given for a few medical objects [7.16]. For exposures of the pelvis, for example, the scattered radiation, at about 85%, is by far the predominant contribution, whereas the contribution of the primary radiation producing the image only amounts to 15%!

7.1.2.3 Reduction of scattered radiation by means of compression and collimation

The large reduction in contrast brought about by scattered radiation necessitates appropriate measures to reduce it. Since the percentage of scattered radiation depends on the volume irradiated (see Fig. 7.32), it is advisable to keep the scattering volume small; this may be done by compression and collimation of the object to be imaged. In the case of larger field sizes and thicknesses of the object, the percentage of scattered radiation is nonetheless unacceptably high: one then has to ensure that, as far as possible, the resulting scattered radiation does not reach the image recording system.

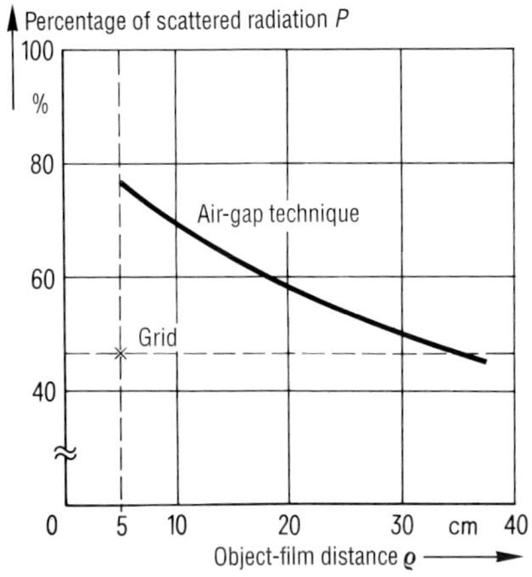

Fig. 7.33
Percentage of scattered radiation P as a function of object-film distance ϱ, water phantom 20 cm × 20 cm × 20 cm. The single measurement at $\varrho = 5$ cm holds when a secondary radiation grid is used.

7.1.2.4 Reduction of scattered radiation by increasing the distance

A well-known method for reducing scattered radiation is to use a greater distance, e.g. 30 cm, between the object and the image recording system. The scattered radiation emerging from the near object is reduced more strongly by this increase in distance than the primary radiation emerging from the more distant focal spot of the x-ray tube. From Fig. 7.33, one can see how the percentage of scattered radiation decreases with increasing object-film distance [7.17, 7.18]. Comparing this technique with the use of a scattered radiation grid (see section 7.1.2.5) shows that it only achieves the effectiveness of grids for large object-film distances. The limits of an enlarged object-film distance are set by the geometrical blurring and the x-ray tube rating.

Instead of air-gap technique, the term Groedel technique is often used. By this is meant more precisely an exposure technique where, apart from the object-film distance, the focus-object distance is also enlarged. It is still used in high-kV techniques for the lungs.

7.1.2.5 Reduction of scattered radiation by grids

The most important and most effective means of reducing scattered radiation is the focussed scattered radiation grid. It consists of thin absorber strips with spaces in between, covered above and below by a sheet which is as radiolucent as possible. By focussing this 'collimator system' on the focal spot of the x-ray tube, the primary radiation emerging from the focal spot is let through, but

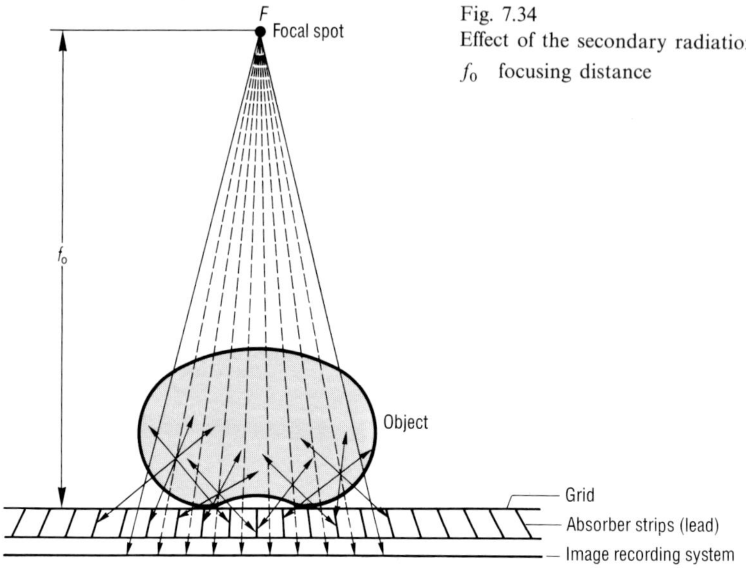

Fig. 7.34
Effect of the secondary radiation grid
f_0 focusing distance

the scattered radiation from the object hitting the absorber strips at various angles is largely absorbed (Fig. 7.34). The absorber strips consist mainly of lead, which has a high absorption capacity. The spacing material is usually paper or aluminum.

Geometrical grid characteristics

Important characteristics of the geometrical relationships in scattered radiation grids are the following (Fig. 7.35):

- *D* Width of the spacing material
- *d* Width of the absorber strips
- *h* Height of the absorber strips

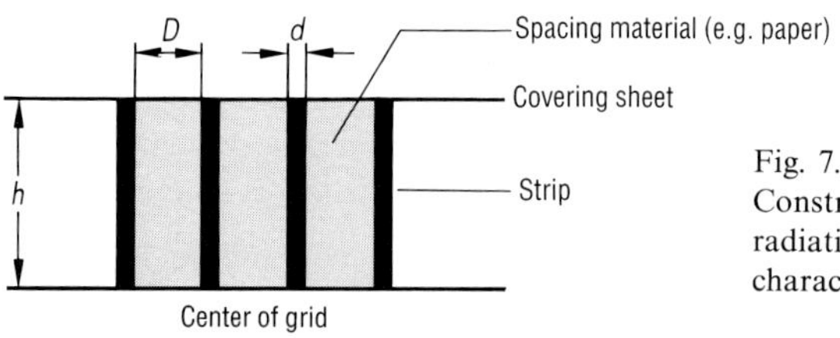

Fig. 7.35
Construction features of scattered radiation grids (geometrical grid characteristics)

From these basic data, the following quantities characterizing the grid properties may be derived [7.19]:

Grid ratio $r = \frac{h}{D}$,

Number of lines $N = \frac{1}{d+D}$ (7.16)

(Number of strips per unit of length)

Lead content $p = dhN\frac{1}{l_0}$ (7.17)

(Lead content per unit length l_0)

Some typical values for these:

The width d of the absorber strips for standard grids is around 0.07 mm, the width D of the spacing material, e.g. paper, around 0.18 mm, the height h of the strips 1.4 mm, for instance. These result in a grid ratio of $1.4{:}0.18 \approx 8$ and a number of lines N of $\frac{1}{0.18\,\text{mm} + 0.07\,\text{mm}} = 4$ lines/mm, or 40 lines/cm. The lead content for this grid is $0.07\,\text{mm} \cdot 1.4\,\text{mm} \cdot 4 \approx 0.4\,\text{mm}$ per 1 mm grid, i.e. 40%.

As can be seen from Fig. 7.36, the efficiency of the grid increases with increasing grid ratio because the angle of incidence for scattered radiation that will be admitted is reduced. However, mainly for practical reasons it does not make sense to raise the grid ratio beyond a certain level because this makes directing the grid onto the focal spot, i.e. focussing, increasingly difficult.

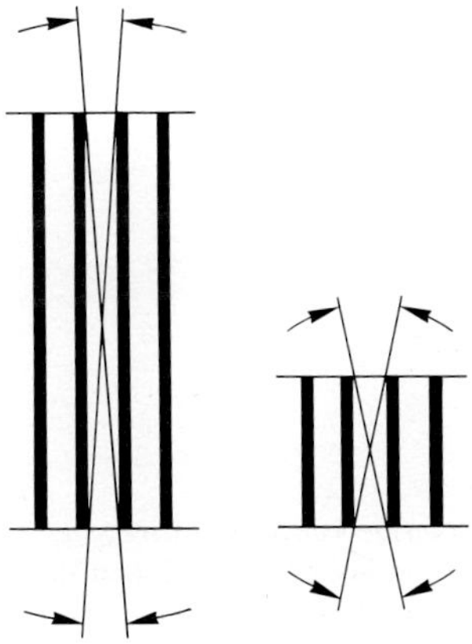

Fig. 7.36
Effect of the grid ratio on the angle of incidence of the scattered radiation

The number of lines per cm and the lead content are closely linked to the grid ratio. It is desirable to achieve a high number of lines per cm because then the image of the grid strips on the radiograph is less distracting. However, if by reducing *D* and *d* by half one were to go to twice the number of lines per cm, then, whilst it is true that one would have doubled the grid ratio, there would be the aformentioned drawbacks. The lead content in the two grids, and thus also their efficiency, would be the same. If we were then to halve the height of the strips, we would have the original grid ratio again, but the lead content would be reduced by half (Fig. 7.37). This means that the efficiency of the grid would be reduced since, other things being equal, a grid is more efficient the higher the lead content. If the lead content is reduced, either by altering the height or the width of the strips, the grid becomes more transparent to scattered radiation.

A further geometrical characteristic of the grid is the focussing. In a focussed grid, the strips are more or less inclined depending on the distance from the center (see Fig. 7.34). The extensions of the strips intersect in a straight line (in Fig. 7.34 perpendicular to the plane of the drawing) which passes through the focal spot *F*. The distance of this line of intersection from the plane of the grid is the focal distance *f*.

A grid only displays its optimum properties if the focal spot of the x-ray tube lies in this imaginary line of intersection.

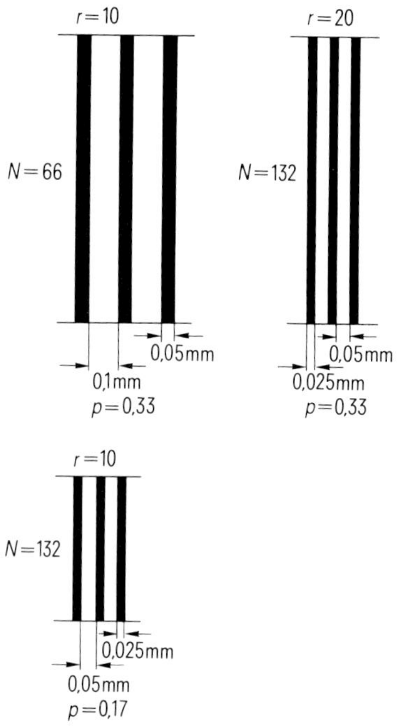

Fig. 7.37
Relationship between grid ratio *r*, number of lines per cm *N*, and lead content *p* (schematically)

Physical characteristics

Selectivity

The transmission of *primary radiation* T_p is the intensity of the primary radiation let through by the grid J_p' divided by the intensity of the primary radiation without a grid J_p, i.e.

$$T_p = \frac{J_p'}{J_p}. \tag{7.18}$$

The transmission of primary radiation may be found approximately from the grid geometry, from the width of the spacing material D, e.g. 0.18 mm, and from the width of the lead strips d, e.g. 0.07 mm, according to the formula $\frac{D}{d+D} = \frac{0.18}{0.25} = 0.72$, i.e. roughly 70%.

In the standard diagnostic voltage range, T_p only has a slight dependence on the tube voltage.

For the efficiency of grids it is important that the transmission of primary radiation is as great as possible (i.e. tending towards 1), whereas the transmission of *scattered radiation* $T_s = \frac{J_s'}{J_s}$ should be as small as possible (high absorption of the scattered radiation).

The aim is a large ratio

$$\Sigma = \frac{T_p}{T_s}. \tag{7.19}$$

Σ is called the *selectivity*. It is a measure of the efficiency of grids. A typical value for a good grid would be, for example, $\Sigma = 10$ (at 75 kV).

The introduction and measurement of physical characteristics such as selectivity is necessary because a grid is not sufficiently well described by its geometrical characteristics. These do not indicate the increasing permeability of the absorber strips to the harder radiation at increasing tube voltage or the technological difficulties such as the exact alignment of the strips [7.20].

The increasing permeability to radiation of the strips implies a decrease in selectivity. Fig. 7.38 shows this for grids with grid ratios of 8 and 12 [7.20]. The selectivity also depends on the grid ratio and on the strip width (or the lead content). Curve 3 in Fig. 7.38 refers to a grid with narrower lead strips. The stronger decline in selectivity is caused by the reduced absorption of scattered radiation with increasing tube voltage for narrower lead strips.

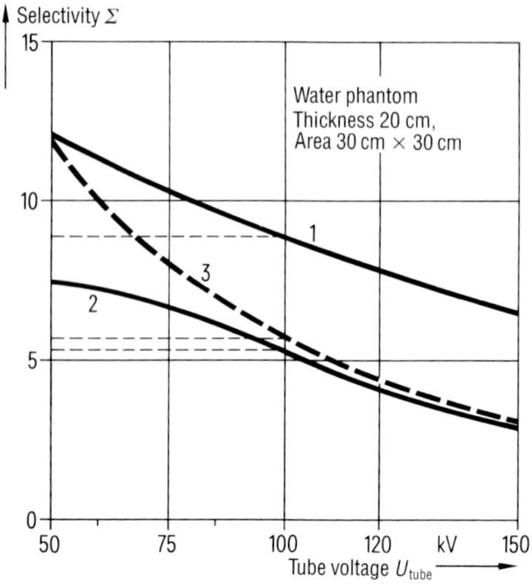

Fig. 7.38
Selectivity of various grids as a function of the tube voltage and the geometrical data

r Grid ratio (h/D)
d Width of the absorber strips

Grid 1: $r=12$, $d=0.07$ mm
Grid 2: $r=8$, $d=0.07$ mm
Grid 3: $r=12$, $d<0.07$ mm

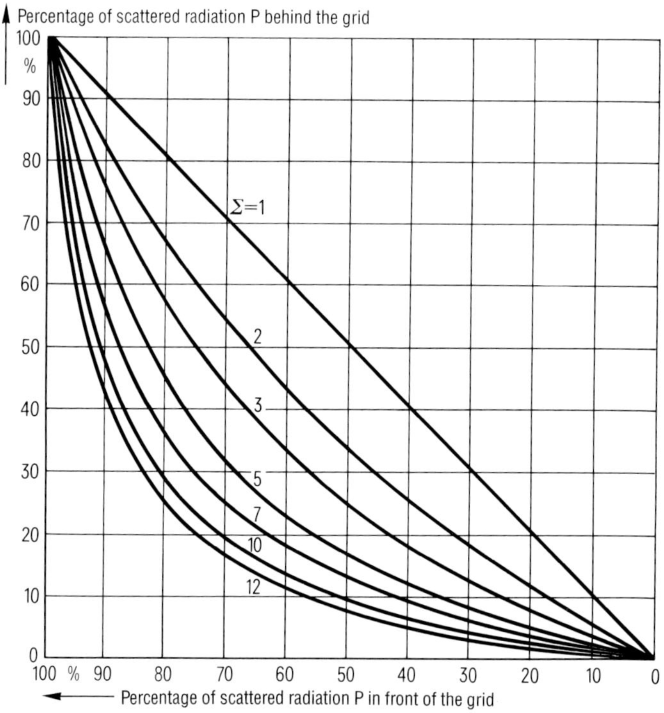

Fig. 7.39
Diagram for determining the reduction in scattered radiation by means of a grid of selectivity Σ

Fig. 7.39 shows how the percentage of scattered radiation P is reduced when using a grid with a higher selectivity Σ (e.g. for $\Sigma=12$, from 80% to 25%) [7.16].

Selectivity is one of the most important characteristics of a grid. Its measurement has been laid down in IEC- and DIN standards and its value should be given for 100 kV.

Contrast improvement ratio

It is useful to indicate the contrast enhancement due to grids by means of a contrast improvement ratio K. This is defined as

$$K=\frac{\text{contrast with grid}}{\text{contrast without grid}}$$

and one has

$$K=\frac{T_p}{T_t}. \tag{7.20}$$

T_t Transmission of total radiation

Compared to the selectivity, the contrast improvement ratio depends to a far greater degree on the dimensions of the phantom [7.20 to 7.22]. For a given phantom, there is a clear relationship with the selectivity.

Grid exposure factor

In x-ray diagnostics, an improvement in the image quality is often accompanied by a lengthening of the exposure time and thus inevitably by a higher dose for the patient. This is also the case with the use of scattered radiation grids: the reduction of the percentage of scattered radiation requires correspondingly more primary radiation in order to achieve the same optical density in the radiograph. A *grid exposure factor or Bucky factor V* is defined for grids as

$$V=\frac{\text{Intensity of the total radiation without grid}}{\text{Intensity of the total radiation with grid}}=\frac{J_t}{J_t'}=\frac{1}{T_t} \tag{7.21}$$

This lengthening of the exposure time (see Table 7.1) results for the various grids in the addition of between 4 and 6 to the exposure points in the familiar x-ray exposure tables. In this context, two aspects should be taken into account;

the scattered radiation absorption as well as

the primary radiation absorption due to the grid.

Example: Suppose the radiation emerging from the object consists of 80% scattered radiation and 20% primary radiation and that T_s is 0.05, T_p is 0.60 and thus $\Sigma = 12$, then one has:

	Scattered radiation	Primary radiation	Total radiation
Without grid	80%	20%	100%
With grid	4%	12%	16%

The necessary lengthening of exposure time is thus 100%/16% = 6.25; so apart from depending on the grid characteristics, the factor also depends on the ratio of scattered radiation to primary radiation. If the ratio of scattered radiation to primary radiation were 50:50, then for the same grid one would only need a threefold lengthening of the exposure time. The dependence of the grid exposure factor on the grid characteristics (T_p, Σ) and on the proportion of scattered radiation P may be represented by

$$V = \frac{1}{T_p} \cdot \frac{\Sigma}{\Sigma - P(\Sigma - 1)}. \tag{7.22}$$

The lengthening of exposure time made necessary by the grid is not a constant for specific grid data and specific tube voltage, but takes various values depending on the scattered radiation originating in the object.

The physical quantities of contrast improvement ratio, transmission of total radiation and Bucky factor are defined by the international standard IEC 627 – 1978. They were not, however, taken over for use in the German DIN standard 6826 because they depend strongly on the field size and thus are not to be regarded as grid characteristics but as technical specifications relating to exposures.

Application

The best practical application of different grids can only be touched upon here. In general, one uses a grid with a grid ratio of $r = 8$. For larger image fields, an improvement in image quality can be achieved with an acceptable lengthening of the exposure time by using grids with $r = 12$. Likewise grids with a large grid ratio are employed at higher tube voltages. If, because of a high percentage of scattered radiation, one has to make use of a grid for exposures of moving structures, the lengthening of the exposure time may be profitably compensated for by means of a correspondingly higher tube voltage. When using grids in spotfilm devices which have a variable focus-film distance, only grids with a grid ratio in the middle range can be employed because of defocussing [7.21, 7.22].

In order to avoid the distracting appearance of the grid strips on the image, grids with a number of lines up to about 50 lines/cm are in general moved perpendicularly to the direction of the strips.

Defocussing

A grid efficiency which is uniformly good over the field of the image is achieved by arranging the tube focal spot at the focal distance perpendicularly above the center of the grid. If the distance of the grid from the focal spot is not equal to the focal distance, then the strips towards the edge of the grid appear broader in the image, resulting in a reduction in blackening on the radiographs. This effect is more pronounced for higher grid ratios. In practice, deviations from the focal distance frequently cannot be avoided, e.g. in spotfilm devices. In these situations one tolerates (somewhat arbitrarily) a decrease in dose at the edge of 40%. From this, the permissible limits to application are obtained for a particular focal distance.

Example: Suppose a moving grid has a grid ratio 8, f_0 is 115 cm and the film width 40 cm. Experience shows that this implies a range of application of 95 to 150 cm focus-film distance.

Decentering

If the tube focal spot (with correct focussing) is not located over the center of the grid, all the absorber strips appear broader in the plane of the film. Besides the necessary lengthening of the exposure, the efficiency of the grid is reduced.

In the case of simultaneous decentering and defocussing, the uniform and lateral shadows are superimposed in an adverse manner (Fig. 7.40).

Other types of grid

Multiline grids

Technological advances in the manufacture of grids in recent years have made it possible to progress from 40 lines/cm, for a long time the standard number, to 60 to 70 lines/cm, whilst aluminum has come to be used as the main spacing material. The advantage of such grids lies in the fact that they do not have to be moved during the exposure; 70 lines/cm can only be detected in the image by using a magnifying glass. The selectivity and hence the image contrast are comparable to the corresponding quantities in the case of moving 40-line grids; as the number of lines per cm increase, however, higher grid ratios results because of the narrower lead strips and interspaces (see Fig. 7.37). Since, because

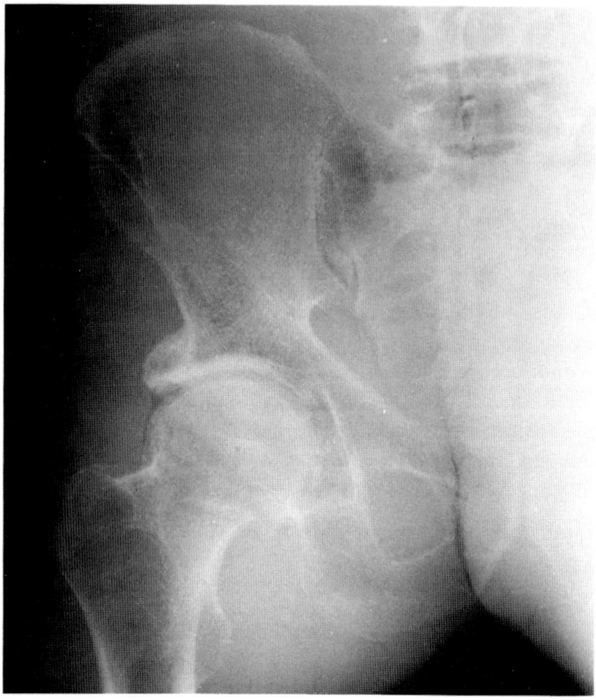

Fig. 7.40
Picture of a pelvis phantom using a grid with grid ratio 12 and focussing distance 115 cm; defocusing −15 cm, decentering 5 cm; 75 kV tube voltage

of the need to adjust the grid correctly in relation to the recording apparatus, the grid ratio cannot be enlarged ad infinitum, it is necessary to achieve a favorable balance between lead content and grid ratio. Roughly the same image contrast is obtained by replacing a standard Pb 8/40 grid by a 60-L to 70-L grid with grid ratio 12.

Parallel grids

In parallel grids the absorber strips are arranged in a parallel fashion, i.e. they are not focussed. Since the primary radiation radiates through the grid structure at an increasingly oblique angle towards the edge of the grid, this means there will be an increased shading towards the edge until finally at a certain angle no primary radiation at all can penetrate the channels between the absorber strips [7.14]. From this there results a certain minimum distance between the focal spot and the grid as well as a certain maximum field size. An advantage of the parallel grid is that it is insensitive to decentering.

Cross-grids

A cross-grid consists of two (focussed) grids lying on top of each other at right angles. The use of cross-grids, where each grid has a grid ratio of 8 or 12, allows high selectivity values (≈ 50), and thus high reduction of scattered radiation. However, this involves a large lengthening of exposure time, to which the reduced transmission of primary radiation due to the crossed strips also contributes. If one replaces a grid with grid ratio r by a cross-grid consisting of two grids each with a grid ratio of $r/2$, the efficiency of this cross-grid is slightly higher compared to the grid with grid ratio r. A disadvantage is that when using cross-grids it is always necessary to have a perpendicularly incident beam, whereas in the case of ordinary grids the tube focal spot may be shifted in the direction of the strips.

7.1.2.6 Reduction of scattered radiation by filters and slot diaphragms

Filters

A certain reduction of the scattered radiation can also be achieved in principle by means of homogeneous filters between the patient and the recording system. The effect of such filters is essentially based on the longer path which the scattered radiation has to traverse because of the fact that it usually hits the filter obliquely. To a small extent, the spectral distribution of the scattered radiation (slightly lower effective energy) is also responsible for the effect. The selectivity Σ of such filters is very low, about 1.5 to 2.0. This goes hand in hand with a low level of transmitted primary radiation, and thus with a large lengthening of exposure time [7.23].

Moving slot

If from a larger radiation field (e.g. 18 cm × 24 cm) one screens out a narrow slot (e.g. 0.5 cm × 18 cm) in front of and behind the object, the scattered radiation from this narrow slice through the object is very small (see e.g. [7.15, 7.24, 7.25]). The slot must then be moved across the field of the image for the duration of the exposure. In this process, however, the x-ray tube is subjected to a correspondingly higher load. An assembly of such slots, where the individual slots are sufficiently far apart from each other, offers an improved possibility (with respect to the tube load) of reducing scattered radiation (Fig. 7.41).

The slots can also be arranged radially on a rotating disk with its center of rotation outside the exposure field [7.26].

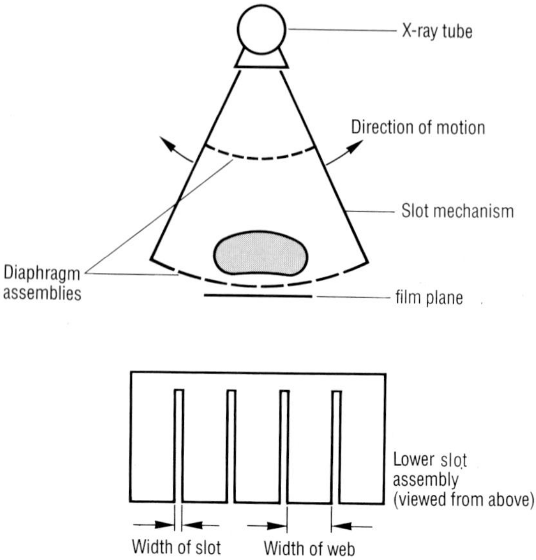

Fig. 7.41
Slot aperture mechanism for reducing scattered radiation

An advantage of this method of reducing scattered radiation is that there is no absorbing spacing material in the path of the radiation. The disadvantages should, however, not be overlooked: such systems are mechanically complicated, require more space, and the tube power must be increased by the ratio of the plate width to the slot width.

7.1.3 Intensifying screens, films, storage phosphor screens

X rays have such a high penetration capacity that when taking photographs only about 1% of the radiation received directly is absorbed by the emulsion layer of the film. In order to arrive at useful results in x-ray diagnostics a relatively high radiation dose would therefore be necessary. Since also those films used in x-ray technology possess a higher sensitivity to visible light, this dose can be substantially reduced if the x radiation is converted into visible light. This conversion is made possible by certain luminescent materials which are applied to screens; these then lie directly on top of the film during the exposure.

What is important for the conversion of the x radiation in a screen film system is the luminescence effect. By luminescence is meant an emission of light from a body, triggered by the supply of energy, without any heat being radiated off. This is called fluorescence if the luminescence rapidly dies away and phosphorescence if there is a lengthy afterglow. In the context of solid state physics, the band model is the standard model for the mechanism of luminescence in inorganic luminescent materials. These so-called crystal phosphors are fine crystalline substances which acquire their luminescent properties when foreign atoms, the activators, are systematically incorporated.

7.1.3.1 Intensifying screens

The films used nowadays, which are covered on both sides with a layer of photosensitive emulsion, are usually placed between two so-called intensifying screens. (This 'sandwich principle' was suggested by M. Levy as early as 1897). Due to the contact exposure on both sides achieved in this way, the luminescent images of the intensifying screens are transferred to the photosensitive layers of the film. Thus for an exposure the pair of intensifying screens contributes a total of 97% to the blackening of the film, i.e., the x radiation only directly contributes to 3% of the blackening.

By using intensifying screens the required x-ray dose in an exposure is reduced by a factor of 10 to 20 compared to an exposure without intensifying screens. Depending on the type of screen, this dose is in the region of 1.8 to 8 μGy in the plane of the cassette. In this way it has been possible to substantially reduce the patient's exposure to radiation.

Because of the shorter exposure times, kinetic blurring is also diminished. In addition, screen technology permits smaller focal spot dimensions in the x-ray tube, which also contributes to a greater image sharpness.

Screen composition

Nowadays, without exception, 250 μm thick polyester films serve as the base for the luminescent layer. Some screens have a thin aluminum layer on the back, which prevents the build-up of static charge.

The luminescent layer is made out of x-ray-luminescent materials whose spectrum is matched to the x-ray films in question. As a binder for the luminescent materials, synthetic resin with a very high transparency is used. The proportion of binder in intensifying screens amounts on average to 10% of the weight of the luminescent materials. The grain sizes of the luminescent materials are between 3 and 10 μm. Depending on the intensifying effect, the thickness of

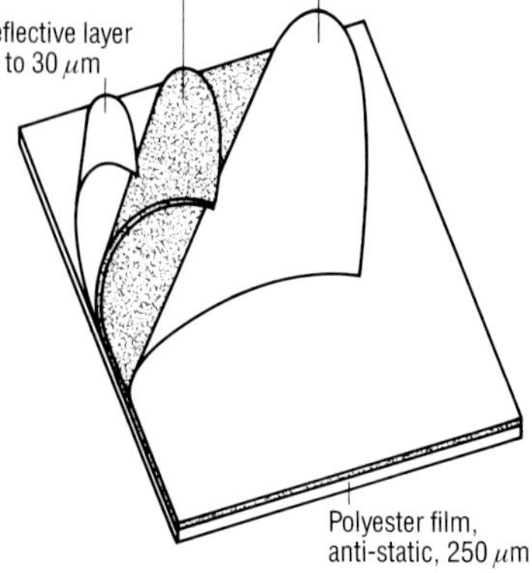

Fig. 7.42
Composition of the layers in an intensifying screen

the luminescent layer is 0.1 to 0.3 mm, which corresponds to a coating of luminescent material of about 30 to 90 mg/cm^2.

In high-speed screens, the luminescent layer is provided with a good reflective background. In high-definition and less strongly intensifying screens the background consists of a layer which absorbs the fluorescent light. The surface of the luminescent layer is protected by a 10 to maximally 15 μm thick protective layer made of a very robust, highly transparent synthetic resin. On account of the image sharpness this protective layer must be as thin as possible.

Fig. 7.42 gives a schematic view of the composition of an intensifying screen.

Luminescent materials

The oldest x-ray-luminescent material for intensifying screens, and one still frequently used nowadays, is calcium tungstate, which was described by Edison [7.28] as long ago as 1896. Under x radiation it has a violet luminescence. The luminescence is brought about by the tungstate doping. Calcium tungstate is a so-called 'pure phosphor' because it does not need activation by foreign atoms. All the other x-ray-luminescent materials listed in Table 7.2 are, however, activated by foreign atoms, especially by rare earths.

The luminescent substances used for intensifying screens have to satisfy the following requirements:

1. highly efficient absorption of x radiation (absorption efficiency),
2. highly efficient conversion of x radiation into visible light (conversion efficiency),
3. an emission spectrum which corresponds to the spectral sensitivity of x-ray films,
4. an emission yield which is as constant over time as possible,
5. an afterglow which is as short as possible.

Of the large number of luminescent materials in use today, only a few were known as x-ray-luminescent materials up to 1969. It was not until after 1972 that a number of new and very efficient x-ray-luminescent materials came to be used (Table 7.2).

Following the successes with rare earths in the sixties with luminescent materials for television, this development continued in the seventies with rare earth compounds for x-ray-luminescent materials. The oxysulfides and oxyhalogenides of lanthanum and gadolinium, in particular, exhibit a higher absorption of x radiation than the previously used calcium tungstate.

The decisive factor leading to their use, however, was their greater efficiency of light emission compared to calcium tungstate. All the x-ray-luminescent materials listed in Table 7.2 are used today in the manufacture of intensifying screens.

It is important for the user to distinguish luminescent materials according to their color of emission, blue (violet, blue-white) or green. Whereas in Europe the emphasis lay for a long time on screens emitting blue light, it appears that here too, as in the USA, screens emitting green light are becoming increasingly popular.

Table 7.2 X-ray-luminescent materials for intensifying screens

Year	Luminescent material	Color of emission	Emission Peak
1896	$CaWO_4$	Blue	420 nm
1949	$(Ba, Pb)SO_4$	Violet	358 nm
1969	LaOBr:Tb	Blue	418, 439 nm
1972	$(BaSr)SO_4$:Eu	Violet	380 nm
1972	Y_2O_2S:Tb	Blue-white	415, 418, 436, 440, 545, 622 nm
1975	BaFCl:Eu	Violet	385 nm
1972	La_2O_2S:Tb	Green	545 nm
1972	Gd_2O_2S:Tb	Green	545 nm

Physical properties of intensifying screens

Intensification factor

The intensification factor (speed) is the numerical value for the effect of intensifying screens on the film. It is defined by the ratio of two exposures B_1/B_2. B_1 is the x-ray exposure which is required to produce an optical density (blackening of the film) above base fog of OD = 1 using a standard screen combination. B_2 is the exposure which one needs to achieve the same optical density of the film as with B_1 using the screen combination under consideration.

Occasionally the exposure factor is given instead of the intensification factor. It represents the reciprocal value of the intensification factor. If, for instance, a screen combination X has the relative intensification factor 2 compared to a reference combination Y, its relative exposure factor is 0.5, i.e. to achieve the same optical density on the film X requires half the x-ray exposure. When indicating the intensification factor, all screen manufacturers always base this on one of their types of screens, usually on their universal screen. The intensification factor of an intensifying screen is affected by the following factors:

the type of luminescent material,
the thickness of the luminescent layer (mg/cm^2),
the proportion of reflected light,
the grain size of the luminescent material,
the transparency of the binder, and
the quality of the radiation.

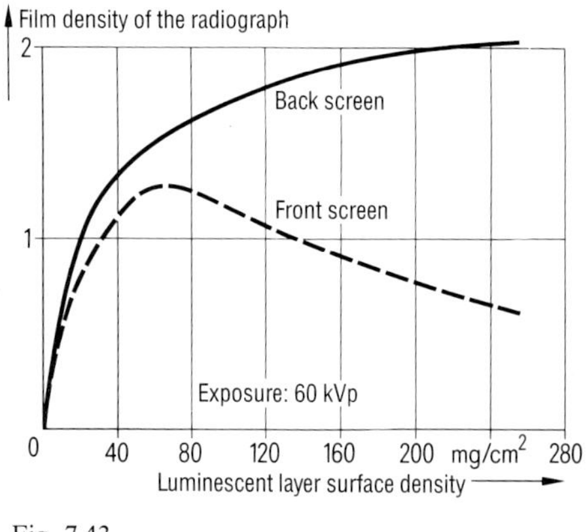

Fig. 7.43
Effect of the thickness of the luminescent layer on the film density of the radiograph

In Fig. 7.43 the optical densities of radiographs taken at 60 kV have been plotted for various thicknesses of the luminescent layer of the screens.

It can be seen that the front screen can be adjusted to have a luminescent layer of optimal thickness. This is because an increase in the thickness leads to a greater absorption of the luminescence in the screen. The relationship between luminescent luminance L and the thickness of the luminescent layer d was described by Gasper [7.29] and Hamaker [7.30].

For the luminance of the front screen L_{VD} one has

$$L_{VD} = \frac{\alpha J_0 \mu}{\mu - K}(e^{-Kd} - e^{-\mu d}). \qquad (7.23)$$

while for the luminance of the luminescent layer of the back screen L_{HD} one has

$$L_{HD} = \frac{\alpha J_0 \mu}{\mu + K}(1 - e^{-(\mu + K)d}). \qquad (7.24)$$

J_0 Dose of incident x radiation
d Thickness of the luminescent layer (coating)
μ Attenuation coefficient of the x radiation
K Attenuation coefficient for the screen light
α Conversion efficiency of x-ray quanta into light quanta

In the latter case, therefore, the optical density of the radiograph (i.e. the intensification due to the screen) increases with increasing thickness of the coating of the back screen.

The two equations (7.23) and (7.24) show that the intensifying effect may be heightened by using types of luminescent substance with a high emission efficiency α and by increasing the thickness of the luminescent layer. Apart from this, minimizing the proportion of binder (reduction of the light absorption) and introducing a light-reflective layer behind the luminescent layer have a positive effect on the sensitivity of intensifying screens.

Image sharpness (spatial resolution)

The resolution of the intensifying screen is of great importance for the perceptibility of detail in a radiograph. Besides this, the properties of the cassette, i.e. the close contact between the film and screen, are very important for good image sharpness.

When considering the MTF, this means that the closer the MTF approaches the value 1 in the spatial frequency range, the better is the image sharpness of an intensifying screen (Fig. 7.44).

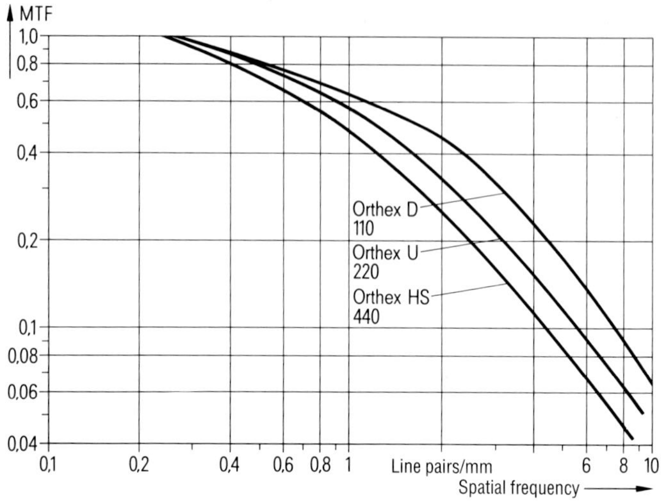

Fig. 7.44
Modulation transfer function (MTF) of Siemens ORTHEX intensifying screens (75 kV, 22 mm aluminum, Ortho-G film)

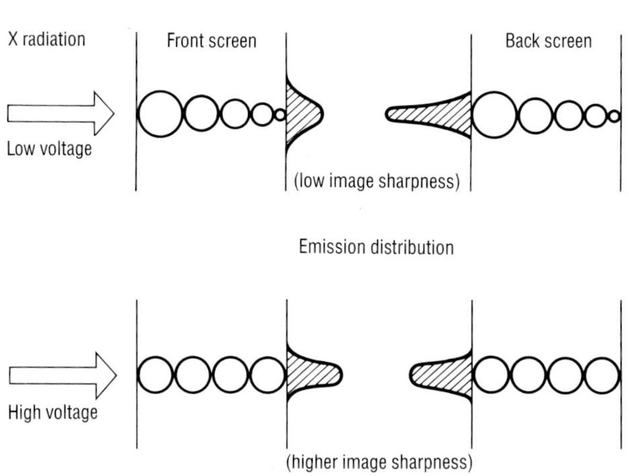

Fig. 7.45
Values of the voltage and emission distribution of luminescent layers (front and back screens have the same thickness)

Listed below are those factors which contribute to an increase in the resolution of the screen:

a thin luminescent layer,

the use of small luminescent crystals,

the avoidance of reflected light at the boundary between luminescent layer and the screen base, best achieved by means of a light-absorbent layer,

the addition of dyes, which reduce lateral scattering of light,

a protective layer which is as thin and transparent as possible.

Apart from the final point, however, all the other factors reduce the intensifying effect of the screen. Thus in order to achieve the greatest possible reduction in dose precisely the opposite properties are relevant.

The intensifying effect and the image sharpness depend on each other in such a way that an increase in one parameter is at the expense of the other. The thickness of the luminescent layer will serve as an example. Increasing the thickness improves the intensifying effect, but at the same time makes the image sharpness worse. In order to cover the entire spectrum of diagnostic tasks, one uses several types of intensifying screens in radiology which are designed with very particular areas of application in mind:

▻ high-definition intensifying screens, which relatively speaking have the least intensifying effect, but allow the imaging of finest details;

▻ high-speed screens with the smallest resolving power to achieve the shortest exposure times;

▻ and finally universal screens, which represent a compromise with respect to intensifying effect and image sharpness.

In particular cases the image sharpness can be influenced by an appropriate adjustment of the radiation quality (kV) values. First consider the distribution of emitted light in an intensifying screen after the absorption of x radiation. The thicker the layer, the weaker the intensity of the x radiation and hence the weaker the partial luminance of the light generated by the intensifying screen. The circles in Fig. 7.45 represent a measure of the partial luminance, and the shaded area indicates the emission distribution. The steeper the sides, the sharper the x-ray image. The shape of the sides, however, depends precisely on how much light from the crystals furthest from the film gets through to the film.

From this one may draw the fundamental conclusion that for a softer radiation quality, the back screen exhibits a sharper emission distribution than the front screen. For harder radiation, on the other hand, the difference in the emission distribution between front and back screen is slight. This has the effect that higher tube voltages yield sharper images.

Fig. 7.44 shows the characteristic spectrum of the new green-sensitive Siemens ortho screens with the MTF and the corresponding intensification factors (speed classes) and dose requirement for an optical density of OD = 1 above base fog.

The combined unsharpness of a radiograph is made up of the geometric unsharpness, the kinetic blurring and the screen-film unsharpness. The geometric unsharpness can be kept small by using a small focal spot and maintaining a large focus-film distance. The kinetic blurring can be reduced by means of a 'fast' intensifying screen (screen with the highest intensification). Some unsharpness, albeit slight, arises because of the absorption and scattering of

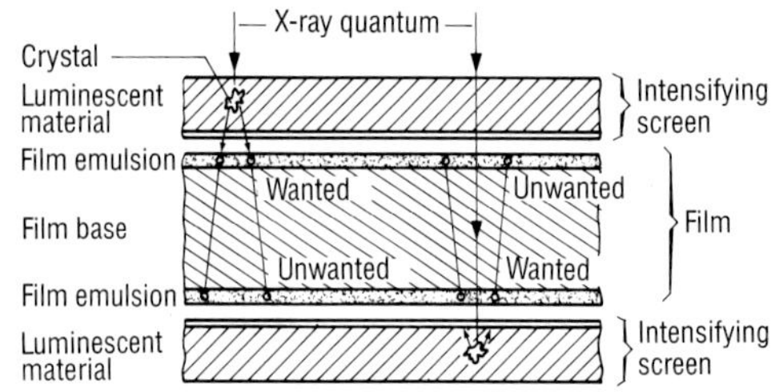

Fig. 7.46
Cross-over effect: unwanted exposure of the opposite film emulsion

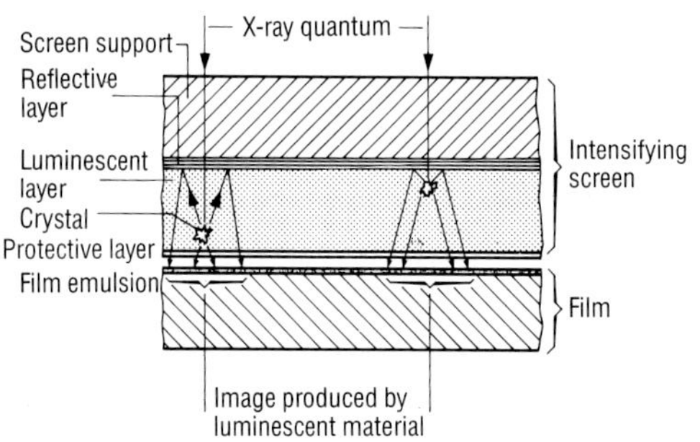

Fig. 7.47
Halation effect in an intensifying screen with reflective layer

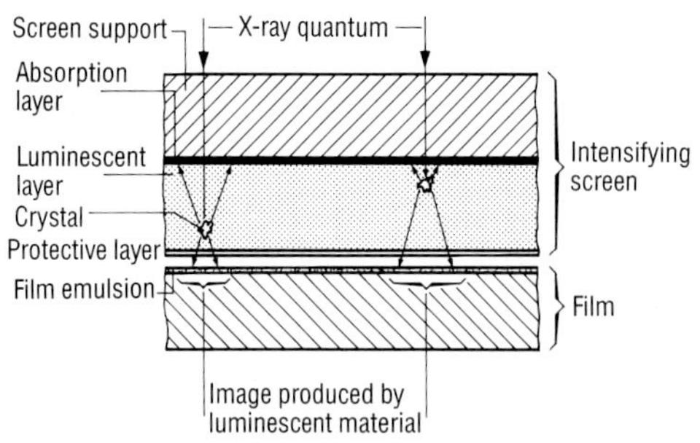

Fig. 7.48
Improved picture sharpness due to intensifying screen with absorption layer

x radiation in the front of the cassette. A further factor contributing to unsharpness is the protective layer of the intensifying screens. A thick protective skin on the luminescent layer of the screen has the same effect on the unsharpness as a poor contact of the screen with the film. In the so-called cross-over effect, blurring comes about through the light of the opposite intensifying screen penetrating the x-ray film or being scattered in the film (Fig. 7.46).

No other parameter, however, produces such a large amount of unsharpness as a thick luminescent layer. With increasing layer thickness, there is also an increase in the scattering of light within the luminescent layer. The luminescence which is radiated by a crystal spreads in all directions. On its way through the luminescent layer, which consists of the three media of luminescent crystal, binder and air, the image producing ray is repeatedly refracted and deflected. In addition, unsharpness arises due to the reflection of the luminescence at the reflective layer (Fig. 7.47). Fig. 7.48 shows the gain in sharpness if this layer is colored black (absorption layer).

Noise

Apart from the image unsharpness, the image quality of radiographs is primarily lowered by statistical disturbances. In high-speed and universal screens, the statistical variations in optical density are mainly caused by the spatially random distribution of the x-ray quanta absorbed in the screen (quantum noise). The proportion of the noise due to the film is negligible here.

In high-definition screens, i.e. those with a thin layer, the so-called grain noise contributes considerably to the total noise. Here, there arises in the first place an uneven, grainy optical density as a consequence of statistical fluctuations in the density of the crystals in the luminescent layer. This can also be caused by differences in the light given off by individual luminescent crystals as well as by grain agglomerations. The second, not inconsiderable source of noise in this case is the grain noise caused by the film. This cannot be neglected especially at high doses, where the quantum noise is reduced because of the large number of absorbed x-ray quanta. In general, however, one can assume that quantum noise is the predominant source of noise in screen-film systems.

The noise may be registered quantitatively by measuring the Wiener spectrum, which describes the noise amplitudes as a function of the spatial frequency. A detailed description can be found in the publications [7.31 to 7.33]. What is important for the radiologist is the relationship between the measured quantity of the Wiener spectrum and the visual impression of noise on the part of the observer. Doi et al. [7.31] have shown that in the Wiener spectrum, roughly speaking, the frequency range between 0.2 and 1 line pairs/mm is relevant. These frequencies are registered visually by the observer and the corresponding spectral values subjectively judged as having ‘more noise’ or ‘less noise’ according to their magnitude.

It is expedient to discuss the dependence of quantum noise on screen and film parameters. To a rough approximation the Wiener spectrum (WS) can be represented by the relationship [7.31];

$$WS(\nu)=\frac{G^2}{\bar{n}}|MTF(\nu)|^2. \tag{7.25}$$

Here $\bar{n}$ is the average number of absorbed x-ray quanta in the screen per unit area. G is the gradient of the characteristic blackening curve of the film (for the gradient, or gamma, see section 7.1.3.2) at OD = 1, and MTF is the modulation transfer function. The consequences of Eq. (7.25) fit in with the experience of radiologists when changing the film or the screen in the screen film system (SFS). For given x-ray exposure conditions, changing the film gradient (by the use of a different film type) or the conditions of development results in a Wiener spectrum which is proportional to the gradient.

Likewise a change in the speed class (sensitivity class) of the SFS has, brought about by the different absorption of the x radiation, an effect on the impression of noise. Thus, the noise is increased by a factor of 2 if the sensitivity class of the film is increased by the same factor, since in this case only half the x-ray quanta are radiated and absorbed.

Screen requirements

At present, intensifying screens may be divided up into conventional screens and rare-earth screens according to the luminescent materials used. A typical example of a conventional screen is the calcium tungstate screen, whereas for rare-earth screens, which were first introduced in 1973 [7.34], oxysulfide compounds of gadolinium, yttrium and lanthanum are used with terbium and europium as activators.

The requirements which intensifying screens should fulfil can essentially be summarized in three key points. The differences between various types of screen will be discussed in the context of these requirements:

1. Maximum capacity to absorb x radiation for a good DQE (detective quantum efficiency) and low quantum noise.
2. Maximum conversion of the absorbed x-ray energy into visible light for a good intensifying effect and reduction of dose.
3. Spectral matching of the film and screen for reduction of dose.

Absorption properties

Conventional screens differ from rare-earth screens with respect to their relative absorption of x rays, their efficiency in converting x-ray energy into visible light and the spectral characteristics of their emission distribution.

Fig. 7.49 shows a comparison of the relative absorption of x radiation of various common intensifying screens as a function of the x-ray energy. In physical terms the absorption of x rays grows with the atomic number of the luminescent materials, whilst the rare-earth luminescent materials such as Gd_2O_2S and LaOBr have the advantage that their maximum absorption capacity is very

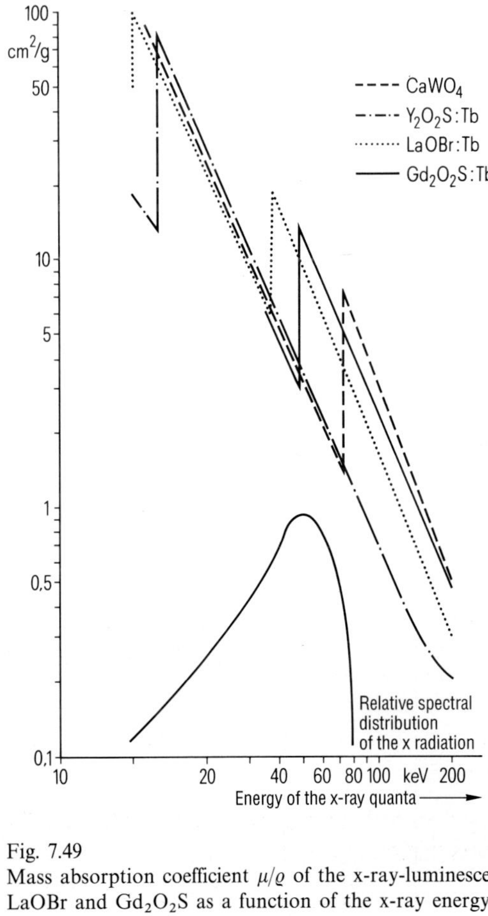

Fig. 7.49
Mass absorption coefficient μ/ϱ of the x-ray-luminescent materials $CaWO_4$, Y_2O_2S, LaOBr and Gd_2O_2S as a function of the x-ray energy

well matched to the relative spectral distribution of the x radiation used in diagnostics. This holds true most of all for Gd_2O_2S, where the K absorption edge is around 50 keV.

Yttrium oxysulfide, whose K-edge lies at 17 keV, is less favorable in this respect. The K-edge for calcium tungstate, at around 70 keV, still just overlaps with the intensity distribution of the x radiation. The x-ray absorption efficiency as a function of the x-ray energy is summarized once again in Table 7.3 for screens 100 μm thick made of various luminescent substances. Here it can clearly be seen that given almost equal resolution of the screens, the absorption and hence the DQE are very different. This then results in very different characteristics with respect to image quality.

Regarding the absorption of x radiation, gadolinium oxysulfide (Gd_2O_2S:Tb) exhibits roughly the same efficiency as the conventional calcium tungstate ($CaWO_4$) material at x-ray energies up to about 40 keV and above 70 keV. In the range in between, the absorption climbs steeply and causes a high DQE and comparatively low noise.

Conversion into light

With respect to the dose requirement, the last column of Table 7.3 is decisive. Here the rare-earth screens with their high conversion efficiency of x-ray energy into visible light quanta demonstrate a clear advantage over $CaWO_4$. Together with the high absorption of x radiation, this is the reason why Gd_2O_2S:Tb screens require a dose which is almost by a factor of 3 smaller than for $CaWO_4$ screens in order to obtain radiographs of the same image sharpness or noise values [7.35].

The emission spectra of the rare-earth luminescent materials are characterized by individual sharp peaks whose position and height depend on the type of

Table 7.3
X-ray absorption percentage of three intensifying screens each with 100 μm layer thickness at three different x-ray energies and their conversion of x-ray energy into visible light

Intensifying screens	x-ray absorption in a 100 μm screen at			Efficiency of light emission
	40 keV	60 keV	80 keV	
	%	%	%	
$CaWO_4$	33	13	27	4
Y_2O_2S:Tb (Titan 2)	32	12	5	24
Gd_2O_2S:Tb (ORTHEX)	37	51	28	19

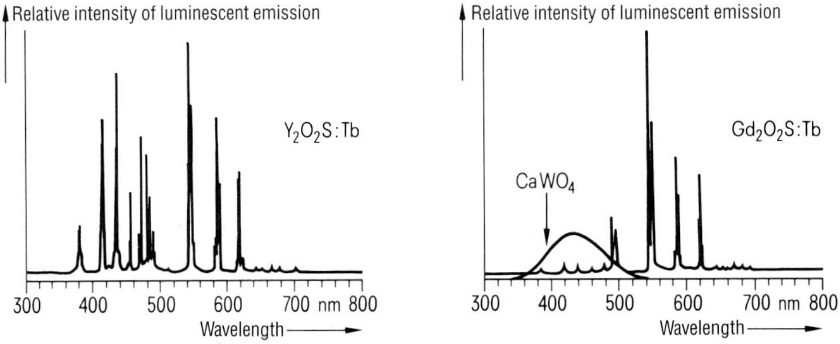

Fig. 7.50
Spectral distribution of three important types of intensifying screen

basic material and activator. The differences in the spectral emission distribution for three important types of screen are shown in Fig. 7.50. On the basis of these emission spectra one distinguishes between blue and green-sensitive screen-film systems. Intensifying screens which emit blue light with luminescent materials such as $CaWO_4$, Y_2O_2S:Tb, LaOBr:Tb or BaFCl:Eu are used to-

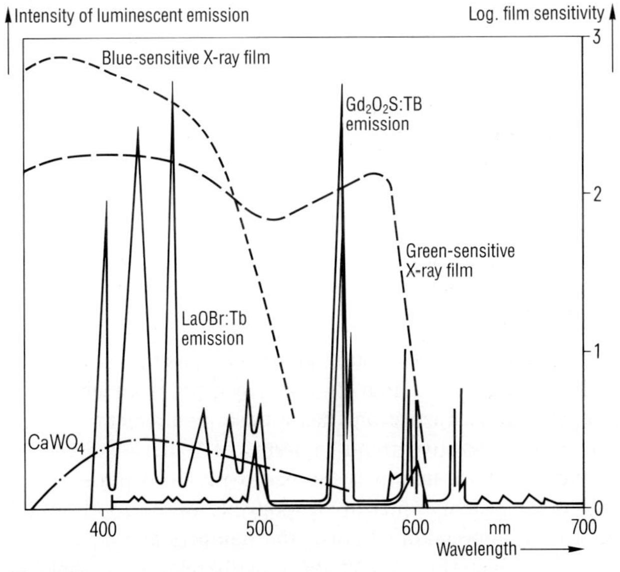

Fig. 7.51
Spectral emission of $CaWO_4$, LaOBr, Gd_2O_2S and their matching to the x-ray film in question

gether with blue-sensitive films whilst screens emitting green light such as Gd_2O_2S:Tb screens are used with orthochromatic films.

Matching to the film

Achieving optimum optical density in a radiograph also involves matching the spectral emission of the intensifying screens to the x-ray film in question, and vice versa (Fig. 7.51). The screen manufacturers are concerned to make their types of screens universal so that they can be used for as many types of film as possible. The blue-sensitive, conventional x-ray films commonly used hitherto are now increasingly being joined by green-sensitized x-ray films which are used in conjunction with the green-luminescent rare-earth screens, in particular gadolinium oxysulfide screens. In high-speed film-screen combinations, efforts are being made nowadays to reduce the graininess of the image and the quantum noise of the radiographs by using very fine-grained x-ray films. The quantum noise can also be suppressed by using less sensitive x-ray films at the expense of the intensifying effect. Thus, the palette of films on offer ranges from highly sensitive x-ray films with somewhat more noise to less sensitive films with the finest grain and reduced noise.

Siemens intensifying screens

The basic physical data for x-radiation absorption and conversion into light shown in Fig. 7.49 and Table 7.3 are reflected in the specifications of the corresponding intensifying screens. Thus, the comparison of Siemens intensifying screen systems in Fig. 7.52 shows the differences in dose requirement for OD = 1 (ordinate, spatial resolution abscissa) and noise values (at the tops of the bars) between $CaWO_4$, Titan 2 (Y_2O_2S:Tb) and ORTHEX screens (Gd_2O_2S:Tb) for three models respectively: high-speed, universal and high-definition.

The results shown there make obvious sense: $CaWO_4$ screens have the largest dose requirement because of the low absorption and light emission values mentioned in Table 7.3. In contrast, the Titan 2 system benefits from its higher light yield (24%) here; as a consequence one has a dose requirement reduced by about a factor of 2. This positive trend in terms of 'radiation hygiene' is continued in the Orthex system; here it is the best x-ray absorption values in comparison with the other systems which are responsible for the good specifications. With respect to the impression of noise, the numbers above the bars indicate the values of the Wiener spectrum at the visually relevant spatial frequency of 0.6 line pairs/mm. These directly reflect the absorption ratios of the three luminescent materials from Table 7.3.

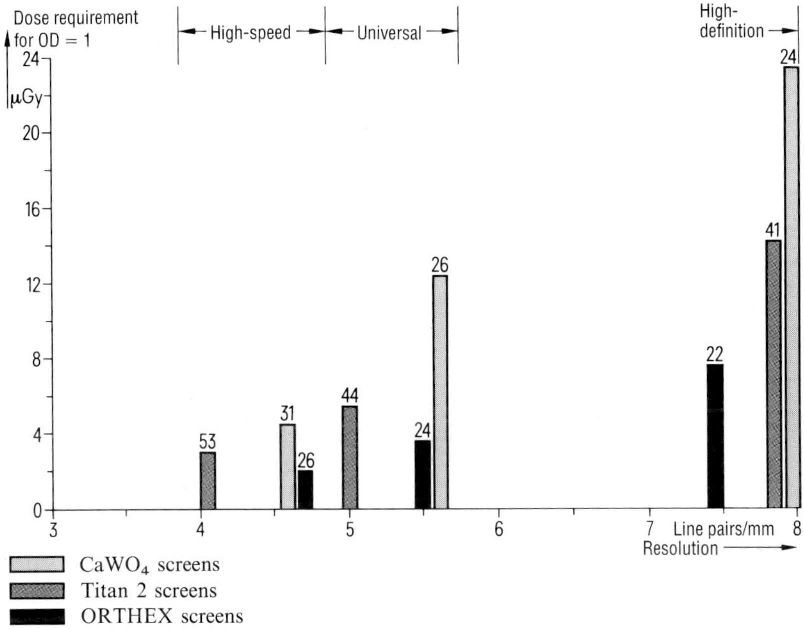

Fig. 7.52
Dose requirement and resolving power of Siemens intensifying screens (The numbers above the bars give the values of the noise amplitudes of the Wiener spectrum at 0.6 line pairs/mm in units of 10^{-6} mm^2)

Using high-speed rare-earth screens offers the following advantages:

- ▻ a lower dose requirement for the patient
- ▻ reduced kinetic blurring through shorter exposure times
- ▻ gains in spatial resolution and image sharpness through reduction of the focal spot size.

7.1.3.2 Films

The most important component when taking photographic exposures in x-ray diagnostics, the film, makes it possible to record as an image the varying intensities of rays which have passed through an object (after converting them into visible radiation). To sensitize the film, silver halides are used. Since their discovery more than 140 years ago they have remained the first choice amongst photosensitive substances because of their simplicity of use, their stability during storage and their reproducibility.

Composition of the film

A diagram of the composition of an x-ray film is shown in Fig. 7.53.

As a rule, x-ray films are provided on both sides with a photosensitive emulsion. This consists of a suspension of silver bromide crystals in gelatine. If such

Table 7.4
Differences between conventional black-and-white films and x-ray films

	Properties	Conventional black-and-white film	Medical x-ray film (cutfilm)
Structure	Thickness of photo-sensitive layer	15 to 20 μm	5 to 9 μm
	Coating	single-coated	double-coated
	Thickness of base	100 to 200 μm	170 to 200 μm
	Backing	present	not present
	Color of base	colorless	blue
Performance	Sensitivity ASA/ISO	100/21°	60/19° to 80/20°
	Contrast (Y)	0.7 to 0.9	2.5 to 3.0
	Grain	0.6 to 0.8 μm	2.0 to 2.3 μm
	Color sensitivity	panchromatic	orthochromatic or blue-sensitive
	Resolution	70–120 lines/mm	40 lines/mm
	Tone of silver	medium gray to pure black	pure black
Processing	Type of developer	fine grain developer	highly active developer
	Developing temperature	20 °C	20 to 35 °C
	Developing time	8 to 10 minutes	24 s to 5 min
	Fast processing system	not available	available
	Object contrast	1:32 to 60	1:5 to 8

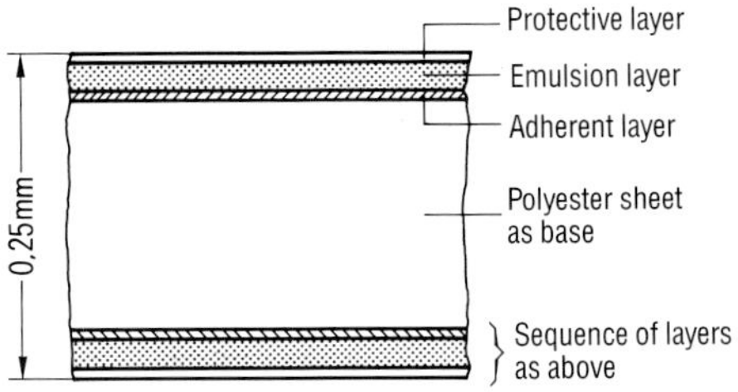

Fig. 7.53 Composition of a double-coated x-ray film

an x-ray film is placed between two intensifying screens, both sides of the film are exposed during irradiation by the luminescence of the intensifying screens.

When the film emulsions are subjected to the luminescence, the silver bromide particles absorb energy. On introducing the film into a reducing medium the exposed silver bromide crystals are reduced to metallic silver, the density of the crystals being greatest at those places which have absorbed the greatest amount of energy. Metallic silver is opaque and, finely distributed, causes the blackening of the film. Table 7.4 lists the differences between conventional black-and-white film and x-ray film.

Optical density (blackening) of the film and gradation

The optical density S is defined as the logarithm to the base 10 of the ratio of the intensity J_0 of the incident light to the intensity J_1 of the transmitted light:

$$S = \log \frac{J_0}{J_i} = \log J_0 - \log J_1 . \tag{7.26}$$

If, for instance, 1/10 of the incident light is let through, this gives an optical density of 1; if 1/100 is let through, the optical density is 2.

The blackening characteristic, also known as the gradation characteristic, is shown in Fig. 7.54. It clarifies the relation between the exposure E and the resulting optical density S. By exposure is meant the product of the intensity of illumination and the exposure time. The logarithm to the base 10 of the exposure $\log E$ is plotted along the abscissa, and the optical density S along the ordinate.

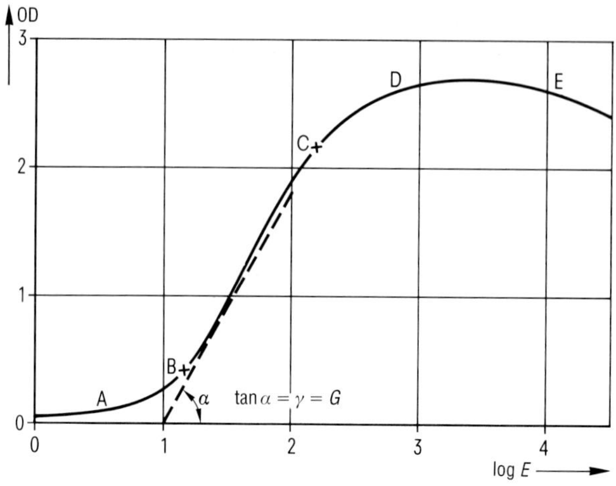

Fig. 7.54
Film density curve with respect to the exposure E (relative units)

Table 7.5
Factors affecting contrast in radiographs
Logarithm of the object contrast[1] × film contrast = x-ray image contrast

Logarithm of the object contrast[1]	large	←	Thickness difference in object	→	small
	low	←	Kilovoltage	→	high
	small	←	Amount of scattered radiation	→	large
	thin	←	Filter	→	thick
	yes	←	Lead film	→	no
	yes	←	Movable secondary radiation grid	→	no
	high	←	Total contrast	→	low
Film contrast	high	←	Contrast potential of film	→	low
	high	←	Contrast potential of developer	→	low
	high	←	Developer temperature	→	low
	long	←	Developing time	→	short
	great	←	Developer exhaustion	→	slight
	strong	←	Agitation of developer	→	slight
	high	←	Density level	→	low
	high	←	Total contrast	→	low
X-ray image contrast	high	←	Contrast in x-ray image	→	low

[1] Object contrast refers to the radiation contrast. If arises when the x rays pass through the object because of the differential absorption of the radiation.

The optical density is defined as a logarithm because the human eye also sees logarithmically. At an exposure 0 the optical density of the film is given by the base fog of the film. The tangent of the angle α formed by the linear part of the curve is known as the gradation or gamma of the film. The non-linear parts at each end of the curve have a less steep slope and are thus not suited for radiographic purposes. The 'toe' of the curve is the area of underexposure and the 'shoulder' the area of overexposure. In both areas there is a loss of contrast. A film with a steep characteristic curve converts contrast in radiation (difference of the logarithms of two exposures) into a larger difference in optical density than a film with a less steep characteristic curve. In other words: a 'steep' film produces more contrast. This guarantees that slight differences in the absorption of x rays in the body which indicate pathological changes are converted into densities (differences in blackening) which are still perceptible.

Given the same intensity of x radiation, a double-coated film displays almost twice the optical density of a single-coated film. Thus, by using double-coated x-ray films, a significant increase in contrast is achieved. However, the contrast of processed x-ray films also depends on various other factors (Table 7.5).

7.1.3.3 Storage phosphor screens

Storage phosphor screens are composed in a similar way to intensifying screens. Besides being able to detect radiation, however, they are also able to store the latent images over a long period. This storage capability (Fig. 7.55) has

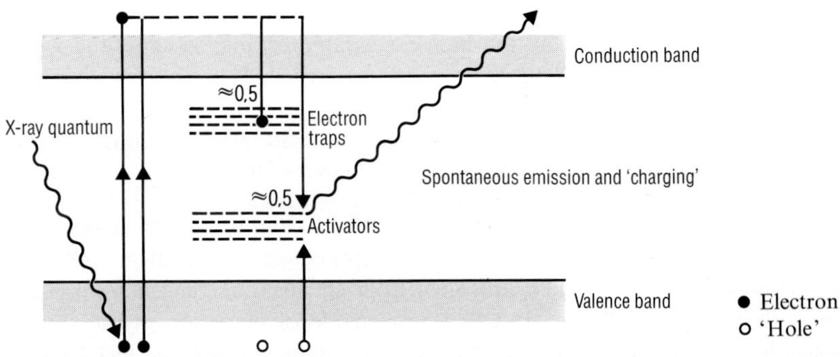

Fig. 7.55
X-ray excitation (charging) of the storage phospor

been achieved by additionally producing electron traps in the band gap through suitable doping, i.e. by the deliberate incorporation of lattice defects. Excited electrons in the conduction band now fall either into the deeper recombination centers whereby the spontaneous emission familiar from intensifying screens occurs, or else they are caught by the electron traps which are present. Depending on the type of luminescent substance used, these excited electron trap states remain stable for days or even weeks. When stimulated by light of a certain wavelength – this usually lies in the red to green region of the spectrum – the electron traps can be read out within a few microseconds. The readout process itself is shown in Fig. 7.56. The incoming light lifts the electrons collected in the electron traps back into the conduction band. A number of these electrons is caught again by electron traps (retrapping), others, however, fall into lower energy levels emitting light at the same time. The spectral maximum of the emitted light is typically around 390 nm and can therefore easily be distinguished from the stimulating light by means of optical filters.

Fig. 7.57 shows a diagram of the sequence of events when taking a radiograph with cassette storage phosphor systems. First of all, a storage phosphor screen which is inside a cassette (as is also used similarly for intensifying screen exposures) is exposed with a standard x-ray unit. The stored image information is then read out in a special readout station – a laser scanner. For this, the cassette is opened, the screens taken out and placed under a scanning laser beam. In this way the image information can be read line by line and after suitable amplification and digitalization can be transferred to an imaging computer. After the screens have been scanned, the residual image is erased.

For this, the screen is briefly subjected to a very intensive light source. This completes the processing cycle of the storage phosphor screen; now it can be loaded, exposed and read out again.

The lifetime of a single screen is comparable to that of an intensifying screen, i.e. with careful treatment it ought to be able to go through several thousand of these cycles. The image information itself emerges in this system in digital form, i.e. in order to display the image, a computer able to show the whole image or parts of it on a television monitor is needed. In contrast to a film exposure, with this method one does not obtain in the first instance an image which can be kept in the records. Thus, the necessity arises to either transfer the images to an 'optical disk' or document them on film.

A storage phosphor screen is very similar in its composition of layers to an intensifying screen (see Fig. 7.42). The phosphorescent material is applied to a polyester base, and is then protected from chemical and mechanical effects by a thin protective layer. Because of the mode of operation of the storage phosphor system, a number of important requirements must be met by such a screen. To optimize the image sharpness, it is desirable to minimize the scattering of light in the luminescent layer. This is achieved on the one hand by

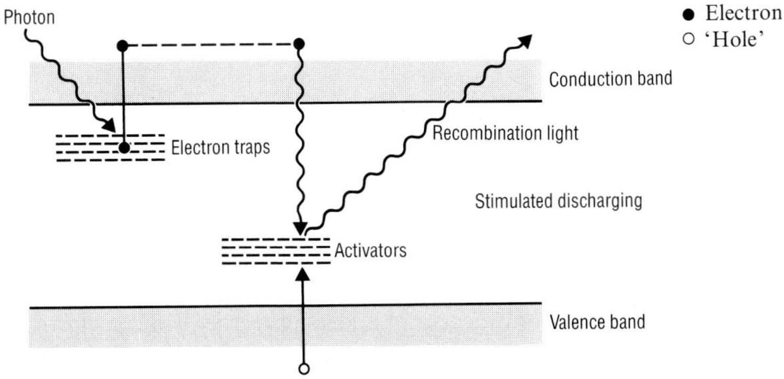

Fig. 7.56
Optical readout (discharging) of the image information from the storage phosphor screen

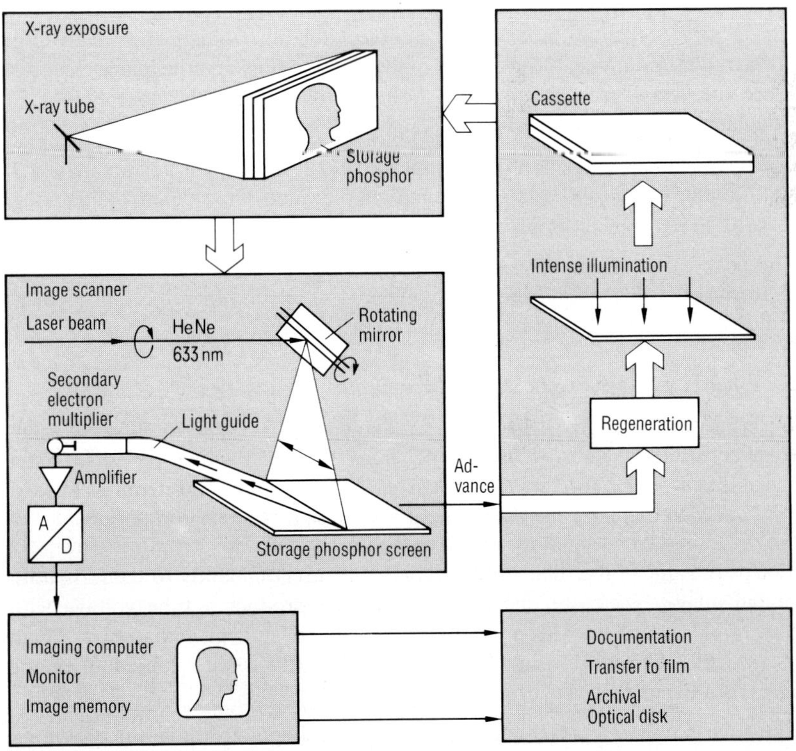

Fig. 7.57
Schematic representation of the sequence of an x-ray exposure with a storage phosphor screen

coloring of the base or the luminescent layer, and on the other hand by using modern so-called synthetic resin varnishes as a binder in the luminescent layer.

7.1.4 X-ray generators and control circuits

The contrast and the perceptibility of details in a radiograph are determined, among other things, by the x-ray generator and its properties. Kinetic blurring, in particular, is affected by the parameters of the generator. The tube voltage U (peak value in kV), tube current I (as the arithmetic mean in mA), and exposure time T (in s) determine the image-producing dose D [7.36, 7.46].

$$D = k_0 \cdot U^n \cdot I \cdot T \tag{7.27}$$

The factor k_0 depends on the irradiated object, the tube voltage, the prefiltration at the radiation source, the geometry of the x-ray system, and the image receptor. Since the x-rays are not coherent, the absolute value of the dose cannot be calculated by means of equation (7.27).

The exponent n is a function of the tube voltage; at 150 kV it is approximately 3. As the value of the tube voltage is decreased, the value of the exponent increases; thus, at 50 kV it is about 5 [7.37].

The peak tube voltage determines the radiation spectrum and thus the image characteristics. Therefore, the tube voltage is selected with respect to medical indication and determined by the required procedure:

a) What is the object to be examined, and

b) What contrast range is necessary for diagnosis?
(For instance, an exposure of the 'bony thorax' requires 66 kV in order to diagnose the bone structure, whereas a chest radiograph requires at least 125 kV to diagnose the lung structure, even that lying behind the ribs.)

The peak value of the tube voltage contributes predominantly to the formation of the image. Therefore, the generator should produce a tube voltage with low ripple in order to keep the proportion of low-energy radiation as small as possible. The ideal would be direct current (DC) voltage because of the impact of the exponent n.

The tube power ($P = kUI$) converted at the focal spot to radiation is, among other things, an indication for the size of the focal spot. It determines, in connection with the other parameters of the system, the spatial resolution of the examined object.

A moving object can only be depicted sharply with a sufficiently short exposure time *T*. Minimizing total blurring is accomplished by taking into account film-screen, geometric blurring and kinetic blurring. Organ motion, especially in the heart and the lung, can well amount to a speed of 200 mm/s [7.38]. Arterial vessels pulsate similarly, and even more so in pediatric applications.

The dose is proportional to both the tube current *I* and the exposure time *T*. Therefore, the value *Q* ("mAs product") is selected and switched in proportion to the examined object.

The reproducibility of generator parameters contributes to the consistency of image quality. A tolerance of 10–20% in generator parameters is barely within acceptable limits for qualitative recording of morphology and organ functions. Tolerance values below 1–5% are necessary for special examinations such as CT, DSA, or quantitative evaluation.

Relevant regulations regarding "radiation hygiene" should be followed. This means that only the medically indicated level of radiation should be applied in diagnostic x-ray procedures. Therefore, the generator must produce the desired value of tube voltage quickly and with as little overshoot as possible. Once the dose for proper image density is achieved the generator must switch off with minimal delay.

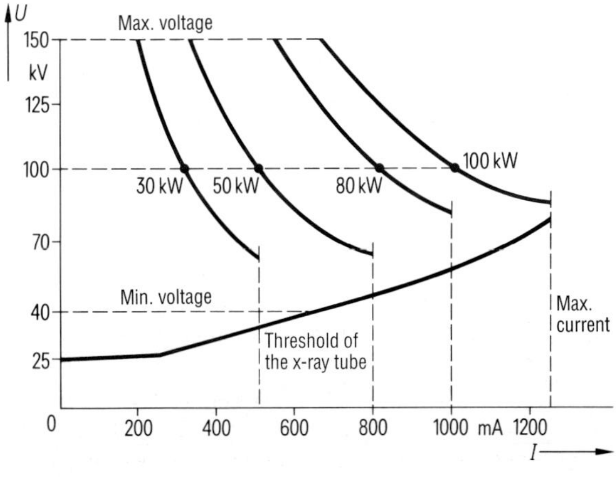

Definition of generator power according to IEC/DIN 6822:
$P = kUI$ (k characterizes the magnitude and form of the ripple)

Hard radiation range: 110 to 150 kV
Normal range: 40 to 125 kV
Soft radiation range: 25 to 49 kV

Fig. 7.58 Range of operation of a generator for an x-ray installation

Considerations of radiation hygiene and image quality led to the development of automatic control systems for various types of examinations, e.g. for fluoroscopy, spot filming, or indirect techniques in order to be able to carry out the examination quickly and safely for both patient and examiner.

Figure 7.58 shows the range of operation of a generator with its voltage ranges. The minimum tube current is about 0.1 mA for fluoroscopy, and the maximum tube current about 1200 mA for radiography. The current is determined by the maximum output of the generator and/or the type of x-ray tube assembly. Output of up to 100 kW are common today. Higher output results in an increase of geometric blurring and inferior image quality. A power of 100 kW is basically sufficient for high speed film-screen combinations with good resolution.

Figure 7.59 shows a block diagram of a generator with its components for general diagnostics.

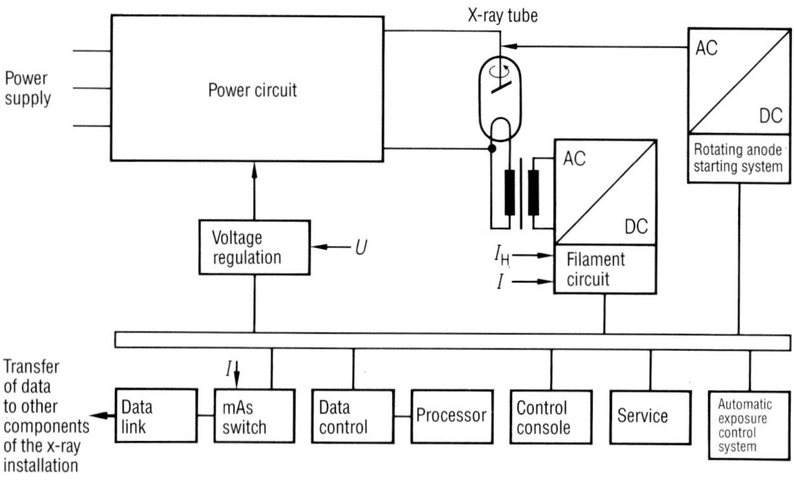

Fig. 7.59
Block diagram of the assembly of a processor-controlled generator with its components

7.1.4.1 Power circuits

The dose rate necessary for production of an image is generated by the tube voltage U and the tube current I. The power circuit transforms the line voltage into these "technique factors". The following sections explain the operation of three different power circuit designs.

Conventional generators from single-pulse to 12-pulse

Figure 7.60 shows the power circuit of a 6-pulse generator in which the three-phase alternating current from the line supply, e.g. 480 V is transformed into a tube voltage of 40 to 150 kV. The total internal resistance R between the power line voltage (U_0) and the x-ray tube plays a decisive role, as can be seen in Figure 7.61.

The specific features of a conventional power circuit are:

▻ The line supply can be single-phase (110 or 220 V) or three-phase (220 to 480 V).

▻ An auto or step transformer allows adjustment to changes in the line supply voltage (line compensation) manually or automatically, as well as setting of the reference value U_{ref} of the tube voltage:

$$U = U_0 - I \cdot R_i \tag{7.28}$$

The no-load voltage U_0 may easily be in the region of 200 kV. The internal resistance R_i is approximately 100 kΩ or more.

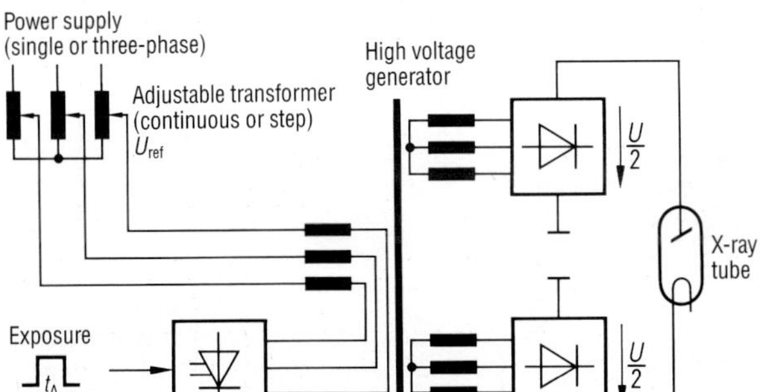

Fig. 7.60
Power circuit of a conventional generator: three-phase principle for 6-pulse rectification

Since the tube voltage following equation (7.28) and Figure 7.61 depends on the tube current, the latter has to be adjusted before the start of the exposure by presetting the cathode filament current as precisely as possible (see section 7.1.4.2). This interdependence can in fact also be used to adjust the tube voltage by changing the tube current via the cathode filament current for a fixed setting of internal resistance R_i and a fixed no-load voltage U_0.

This method of setting the tube voltage can also be combined with several internal resistances R_i and/or no-load voltages U_0.

The reproducibility of the tube voltage is only ensured under stable line supply conditions. It can be improved by using an autotransformer with motorized adjustment, and/or electronically controlled tube current. Since such controlled mechanisms operate in the 100 ms range, rapid changes in the line supply voltage are still immediately transferred to the tube voltage.

Switching on and off takes place in the primary supply leads to the high voltage transformer by means of electro-mechanical switching devices (relays or contactors) or thyristors (as shown in Figure 7.60). The switching-on process usually requires a delay of up to 20 ms – known as the phase-in time – so that the tube voltage assumes the correct form, i.e. without overshooting or undershooting the voltage.

The high voltage generator consists of an oil filled container. It contains the transformer (iron core, primary and seocndary coils), the high voltage rectifiers,

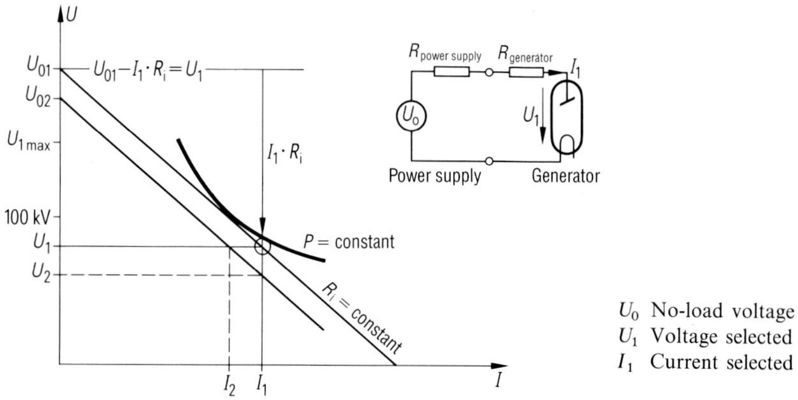

Fig. 7.61
Internal resistance line ($R_i = R_{power\ supply} + R_{generator}$) for a conventional generator in range of operation determined by U_{01}, U_1, I_1. For the same R_i but smaller no-load voltage U_{02}, other operational parameters e.g. U_2, I_1 or U_1, I_2 can be set.

the filament transformer for the cathode of the x-ray tube, the high voltage switches, and the receptacles for the high voltage cables. All Siemens high voltage generators are additionally equipped with a measuring device for registering the actual values of tube voltage and tube current.

High voltage generators and x-ray tube assemblies usually have a two pole design so that the insulation is only subjected to half the value of the tube voltage $U/2$ (i.e. symmetric to ground potential).

Criteria such as power, ripple of the tube voltage, volume, and costs led to the design of generators with various pulse numbers:

- ▻ Single-pulse generators produce only one tube voltage pulse for each cycle of the line supply voltage. They are very low powered ($P \leq 2$ kW) and are only intended for dental and mobile x-ray units.
- ▻ Two-pulse generators produce two tube voltage pulses for each cycle of the line supply voltage through bridge rectification; for low and medium power ($P \leq 50$ kW).
- ▻ Six-pulse generators produce six tube voltage pulses for each cycle of the line supply voltage through three phase bridge rectification; for medium to high power ($P \leq 100$ kW).
- ▻ Twelve-pulse generators produce 12 tube voltage pulses for each cycle of the line supply voltage from two shifted six-pulse circuits; for high power ($P \leq 150$ kW).

The higher the pulse number of the tube voltage, the higher the yield of image producing dose. This means shorter exposure time and hence less kinetic blurring. Furthermore, the portion of low energy radiation is reduced.

The actual ripple of the tube voltage is derived from the accumulation of technical tolerances and the asymmetry in the three phases of the line voltage. It amounts to:

	100%	in single- and two-pulse generators
around	25% (theoretically 13.4%)	in six-pulse generators, and
around	10% (theoretically 3.4%)	in 12-pulse generators.

The ripple or pulsation [7.46] of the tube voltage is given as a percentage of the peak value:

$$w = [(U - U_{\text{min}})/U] \cdot 100\%.$$

Direct current generator

Since the reproducibility and consistency of the tube voltage has a substantial effect on image quality, an especially fast voltage control system was designed in which fluctuations both in the line supply voltage and the tube current have no effect on the tube voltage.

Figure 7.62 shows the principle of the power circuit of a direct current generator. Special features are:

▻ The high voltage generator can be directly connected to the line supply.

▻ Two high voltage electron tubes (triodes or tetrodes) serve for both switching the tube voltage on and off, as well as adjusting it via closed loop control circuit [7.39, 7.40].

▻ The tube voltage can be switched on and off at any point in time (no phase-in time).

▻ The tube voltage is preset as a reference value U_{ref} and is completely independent of the value of the tube current, as well as any changes in it.

▻ The response time for this method of fully electronic voltage closed loop control is approximately 20 µs.

This elaborate system of voltage control has proven its value for all types of examination technique, with the most stringent requirements being image quality and reproducibility. The very high speed of adjustment permits both fast repetition rates of 500 frames per second or more – irrespective of the tube power – as well as rapid adaptation of the tube voltage to the image quality requirements. The actual ripple of the tube voltage is less than 1%. The result is virtually pure DC voltage. Extremely short exposure time and the lowest possible portion of low energy radiation are now achieved.

The advantages of the direct current generator are obtained at the expense of a bulky unit, inefficient power consumption, and relatively high costs.

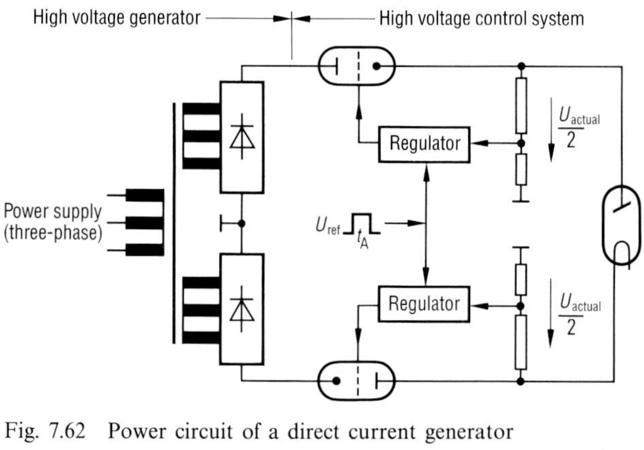

Fig. 7.62 Power circuit of a direct current generator

High frequency generator (multipulse generator)

This type of generator combines the advantages of the direct current generator, however, with very small volume and lower costs. The reproducibility and consistency of tube voltage is enhanced by a relatively fast closed loop control circuit, and is virtually independent of changes in both the line voltage and tube current.

Figure 7.63 shows the power circuit of a high frequency generator. Unique features are:

- ▻ The line supply can be either single-phase or three-phase (220 to 440 V).
- ▻ Controlled or uncontrolled generation of the intermediate DC voltage U_z.
- ▻ Series *oscillator circuit* (inverter) [7.41], which generates a high frequency alternating current from the DC voltage of the intermediate circuit U_z.
- ▻ The tube voltage can be switched on and off at any point in time (no phase-in time).
- ▻ The tube voltage is preset as a reference value U_{ref} and is virtually independent of both the tube current and any changes in it.
- ▻ The response time for this method of fully electronic voltage closed loop control is approximately 250 µs.
- ▻ Extremely compact high voltage generator accomplished by raising the operating frequency f. This allows reduction of the cross-section A of the core and the number of turns n on the coils ($U \sim A \cdot n \cdot f$).

The method to control the tube voltage is shown in Figure 7.64. The actual measured tube voltage U_{act} is compared with the reference tube voltage U_{ref}. The controller fires trigger pulses to the thyristor gates as long as both tube values are not in equilibrium.

The response time of the closed loop control circuit depends on the trigger frequency. It is approximately 250 µs, which is slower than that of a direct

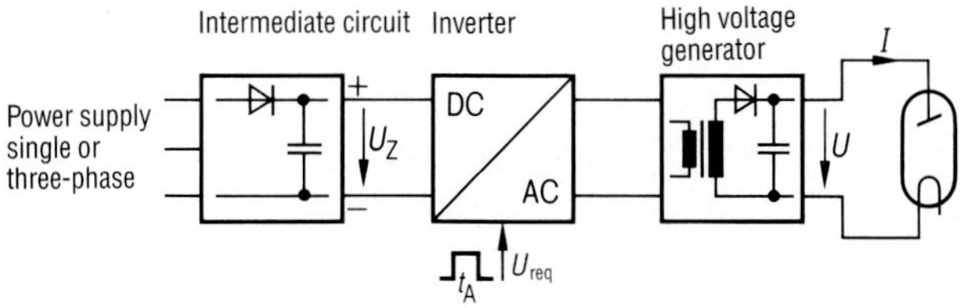

Fig. 7.63 Power circuit of a high frequency generator (multipulse generator)

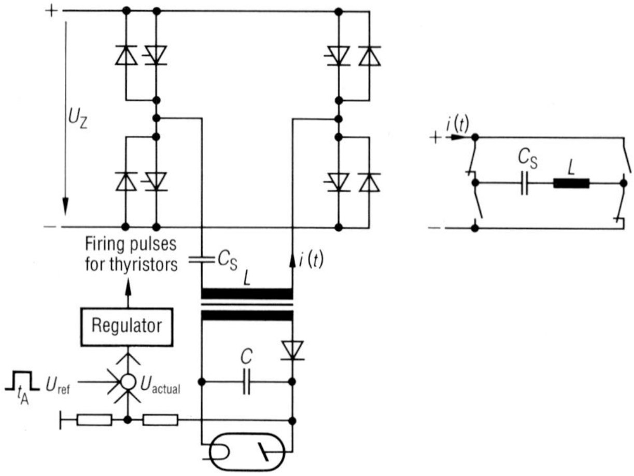

a) Basic circuit diagram

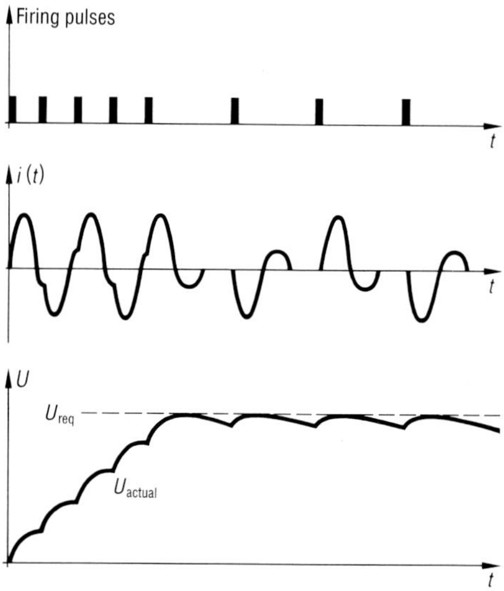

b) Temporal course of the firing pulses, the oscillating current $i(t)$ and the tube voltage U

Fig. 7.64
Functioning of the tube voltage control with a series oscillator circuit inverter

current generator but is by far faster than the response time of a conventional generator.

The actual ripple depends on the technique factors (power), the smoothing capacity C parallel to the x-ray tube, and the value of the voltage U_z of the intermediate DC circuit. The ripple is typically

13% for medium power (30 to 50 kW) and
4% for high power (50 to 100 kW).

High frequency generators produce many tube voltage pulses during each cycle of line voltage. Their number depends on the firing frequency of the inverter system. This led to the name 'multipulse generator'. It delivers a dose rate which is better than that of a conventional 12-pulse generator. Therefore, the low energy radiation produced is at a fairly low level.

Thanks to power electronic components for high frequencies the volume of the generator is about 80% less, the space requirement about 85% less, and the weight about 75% less than the corresponding values of a direct current generator.

For serial and cine operation each focal spot up to 100 kW can be operated at all relevant frame rates up to 120 frames per second.

Types of design

Since generators belong to the class of products with a long lifetime, it is necessary to pay particular attention to the growing demands regarding image quality when making such a purchase decision. Less than 5% tolerances for tube voltage, tube current and exposure time is state-of-the-art today. Conventional generators at best achieve tolerances of 10–20%, however, they will continue to serve for many years.

Figure 7.65 shows the measuring and closed loop control circuits of a modern generator which meet the requirements for consistency and reproducibility of tube voltage and tube current.

The direct current generator is still intended for use in the small field of radiological research where the emphasis is on extremely low ripple, extremely fast tube voltage control, pulse widths of less than 2 ms, and frame rates of more than 120 frames per second.

The high frequency generator represents state-of-the-art technology. For exposure power up to and including 50 kW the high voltage generator and the x-ray tube are built into the same housing assembly. This method of construction is called a 'single-tank generator' and does not require high voltage cables. The size and weight roughly correspond to that of a conventional x-ray tube assembly. A focal spot of 1.0 for 50 kW can be achieved by using a CALOREX anode disk rotating at high speed (see section 7.1.1 also). Two single-tank gener-

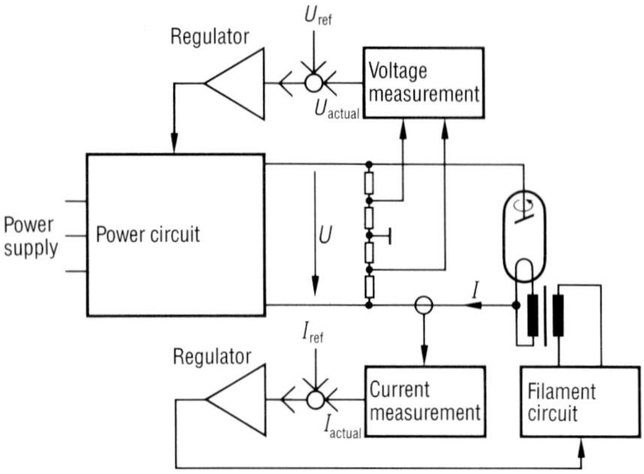

Fig. 7.65
Independent, electronic control circuits for the tube voltage U and the tube current I of a generator

ator assemblies can be connected to one generator control console for spot filming and Bucky operation.

For a high generator power of 50 to 100 kW we separate the tube housing assembly and the high voltage generator. Normally up to four different x-ray tubes can be connected and operated in time-sharing mode.

On their merits high frequency generators are not only suitable for routine procedures, but also for all types of angiography, including digital subtraction angiography (DSA). Thus, they are probably the most economical solution for interventional procedures.

7.1.4.2 Filament circuit

The tube voltage U is determined by the character of the image (contrast) and the resolution of the image by the size of the focal spot. The tube current I is determined by the permissible output $P(t)$ of the focal spot:

$$I = \frac{P(t)}{U} \tag{7.29}$$

The tube current can be obtained via the filament current I_F of the directly heated cathode as a function of the output and the tube voltage as shown in section 7.1.1. Figure 7.67b shows the relationship $I = f(I_F)$ at a selected tube voltage. Each pair of technique factors I, U has its filament current I_F.

There are three distinct ranges of filament current:

1. Preheating with about 2 to 4 A to keep the cathode filament warm without emission of any tube current I;
2. Fluoroscopy heating for $I = 0.1$ to 4 mA, under certain conditions up to 25 mA;
3. Exposure heating for $I \leq 1600$ mA; due to the gradient characteristics of $I = f(I_F)$ exact presetting of the filament current is required. A deviation of 1% I_F leads to a high deviation in tube current I. A short transition time from fluoroscopy to exposure and back during spot filming is very important. The reduction of I_F after the exposure to the preheating value or fluoroscopy heating prolongs the life of the cathode.

Exposure heating can be kept constant during the exposure time (constant load) or be reduced by a closed loop control kV and mA circuit (continuously falling load, initial load). The reduction of exposure heating is based on keeping the focal spot temperature constant over the exposure time. If the highest possible temperature is used the exposure time will be the shortest possible, and thus, the kinetic blurring will be minimal. Figure 7.66 shows the timing diagram of tube voltage U and tube current I using continuously falling load operation.

The filament current I_F can control the dose rate value during fluoroscopy in automatic exposure control mode (see section 7.1.4.5 Fluoroscopy)

Figure 7.67a shows the functional diagram of a conventional filament circuit with three-point adjustment. Figure 7.67b illustrates the relationship between filament current I_{F1}, I_{F2}, tube current I_1, I_2, and no-load voltage U_{01}, U_{02}, for a selected tube voltage U_1.

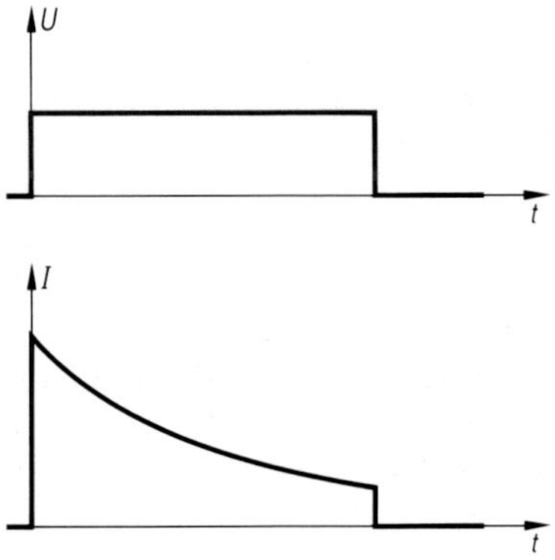

Fig. 7.66
Evolution of tube voltage U and tube current I for falling load operation

The filament current is adjusted by a three-point technique:

R_1 at low kV and high mA settings,
R_2 at low kV and low mA settings, and
R_3 at high kV and low mA settings.

The primary filament current is monitored with a current relay hr to protect the x-ray tube assembly.

An exact presetting of the filament current value is absolutely necessary since the closed loop kV control can only have an effect after the exposure has been turned on. Incorrect filament current settings cannot be corrected within a short exposure time because of the inertia of the filament itself.

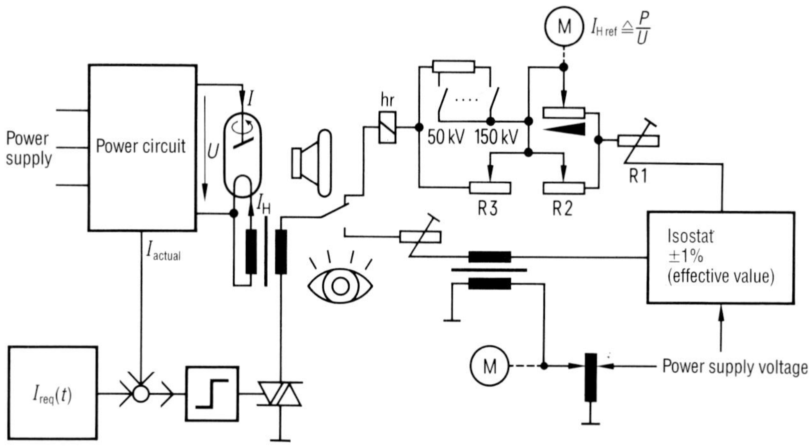

a) With three-point equalization of the heating for exposure operation

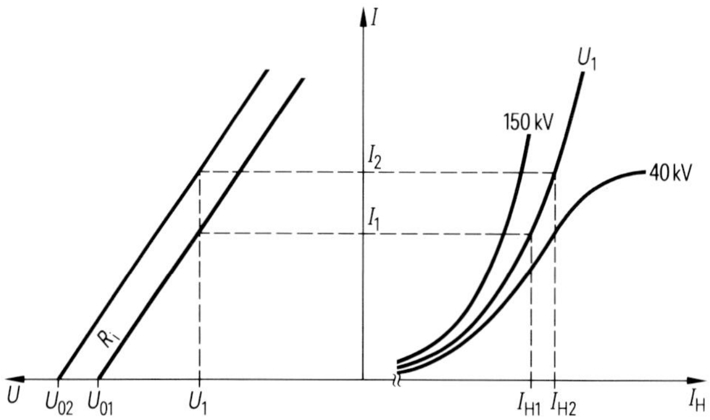

b) Relationship between filament current I_{H1}, I_{H2}, tube current I_1, I_2 and no-load voltage U_{01}, U_{02} for a selected tube voltage U_1

Fig. 7.67
Functioning of a conventional filament circuit

The filament current is an alternating current operated at line frequency. Therefore, the cathode temperature changes at twice the frequency, which results in a tube current ripple of about 10% during the exposure. This ripple is superimposed over the ripple of the tube voltage and results in a relatively high ripple of the dose rate (see Eq. (7.27)). Due to this phenomenon, inverter based

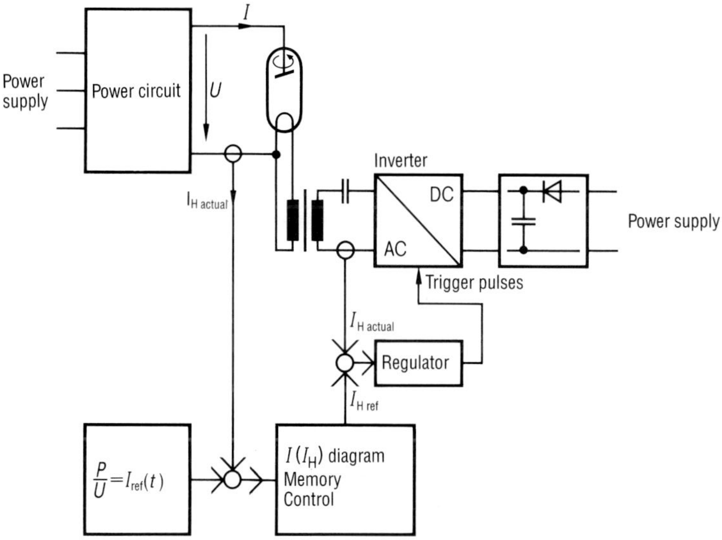

a) Basic circuit diagram

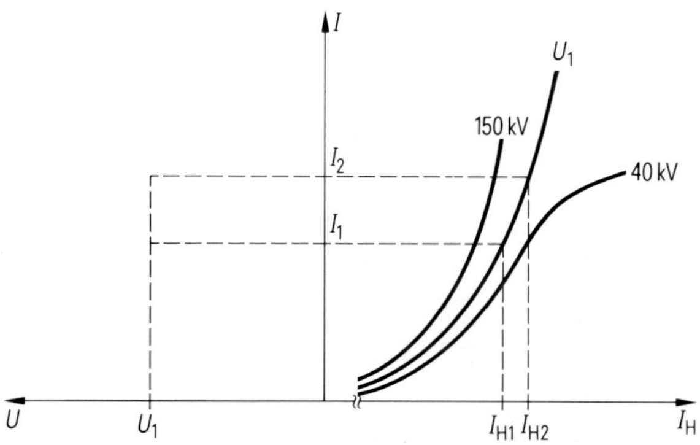

b) Relation between filament current I_{H1}, I_{H2} and tube current I_1, I_2 at a selected tube voltage U_1 when a rapid tube voltage control circuit is present

Fig. 7.68
Functioning of a high-frequency filament circuit with pulse-frequency modulation and tube current regulation

filament circuits were developed which operate at higher frequencies and therefore avoid temperature changes.

Figure 7.68 shows the functional diagram of a high frequency filament circuit with pulse-frequency modulation and closed loop tube current controls. The filament current values $I_F = f(U, I)$ are electronically stored in the computer memory of the generator for each focal spot. The real required value I_F varies by a few percent due to production tolerances of the cathodes. This is not crucial for direct current generators and high frequency generators because the tube voltage is independent of the tube current due to fast closed loop control systems. In addition, the mAs switch ensures the correct dose value at the image receptor (see section 7.1.4.4).

Furthermore, the pulse-frequency modulated closed loop control circuit for the tube current regulation can compensate for deviations of the actual value within approximately 50 ms once the tube voltage has been switched on. In this way the tube current is independent of line voltage regulation and can be kept within a narrow tolerance band of 5%. The only ripple of the tube current is that generated by the tube voltage influenced by the space-charge characteristics.

Modes of operation (see section 7.1.4.5) which require a change of the tube current over time are now easily accomplished. The speed of tube current change depends on the thermal time constant of the cathode filament and ranges from 50 to 200 ms.

7.1.4.3 High speed starter

A rotating anode offers considerable increase in output compared to a stationary anode (see section 7.1.1). This improves the image quality. The high speed starter drives an asynchronous motor. The unique property of this motor is the large air gap between rotor (anode potential) and stator (ground potential). The slip is correspondingly large. The number of revolutions per minute (rpm) for the drive frequency f_A is:

$$n < n_{\text{synchron}} = 60 \cdot f_A \tag{7.30}$$

The bearings of a x-ray tube run 'dry' in a vacuum, therefore, the anode is only accelerated before each exposure (acceleration) and thereafter this is brought to a standstill (braking circuit) to extend its life. The inertia of the anode disk caused by weight and torque determines the acceleration time. It can be shortened by supplying a variable frequency f_A instead of a fixed frequency.

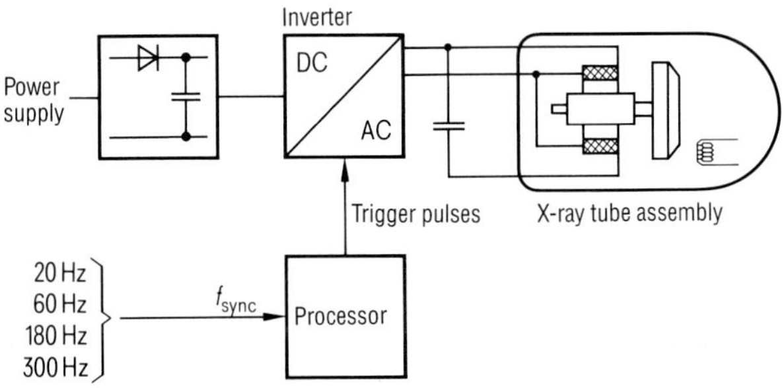

Fig. 7.69 High speed starter with variable drive frequency

Conventional high speed starters use either the line frequency directly (e.g. 50 Hz: $n_{synchron} = 3000$ r.p.m), or its third harmonic (e.g. 150 Hz: $n_{synchron} = 9000$ r.p.m). This is produced from a three-phase line voltage by means of three saturated transformers.

Figure 7.69 shows the high speed starter with variable drive frequency f_A. This device allows operation of different types of x-ray tube assemblies with variable frequencies from a single generator. Synchronous frequencies used today are 15 to 20 Hz for fluoroscopy, 50 to 180 Hz for radiography, and in special cases up to 200 or 300 Hz.

Circuits monitoring the number of revolutions per minute are used in order to protect the x-ray tube assembly. If a fault is indicated it prevents the system from switching on the radiation. The cause may also be a worn bearing, in which case the x-ray tube assembly should be replaced.

7.1.4.4 Timer circuits and exposure circuits

The desired dose is proportional to the exposure time T according to equation (7.27) with the prerequisite of constant and corect tube voltage and tube current values. Conventional generators kept the tube voltage constant by changing the tube current as shown in sections 7.1.4.1, Power Circuits, and 7.1.4.2, Filament Circuits.

Therefore, the tube voltage was constant but not the tube current. Applying equation (7.27) led to switching of the mAs product, Q [7.46]; that is, the product $I \cdot T$ (called mAs switching), or even to switching the dose value itself (automatic exposure control). This provides excellent reproducibility of dose values.

Timing devices

Timing devices are not used any longer in diagnostic equipment with the exception of dental exposures, pulse width switches in cine operation, tomography operation, and as time limiting switches for safety purposes. This is due to improvements in mAs switching and automatic exposure control systems. Therefore, it is not necessary to discuss timers at length here.

'mAs switching'

It is clear from equation (7.27) that the necessary mAs product, Q, must be preset in order to achieve the appropriate optical density. After switching on the tube voltage, the tube current I_{act} is measured as shown in Figure 7.70 and integrated over the exposure duration t_A (see Figure 7.71). Once the mAs product reaches its preset value Q_{ref} the tube voltage and thus the radiation must be switched off immediately. The mAs product Q is:

$$Q = \int_0^{t_A} I(t)\,dt \tag{7.31}$$

It is measured in milliampere seconds, called mAs.

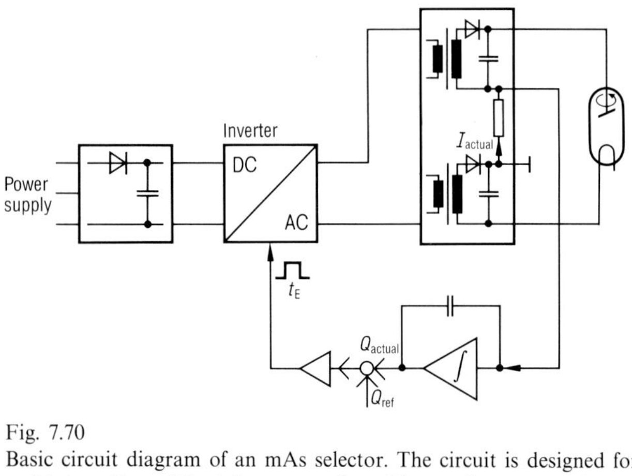

Fig. 7.70
Basic circuit diagram of an mAs selector. The circuit is designed for the measurement and integration of the tube current $I_{actual}(t)$ as well as comparison of the required and actual value of the mAs product Q

Figure 7.71 contains the definition of the exposure time according to IEC/DIN 0750. It also clearly shows that the actual mAs value triggering the switch is always slightly higher than the preset one. This is a result of the current discharging the capacitances via the x-ray tube after terminating the exposure. Not only in conventional generators, but also in modern high frequency generators the switchoff command can come shortly before or after a triggering pulse for an energy package. However, it contributes to a further ΔQ or ΔD. The quantity ΔQ only has a negative impact at low mAs reference values.

Reproducibility of the mAs value: a 25% change in mAs for an exposure leads to a clearly visible change in optical density of an x-ray film. This value represents one exposure point according to the exposure tables [7.42].

In order to avoid problems caused by ΔQ or ΔD, the tolerances given in Figure 7.71 for different operating modes such as film, cine, and DSA must be adhered to. The smallest mAs product Q_{min} for film-screen systems which can be switched in a reproducible way is therefore expressed as:

$$Q_{min} = 10 \cdot \Delta Q. \quad (7.32)$$

Due to the fact that the image is only affected by about 25% of the total electric charge ΔQ stored in the high voltage capacitances C_H,

$$\Delta Q_H = 0.25\, U \cdot C_H. \quad (7.33)$$

(e.g.: $\Delta Q_H = 0.25 \cdot 100\text{ kV} \cdot 6\text{ nF} = 0.15\text{ mAs}$).

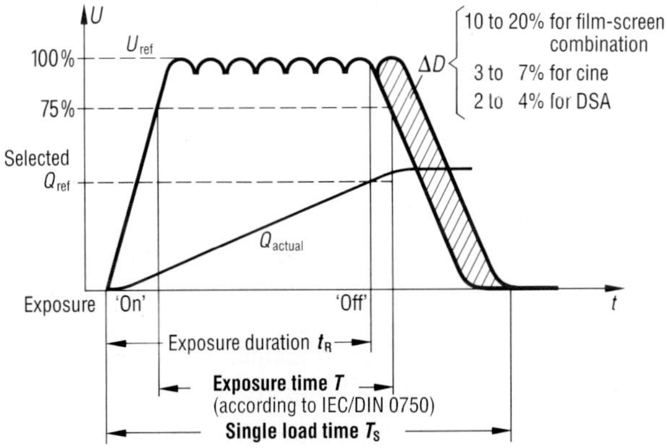

Fig. 7.71
Exposure time, exposure duration and single load time for an x-ray exposure. Admissible tolerance of the dose in ΔD.

The charge, which depends on the tube current I and the switching frequency f_A at the operating point of the inverter, is called ΔQ_f, and is expressed as:

$$\Delta Q_f = \frac{I}{2 f_A} \tag{7.34}$$

$$\left(\text{e.g.: } \Delta Q_f = \frac{1000 \text{ mA}}{2 \times 5 \text{ kHz}} = 0.1 \text{ mAs}\right).$$

The larger of the two values ΔQ_H and ΔQ_f is assigned to ΔQ, according to equation (7.32). Using our example:

$$\Delta Q_H = 0.15 \text{ mAs} > \Delta Q_f = 0.1 \text{ mAs: therefore, } Q_{min} = 10\, \Delta Q_H = 1.5 \text{ mAs}$$

The idea of counting the number of energy packages and thus always switching the same number of pulses would only work at a constant pulse width and constant switching frequency. However, this is contradictory to the concept of the closed loop tube voltage control circuit as described in section 7.1.4.1.

Automatic exposure control system

The region of an object which is of diagnostic interest is called the dominant. In a radiograph this region should maintain a specific average optical density. The measuring field of the sensor (ionization chamber, solid state radiation detector, or photomultiplier) must coincide with the dominant when positioning the patient. Thus, automatic exposure control systems are suitable for all types of exposures where the equipment allows alignment of the measuring field and dominant, and the collimated x-ray field is not smaller than the measuring field. They are applied in fluoroscopy, Bucky exposure techniques, spot filming, film changer techniques, all indirect operation (DSA, 35 mm or 100 mm techniques), and in mammography.

Automatic exposure control systems operate on the principle of dose rate measurement (Figure 7.72). By means of integration, a signal is obtained which is proportional to the actual dose D_{actual} accumulated at any point in time. A preset reference dose value D_{ref} eliminates the necessity of guessing the mAs value, which has to be selected by the operator in manual mode on the basis of his experience and by estimating the patient's transparency [7.43].

Three different types of sensors are used: an ionization chamber is placed in front of the film cassette. A current proportional to the dose rate $\dot{D}$ is generated by the radiation in an air capacitor charged with 300 or 1000 V. The order of magnitude of the ionization current is in the picoampere range (10^{-12}).

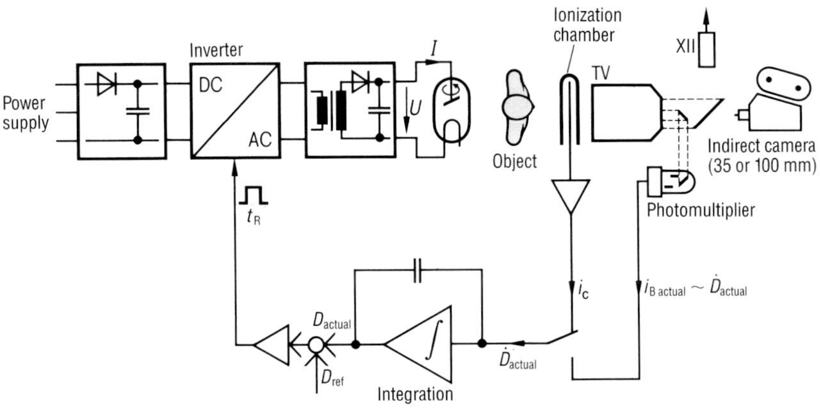

Fig. 7.72
Basic circuit diagram of an automatic exposure control system
Sensor: Ionization chamber or solid state radiation detector for x-rays, photomultiplier for light at the x-ray image intensifier output

The ionization chamber should be as narrow as possible, and should not create a shadow on the film.

The solid state radiation detector (SSRD) is placed behind the film cassette or in film changers behind the film screen combination because it would create a shadow on the film if it were placed otherwise. Its advantage over the ionization chamber is that the dose can be kept at a somewhat lower level due to reduced absorption in front of the film (e.g. mammography, pediatrics). The current of the SSRD is proportional to the dose rate behind the cassette and not to that in the plane of the film. Therefore, the optical density is no longer directly proportional to the SSRD current.

The photomultiplier operates on the principle of an electron multiplier tube. The multiplier current is directly proportional to the dose rate at the input screen of the image intensifier and therefore, to the brightness of the image intensifier output screen.

Optical density correction

Since the proportion of scattered radiation depends on the irradiated volume, more scattered radiation occurs in a thick object. The sensor of the automatic exposure control system measures the total radiation emerging from the object. It includes the scattered radiation, and therefore the reference dose value is reached sooner in the case of thick objects. The film thus exhibits a lower optical density than the preset one.

Experienced doctors and technicians alter the reference dose value D_{ref} by means of an optical density correction switch depending upon the object to be examined. This switch is graduated in plus and minus exposure points. In organ-programmed exposure techniques this adjustment may already be pre-programmed in the organ key. Preference should be given to organ-programmed operation because the choice of sensor is also included.

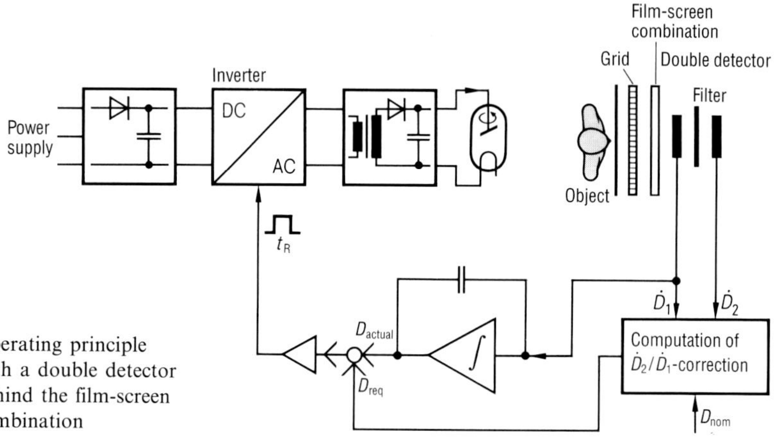

a)
Operating principle with a double detector behind the film-screen combination

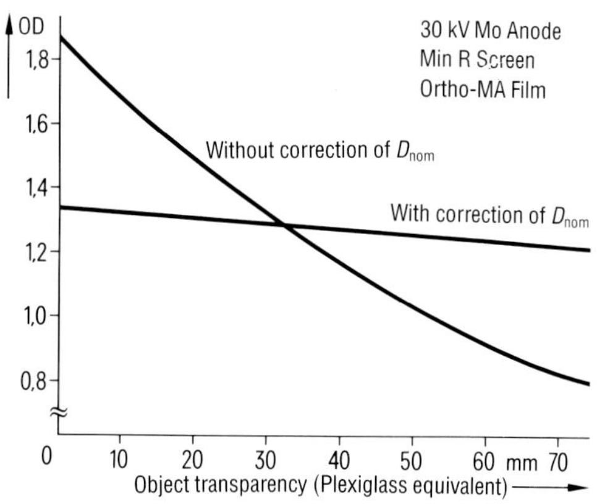

b)
Dependence of the optical density S of the film on the object transparency with and without correction of the nominal dose value D_{nom}

Fig. 7.73
Automatic exposure control system for mammography with automatic transparency equalization

Transparency compensation

The ratio of quanta according to equation (7.35) is called the transparency. N_e denotes the number of quanta which enter an object, while N_a indicates the number of quanta which emerge from the object:

$$\text{Transparency} = \frac{N_a}{N_e} \tag{7.35}$$

The transparency depends on both the density and thickness of an object. For very low tube voltages (e.g. in mammography 25 to 40 kV) the sensor for the automatic exposure control system is placed behind the film-screen combination. The optical density, therefore, depends on the transparency of the object at identical tube voltage values and identical object thickness.

It is very difficult for the technician to correctly compensate using the optical density correction switch. A modern automatic exposure control system (Figure 7.73) using microprocessor technology and a double detector sensor can correct optical density within a tolerance of half an exposure point.

In examinations where the shortest possible exposure time is imperative, the automatic exposure control system and the generator operate with continuously falling load (see section 7.1.4.2).

The exposure time and the actual mAs value can be displayed after an automatic exposure for the technician's information.

Time-controlled exposures

Tomography

The single load time (see Figure 7.71) is predetermined by the movement of the x-ray tube assembly in tomography. The correct exposure is obtained at a given tube voltage in free operation via the selected mAs product Q. The tube current I_{ref} is calculated and automatically set (see also Figure 7.80):

$$I_{ref} = \frac{Q_{ref}}{T_L} \tag{7.36}$$

Automatic exposure controlled tomography requires the setting of a reference value for the dose rate $\dot{D}_{ref}$.

$$\dot{D}_{ref} = \frac{D}{T_L} \tag{7.37}$$

The maximum permissible 'kWs' value corresponding to the dose D is reduced by the automatic exposure control system during the exposure until the actual dose rate coincides with the dose rate reference value. The automatic exposure control system works by means of phase control in the power circuit of a conventional generator. It works by means of pulse modulation in high frequency generators.

Exposures with intentional blurring

The examination of the cervico-vertebral spine (anterior-posterior) should not be performed with the shortest possible exposure time because the lower jaw would be superimposed onto the vertebrae, causing some distraction. Therefore, the exposure is performed with a longer exposure time and wagging jaw.

Similarly, examinations of the lateral thoracic spine are performed with suspended or quiet respiration. Here the superimposed lung tissue is intentionally blurred.

In manual operation the correct exposure for these examinations is achieved by presetting the tube voltage, required single load time T_L, and the mAs value. The tube current is automatically calculated and set according to equation (7.36).

Using automatic exposure control the examination is done similarly, except the selected mAs value is increased by a factor of 1.5 to 2. Then the automatic exposure control mode is selected and the exposure will be terminated within the single load time T_L.

Serial techniques
(Film changers, indirect exposure techniques with cut-film or rollfilm cameras, and cine cameras)

Here, the most important condition using automatic exposure control is that the single load time T_L must be shorter than the shutter-open interval. By shutter-open interval we mean the time which is defined by the cycle time of the selected frame rate minus the film transport and settling down time of the system. If the shutter-open interval turns off the radiation before the right optical density has been reached the resulting image is underexposed. This may be the case when working with a power lower than 20 kW and/or very small focal spots (focal spot ≤ 0.3 for magnification).

The reference tube current is calculated according to equation (7.36) in manual operation. One must ensure that:

$$T_L \leq T_{\text{shutter-open}}.$$

When using automatic exposure control various automatic exposure control systems are designed to meet this requirement (see section 7.1.4.5).

7.1.4.5 Automatic control systems and operation

The physician needs a specific image character for the examination and therefore for the radiation dose. For this purpose the generator transforms electrical energy from the line supply to the x-ray tube. However, the x-ray tube must not be overloaded while, at the same time, the load must be chosen as high as possible within the permissible range so that kinetic blurring is avoided via short exposure times. The high load is concentrated in a small optical focal spot in order to keep the geometric blurring low and ensure the diagnostically required spatial resolution. However, a single exposure is not enough for some examination techniques. A series of exposures of particular scene duration is necessary, in some instances up to 150 frames per second as in pediatric cardiology. Various types of outputs of focal spots and x-ray tube assemblies were discussed in section 7.1.1 in the form of diagrams and tables.

It is necessary to free the operator from routine technical procedures with the aid of automatic control systems and user-friendly operating instructions. In this way, the operator obtains the best image quickly with minimal strain to the patient.

The operation of the generator is part of the automatic control systems, which are designed to suit each particular examination. A few examples will illustrate this concept.

Fluoroscopy

Fluoroscopy is used by the physician for the purpose of orientation and recognition of physiological functions. Here radiation of low output is produced at the focal spot. The setting of the tube voltage and tube current must take into account the required contrast and the lowest possible dose for patient and operator.

Figure 7.74 shows the operational range for fluoroscopy with an image intensifier TV chain. It can be operated within this range by an automatic exposure control system and therefore does not require that the technique factors be set manually (see Figure 7.75). Due to image character and dose, tube voltages over 110 kV and below 50 kV should not be used.

Isowatt fluoroscopy (curve 1 in Figure 7.74) cannot be used for imaging modalities. The reasons are: the transparency range of an object is not sufficient, the dose is too high, and the tube voltage would have to go below 40 kV.

Anti-isowatt fluoroscopy (curve 2 in Figure 7.74) represents a characteristic which is technically simple to achieve and does not require any technique factor selection. It offers a good compromise between contrast and dose for all objects. The brightness of the image intensifier output screen is measured and used by the automatic exposure control system during fluoroscopy (Figure 7.75). It is measured with a photomultiplier ($i_{B\,actual}$) and compared with the reference value $i_{B\,ref}$. The brightness is kept at a constant value by the reference values for tube voltage U_{ref} and tube current I_{ref} when the transparency changes.

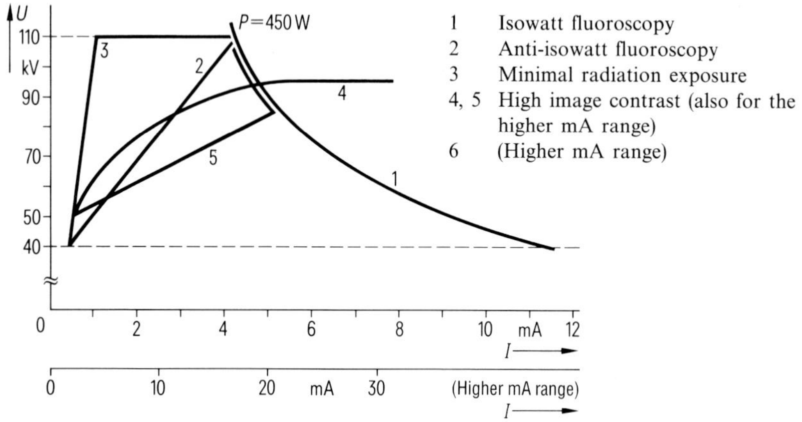

Fig. 7.74
Operational range for fluoroscopy. Characteristic curves of tube voltage U and tube current I

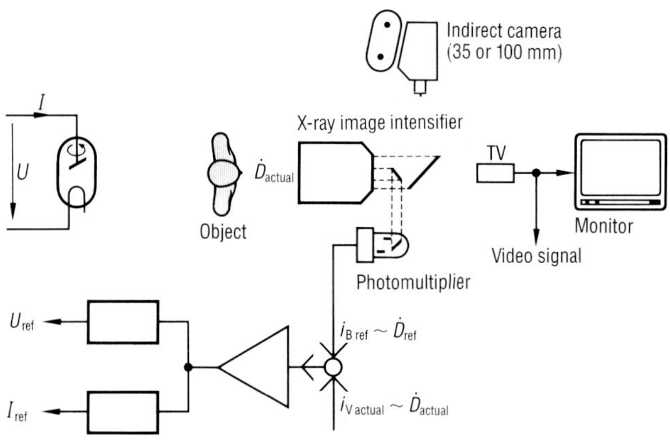

Fig. 7.75
Basic circuit diagram for fluoroscopy with automatic exposure control system (ADC)

Minimal radiation exposure (curve 3 in Figure 7.74) is used mostly in pediatric radiology because special attention must be paid to minimal dose. Therefore, a certain loss of contrast may be acceptable. Application of equation (7.27) means operation at the highest possible tube voltage and low tube current.

High image contrast (curve 4, 5 Figure 7.74) is necessary in interventional radiology procedures. In small vessels the catheter is only visible with high contrast. This contrast is achieved by means of applying low tube voltage and higher tube current. Curve 5 allows high image contrast without exceeding the permissible power P by following the isowatt curve at higher kV values up to 110 kV.

Even higher contrast can only be achieved, among other methods, by extending the tube current range to higher values.

The relationship of tube voltage and tube current shown in curve 4 or 5 is technically complex and requires independent tube voltage and closed loop tube current regulation systems.

Pulsed fluoroscopy is used to reduce dose and improve image quality, especially in interventional cardiology.

The value of tube voltage and tube current relate directly to the transparency of the examined object because the dose rate at the input screen of the image intensifier is adjusted to a fixed value (e.g. 0.175 μGy/s) at the time of installation. This information is used in various automatic control systems to automatically preset technique factors when recording images. This is called the 'automatic data transfer' of technique factors from fluoroscopy.

Indirect exposure techniques

100/105 mm techniques with up to 6 frames per second

Image intensifier photography with 100/105 mm spot film cameras which can record up to 6 frames per second were made possible by the introduction of the image intensifier television chain. The advantages of this technique are the reduction of radiation dose (about 0.9 μGy per frame), lower film costs due to size, and reduced archive capacity requirements.

Organ-programmed techniques are used to set all exposure parameters which include the required frame rate for the medical indication. The tube voltage for spot filming is retrieved from the fluoroscopy tube voltage and corrected depending upon the organ: a gall bladder exposure needs a 10% lower kV value, a double contrast examination of the stomach is done at a 10% higher level, etc. The spot filming exposure is made in continuously falling load operation using the photomultiplier as a sensor for the automatic exposure control system (see Figure 7.72).

35 cm cine technique

Cine technique is necessary to show rapidly moving organs or functions. The images are recorded from the image intensifier output screen on cine film (constant dose value per frame).

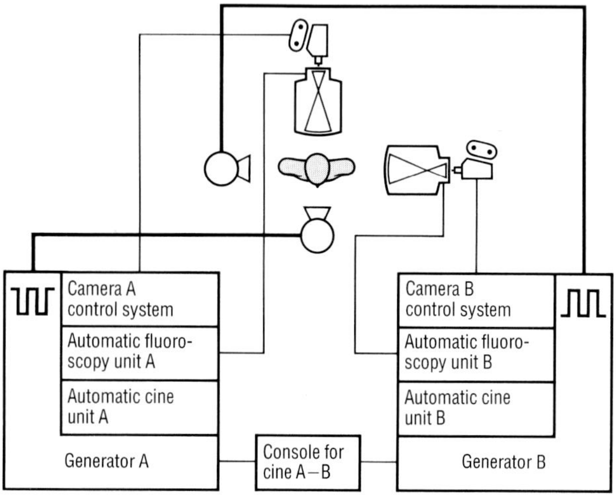

a) Schematic view

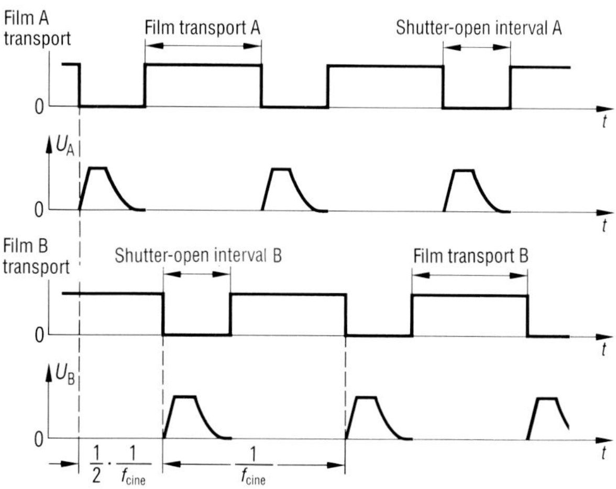

b) Alternating pulse sequence

Fig. 7.76 Biplane cine system

Frame rates f_{cine} of up to 90 or 150 frames/s can be attained depending on the type of cine camera. The drive control of the camera is part of the generator and must be able to run at a selected frame rate in a reproducible way. In addition, the synchronization between the shutter-open interval (when the 35 mm film in the camera is stationary) and the x-ray pulse must be maintained. It is mandatory to avoid any radiation during the transport phase of the film as this kinetic blurring would reduce image quality, increasing at the same time radiation to the patient and operator.

Examinations of the heart (cardiology) are routinely done using cine techniques, especially with biplane cine systems. Figure 7.76a shows the schematic view of a biplane cine system with its controls and figure 7.76b the alternating pulse sequence. The volume of a ventricle can be calculated from cine scenes acquired in both planes. It would be desirable to have simultaneous display of the images. The quality of simultaneously acquired images is, however, very poor due to the scattered radiation produced by plane A or plane B. Therefore, alternating biplane operation is commonly applied.

The principle of the automatic cine system is illustrated in Figure 7.77a. The reference tube voltage for cine is retrieved from fluoroscopy and corrected depending upon the transparency of the patient. A function key contains several pieces of preset information: the focal spot size and power P, the pulse width T_P, the scene duration T_S, and the frame rate f_{cine}. The maximum permissible tube current I_{ref} is calculated and set from the respective tube load data of the focal spot.

Another type of automatic cine system employs the photomultiplier as a sensor to achieve a shorter pulse width rather than to use a preset pulse width. The radiation for each individual cine frame is switched off by the automatic exposure control system.

Geometric blurring can be reduced by an automatic system which always applies the smallest possible focal spot under the condition that a tube voltage range for best contrast is maintained. Figure 7.77b shows the change of focal spot depending on the object transparency. The criterion is the tube voltage U_{CF} determined by the operator, which depends on image contrast. A tube voltage which is too high has a negative effect on image contrast. Therefore, the system automatically switches to the next larger focal spot with increasing transparency and vice versa. The result is a higher tube current at a lower tube voltage.

A lock-in function is applied to prevent an automatic dose increase per frame when the contrast medium is injected into the vessels. It freezes tube voltage and tube current if selected. The lock-in function starts to work beyond the start of the cine scene either immediately, after a programmed time (e.g. two seconds), or a predetermined number of cine frames (e.g. seven frames). The availability of this function is determined by the type of automatic system.

Figure 7.78 shows three conditions under which cine operation may be used. A special x-ray tube with a small grid-controlled focus must be connected to a conventional generator for cine because it is limited to switching 6 to 12 frames/s without grids. The grid interrupts the tube current electronically and is controlled by a pulse attachment.

Timing of the frame rate should be synchronous to the line frequency to achieve reproducibility of dose values. The reproducibility cannot be maintained due to the ripple of the tube current (see section 7.1.4.2, Filament Circuit) if operated in an asynchronous manner.

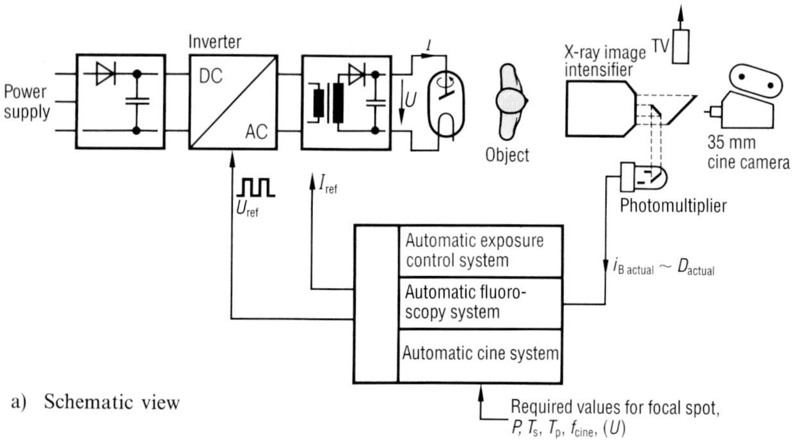

a) Schematic view

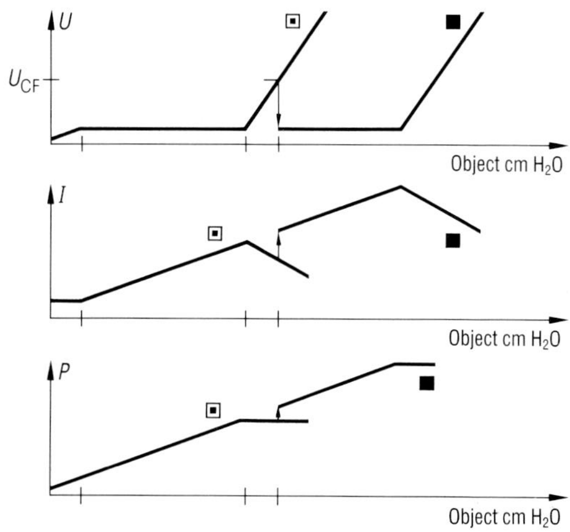

⊡ Small focal spot
■ Large focal spot

b) Method of operation depending on object transparency

Fig. 7.77 Automatic cine system

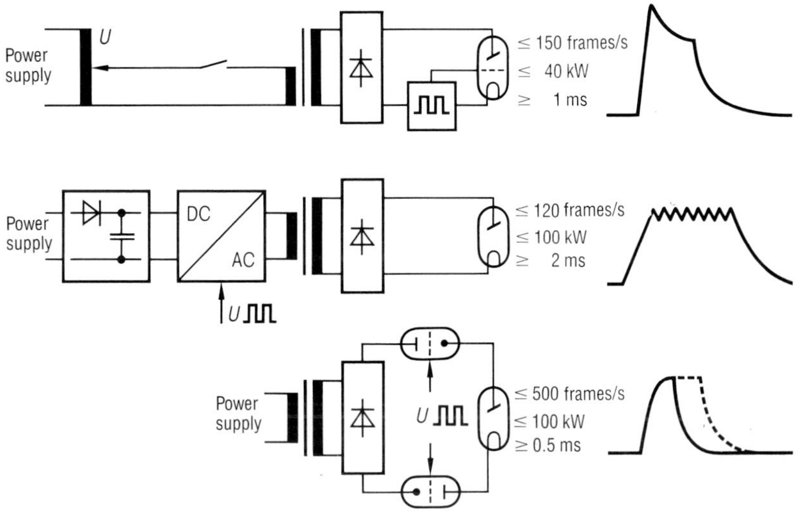

Fig. 7.78 Generators for cineradiography

Top: Generator with grid-controlled x-ray tube assembly and pulse attachment
Middle: High frequency generator
Bottom: Direct current generator with secondary regulation

The power circuits of the high frequency generator and the direct current generator offer cine frame rates for every focal spot up to 100 kW. If the filament circuit is designed as a high frequency circuit (see section 7.1.4.2), pulsing synchronously with the line frequence is no longer necessary.

Digital subtraction angiography (DSA)

Vessels can only be seen in an x-ray image if they are filled with a contrast medium. The quantity of contrast medium may be substantially reduced if the technique of digital subtraction is applied. An unfilled image of the vessel, called a mask, is subtracted from an image filled with contrast medium. The result is an image which contains only the vessel and not the background. An automatic control system for DSA (Figure 7.79) adjusts the technique factors and the iris diaphram so that the tube voltage is kept at a value of $U_{IC} = 63$ kV. This tube voltage is optimum, because the absorption edge of iodine contrast is 33.2 keV.

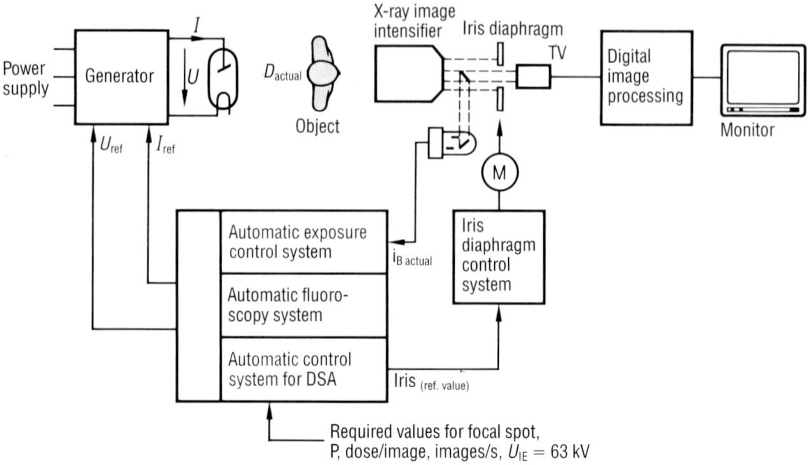

Fig. 7.79 Automatic control system for digital substraction angiography (DSA)

The transparency of an object is obtained from fluoroscopy and automatically transferred into technique factors. The fine tuning of technique factors is performed by the automatic exposure control system.

Hybrid subtraction eliminates motion artifacts or displays soft tissues and bone structure separately [7.44]. To achieve this the generator must produce two x-ray pulses in quick succession with different tube voltages, but at the same dose.

Even small fluctuations of a few percent in dose have a distracting effect on the image in DSA. Therefore, only direct current generators or high frequency generators with a fast closed loop tube voltage control system should be used in this application. Line regulation of 1 to 2% changes the tube voltage of a conventional generator so that DSA images produced are useless (see section 7.1.4.1).

Direct exposure techniques

All exposures where the photographic effect of radiation is used in a film-screen system require a fixed dose value in accordance with equation (7.27). The same is true for xeroradiography and reusable memory screens. The dose value is achieved by the tube voltage U and the mAs product Q. Figure 7.80 shows the principle used by the automatic system to calculate the reference tube current from permissible tube output data and technique factors. In the early days

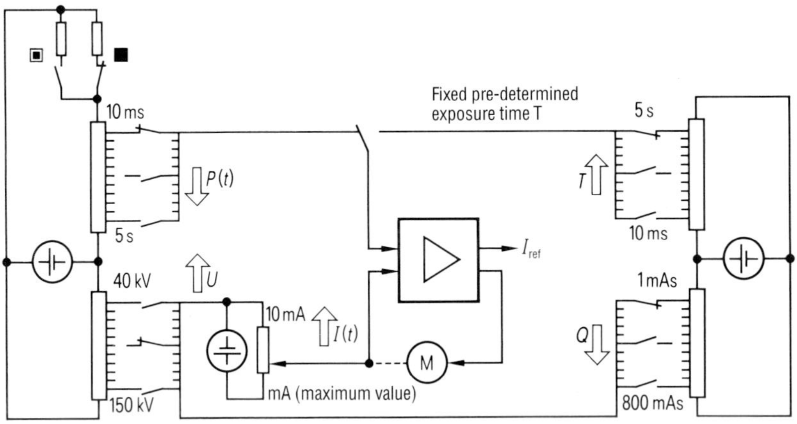

$\log(I/\text{mA}) = \log(Q/\text{mAs}) - \log(T/\text{s}) \leq \log(I(t)/\text{mA})$ $\qquad$ $\log(I(t)/\text{mA}) = \log(P(t)/\text{kW}) - \log(U/\text{kV})$

Fig. 7.80 Automatic control system for direct exposure technique
Analog implementation: For simpler processing, the operational values are converted to their logarithms in a mechanical calculating machine or electronic calculator.
Digital realization: Microprocessor

of radiology the operator had to use several diagrams to set the technique factors. Later mechanical calculators were designed and used according to this principle. More recent advances led to an electronic calculator, and today it is the job of microprocessors.

The operator selects the focal spot and tube voltage to insure spatial resolution and contrast. If an automatic exposure control system is used the selection of the mAs product, Q, is not necessary.

The technique factors pertaining to particular organs can be stored and thus recalled at any time by the 'organ programmed' key. The reproducibility of image quality is increased and retakes are avoided due to elimination of human error. This reduces cost and unnecessary radiation exposure to the patient. Thus, the operator's workload is made easier.

Functional studies require direct exposures of up to 6 frames/s. This type of examination with film changers is called serial technique. Automatic exposure control can be used with film changers.

The image receiver system (the grid contact or film changer control) triggers the exposure for both the direct exposure technique and serial technique. The signal is sent from the receiver to the generator, where exposure is initiated.

The automatic control system used to calculate the reference tube voltage (Figure 7.80) does not take into consideration the thermal state of the x-ray tube assembly. Therefore, the operator must observe the recovery time of the x-ray tube assembly after each exposure (see next section).

Tube load indicator

As described in section 7.1.1 a certain mean continuous power of the tube may not be exceeded. All automatic control systems described above take into consideration the thermal condition of only one examination. The operator must be aware of the cooling break required between examinations. This was in the past never a problem, because the work performed between two successive examinations was longer than the cooling break needed. The time span for an examination and the time between examinations are drastically reduced by automation in table and stand handling, generator techniques and increased routine in performing the examination, as well as cost constraints mandating greater patient throughput. Thus, the neglect of recovery time causes the greatest problem. The consequence is a blown x-ray tube due to thermal overload occurring after only a few examinations.

The thermal state of the anode can be determined by means of measuring or computing:

By measurement – A light sensor built into the tube housing assembly recognizes the red coloration on the back of the anode disk. After amplification the signal is displayed to the operator according to the traffic light principle [7.45]. This technique permits the physician to decide whether it is necessary to risk damage to the tube or not; a green signal lets him know there is no risk of damage, while an amber signal indicates it may be possible to complete an exposure or series without damage to the tube, and red indicates an overload condition exists and damage will probably result.

As a rule, the intervals between amber and green signals are short, lasting only a few seconds or minutes depending upon the tube assembly. Therefore, these hardly disturb the examination.

By computation – From the accumulated loads and the cooling curve, a computer continuously determines the current thermal state of the anode disk and displays this information in HU (heat units) percentage points or waiting time.

The waiting time can also be shortened by means of a reduction in tube power, i.e. from 100% to 80%, if the requirements of the examination permit this. Operation with reduced power and careful observation of the waiting time can substantially increase the life of an x-ray tube, as shown by experience.

A tube load indicator should warn the operator visually and/or acoustically of situations which are dangerous to the x-ray tube assembly. The decision of whether or not to switch off the radiation must be left to the operator's discretion.

Control circuits and safety circuits

Control circuits and safety circuits are the systems for information processing and condition monitoring. Pieces of information are indicated and partially used as signals for control systems in the generator. Measuring points, optical display of functions, and error messages are provided to help the service technician. He can quickly identify errors in the system and keep the 'down-time' low and the 'up-time' high, which is an important prerequisite for good image quality. Good image quality can only be achieved if the operator is familiar with the handling and technical capabilities of the system.

7.1.4.6 Documentation

Relevant generator parameters are provided for documentation. A data plotter or data link to a computer system in the doctor's office or clinical data processing network is helpful for complying with the law. Certain tasks, such as radiation protection for patient and staff, data management for planning and billing, and statistics for administrative and scientific analysis, can be provided by the documentation system.

The simplest form of documentation is taking a manual record of displays. Figure 7.81 shows a serial data link to a printer or a clinical data network for documentation functions or service support. Such a data link is not intended for image transfer.

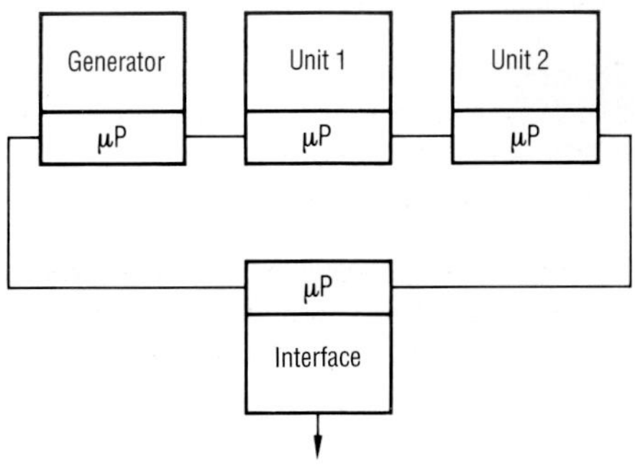

μP Microprocessor

Fig. 7.81
Serial data transfer for documentation

7.1.5 X-ray image intensifiers

As opposed to the x-ray *exposure*, which achieved a useful technical level relatively soon after the discovery of x-rays, x-ray *fluoroscopy* remained virtually unchanged right up until the fifties: the radiologist viewed the fluoroscopic screen after suitable dark-adaptation of his eyes. For normal dose rates in fluoroscopy, the luminance of the screen is in the pure rod vision range, i.e. the viewing conditions are poor (see chapter 1). The mismatch between the flow of x-ray quanta supplied (behind the patient) and the flow of visually recorded information had been recognized for a long time; an effective remedy was not found, however, until the introduction of the electron-optical x-ray image intensifier tube in 1948 [7.47].

In the early years of x-ray image intensification the bright, but extremely scaled-down output image of the x-ray image intensifier was viewed with an optical magnifier. Then, in the sixties, image intensifier television became established which brought further substantial advantages compared to viewing with optics magnifying. Modern x-ray image intensifiers are manufactured with an input field diameter between 15 and 57 cm. Fig. 7.82 shows a modern 40 cm x-ray image intensifier. Here the x-ray input window is made out of a 1.2 mm thick aluminum sheet, the tube housing out of stainless steel, and the insulating ring surrounding the output window of aluminum oxide ceramic material.

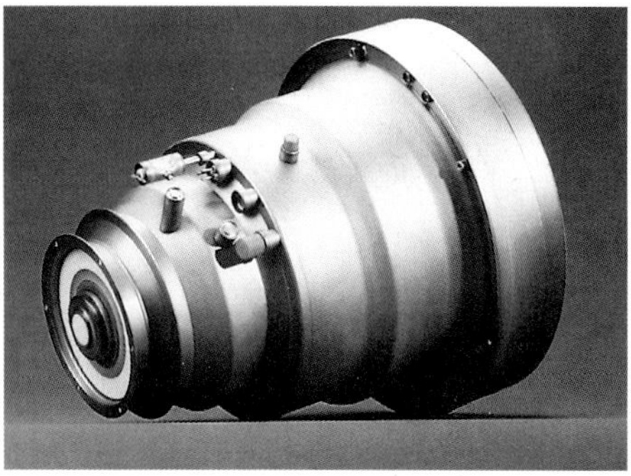

Fig. 7.82
X-ray image intensifier tube with 40 cm input diameter. By changing the focusing voltages whilst retaining the anode voltage of 35 kV, it is possible to switch to input field diameters of 28 cm, 20 cm and 14 cm. In this process the conversion factor decreases (i.e. the output screen luminance relative to the dose rate in the input plane); the resolution increases

In order to be able to use fluoroscopy with bright-adapted eyes even without x-ray television (for the simpler types of examination equipment or in restricting circumstances), an image intensifier of a flat construction was developed in 1980, producing an output image having true dimensions (see section 7.1.5.9).

7.1.5.1 Principles of operation of the x-ray image intensifier

An x-ray image intensifier (x-ray I.I.) is a vacuum tube in which an x-ray image is transformed into a visible image of high luminance. Fig. 7.83 shows a longitudinal section through an x-ray I.I. tube in which only the essential components are depicted. It works as follows:

The x radiation which has been spatially modulated by the object under examination penetrates the *radiolucent input window* of the tube and strikes an *x-ray fluorescent screen*. This converts the x-ray image into an optical image. A very thin photosensitive layer, the *photocathode*, is in optical contact with the fluorescent screen. This photocathode transforms the brightness distribution of the optical image on the screen into an electron flux density distribution. In the half-space in front of the photocathode, the photoelectrons are emitted in all directions. The x-ray screen and the photocathode are situated on a curved base which for electron-optical reasons has approximately the shape of a spherical dish.

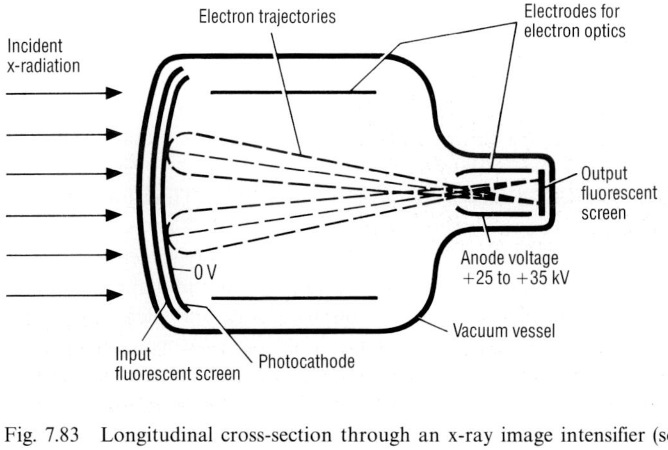

Fig. 7.83 Longitudinal cross-section through an x-ray image intensifier (schematic)

As shown in Fig. 7.83, the electrons emitted in various directions from a point in the photocathode are deflected by the *electrical field* in the interior of the image intensifier in such a way that together their trajectories form a lobar bundle which attains its greatest thickness near the photocathode and becomes progressively narrower towards the anode. At the *output fluorescent screen*, the electron trajectories come together again at one point, the image point. During their motion in the externally applied electric field, the electrons pick up kinetic energy. After traversing a potential difference of about 25 to 35 kV, the energy of an electron is sufficient to generate roughly a thousand light quanta in the output screen.

The electric field in the x-ray image intensifier has a similar effect on the electrons as a focussing lens has for light rays: there arises an inverted, in this case substantially reduced, image. Since *all* the photoelectrons emitted into the half-space are caught by the electron lens, electron-optical imaging is very 'efficient'. The high luminance at the output fluorescent screen is achieved, on the one hand, by the acceleration of the photoelectrons, and, on the other hand, by the concentration of the electron flux from the large photocathode area onto the very much smaller output screen area. The total *luminous flux* is not increased by this second effect, but the *luminance* is. The small, bright output image is very well suited for image transfer to the connected systems (television camera, single-frame or cine camera), because further recording can now take place through lenses with short focal lengths and wide apertures (see section 7.1.5.8).

A numerical example will now be given for the flux density of the respective information-carrying quanta in the various transformation stages. The example uses the dose rate of 0.2 μGy/s ($\approx$20 μR/s) at the image intensifier input, this being normal for x-ray fluoroscopy. With a radiation quality corresponding to a half value thickness of 7 mm aluminum and given this dose rate, roughly 5×10^5 x-ray quanta per square centimeter and second arrive at the image intensifier input. In the input window there is a loss due to absorption of the order of 10%. The absorption in the x-ray fluorescent screen which can be used for generating the image ('effective' absorption) depends on the material of the screen and the thickness of the coating as well as on the radiation quality. For screens of a more recent design made from sodium-doped cesium iodide, one can assume an effective absorption level of 50 to 70%. Thus, for the actual image intensification only a flux density of about 2×10^5 x-ray quanta per square centimeter and second remains available. In the x-ray screen every effectively absorbed x-ray quantum generates several thousand light quanta, of which, however, only a fraction reach the photocathode and there lead to the emission of photoelectrons with a quantum yield of a few percent. In total one obtains about 250 photoelectrons per absorbed x-ray quantum, i.e. roughly 5×10^7 electrons per square centimeter and second. Each electron accelerated, e.g. to 25 kV, finally produces about 1000 light quanta in the output screen.

Thus, one obtains a photon flux of 5×10^{10} per square centimeter of *input area* and second.

This numerical example shows that the flux of the quanta transmitting the image information is clearly smallest at one particular part of the chain, namely when the *effective absorption* of the x-ray quanta occurs in the x-ray fluorescent screen. The following considerations show that this so-called quantum bottleneck acquires fundamental importance with respect to the achievable image quality.

If, for the resolving power of an image intensifier television combination, one assumes a value of 2.5 line pairs per millimeter – in the input plane – then one obtains 2500 resolution elements per square centimeter of input area. The integration time of the entire transmission chain (including the eye) is about 0.2 s. The above-mentioned flux density effectively contributing to the image transformation (in the image intensifier input plane) of 2×10^5 x-ray quanta per square centimeter and second is thus distributed over 2500 spatial and five temporal resolution elements, with the result that on average only 16 x-ray quanta contribute effectively to each spatiotemporal resolution element of the fluoroscopic image.

From statistics one learns that the frequency of occurrence of statistically independent events – in this case the incidence of x-ray quanta – forms a Poisson distribution. If N is the mean value of this distribution, then the standard

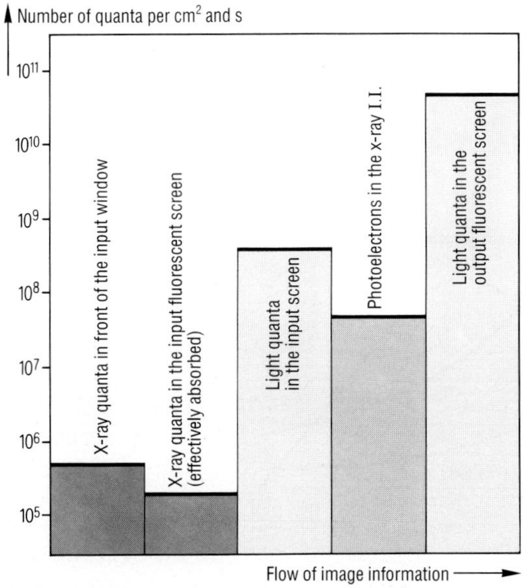

Fig. 7.84
Flux densities of the information-carrying quanta in the various transformation stages of the x-ray image intensifier (x-ray I.I.) for fluoroscopy

deviation σ is equal to $\sqrt{N}$ (mean fluctuation). In 68% of all cases, the number of events lies within the frequency range between $N-\sqrt{N}$ and $N+\sqrt{N}$, and in 32% of all cases outside it.

In the numerical example, $N=16$ and the standard deviation $\sqrt{N}=4$, i.e. a full quarter of the mean value. This numerical example illustrates the statistical graininess of the x-ray fluoroscopic image known as *quantum noise*. As already mentioned, this is caused by the relatively low number of effectively absorbed x-ray quanta. At the same time it becomes clear that in the case of less good spatial or temporal image resolution (the latter e.g. due to a 'slow' television camera tube) the impression with respect to noise is more favorable, i.e. the picture is steadier. A more detailed discussion of quantum noise can be found in [7.48].

7.1.5.2 X-ray fluorescent screens (input screens)

The properties of input phosphors have a crucial influence on the quality of the image transmission of the x-ray image intensifier as a whole. The input phosphor determines to what extent the x-ray quantum flux, which for reasons of radiation protection and often also for technical reasons (see section 7.1.1) is kept small, can be exploited for the generation of images. A compromise must be found between the conflicting requirements for a higher absorption of quanta (*large* thickness of the x-ray fluorescent layer) and for high resolution – or more generally: high MTF values – (*thin* fluorescent layer). Since the resolution limit is more immediately noticeable than a little more or a little

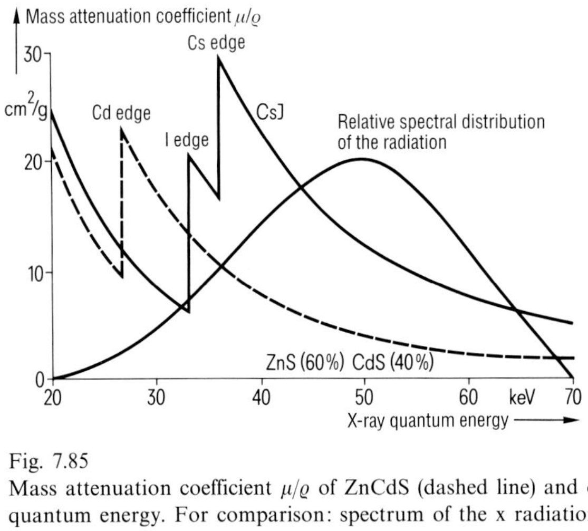

Fig. 7.85
Mass attenuation coefficient μ/ϱ of ZnCdS (dashed line) and of CsI as a function of quantum energy. For comparison: spectrum of the x radiation behind a patient submitted to fluoroscopy, simulated by a 15 cm water layer, at 70 kV x-ray tube voltage.

less quantum noise, one has to consciously resist the temptation to give preference to the resolution at the expense of the absorption of the quanta. The aim must be the optimization of the *diagnostically significant* image quality at the end of the entire information chain, and, moreover, in conditions corresponding to those found in clinical practice with respect to focal spot size of the x-ray tube, dose rate, radiation quality, organ motion, geometric magnification, lag of the television camera tube, and MTF of the connected systems, to mention just the most important factors.

In the case of the x-ray-fluorescent material zinc cadmium sulfide (ZnCdS:Ag) generally used for input screens up to the beginning of the seventies, the above-mentioned compromise was a very unsatisfactory one. It was not until the introduction of the new x-ray-fluorescent material cesium iodide (CsI:Na) that the breakthrough was made to the high image quality standard usual today.

The x-ray fluorescent material CsI:Na combines several desirable properties in an almost ideal way:

- ▻ favorable absorption values for x-ray quantum energies above the *K* absorption edges of Cs (33 keV) and I (36 keV) (Fig. 7.85),
- ▻ good spectral matching to $SbCs_3$ photocathodes (Fig. 7.86), chemical compatibility with this photocathode,
- ▻ good vacuum properties (withstands the degassing temperature),
- ▻ screen manufacture by vapor deposition, producing
- ▻ packing density almost equal to that of the bulk material (in contrast to screens made by sedimentation with a substantially lower packing density), and
- ▻ good adhesion of the vapor-deposited screen to aluminum sheet – thus ease of manufacturing any shape of screen to within narrow tolerances (important for the electron optics).

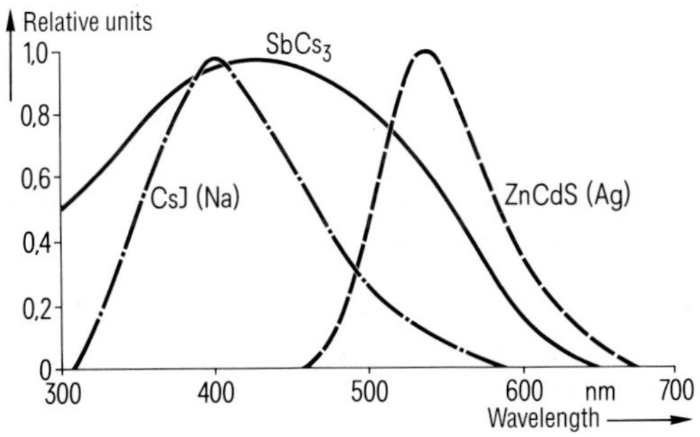

Fig. 7.86
Spectral matching of ZnCdS:Ag and of CsI:Na to the sensitivity distribution of the cesium-antimony photocathode

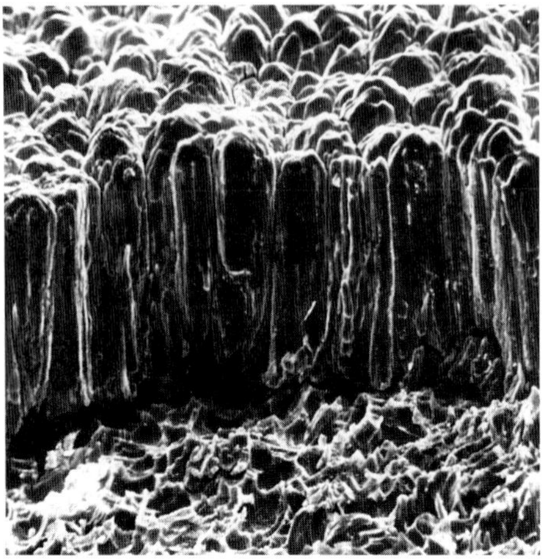

Fig. 7.87
Picture of the broken edge of a CsI x-ray screen taken with a scanning electron microscope

Top: Surface of the x-ray screen

Middle: Broken edge of the CsI crystallites (height about 150 µm)

Bottom: Chemically roughened aluminum substrate

If the vapor deposition process is carried out in a suitable way, the screen consists of continuous crystallites partially separated by fissures which are perpendicular to the substrate and help to conduct the light in the desired direction (Fig. 7.87).

With the CsI screen, the long-standing wish for a screen with a high quantum yield *and* a high resolving power was largely realised.

7.1.5.3 Photocathode

The photocathode in the x-ray image intensifier is a transparent cathode. It is made out of antimony and one or more alkali metals, preferably cesium, which are deposited simultaneously or sequentially by vaporization in a thin layer (about 10 to 30 nm) [7.49]. Its substrate is the x-ray screen, itself, with or without a transparent intermediate layer. The spatial distribution of the photoelectron emission is thus a 'contact print' of the instantaneous distribution of luminescent light in the x-ray screen.

The life of the photocathode – and thus of the x-ray image intensifier tube – is many years at room temperature and with a good vacuum (about 10^{-6} mbar; if necessary, it must be regettered). Long-term exposure to temperatures above approximately 35 °C has an adverse effect on its life.

7.1.5.4 Electron-optical imaging

The electron-optical system in the x-ray image intensifier (x-ray I.I.) is intended to accelerate the photoelectrons that emerge from each point on the photocathode in all directions into the half-space in front of it and to form as point-like an image of these as possible on the output screen. This is only possible to a limited extent, especially as the photoelectrons, apart from the distribution of directions, also have an initial energy between 0 and approximately 1.3 eV. This is small in comparison to the acceleration voltage of 25 to 35 kV, but it is not negligible. Furthermore, the pincushion-shaped distortion must be kept small, and the depth of the x-ray I.I. tube should be as short as possible. And finally, for further imaging on to the connected cameras a *planar* output image is required, unless one decides to let the output image be formed on the hollow-ground inner surface of a fiber optic plate coated with fluorescent material and to level it out with its flat-ground outer surface.

The imaging takes place by means of an axially symmetric electrostatic potential distribution which is produced by the photocathode, several auxiliary electrodes

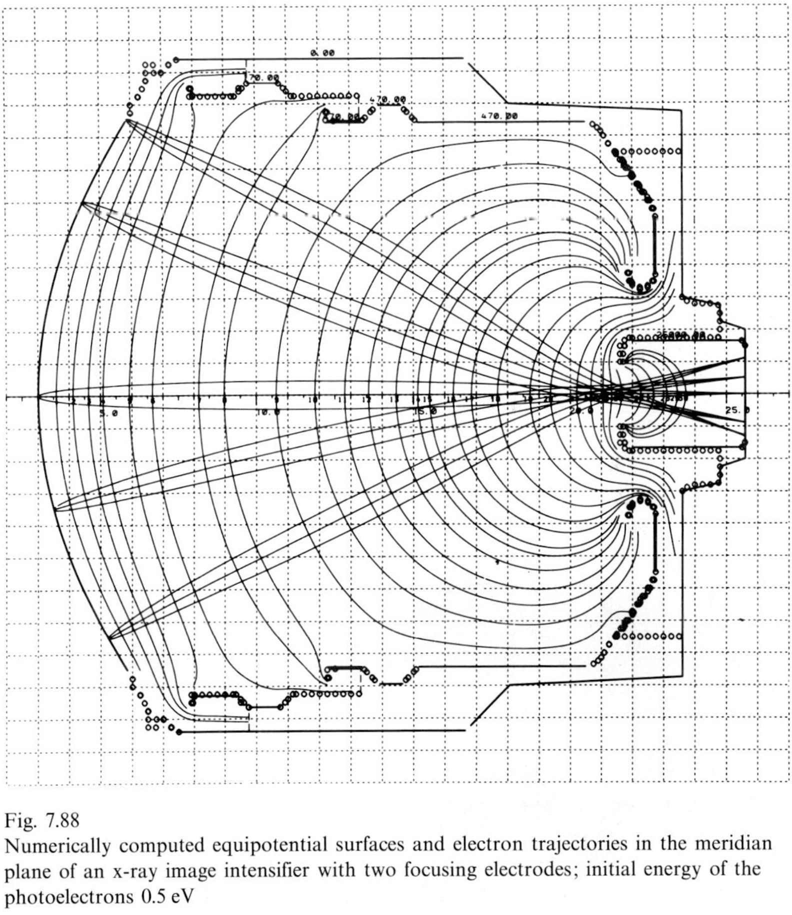

Fig. 7.88
Numerically computed equipotential surfaces and electron trajectories in the meridian plane of an x-ray image intensifier with two focusing electrodes; initial energy of the photoelectrons 0.5 eV

and the anode with the output screen. The calculation of the potential distribution and the electron trajectories for the various initial conditions requires a large computer system [7.50]. Favorable imaging properties result if the photocathode has the shape of a hyperboloid of rotation, whose contour, however, only deviates slightly from that of a spherical cap. In this way a good flattening out of the output image is achieved. Fig. 7.88 shows such a computed potential distribution with a few electron trajectories.

Deviations from the axially symmetric potential distribution lead to imaging errors (astigmatism). Dimensional stability of the electrodes is therefore important, and for large diameters this can only be maintained with a great deal of effort. Fig. 7.89 shows two interlocking cylindrical electrodes made of stainless steel which have several rings to make them stiffer.

Electron-optical imaging is very sensitive to external electric and magnetic fields. In the protective casing a magnetic shield is therefore provided, which is made out of highly permeable sheet-metal and sealed as well as possible. This at least largely excludes the geomagnetic field. Nonetheless, it is advisable that coils, magnets and larger electrical alternating fields (such as those which occur for example near electric cables carrying a heavy load) be kept away from the image intensifier.

The majority of modern x-ray image intensifiers, especially the large-format ones, offer the possibility of electron-optical *format switching* ('zoom'). In this process the anode voltage remains constant, but by changing the focussing voltages only a (concentric) part of the input field is imaged on the whole output screen, i.e. the electron-optical minification is lessened. Because of this, the image resolution is increased; however, the conversion factor is reduced (see sections 7.1.5.6 and 7.1.5.7). Format switching is above all desirable so that the smallest possible image field for the particular radiological task can be projected on to the film or the television monitor so that it *fills the format.*

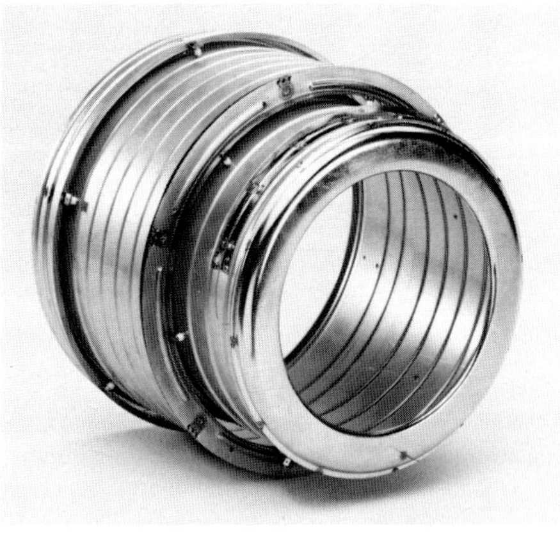

Fig. 7.89
Two concentric interlocking cylindrical focusing electrodes from a 27 cm x-ray image intensifier

7.1.5.5 Output screens

X-ray image intensifier output phospors consist of a fluorescent layer (generally ZnCdS:Ag) just a few micrometers thick and as uniform as possible, on a glass base which may simultaneously by the image output window of the vacuum envelope. Feedback of light to the photocathode is prevented by the fact that the surface of the fluorescent layer is covered with an aluminum skin which is opaque to light but allows the high-energy electrons through. It also serves as an equipotential surface and as an electrical connection to the anode.

Multiple reflection in the output screen base causes stray light which deteriorates the image contrast. The contrast can be improved by using tinted glass as the screen base; the useful light, which only passes through the base once, is attenuated less in the glass than the stray light, which has to go through the glass base at least three times. An expensive, but effective measure for selective attenuation of the stray light is the use of a fiber-optic disk for the output screen base.

There is a new development which enables the interference light to be suppressed *without* the concomitant attenuation of the useful light: one makes the glass base of the output screen roughly as thick as its radius. Then the totally reflected part of the stray light – which makes by far the biggest contribution – is not directed back towards the fluorescent layer but to the blackened edge of the screen base where it is absorbed.

7.1.5.6 Total gain factor, conversion factor

According to the above estimates (see also Fig. 7.84), one obtains about 100 light quanta in the output half-space for every light quantum emitted by the x-ray screen into the photocathode half-space. This factor is called the *lumen gain*, although the term is slightly dubious because of the different luminescence spectra. The *luminance* (unit: cd/m^2) is increased additionally by the factor corresponding to the ratio of the areas of the input and output screens, i.e. for standard x-ray image intensifiers by a factor of 50 to 200, so that there results a total luminance gain of about 10^4.

It is more useful to give the *conversion factor* G_x (old unit: cd/m^2/mR/s; new unit: cd/m^2/μGy/s), which states the ratio of the luminance obtained at the output phosphor to the dose rate of the incident radiation (for standardized ICRU[1] radiation quality, i.e. 20 mm Al-prefiltration and 7 mm aluminum first half value thickness).

[1] International Commission on Radiological Units and Measurements (see also DIN 6814 Part 2)

7.1.5.7 Resolving power, modulation transfer function (MTF)

The resolving power of an x-ray image intensifier is determined by the two screens and the quality of the electron-optical imaging, in particular the electron-optical minification ratio. In x-ray image intensifiers with an input field which can be switched electron-optically, i.e. with a variable image ratio, the resolving power increases with the reduction of the input field used.

Example: In Fig. 7.90, the MTF of a 27 cm x-ray image intensifier with *full* input field is compared to the MTF with the input field *switched* to a diameter of 17 cm. Experience shows that the limit of resolution corresponds to the spatial frequency at which the MTF value has dropped to about 0.04; here this is slightly over four line pairs/mm for the full input field, and about five lines pairs/mm for the 17 cm input field. As recently as 1970, a resolution of two line pairs/mm could only be achieved with difficulty [7.51, 7.52].

7.1.5.8 Further processing of the x-ray image intensifier output image

The output image of the x-ray image intensifier is transmitted with special large-aperture lenses in a *tandem optical arrangement*. By this is meant an arrangement consisting of two lenses, whereby the *object* (x-ray I.I. output phosphor) lies in the focal plane of the first (the so-called collimator) lens, whilst

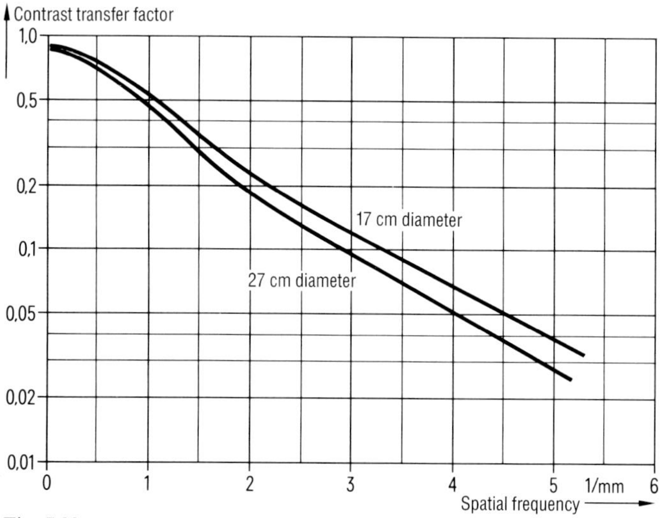

Fig. 7.90
Modulation transfer function of a 27 cm x-ray image intensifier for the full input field, and an input field switched electron-optically to 17 cm respectively

the *image* (on the film or in the television camera) is created in the focal plane of the second (the so-called camera) lens. In between the two lenses of the tandem arrangement, the light rays run parallel. The lenses can therefore be pulled apart and can each be focussed individually. The lateral magnification is equal to the ratio of the focal lengths of the two lenses. The relatively narrow emission spectrum of the output phosphor (e.g. emission maximum of 535 nm, width about 100 nm) permits aperture ratios up to 0.75 for a focal length of 50 mm.

Because of the image quality achieved nowadays with x-ray image intensifiers, *indirect radiography* (using a film format of 100 mm × 100 mm), which allows the more economical use of dose and film, is becoming more and more widely used. Rapid processes, e.g. in cardiology, are investigated with the aid of *x-ray cine*. Since both procedures are always linked to fluoroscopy, an image distributor is used, which guides the light beam to the desired systems by means of mirrors (in certain circumstances semi-transparent ones for simultaneous television observation). Because the rays run parallel behind the collimator lens the position of the deflecting mirror and the respective camera lens is not critical. Fig. 7.92 shows schematically a 3-channel image distributor.

Whereas in the past the 'indirect' radiographs taken through the image intensifier were only accepted out of necessity (because of their poorer image quality) when it was important to have very short exposure times and a rapid image sequence as in cardiology, the indirect images exposed with present-day high-

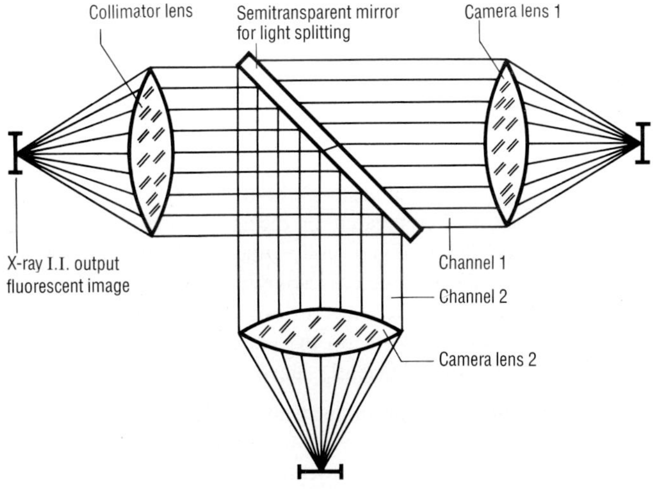

Fig. 7.91 Tandem optical arrangement with 2-channel image distributor

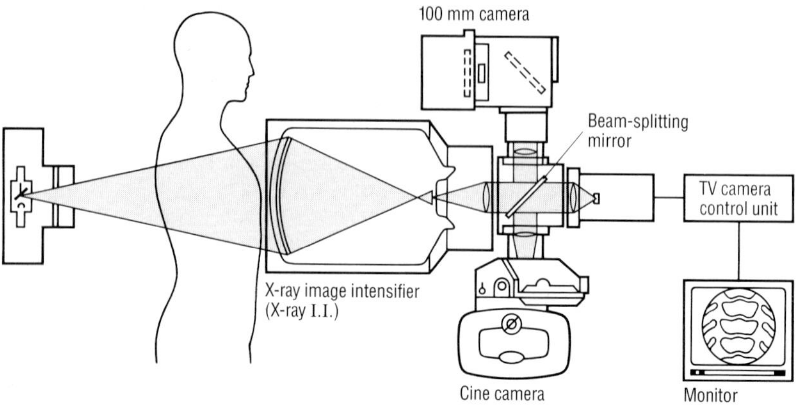

Fig. 7.92
Schematic view of an x-ray unit with a 3-channel image distributor. The semitransparent image-distributor mirror in the parallel path of the rays allows simultaneous television observation during cine or single frame fluorography.

resolution image intensifiers are definitely comparable in image quality with conventional radiographs. The dose requirement for an indirect image at about 75 μR (0.66 μGy) is still considerably less than that for a full-size radiograph with rare-earth screens. Thus it is also possible to have very short exposure times to avoid kinetic blurring.

7.1.5.9 Panel-type image intensifiers

In contrast to the x-ray image intensifiers described up to now, the panel-type image intensifier produces a non-inverted true-size image. In a panel-type image intensifier the electron-optical imaging discussed in section 7.1.5.4 is replaced by so-called *proximity focussing* of the photoelectrons (Fig. 7.93). Here the photocathodes and the fluorescent screens are situated opposite to each other in parallel planes with a voltage difference of about 15 kV, with the result that a homogeneous electric field is created in the space between them. In this space the photoelectrons describe parabolic trajectories. Because of the small distance between the plates and the correspondingly high field strength, however, the 'opening' of the parabolic trajectories remains so small, i.e. the bundle of electrons emerging from a point on the photocathode is so narrow, that the resulting 1:1 imaging is still sufficiently sharp.

In order to achieve the roughly 3000-fold intensification of luminance required, two such intensification stages are necessary. A transparent support transfers the image of the intermediate screen to photocathode 2, and the imaging by proximity focussing is repeated. Nonetheless, the panel-type image intensifier

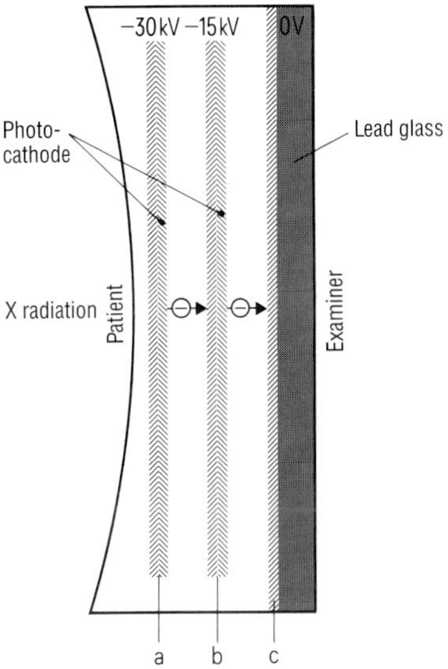

Fig. 7.93
Construction of a 1:1 recording ratio, two-stage x-ray image intensifier of flat design. Input screen (a), intermediate screen (b), and output screen (c) are flat, but otherwise similarly constructed as in a conventional (minifying) x-ray I.I.

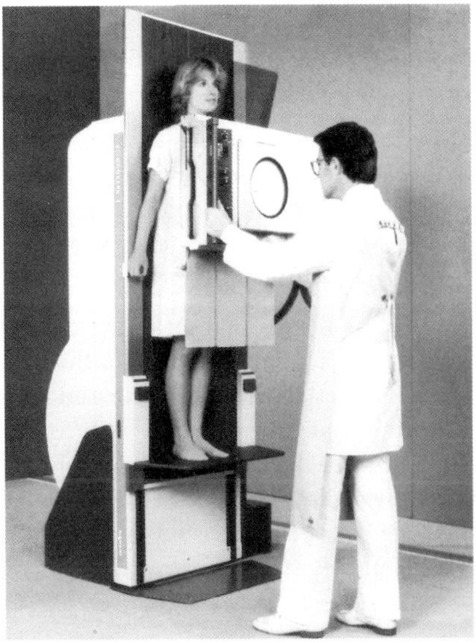

Fig. 7.94
KLINOGRAPH 4 examination unit with the PLANICON. Panel-type x-ray image intensifier
The round image field has a diameter of 20 cm.

attains a resolving power of about 2 line pairs/mm, which roughly corresponds to that of x-ray television. Imaging in a panel-type image intensifier is practically inertia-free. Fig. 7.94 shows an examination unit with a panel-type image intensifier.

7.1.6 X-ray television

7.1.6.1 Television camera tubes (pick-up tube)

The television camera tubes which are used to transform the light from the x-ray image intensifier into an electric signal current are all of the Vidicon type. Thus, the construction and operation of the Vidicon will be described below as being representative for all camera tubes. Tubes like PLUMBICON, SATICON, PASECON, NEWICON and VIDICON (or HIVICON) differ from each other only in the type and the construction of their photoconductive layer (photo-semiconductor, hereafter called 'the layer' for short).

The tubes may be classified according to their dimensions and type of layer.

For high quality requirements in x-ray diagnostics one mainly uses tubes with a nominal external diameter of 1 inch (Fig. 7.95).

More important than the external diameter is the useful layer diameter. This is decisive for the image quality, in particular for the resolution (MTF) to be achieved. For 1-inch tubes the useful layer diameter is usually 16 mm; by means of special design and appropriate manufacturing methods it is possible to increase the useful diameter up to 19 mm.

Fig. 7.96 shows a diagram of the construction and working of a camera tube. A deflecting system takes care of the deflection of the beam of electrons emitted by an indirectly-heated cathode and accelerated by a system of electrodes. This deflecting system guides the electron beam line by line and with a vertical shift over the layer. Focussing coils together with a suitable voltage on the focussing cylinder see to it that the electron beam is sharply focussed onto the layer. In x-ray television units with high quality requirements, this focussing is dynamically modified towards the edge so that each pixel is displayed with optimum sharpness (dynamic focussing).

The photoconductive layer is in principle a capacitor whose dielectric is made out of the material typical for the various types of tube (see Table 7.6). A thin, transparent conductive layer which is mounted on the inside of the glass faceplate (target) forms one of the plates. The plate voltage is applied to this

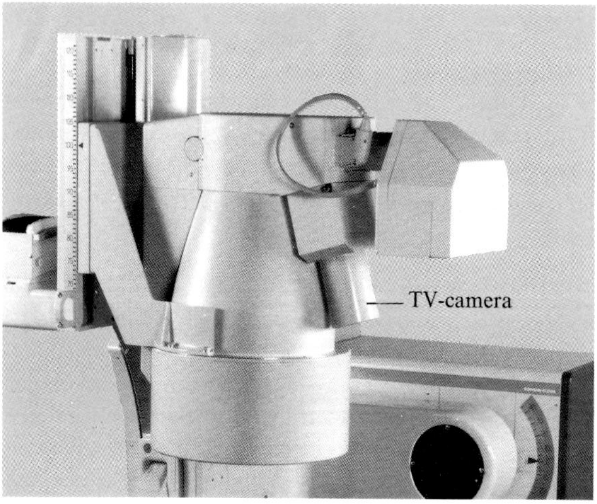

Fig. 7.95
X-ray image intensifier SIRECON 40-4 HD with attached television camera for a 1-inch television camera tube

conductive layer. This voltage is 15 to 50 V depending on the type of tube. The other plate of the capacitor is the free surface of the layer which for a brief moment is brought pixel by pixel to cathode potential (0 V) by means of the deflected electron beam. The capacitor is thus charged up to the potential of the plate voltage.

The individual fictitious pixel represents a parallel connection of a small capacitor with a resistor. This resistance is modified by the intensity of illumination occurring at the pixel. With increasing intensity of illumination the resistance decreases with the result that in the time interval between two scans, the capacitor is discharged more than at a pixel with a lower intensity of illumination. Thus, the electron beam (0 V potential) recharges each pixel with a charge corresponding to the local intensity of illumination. This recharging generates a displacement current, which causes a voltage drop across the resistance (about 2 MΩ) in the plate voltage lead. This voltage drives an amplifier. The displacement current, also called the signal current, is about 100 nA for a pixel of average brightness, whilst the maximum current for the corresponding maximum luminance can be as much as 2000 nA depending on the type of tube (high dynamics of the x-ray image).

The signal current I_S approximately obeys a power function:

$$I_s = CE^{\gamma} + I_d$$

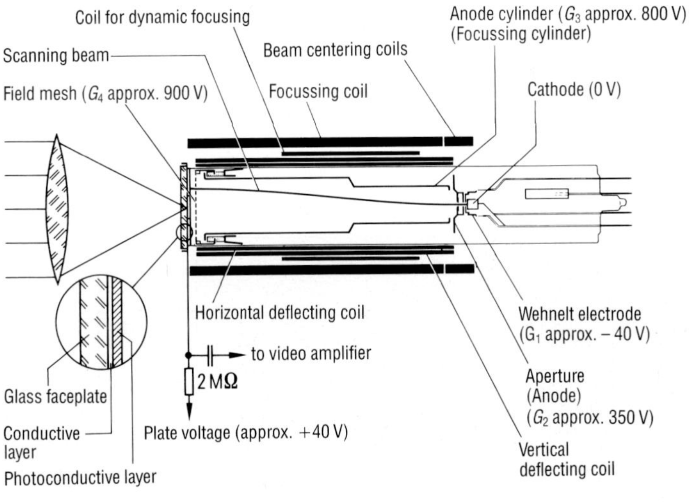

Fig. 7.96
Schematic view of the construction of a Vidicon with deflecting/focusing coil system

Here E is the intensity of illumination (e.g. 1 lx) and C is a constant corresponding to the sensitivity (e.g. 100 nA/lx). The gamma (γ) indicates the slope of the transmission characteristic (I_s/lx), while the dark current I_d is an unwanted and highly temperature-dependent signal current which arises without illumination.

The type of layer is the key factor determining the properties of the camera tube. Inertia (transmission behavior in time) is one of the most important characteristic quantities and essentially determines whether it can be used in x-ray diagnostics. A tube with high inertia (e.g. HIVICON) cannot accurately transmit processes involving rapid movement, but, on the other hand, operates in such a way as to strongly integrate the quantum noise. The PLUMBICON, on the other hand, exhibits a very low inertia, which is accompanied by clearly visible quantum noise in the fluoroscopic image. The SATICON lies between the two types as regards inertia.

Further important properties of the layer are the sensitivity, the MTF, the dark current (the storage capacity during pulsed operation depends on this), the gamma, the spectral sensitivity and the maximum signal current. These characteristic quantities are listed in Table 7.6.

Table 7.6 Characteristics of various types of camera tubes

Type	PLUMBICON		HIVICON	SATICON		PASECON	NEWICON
	1 inch	2 inch	1 inch	1 inch	1 inch	1 inch	1 inch
Type of layer	PbO	PbO	Sb_2S_3	SeAsTe	SeAsTe	CdSe	CdZnTe
Useful diameter (mm)	16.6	26	16.6	16.6	19	16.6	15
Max. signal current µA	1	3.5	1.4	1.4	1.4	1.4	1
Dark current nA	1	3	30	1	1	1	15 … 30
Storage capacity	yes	yes	no	yes	yes	yes	no
Gamma (mean)	1	1	0.7	1	1	1	1
Residual signal after 20 scans (inertia) %	1	1	8 … 16	5.5	6	11 … 14	3 … 8
Sensitivity (relative)	0.85	0.4	1	0.75	0.95	1.5	1.4
MTF (400 line pairs per height of image)	0.2	0.65	0.55	0.53	0.74	0.52	0.39
Max. spectral sensitivity nm	460	490	520	430	430	700	700

7.1.6.2 Video amplifiers

The television camera tube is a very high-resistance signal current source with an internal resistance of several megohms. Fig. 7.97 shows schematically the frequency-response characteristics for a camera input video amplifier. For good matching to the Vidicon, the input resistance (R_I) of the video amplifier has to be as large as possible. In parallel with this input resistance, there are, however, harmful capacitances, e.g. the capacitance of the signal plate of the Vidicon related to the other Vidicon electrodes, the inevitable amplifier input capacitance as well as various other unwanted circuit capacitances. In Fig. 7.97 these capacitances have been collected together in the input capacitance C_I. The voltage at the input of the video amplifier therefore drops strongly with increasing frequency due to R_I and C_I being in parallel. The inverse frequency response of the video amplifier corrects this frequency response in such a way that the output voltage of the video amplifier no longer shows any frequency dependence. The amplification factor (A) of the video amplifier in Fig. 7.97 is thus a function of the frequency f with the parameters C_I and R_I.

Even for conventional x-ray television units, the electric bandwidth of the video amplifier is about twice as large as that in frequency-modulated television broad-

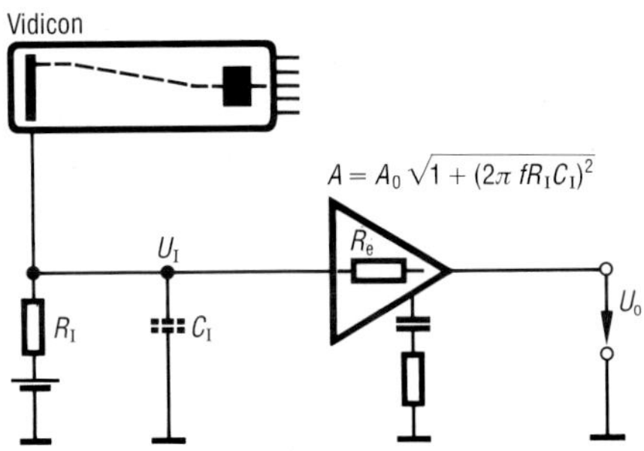

Fig. 7.97
Electric frequency-response characteristics of input and output voltage as well as amplification factor of the camera video amplifier

(R_e is the equivalent noise resistance of the first amplification stage)

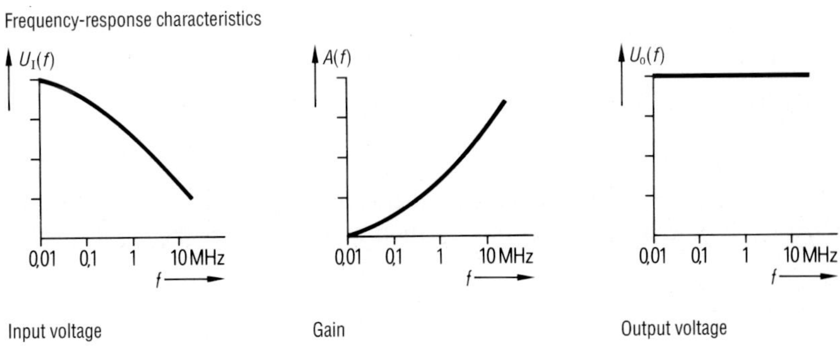

casting. In the case of high-resolution 1249-line x-ray television units, the bandwidth is actually five times as large (25 MHz) as the television broadcasting bandwidth.

Electric noise

The components of electric noise at the output of the video amplifier consist of a part which comes from the input resistance R_I and a part which is determined by the video amplifier. The latter is indicated by the equivalent noise resistance R_e in Fig. 7.97. The contribution to noise of the input resistance R_I is frequency-independent at the output of the amplifier. The noise of the video amplifier, i.e. of the equivalent noise resistance R_e, is not affected by the input capacitance C_I so that the frequency enhancement of the amplifier is fully active. The amplifier noise therefore increases strongly with the frequency.

When dimensioning a camera video amplifier it is important to have the smallest possible circuit capacitances (C_I) and to use amplifier input transistors with low noise and high gain. The result of the high gain is that the subsequent amplification stages no longer have any effect on the noise.

The signal-to-noise ratio (S/N) of a camera video amplifier, which is defined as the ratio of the maximum useful video signal to the effective value of noise, decreases strongly with the frequency because of the frequency dependence of the amplifier noise.

For this reason it was necessary to develop improved video input amplifier circuits for high-resolution 1249-line x-ray television units because of their high electric video bandwidth [7.53]. Compared to conventional x-ray television units, these have improved signal-to-noise ratios by about a factor of 2 over the whole frequency range.

Methods of measurement for obtaining the signal-to-noise ratio (S/N)

There are two methods for determining the signal-to-noise ratio S/N, based on two different principles. On is the integral method of measurement suggested by the CCIR[1] which characterizes the S/N in the frequency range up to 5 MHz by a resulting numerical value. On the other hand, there is the selective measurement method, which describes the variation of the S/N over the full frequency range.

[1] Comité Consultatif International des Radiocommunications

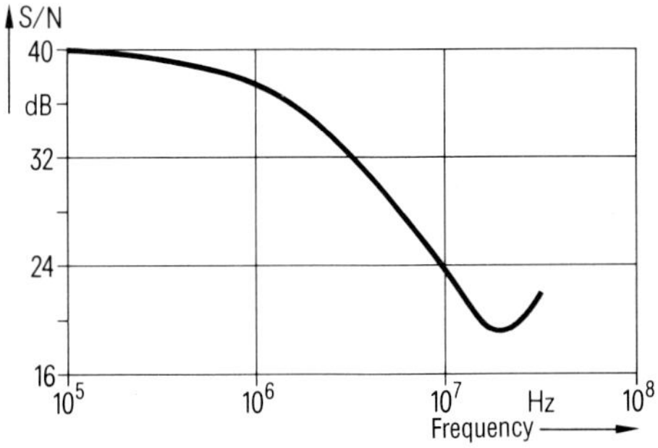

Fig. 7.98
Selective signal-to-noise ratio S/N for a high-resolution television system

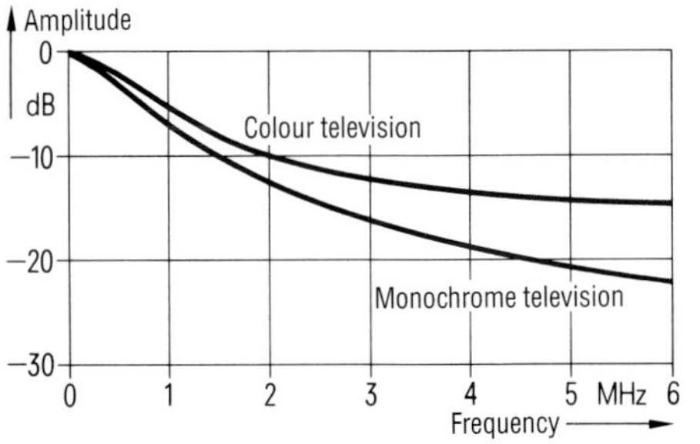

Fig. 7.99
Amplitude responses of the weighting filters

The result of the selective measurement method can be translated into the result of the integral measurement method with the aid of a conversion formula, but not the other way round.

In the selective measurement method, the effective value of the noise voltage is measured at different frequencies with a selective microvolt meter (bandwidth 5 kHz) and compared to a signal which is imposed. The result is the S/N curve as a function of the frequency (Fig. 7.98).

In the integral method of measurement, on the other hand, the total effective noise voltage is measured in a frequency range of 0 to 5 MHz and the ratio to the maximum possible useful output voltage formed. Here attention must be paid to the fact that according to CCIR there is a non-weighted and a weighted measurement. In the weighted case, the measurement of the noise voltage is carried out via a so-called noise weighting filter (Fig. 7.99), which takes into account the subjective assessment of noise by the human eye.

Video signal control

The absorption of the x radiation depends on the transparency of the object and is thus subject to large variations. For routine examinations it is, therefore, necessary that for the physician the average image brightness of the fluoroscopic image at the monitor remains the same. In this way laborious and time-consuming adjustments to the unit are avoided.

Regulation can be realized by means of two different designs

1. automatic *dose rate control* through changing the intensity of the x radiation (ADC),
2. automatic *gain or brightness control* of the television transmission (AGC), (ABC).

For optimum adjustment to the object transparency a combination of the two types of regulation is advisable.

Fig. 7.100 shows the various possibilities of registering the controlled value. Methods where the measurement takes place behind the image intensifier have the advantage that the conversion factor of the image intensifier, which within certain limits depends on the radiation quality, is also registered by the control system.

Dose rate control is a prerequisite for the patient's only being exposed to the dose rate which is absolutely necessary for the desired image quality.

For adjusting to the large range of object sizes which occur in practice, combined control of tube voltage and current is advantageous (see also section on generators).

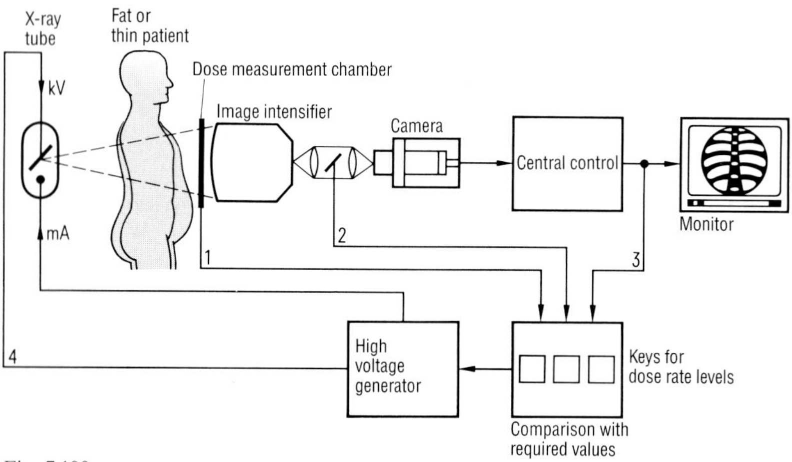

Fig. 7.100
Brightness control of a x-ray television chain by means of keeping the dose rate at the image intensifier input constant. Changes in transparency of the patient are passed to an automatic regulator by a dose measurement chamber (1) or a branched-off light flux (2) or via the output signal (3), which causes a corresponding change in the dose rate (4).

Brightness and gain control

Apart from dose rate control, which attempts to keep the light in front of the television camera tube constant, a second control circuit is incorporated in the television system itself, which ensures correct modulation of the monitor even when the maximum tube power (high object absorption) is reached. Increasing the sensitivity or the gain is, however, also accompanied by an increased impression of noise.

The control the video signal can be done through a *brightness control system* (number 2 in Fig. 7.101) with the aid of the plate voltage in pick-up tubes of the HIVICON type or, alternatively, via the objective diaphragm (iris diaphragm) in all types of camera tube as long as there is a sufficient reserve of light available.

The more common procedure for holding the brightness constant, however, is adjustment of the video signal through *gain control* (number 1 in Fig. 7.101) in the television control unit, since it is independent of tube type and the reserve of input light.

Dominant

To avoid the control systems by being affected by the object areas which are irrelevant to the image, e.g. the occurrence of direct radiation in the case of the extremities or the cervical spine, the controlled value is derived only from

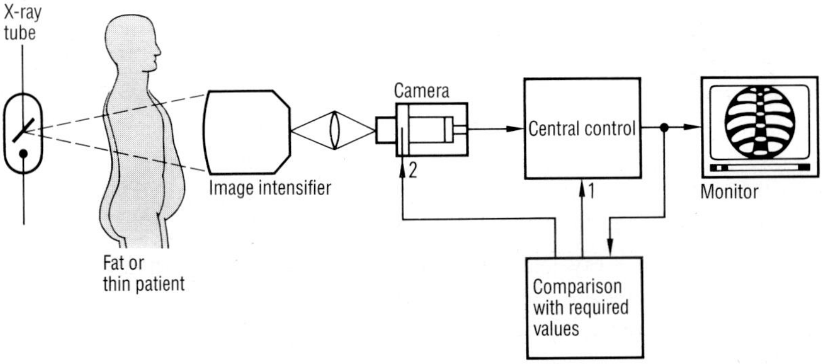

Fig. 7.101
X-ray television chain with gain or brigthness control. The video signal at the monitor is kept constant either via the gain in the transmission channel (automatic gain control (1)) or via the sensitivity of the Vidicon (plate voltage control (2)) irrespective of fluctuations in brightness at the image intensifier.

a part of the visible area, the region of interest (ROI). This part is called the dominant. As a rule the central part of the visible area is used for this purpose. In this way, any direct radiation which may still occur in the peripheral area with optimum positioning of the object does not affect the control mechanism.

Whenever direct radiation strikes the dominant area, this leads, if the object is moving, to large changes of brightness in the object, and the observation of important details is hindered.

Weighting within this area can be done:

a) with reference to the maximum signal value, i.e. peak value,

b) with reference to the minimum signal value, and

c) with reference to the mean value.

Weighting the peak value avoids any overdriving, even locally. On the other hand, it leads to parts which are important to the image becoming too dark when there are only locally confined peak light values.

The control of the dose rate on the basis of the video signal can take place according to any of the three above-mentioned procedures. Control via a dose measurement chamber or a branched-off light flux (multiplier) can only assess the mean value in the dominant.

It should be borne in mind that in a dose rate measurement which compares the two types of control system, the nature of the test phantom (homogeneous or graduated transparency) leads to differing results.

7.1.6.3 Monitors

Operating principle

In modern x-ray diagnostics the fluoroscopic image is observed exclusively on a monitor. Images are increasingly being stored electronically and displayed on the monitor. Thus, the properties of the monitor acquire central importance and will be described in more detail below. Fig. 7.102 shows a very simplified schematic circuit diagram of a monitor.

The monitor of an x-ray television system receives its picture (video signal), also called the composite video signal (BAS-Signal), via coaxial cables with a characteristic wave impedance of 75 Ω.

There are two monitor versions in x-ray television systems: the standard version with 625/525 lines (50 or 60 fields/s respectively) and the high-resolution multi line version with 1249/1023 lines (50 or 60 fields/s respectively). In accordance with the standards, the width-to-height ratio of the scanned area in the standard model has been fixed at 4:3, despite the fact that because of the x-ray image

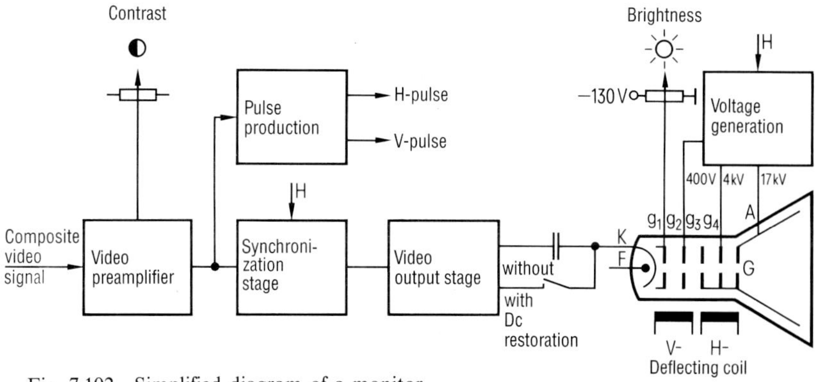

Fig. 7.102 Simplified diagram of a monitor

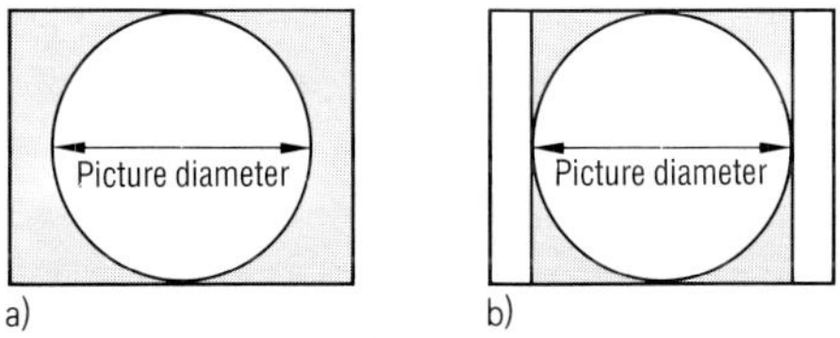

Fig. 7.103
Width-to-height ratio of the scanned area for (a) standard specification: 625 lines (50 Hz) or 525 lines (60 Hz) and for (b) high-resolution model:
1249 lines (50 Hz) or 1023 lines (60 Hz)

intensifier, only a circular image is reproduced (Fig. 7.103 a). The high-resolution model with a square width-to-height ratio of the scanned area of 1:1 achieves a better matching of the amplifier bandwidth to the useful picture format (Fig. 7.103 b). The most commonly used monitor size has a screen diagonal of 44 cm.

Color tone

The transmitted x-ray pictures only encompass gray levels. When they are displayed on monitors a slight color tone appears on the screen depending on the phosphor used. P4 screens produce a grayish-brown impression, and P45 screens a bluish tone, which comes very close to that of x-ray pictures on film. Fig. 7.104 illustrates the spectral distribution of the emitting wavelengths

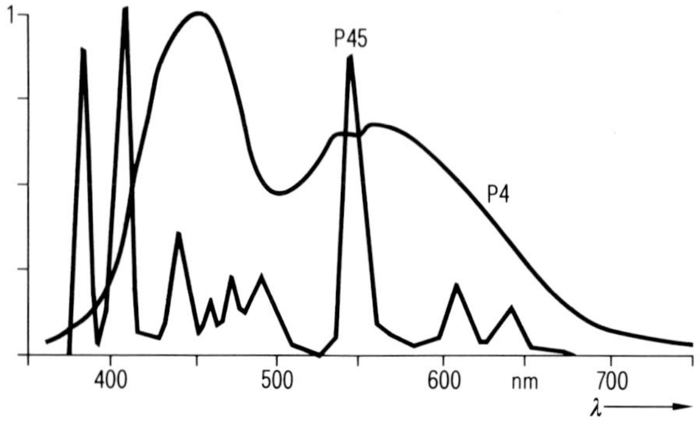

Fig. 7.104
Spectral distribution of phosphors

of P4 and P45 phosphors. The line spectrum for P45 differs strikingly from the smooth spectrum for P4. In this way a color tone with less spread can be achieved.

Contrast and brightness adjustment, picture tube characteristic

To be able to adapt to the object to be displayed to the individual viewing habits of the observer and to the brightness of the room, contrast and brightness control of the monitor is necessary. This can be done by means of two controls on the monitor itself or via remote control from the console.

The correct adjustment of these two quantities is of key importance for the subjective picture impression. To give two examples: A contrast set too high leads to an unsteady picture due to the accompanying increase in quantum noise, making it difficult to recognize fine details. Selecting too high a brightness produces a subjectively flatter picture, since the human eye has a low ability to perceive contrast in bright surroundings.

Setting a higher brightness causes a reduction at the monitor of the negative bias on grid 1 (Wehnelt electrode) of the picture tube with respect to the cathode potential (Fig. 7.105). In this way more beam current is able to flow and the screen brightness increases. Changing the contrast means changing the gain and thus raising or lowering the video signal amplitude at the cathode which controls the beam current.

Because of the picture tube characteristic (Fig. 7.105), setting a higher contrast also means raising the mean brightness in the same way as increasing the brightness also affects the contrast (as a result of the effect of the varying slope of the curve). It should be remembered that when changing one quantity, the other one should also be adjusted so that the desired picture impression is achieved.

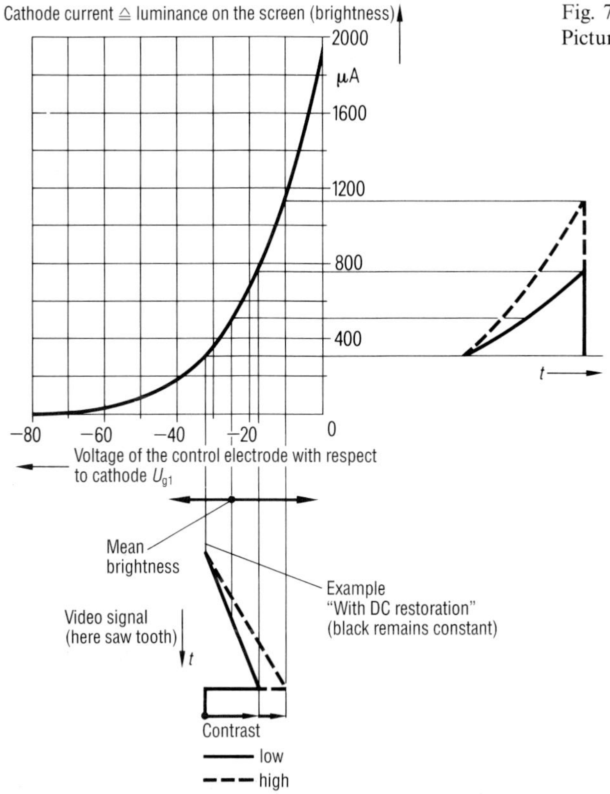

Fig. 7.105
Picture tube characteristic

DC restoration

Monitors can be operated in the mode 'With DC restoration' or 'Without DC restoration' (see Fig. 7.102).

The operating mode 'With DC restoration' (direct current coupling in the amplifier) has the effect that the darkest area of the image retains a certain brightness once it has been set, irrespective of how many white parts of the image there are and how intensive they are (fluctuating picture mean value).

In the operating mode 'Without DC restoration' (alternating current coupling in the amplifier), the mean brightness is kept constant at the value preset on the brightness control.

The mean value in the image can, however, assume quite different values. Fig. 7.106 shows two types of extreme case:

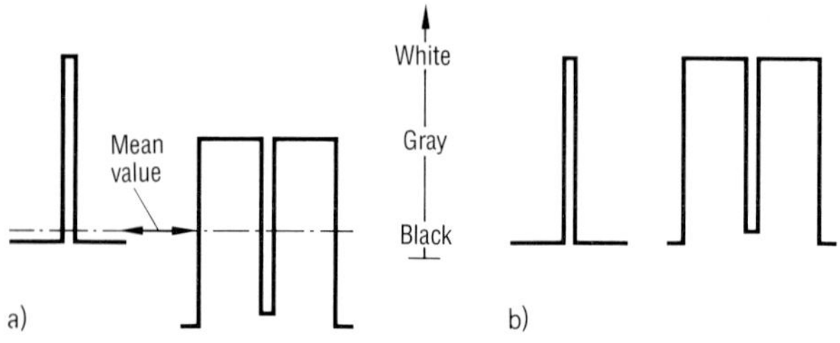

Fig. 7.106
Video signal at the cathode of the picture tube (a) 'Without DC restoration' and (b) 'With DC restoration'.

Fig. 7.106a shows on the left the video signal (line) of a dark image with a white point (low mean value) and on the right the signal of a bright image with a black point in the operating mode 'Without DC restoration. Fig. 7.106b shows the same video signals 'With DC restoration'.

Depending on the examination technique, one or the other mode of operation can be more advantageous:

In coronary angiography, for example, it is appropriate to use DC restoration since in this case, depending on the projection, differing amounts of high-intensity white areas (pulmonary fields) occur in the picture which, however, must not be allowed to change the gray level of the region of interest, the heart.

Measures for enhancing the contrast

Light reflections on the monitor screen have a distracting effect on the image quality. An effective procedure for reducing such reflections is provided by $\lambda/4$ anti-reflective coating. In this process a thin transparent coating is deposited by vaporization on the front screen of the monitor. In this way distracting light incident at a certain range of angles is phase-shifted by the $\lambda/4$ coating by the magnitude of a $\lambda/4$ wavelength. At the glass surface or the luminescent layer the light is reflected and leaves the picture tube through the $\lambda/4$ coating. In this process there is once again a phase shift of $\lambda/4$ so that the sum total of the shift is $\lambda/2$. Ideally this leads to the complete elimination of the distracting light reflection.

A further measure for reducing contrast-diminishing distracting light (brightness of the room) is the use of gray-tinted glass. Whilst tinting the screen glass of the monitor picture tube gray causes an attenuation of the useful light from the screen, it also has the effect of doubly attenuating the distracting light, i.e. when it is incident from outside as well as when it reemerges from the front glass after reflection at the luminescent layer.

7.1.6.4 Spatial modulation transfer function (MTF)

The MTF has proved to be an important and recognized criterion of image quality in x-ray television as well. When the first high-resolution x-ray image intensifier was introduced, it transpired that there was a large increase in image quality associated with the 70 mm or 100 mm x-ray image intensifier image, due above all to its better MTF. Likewise the television fluoroscopic image had become better with the new generation of image intensifiers, but the gain was distinctly less than was the case for x-ray image intensifier images. An

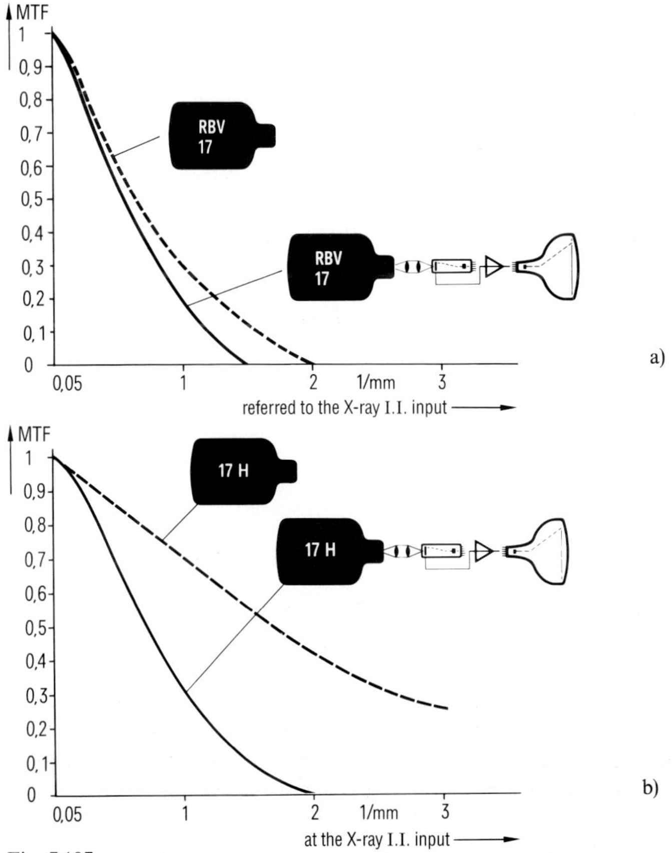

Fig. 7.107
Resulting modulation transfer function of a conventional 625-line x-ray television system together with (a) an older 17 cm x-ray image intensifier RBV 17 (with ZnCdS input phosphor) and (b) a high-resolution x-ray image intensifier RBV 17H (with CsI input phosphor).
The dashed curves are the modulation transfer functions of the x-ray image intensifier alone, i.e. without television chain.

important reason for this was that conventional x-ray television systems, because of the 'poor' MTF of their individual components, were not capable of transmitting the high quality of the image intensifier image without considerable losses in sharpness [7.54, 7.55]. Fig. 7.107 illustrates these relationships with the aid of the resulting MTF of an x-ray image intensifier television system (with a conventional television unit) compared to the MTF of an x-ray image intensifier alone, both with an older x-ray image intensifier with zinc cadmium sulphide phosphor as well as with a high-resolution x-ray image intensifier with cesium iodide input phosphor. The difference between the modulation transfer functions which results using the same conventional x-ray television unit becomes distinctly larger for the high-resolution x-ray image intensifier.

The MTFs of the individual components of the x-ray television chain which determine the image quality can each be measured separately. Fig. 7.108 shows examples of such MTFs for a high-resolution image intensifier and the components of a conventional high-resolution x-ray television system.

In fact the MTF is only defined for linear systems. However, not all the components of x-ray television systems are linear over the entire range of modulation. For sufficiently small deviations around certain averages, linearity can, however, be assumed. Thus, one has for example different MTFs for the image display tube depending on the mean luminance. In Fig. 7.108, therefore, for the MTF of the image display tube, for instance, a mean luminance of 40 cd/m^2 is given.

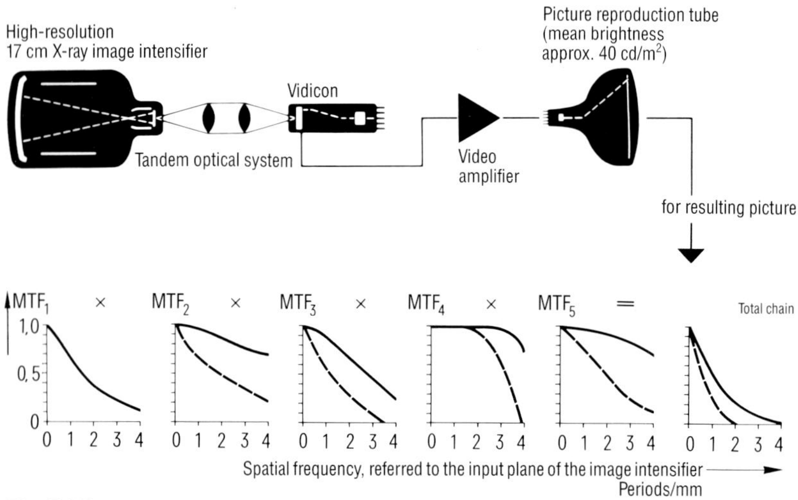

Fig. 7.108
Spatial modulation transfer functions (MTFs) of the components of an x-ray image intensifier television chain and the resulting MTF of the entire chain

The MTF which results with a high-resolution 1249-line x-ray television system is distinctly better than that of a 625-line x-ray television system. With a high-resolution x-ray television system, the MTF which results from the whole chain approaches more closely the MTF of a high-resolution x-ray image intensifier. In this way the image sharpness of the monitor image of a high-resolution 1249-line x-ray television system is no longer so different from the output image of a high-resolution x-ray image intensifier [7.56]. The use in clinical practice of high-resolution x-ray television systems has yielded positive results (e.g. [7.57]). High-resolution x-ray television systems are, indeed, also a necessary prerequisite for high image quality in monitor photography and high-resolution video-storage [7.56].

7.1.6.5 Temporal modulation transfer function (MTF)

The temporal MTF which results from an x-ray image intensifier television chain is essentially determined by the temporal MTF of the television camera tube. Compared to the inertia of the antimony trisulphide Vidicon, a high-resolution x-ray image intensifier with the virtually inertia-free cesium iodide input phosphor no longer has a significant effect, as opposed to older image intensifiers with zinc cadmium sulphide phosphor. The temporal MTF or inertia

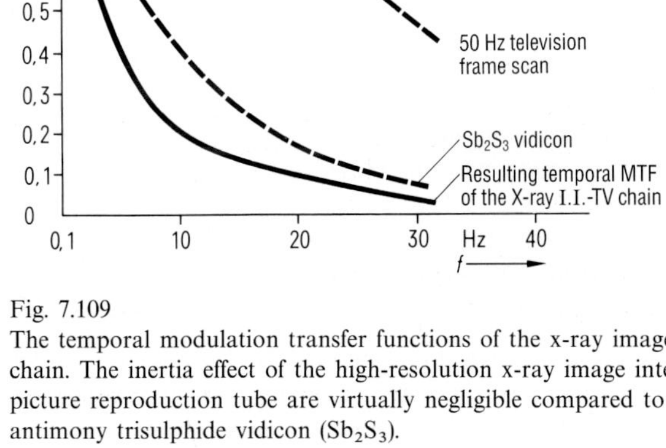

Fig. 7.109
The temporal modulation transfer functions of the x-ray image intensifier television chain. The inertia effect of the high-resolution x-ray image intensifier and that of the picture reproduction tube are virtually negligible compared to the inertia of of the antimony trisulphide vidicon (Sb_2S_3).

of the Vidicon is, as has already been mentioned, dependent on the properties of the photoconductive layers [7.58]. Fig. 7.109 shows the temporal MTF of an antimony trisulphide Vidicon for a particular mean value of the signal current [7.59]. A further contribution is made by the television frame scan with its 50 pictures per second. The corresponding temporal MTF can be given as a function which has the form of sin x/x [7.61].

The resulting temporal MTF of an x-ray image intensifier television chain can be obtained by multiplying the temporal MTF of the Vidicon by the temporal MTF of the 50 Hz frame scan [7.60].

The duration of the after-glow, i.e. the inertia of the picture reproduction tube is so short the phosphor used in the case of x-ray television that the image display tube likewise does not make a contribution of any consequence to the resulting temporal MTF on an x-ray image intensifier television chain.

7.1.6.6 Quantum noise, amplifier noise

For reasons of radiation hygiene, in x-ray television one generally uses very low dose rates, e.g. 5×10^{-9} A/kg $\triangleq$ roughly 20 μR/s. Thus, the number of quanta per unit of time and area is correspondingly small (as already shown in section 7.1.5) with the result that quantum noise makes its presence clearly felt in fluoroscopic pictures. In general, it is the quantum noise that limits the resolution in the fluoroscopic picture.

The question therefore arises of whether a better MTF of the x-ray image intensifier television system still has an effect on the image in the case of the low dose rates encountered in fluoroscopy.

Measurements of resolution at various dose rate values (following Fig. 7.110) show that in fluoroscopic images with high-resolution x-ray television systems even for the lowest dose rates (2.5×10^{-9} A/kg $\triangleq$ roughly 10 μR/s) one still has significantly higher resolution than in television fluoroscopic images with a conventional 625-line television system [7.53].

If one evaluates the output image of a high-resolution x-ray image intensifier with an optical observation instrument, one finds, similarly to Fig. 7.110, higher resolution values than in the monitor image of a high-resolution x-ray television system for the same dose rate values in both cases. This means that with a high-resolution x-ray television system one comes closer to the theoretical resolution limit determined purely by the quantum noise, without however quite reaching it.

For monitor photography, or in the case of the simultaneous storage of spotfilm images, i.e. wherever one has a high image dose, a corresonding further increase in image quality is obtained with a high-resolution x-ray television system.

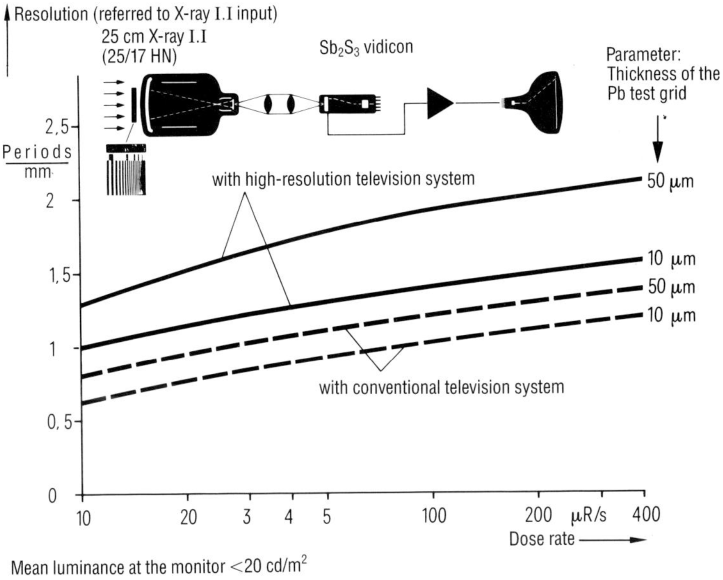

Fig. 7.110
Measurements of resolution with 10 μm and 50 μm lead test grids as a function of the fluoroscopic dose rate. With a high-resolution x-ray television system, even for very low dose rates of 10 μR/s ($\triangleq$ about 2.5×10^{-9} A/kg) one obtains a significantly higher resolution than in a conventional 625-line x-ray television system

In the case of fluoroscopy or video image storage the noise of the video amplifier in relation to the quantum noise in the image only has an effect if the television camera tube is not sufficiently well controlled.

7.1.6.7 Scanning systems

Owing to the increasing use of television systems in electronic recording of images, the necessity arises of implementing other scanning systems besides the standard interlaced scanning procedure, which will be described first.

Interlaced scanning

As is known from cinematography, the frame repetition rate should not lie below 50 frames/s for flicker-free picture reproduction. This, however, would lead to an increased video bandwidth which would have considerable conse-

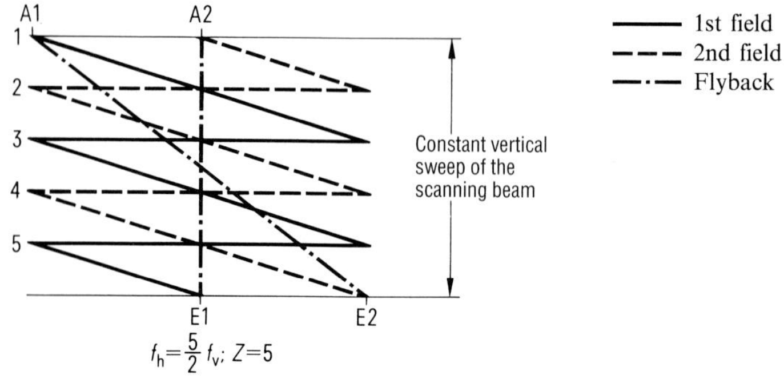

Fig. 7.111
Interlaced scan by tying the horizontal frequency to the vertical frequency (double interlacing). Simple example for a scan with 5 lines

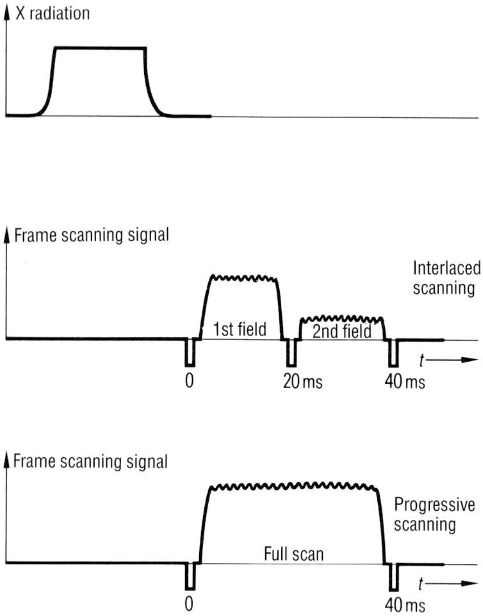

Fig. 7.112
Comparison between interlaced scanning and progressive scanning in pulsed operation

quences, in particular with respect to wireless transmission. For this reason, the procedure of interlaced scanning was generally introduced. The impression of flicker is avoided by the fact that although each individual pixel does not light up 50 times a second, pixels on two neighboring lines are scanned alternately (but each only 25 times per second). The eye merges the two neighboring pixels together and thus gets the impression of scanning at 50 frames/s.

The operation is carried out by dividing up the complete image (frame) into two partial pictures (1st and 2nd fields), which are interlaced as in Fig. 7.111.

Progressive scanning

The introduction of this scanning system became necessary because of pulsed operation (single shot and serial). Scanning following the conventional interlaced procedure would lead to flickering of the brightness. This is due to the nature of the camera tube. In the case of a quantity of charge applied once only to the target, scanning using the interlaced procedure would lead to the amplitudes of the two fields having different levels. In the 1st field, charge from the neighboring line of the 2nd field is also read out (see Fig. 7.112). In progressive scanning, on the other hand, the image is read out line by line in 40 ms.

Since, however, a frame repetition rate of 50 frames/s is required for display, the direct reproduction of a progressively scanned image is not possible. For this reason a digital memory serves as a so-called standard converter (image storage in which the sequence of pixels read out is different from that of those read in). The standard converter reads in the progressively scanned image in 40 ms and reproduces it with the interlaced procedure using 20 ms per field.

Slow progressive scanning

For single images with a high dose and the high quantum signal-to-noise ratio associated with this, it is appropriate to raise the electric signal-to-noise ratio (S/N) of the television system accordingly.

Electric noise increases with the bandwidth of the television system (see section 7.1.6.2 on video amplifiers). An effective measure for improving the S/N is thus limiting the bandwidth. So as not to suffer losses in resolution despite the reduced bandwidth, the horizontal and vertical deflection frequency must be reduced (by a factor of 2 to 5).

Flicker-free reproduction with 50 fields/s of an image scanned using slow progressive scanning is again made possible by a digital image memory operating as a standard converter.

7.2 Digital image storage and image processing

Progress in digital electronics nowadays allows the construction of video image memories which have a high spatial resolution (matrix), and a large dynamic range, that is to say good contrast resolution (quantization width). These digital image memories can store and reproduce the video signals of a high-resolution x-ray image intensifier television chain in real time. Apart from their use for purely storage functions, systems are increasingly being used which simultaneously carry out digital image processing, e.g. noise reduction.

Digital techniques are particularly advantageous in this area because they permit image signal storage, processing and assessment in a manner that is reproducible and with a chosen degree of precision (quality).

7.2.1 Single image storage

7.2.1.1 Principles and technology

For digital image signal storage and reproduction, the following units are necessary:

▻ analog-to-digital converter (ADC)

▻ solid state memory

▻ digital-to-analog converter (DAC)

The analog output signal of the television camera is converted by the ADC into a digital image signal and subsequently stored in the solid state memory.

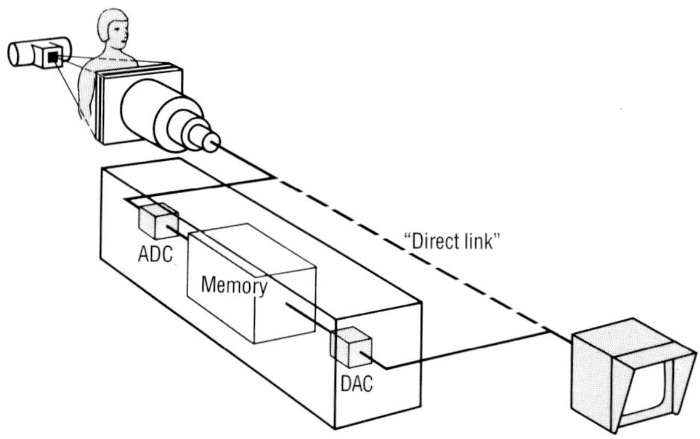

Fig. 7.113 Basic units for digital image signal storage and reproduction

For reproduction the stored pixels are converted back into an analog image signal with the aid of a digital-to-analog converter and displayed on the viewing monitor.

Analog-to-digital conversion

The task of an ADC consists in converting the instantaneous amplitude of the analog image signal into a number proportional to it (Fig. 7.114). This is basically done in three steps:

1. Scanning,
2. Quantization,
3. Coding

Scanning

First of all, the image signal which has already been scanned line by line by the television camera is divided up at equally spaced points in time into single image points called pixels (picture elements).

So that the image signal can be reconstructed without errors from the individual scanning values, the scanning frequency must, according to the sampling theorem, be at least twice as large as the highest frequency appearing in the image signal.

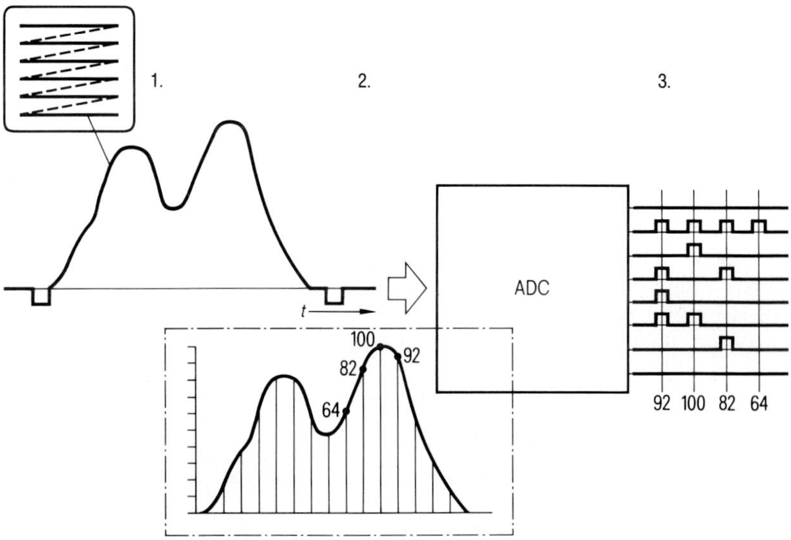

Fig. 7.114 Conversion of the analog image signal

In order to fulfil this requirement, the frequency spectrum of the image signal is restricted before entering the ADC by means of a low-pass filter to half the scanning frequency.

Quantization and Coding

For quantization the entire input amplitude range of the image signal is divided up into 2^N (N is the resolution of the ADC in bits) equal amplitude intervals. Each of the quantization levels is assigned an integer between 0 and $2^N - 1$, e.g. in the case of an 8-bit ADC the numbers 0, 1, …, 255.

The instantaneously scanned image signal is assigned the relevant number in proportion to the amplitude.

This number is turned into binary code by the ADC, represented in a bit-parallel fashion and passed on.

When the analog image signal is converted into an N bit number, there is a loss of information as a result of this limited amplitude resolution, known as a quantization error. Even with an ideal ADC it amounts to $+/-1/2$ the width of a quantization step, i.e. it is as large as half the input signal change which is necessary to change the output code in the lowest place (LSB least significant bit) [7.77].

So as not to reduce the perceptibility of objects with low contrast by the quantization errors, an ADC with an appropriate amplitude resolution should be used, i.e. compared to the quantum noise, the 'ADC noise' should remain negligible. This is ensured if for fluoroscopic operation 8 bits are used, and for images with an x-ray I.I. input dose of e.g. 200 μR at least 10 bits are used.

Solid state memories

For digital storage of single images currently read-write memories (dynamic RAMs – random access memories) are used [7.78]. Depending on the memory capacity and the cycle time of a memory chip, several chips have to be cascade-connected, firstly, in order to reach the required total memory capacity for an image (matrix size times ADC bits), and, secondly, in order to achieve the necessary data transfer rate for real-time image storage by linking memory chips in parallel.

The spatial resolution is decisive for the achievable image quality.

For a resolution of one line pair per mm, 2 pixels per mm are needed. If, e.g. in an image intensifier with a diameter of 270 mm, a spatial resolution of 1 mm is to be achieved, a matrix of 540 × 540 pixels is necessary.

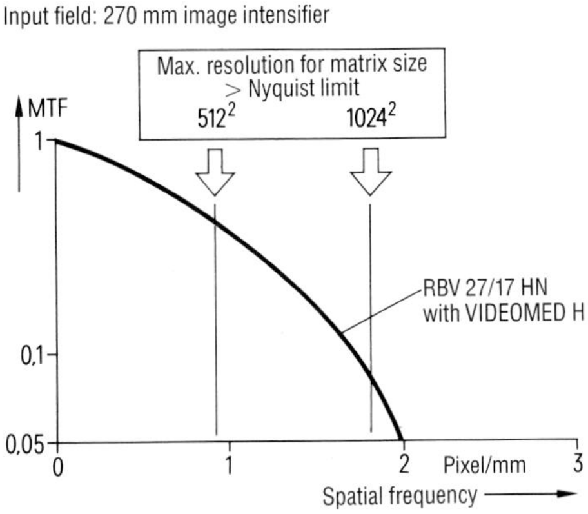

Fig. 7.115
Resulting MTF of an x-ray image intensifier television chain and the resolution limit determined by the matrix

The curve in Fig. 7.115 shows the modulation transfer function (MTF) of an x-ray image intensifier television system with a 27 cm image intensifier and the resolution limit determined by the matrix size.

Digital-to-analog conversion

The digital image signal consisting of individual pixels and stored in the solid state memory has to be converted back into a video-compatible analog signal for viewing on the monitor. To change back a number into a voltage proportional to it, one uses a digital-to-analog converter.

The operating principle of such a converter consists in assigning a weighted current to each bit of a data word. The sum of all the partial currents then yields the analog output voltage, proportional to the digital data word, across the output resistance [7.78].

7.2.1.2 Medical application

Digital single image memories are used to advantage in cases where the possibility of immediate observation of the results of the exposure on at the monitor considerably simplifies the examination procedure (IEI instant electronic image).

A further area of application is the automatic simultaneous storage of the last image of a fluoroscopic scene. This makes it possible to continue to observe on the monitor without radiation and is primarily used in surgical applications.

When simultaneously viewing indirect exposures (cine, 100 mm), the use of a single image memory makes it possible to fill the gaps between two pulses, which would lead to distracting flicker at frame speeds ≤ 25 frames/s, by means of multiple read-out of the memory.

7.2.2 Multiple image storage

The multiple image memory is a central component of a digital image processing system. In contrast to the single image memory it also allows dynamic processes to be registered.

Nowadays a large number of storage media are used as digital multiple image memories:

Solid state memories, magnetic disks, magnetic tape, diskettes and optical disks.

Important features of multiple image memories are:

1. Storage capacity,
   i.e. the number of images which can be stored in a single storage unit
2. Transfer rate,
   i.e. the image frequency (images/s) attainable,
3. Access time,
   i.e. the time required to retrieve a stored piece of information

The data quantities and transfer rates required for the storage of x-ray television images are given in Table 7.6. To obtain these quantities one has to take into account the frame repetition rate, the duration of the scene, the matrix size and the amplitude resolution.

The choice of a storage medium depends, on the one hand, on the above-mentioned three features and, on the other hand, on the cost, the avoidance of errors and the ease of operation.

The various storage media will be discussed below, taking into account the 3 features mentioned above.

Table 7.6 Matrix and image gray level resolution

		512 × 512 × 8	1024 × 1024 × 10
Data quantity per image		256 kbyte	1.25 Mbyte
Transfer rate	4 images/s	1 Mbyte/s	5 Mbyte/s
at image frequency	25 images/s	6.25 Mbyte/s	31.25 Mbyte/s
Data quantity for	4 images/s	8 Mbyte	40 Mbyte
8 s scene duration	25 images/s	50 Mbyte	250 Mbyte

Digital solid state memory

By connecting up digital single image memories one obtains a digital multiple image memory based on semiconductors. With such a memory it is possible to store and reproduce dynamic processes as well as to retrieve single images in real time.

Nowadays digital solid state memories with a storage capacity of e.g. 40 Mbyte can be made. With these it is possible to store 128 images for a matrix of 512×512 and an amplitude resolution of 10 bits.

Digital disk storage (Winchester)

In this storage medium the information is recorded in digital form on one or more magnetic disks arranged on top of each other on a spindle.

Conventional disk storages operate with a mean transfer rate of up to 1 Mbyte/s. This corresponds to an image repetition frequency of 4 images/s for a matrix of $512 \times 512 \times 8$. If suitable measures are taken (parallel connection, data compression) disk storages can achieve image repetition frequencies of 25 images/s for a matrix size of $512 \times 512 \times 10$ and a storage capacity of 4000 images. The access time for stored information is around the 10 ms mark.

Digital magnetic tape

The digital magnetic tape storages common nowadays have a storage capacity of up to 100 Mbytes and a transfer rate of 120 Kbytes/s.

A drawback is the relatively long retrieval time for a stored piece of information. It may be of the order of one minute.

Thanks to the standardization of recording formats, digital magnetic tape is a universal, portable storage medium. Because of this, exchange of image data between different image processing systems is possible.

Floppy disks

Floppy disks are only suitable to a limited extent for digital multiple image memories because of their low storage capacity of 1 Mbyte and their low transfer rate of about 30 Kbytes/s. Floppy disks also belong to the class of portable storage media. In contrast to digital magnetic tape, data exchange between different image processing systems is not straightforward because of non-standardized interfaces.

Digital optical disks

Digital optical disks are especially suited as an archival medium because of their particularly large storage capacity (in the Gbyte range). The transfer rate (throughput) which can be achieved is, however, considerably lower than is e.g. the case with a magnetic disk on account of the thermal recording procedure. In this storage medium, the digital image information is burnt into a specially coated disk with the aid of a laser beam (in a similar way to compact disks). Because of this recording procedure the optical disk can also only be written on once (write-once), i.e. a piece of information once recorded can no longer be erased. In the future, however, with magneto-optical recording procedures, optical disks which can be written on many times will become available.

Comparison of the various types of storage

When comparing the individual types of storage, it becomes clear that the demand for a multiple image memory that simultaneously possesses a large storage capacity, a high transfer rate and a short access time cannot yet be realized by a single storage medium. For this reason, image processing systems are built up out of a combination of different storage types. Such systems are based on the fast solid state memory, which is capable of storing the digitized images in real time. Because of the high specific storage costs ($/bit) the storage capacity is limited. In order to have the solid state memory ready again for the next exposure, all the relevant information is transferred to magnetic disk. Here the magnetic disk has the function of a medium-term storage medium. As the final link in this chain, the optical disk is a suitable medium. It involves the lowest specific storage costs. All the images from the magnetic disk which are to be archived for longer-term availability are stored on optical disk.

Apart from these digital multiple image memories, analog magnetic tape (video tape storage) still has a broad spectrum of applications today. It serves the purpose of storing fluoroscopic scenes and of synchronous storage for x-ray cinematography (cardio-angiography). The advantage of video tape storage is the real-time storage and the large storage capacity (300,000 images) at relatively low specific storage costs.

Disadvantages are the lengthy access time (up to a minute) for a stored scene, the fact that the retrieval of single images is only possible with considerable extra effort, the limited bandwidth of 10 MHz (in particular for cassette models, typically ≤ 5 MHz) compared to a high-resolution TV system (20 MHz), and the lower signal-to-noise ratio.

Data compression

The problem of storing large amounts of data with a high data transfer rate can either be solved by the parallel connection of many disks, which involves high expenditure, or on the other hand by intelligent reduction of the amount of data without losing relevant image information in the process. In reversible data reduction only the redundancy contained in each image is reduced. In practice, in increasing the compression factor one sacrifices fully reversible data compression and tolerates the fact that an irrelevant piece of image information, e.g. noise in the image, is reproduced with a limited gray level resolution. For the purposes of data compression two procedures are used: difference value formation and prediction.

Difference value formation

Instead of storing the absolute digital value of all the pixels, the difference value from pixel to pixel is stored. The absolute value is stored only for the first pixel of each line of the matrix. With this procedure alone a marked reduction in data can be achieved. The compression factor is largest where one has a homogeneous object. No data reduction is achieved if the image presented has a checkerboard pattern and the maximum possible spatial frequency.

Prediction

A further development of the difference value formation procedure is so-called prediction. From the known pixel values surrounding a new pixel a prediction is made concerning the possible value for the latter. The more precise the pixel value to be calculated has to be, the more surrounding values have to be brought into the calculation, which requires a large computational effort. If one only brings one value into the calculation, the computational effort is small, but the result is less exact. Calculating with the aid of three surrounding pixels represents a good compromise between accuracy and speed of computation. The actual and the predicted value are compared and the difference between the two values is processed further. For these difference values an optimum code is calculated according to the Huffman method [7.79], which consists of few bits for difference values close to zero and several bits for larger values. If a code is calculated for every possible difference value one gets a very extensive code table, in which from a certain limit onwards the code requires more bits than the actual difference value. When this happens, the actual difference value is stored directly.

Since in the peripheral areas (outside the circle) the image information usually has zero information content, the difference value zero very frequently occurs in a successive row. In this case one does not code each zero, but the code is transmitted just once together with a multiplier (run-length coding).

This procedure will be illustrated in more detail in an example. Fig. 7.116 shows an extract from an x-ray image with a gray level resolution of 10 bits. The prediction will be made for pixel A taking into account the surrounding pixels X, Y and Z.

The formula for the prediction is:

$$P = X + Y - Z = 820 + 810 - 800 = 830$$

(P predicted value). Subsequently, one forms the difference value D from the actual gray level A and the predicted value P:

$$D = A - P = 840 - 830 = 10.$$

If the frequency of the difference values is determined, one gets a distribution of the type shown in Fig. 7.117. From the distribution one can see that values around zero occur very frequently, and larger difference values more rarely. Using a coding which is optimized to this frequency distribution, the word length of the value to be stored is chosen to be only as large as is necessary to represent the difference value.

Example:

Actual gray level $A = 840$
Required word length in bits $= \mathrm{ld}(A) = \mathrm{ld}(840) = 10$ bits

Difference value $D = 10$
Required word length in bits $= \mathrm{ld}(D) = \mathrm{ld}(10) = 4$ bits

The amount of data required to store pixel A is reduced by a factor of 2.5 by this procedure.

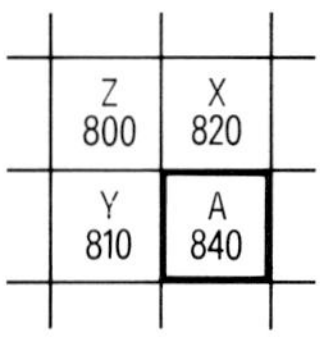

Fig. 7.116
Example of an extract from an x-ray image for data compression by the prediction method

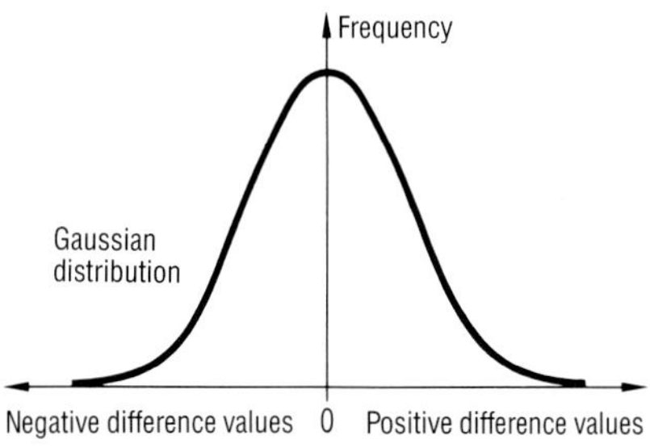

Fig. 7.117
Frequency of the difference values

7.2.3 Digital image processing

The aim of digital processing is the editing of x-ray images by statistical-mathematical methods to facilitate or speed up diagnosis and to reduce the radiation exposure of the patient and the examiner.

A prerequisite for the application of this procedure is that the image is presented in digital form, i.e. that gray levels are converted into numerical values (digitization of the image).

It should be quite categorically stated that there is no method of reconstructing information which is not in some way contained in the raw data of an image or a series of images. It is equally impossible for image processing to relieve the doctor of decisions, not to speak of the responsibility for his diagnosis.

On the other hand, image processing is very well able to function as an intermediary in those cases where a piece of image information is present in a form which is inaccessible to the eye because of the physiological properties of human vision. It can, for example, concentrate the information content of several images into a single one and thus e.g. depict the morphology and functioning of an organ simultaneously, or it can provide aids which compensate for the limited capacity for contrast perception of the eye.

Apart from these procedures for the objective improvement of image quality, there are methods which take account of individual viewing habits or differing diagnostic experience (HP, LP filters, enhancement of particular details, e.g. for teaching purposes).

A selection of current methods of digital image processing will be described below.

Methods of single image processing

Windowing

The present-day level of technology allows the quantization of an image signal with a resolution of 10 to 12 bits. This means that in the digitized image 2048 or 4096 gray levels can be distinguished. In comparison, the human eye is only capable of perceiving about 35 gray levels and thus only a fraction of the information provided.

Here windowing is thus used to purposefully narrow down the range of contrast provided so as to emphasize more clearly details with low contrast.

The windowing technique will be clarified using the example of a 12-bit system (see Fig. 7.118).

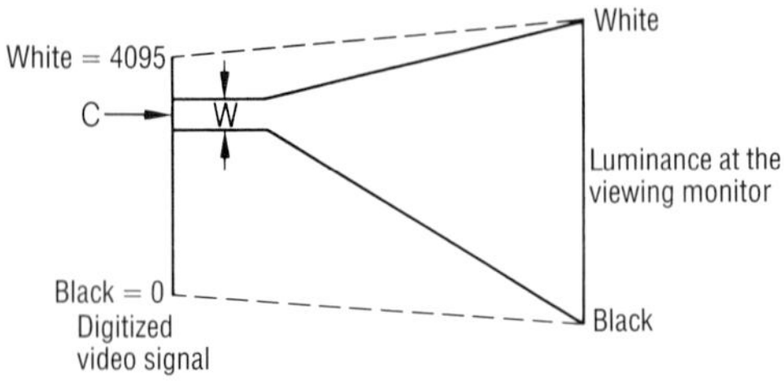

Fig. 7.118
Windowing of the gray level scale of the digitized video signal

The situation without windowing is indicated by the dashed lines, i.e. on the viewing monitor

gray level 0 is represented as black, and

gray level 4095 is represented as white.

By introducing a 'window' within the gray level scale of the digitized video signal (with a center (C) and width (W) which may be freely chosen), and subsequently spreading (amplifying) over the whole luminance range of the viewing monitor, it is possible to represent any gray level ranges of the digitized video signal with maximum contrast resolution on the viewing monitor.

In this case gray levels of the video signal above C + W/2 are shown on the viewing monitor as white and levels below C − W/2 as black.

Look-up Table (LUT)

A LUT is an aid for producing a (non-linear) effect on the amplitude transmission characteristic by digital means. A LUT is realized technically by means of a ROM or a RAM depending on whether the signal conditioning is to

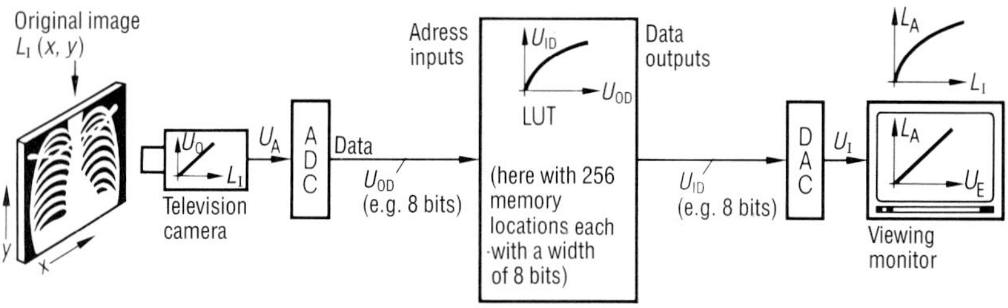

Fig. 7.119
Effect produced by a look-up table (LUT) on the transmission characteristic

proceed according to a fixed or a variable rule. It is located between the ADC and the DAC of a digital image processing system (Fig. 7.119).

The ADC addresses the locations of the LUT memory with the digital gray levels (U_{OD}) of the image signal (U_O).

Each digitized actual gray level on the brightness scale thus addresses its own memory location, which responds with the required value (the previously written location content depending on the application in question).

In this way any input data (U_{ID}) for the DAC can be generated from any digital output code (U_{OD}) of the ADC, i.e. any transmission characteristic can be generated for the total system (see Fig. 7.119).

An example of an application of the LUT is indicated by the transmission characteristics of the simple television chain in Fig. 7.119: let there be a linear relationship for the television camera between input luminance L_I of the original image and the output voltage U_O: let the same be true at the viewing monitor between the input voltage U_I and the output luminance L_A.

If now the LUT is 'written linearly' (i.e., data and addresses of the data in the LUT are identical i.e. $U_{ID} = U_{OD}$), this is equivalent to a direct link between the camera and the monitor: the image impression at the monitor in this case is the same as that of the original image.

If, on the other hand, one wants a change in the contrast characteristic, one loads a suitable characteristic into the LUT: the LUT content indicated in Fig. 7.119 by the characteristic U_{ID}/U_{OD} produces, for example, a compression of contrast in the white region (L_A/L_I).

Spatial frequency filtration (SFF)

By SFF is meant altering the MTF in a linear fashion in order to bring out or tone down certain structures in the image.

Thus, for example, an enhancement of contrast in the case of fine image structures is achieved by high-pass filtering of the image. This is used, for example, in so-called harmonization (which aims to tone down parts of the image covering large areas in favor of fine object structures), or to compensate for the MTF of the image intensifier television chain.

Since, when using high-pass filtering, the high frequency parts of the noise are also amplified, this procedure is most suited to images with a low noise content.

Because of the two-dimensional nature of the image signal (the image brightness is a function of the position coordinates x and y), two-dimensional filter structures (systems) are needed for the filtering of image signals. To describe the effect which a signal (image) undergoes when passing through such a system, two mathematically equivalent procedures are employed: in these, multiplication of the signal $F(k, l)$ (where k and l are the spatial frequencies in the x and y direction) in the frequency domain by the desired correction function $H(k, l)$ corresponds in position domain to a two-dimensional convolution of the spatial signal $f(x, y)$ with the pulse response $h(x, y)$ of the same system in the position domain:

$$G(k, l) = F(k, l) * H(k, l) \quad \text{(Multiplication) corresponding to}$$

$$g(x, y) = f(x, y) \otimes h(x, y) \quad \text{(Convolution)}$$

For the frequency domain:

k, l	spatial frequencies in the x and y direction (in line pairs/mm)
$F(k, l)$	input signal (original image) of the system (filter)
$H(k, l)$	two-dimensional spatial frequency transfer function
$G(k, l)$	output signal of the system (filtered image)

For the position domain:

x, y	position coordinates
$f(x, y)$	input signal of the system
$h(x, y)$	two-dimensional pulse response
$g(x, y)$	output signal of the system

The basic procedure in convolution (to produce a certain behavior of the system in the frequency domain) will be illustrated with the aid of a simple Laplace filter:

Let a two-dimensional convolution kernel for the position domain 3×3 elements in size ($k=3$) be assigned the following weighting factors $W_{\mu\nu}$:

Kernel K1

$$\begin{array}{c|ccc} & & \nu \rightarrow & \\ \downarrow & 1/9 & 1/9 & 1/9 \\ \mu & 1/9 & 1/9 & 1/9 \\ & 1/9 & 1/9 & 1/9 \end{array}$$

$W_{\mu\nu} = 1/9$

$\mu, \nu = 1 \ldots 3$

Kernel K2

$$\begin{array}{c|ccc} & & \nu \rightarrow & \\ \downarrow & -1 & -1 & -1 \\ \mu & -1 & 8 & -1 \\ & -1 & -1 & -1 \end{array}$$

$W_{\mu 1} = -1 \qquad \mu = 1 \ldots 3$

$W_{\mu 3} = -1 \qquad \mu = 1 \ldots 3$

$W_{12} = W_{32} = -1$

$W_{22} = 8$

Let the following image patterns be adopted as test structures (0 black, 1 white):

1 1 1 1 1	0 0 1 1 1	0 0 1 0 0
1 1 1 1 1	0 0 1 1 1	0 0 1 0 0
1 1 1 1 1	0 0 1 1 1	0 0 1 0 0
1 1 1 1 1	0 0 1 1 1	0 0 1 0 0
f_1 (position) Uniformly bright image field	f_2 (position) Horizontal jump in brightness	f_3 (position) Horizontal brightness pulse

Fig. 7.120 shows the pictorial representation of the test structures before and after convolution with kernel K 1 and K 2 respectively in the position domain.

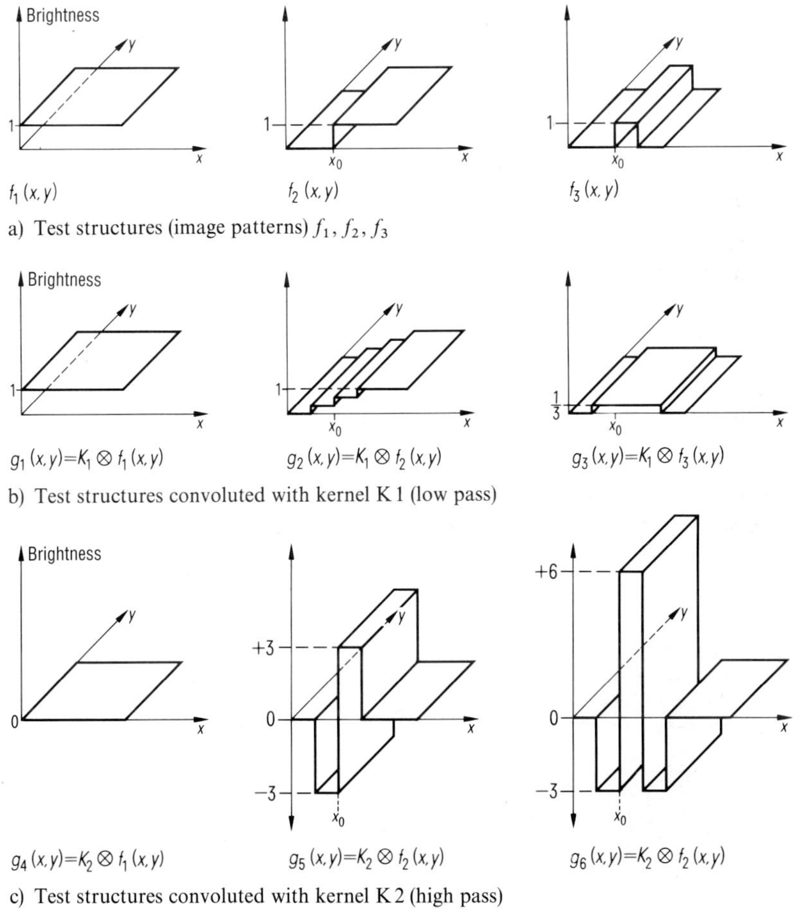

Fig. 7.120 Convolution of test structures with low and high pass

Fig. 7.121
Digital angiographic subtraction images of the cranium (imaging vessels)

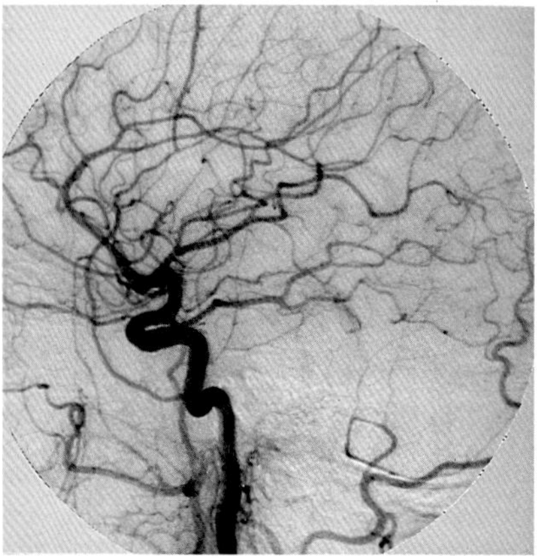

Matrix 512 × 512

a) Original image

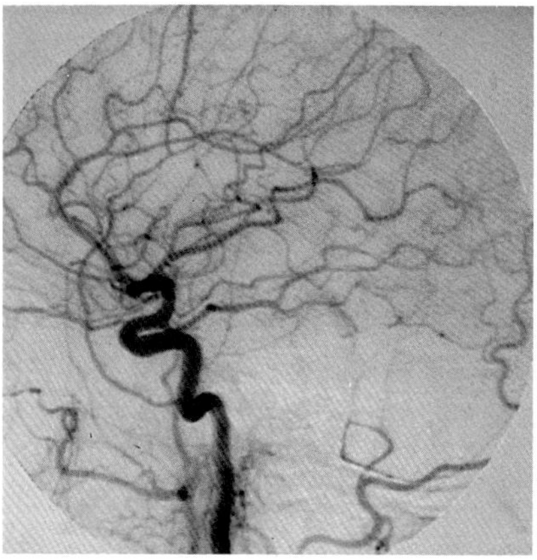

Kernel

$$\begin{matrix} 1 & 1 & 1 \\ 1 & 2 & 1 \\ 1 & 1 & 1 \end{matrix}$$

b) Filtered with low pass (contrast reduction)

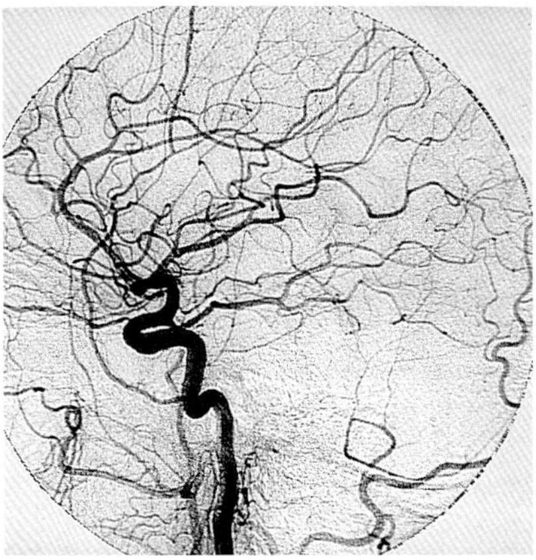

Kernel

$$\begin{matrix} -1 & -1 & -1 \\ -1 & 9 & -1 \\ -1 & -1 & -1 \end{matrix}$$

c) Filtered with high pass (contrast enhancement)

The analytical description of the system response $g(x_0, y_0)$ on convolution of the kernel with the test function f_1, f_2 or f_3 (position) is obtained from the convolution rule for the position x_0, y_0 for an arbitrary kernel to give:

$$g(x_0, y_0) = \sum_{\nu=1}^{k} \sum_{\mu=1}^{k} W_{\mu\nu} f\left(x_0 + \mu - \left(\frac{k+1}{2}\right), y_0 + \nu - \left(\frac{k+1}{2}\right)\right) \tag{7.38}$$

and for the above case ($k = 3$) to give:

$$g(x_0, y_0) = \sum_{\nu=1}^{3} \sum_{\mu=1}^{3} W_{\mu\nu} f(x_0 + \mu - 2, y_0 + \nu - 2). \tag{7.38a}$$

To put it in a more intuitive way, each pixel of the filtered image ($g(x_0, y_0)$) is thus calculated as the sum of the pixel of the original image ($f(x_0, y_0)$) at the same position (x_0, y_0) and the surrounding points encompassed by the filter kernel.

Before addition, each point is weighted with the corresponding factor $W_{\mu\nu}$. Thus, the kernel is 'shifted' uniformly over each point in the original image and incorporated in the calculation according to the convolution rule, i.e. to filter an image matrix of 1024×1024 points, this calculation must be carried out for all points $x_0, y_0 \ldots x_{1023}, y_{1023}$.

Now, the nature of the step or pulse responses (in the position domain) immediately allows one to draw a rough conclusion about the behavior in the spatial frequency domain: thus, a system with a convolution kernel

K1 possesses evidently integrating behavior, i.e. the nature of a low pass (see g_2, g_3, Fig. 7.121b), and a system with a convolution kernel,

K2 describes a high pass (differentiating behavior, see g_5, g_6, Fig. 7.121c).

By an appropriate choice of kernel size and values for the coefficients $W_{\mu\nu}$, limiting frequencies and filter behavior can largely be determined.

One problem of digital filtering should not be passed over at this juncture: the large amount of numerical operations involved. If, for example, an image consisting of 1024×1024 pixels is to be convoluted using a kernel of 15×15 coefficients, at least $1024^2 \times 15^2 \times 2 = 4.7 \times 10^8$ arithmetic operations are needed per image.

Computation times of the order of seconds and less can therefore only be realized with special hardware solutions.

Multiple image processing

Temporal filters, noise reduction

Irregular interference in the form of noise is always superimposed on the image signal. Causes of this are, for instance, quantum noise, electronic noise in the television transmission chain or quantization noise in the ADC. Since in normal circumstances the spectral bandwidth of the noise signal and the useful signal overlap to a large extent, only minimal success can be achieved by analog filtering of the video signal.

Reduction of noise is of particular radiological importance in the case of low-dose images (e.g. fluoroscopy) which by their nature have an unfavorable ratio of useful signal to quantum noise S/N (signal/noise).

An effective method is digital temporal filtration by averaging several images.

The noise-reducing effect of this method can be explained intuitively by the fact that when several images are added together, the correlated useful signals (image) are added up linearly, whereas the noise, which because of its random nature does not show any correlation between the different images, is partially averaged out.

The noise-reducing effect of averaging can be described quantitatively by using the standard deviation σ. For a single image with noise x_i from a series of n images, this is given by:

$$\sigma_i = \pm\sqrt{\frac{\sum(x_i - \bar{x})^2}{n-1}}; \quad \text{with } \bar{x} = \frac{1}{n}\sum_{i=1}^{n} x_i \tag{7.39}$$

For the standard deviation $\sigma_{\bar{x}}$ of the average formed from n images, one has, on the other hand:

$$\sigma_{\bar{x}} = \frac{\sigma_i}{\sqrt{n}}. \tag{7.39a}$$

Since the standard deviation and the effective value of the noise are synonymous in this context, it can immediately be seen on comparing σ_i (noise of a single image) with $\sigma_{\bar{x}}$ (noise of the average of n images) that there is an improvement of the noise behavior by a factor $\sqrt{n}$. Thus, for instance, averaging over $n = 16$ images produces a reduction in noise by the factor of $\sqrt{16} = 4$.

A recursive variant of averaging which allows continuous image display is moving weighted averaging. Here the noise-reduced image $Y(t)$ is calculated not from n images fixed in advance but from all the past images according to the rule (see Fig. 7.122)

$$Y(t) = \frac{1}{k}(x(t) + (k-1) \cdot Y(t-1)).$$

The instantaneously displayed image thus contains all the previous images ($Y(t-1) \ldots Y(t-n)$) with a contribution which decreases proportionally with time. This type of averaging likewise produces a reduction in noise, in this case by a factor of $\sqrt{2k-1}$.

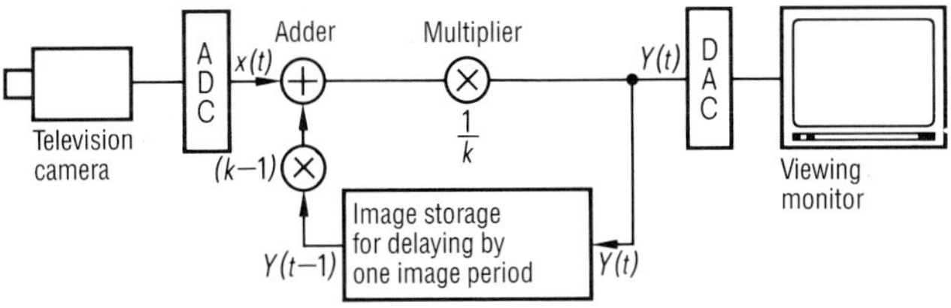

Fig. 7.122 Schematic representation of recursive averaging

This method is accompanied by a reduction in the temporal resolution (inertia of the image, 'streaking' in the case of moving objects). This effect increases with the degree of noise suppression (i.e. with increasing k factor).

This drawback of moving weighted averaging can be partially or totally removed by means of a so-called motion detector:

By a motion detector is meant a numerical process which recognizes moving image regions by a pixel-oriented comparison of successive images and reduces the k factor specifically for the location and the duration of the motion. A process can, however, only be recognized as motion if the difference signal and hence the contrast of the moving object stands out clearly from the noise.

7.2.4 Digital subtraction angiography (DSA)

Basic principle

Subtraction angiography is an x-ray diagnostic procedure for representing images of vessels in isolation. To this end two images, separated by a time interval, are taken of the same region after injection of a contrast medium. The first, the so-called mask, is taken when the contrast medium has not yet reached the target area, the second, the contrast image, is an image of the vessels filled with the contrast medium. The two images are subtracted from one another eliminating the coincident parts of images containing bones and soft tissues so that only the vessel filled with the contrast medium is displayed (Fig. 7.123).

The idea of subtraction angiography goes back to the '30s. As early as this the Dutch radiologist Ziedses des Plantes had described the principle of film subtraction by which two film images, the mask and the contrast image, were produced in a simple way. From the mask a positive was made by producing a copy. If this positive and the contrast image are placed one on top of the other so as to coincide exactly, only the vessels can be seen.

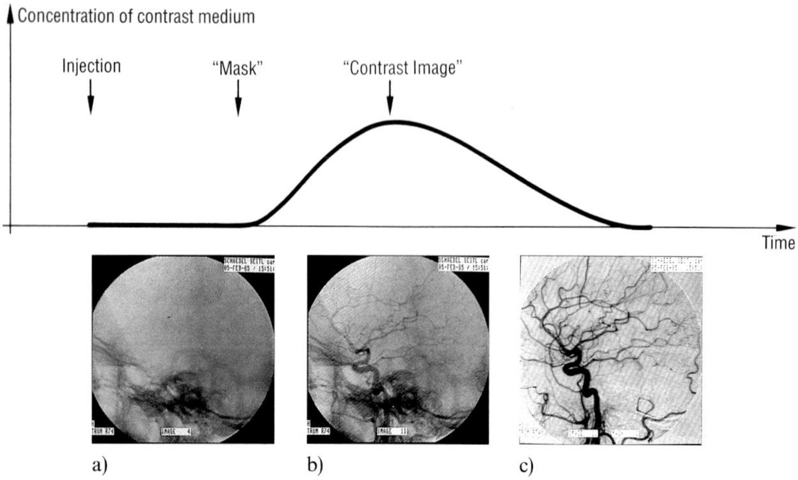

Fig. 7.123
Evolution over time of the concentration of contrast medium with the corresponding images: (a) mask, (b) contrast image and (c) subtraction image

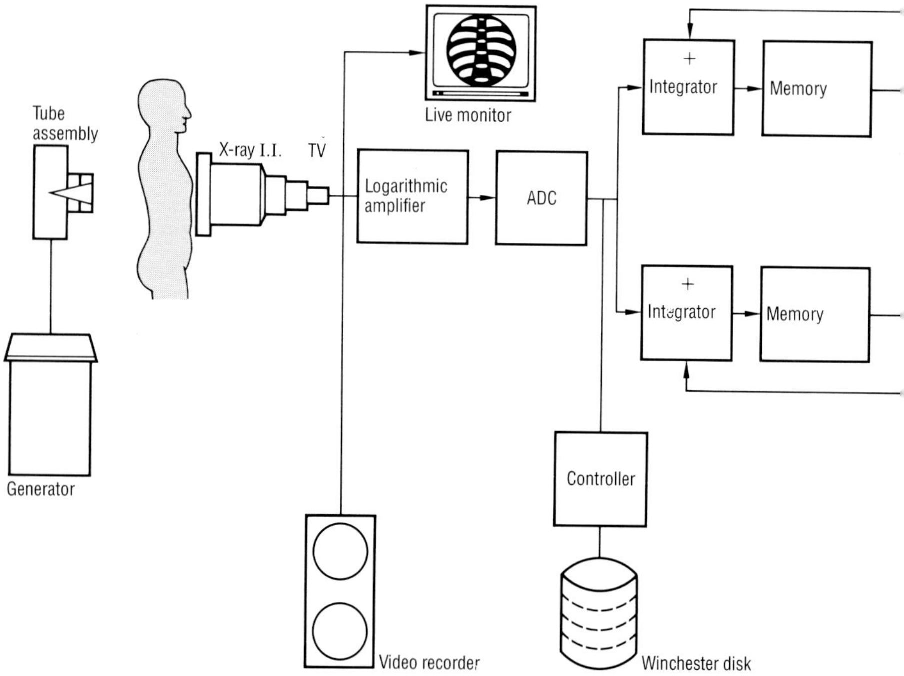

In the '60s and '70s technical procedures were developed for electronic film subtraction. All these procedures yielded useful results, but in spite of this they did not become established because of the effort which was still required to process the film.

It was not until it became possible to digitize, store and process television images in real time that the procedure became widely used (Fig. 7.124). Digital technology permits signal processing which is reproducible and whose precision can be selected in advance. In particular, the technique of intravenous injection which is characterized by an extremely low concentration of contrast medium in the target area, could now be used because of the large signal amplification which had become possible. However, it was also the electronic instant image, i.e. the display of the clinical situation during or immediately after the end of the scene, as well as the possibility of integrating over several images and the accompanying improvement of the S/N (signal-to-noise ratio), which allowed DSA to become an established part of angiographic practice.

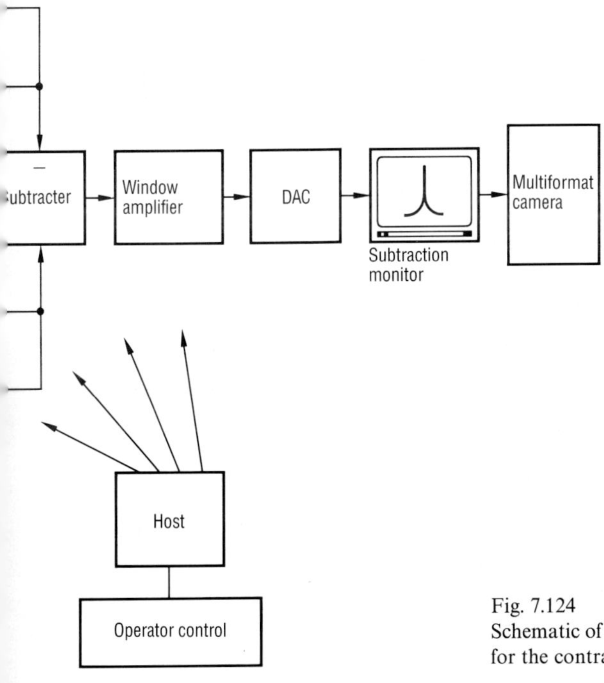

Fig. 7.124
Schematic of a DSA system with two memories for the contrast image and the mask image

Technical realization

The video signal obtained via the image intensifier television chain is converted to its logarithm (see 'Conversion to the logarithm') and subsequently transformed from analog to digital (ADC).

Two memories serve the purpose of holding the mask and the contrast image. The memory contents are subtracted in another arithmetic unit, pass through a digital amplification stage (windowing) and are finally shown on the monitor after digital-analog conversion (DAC). In addition to the chosen mask and contrast image, all images of a scene are stored in a so-called raw data memory. This can be a video recorder with a high S/N, a digital disk storage (Winchester disk) or a large semiconductor memory (>20 Mbyte).

A control system (host processor) makes sure events proceed as required, parameterizes the high-speed arithmetic units for processing the actual image data and organizes the images in the raw data memory.

Postprocessing

Apart from the procedures for postprocessing already discussed in section 7.2.3, such as windowing, temporal and spatial filtering, a special role is played by measures for reducing motion artifacts (coincidence errors). This is done by choosing a mask or contrast image which has been taken at a different time and coincides more exactly, or alternatively by shifting the mask or extracts from it with respect to the contrast image (pixel shift). Often it is sufficient to make a shift by a fraction of a pixel (subpixel shift).

Conversion to the logarithm

An essential prerequisite for DSA is that the contrast signal obtained by the subtraction has a linear correspondence with the concentration of contrast medium. This means that the image of the vessel displayed is a true representation of the concentration of contrast medium and is not distorted by the local amount of total absorption e.g. by superimposed bones.

The intensity of the absorbed x radiation depends on the input intensity, the attenuation coefficient and the thickness of the object; it has the form of an exponential function.

Making the simplifying assumption of monochromatic radiation, one has for the mask image

$$I_M = I_0 \cdot e^{-\mu \cdot d}. \qquad (7.40)$$

I_M Intensity behind the object without contrast medium
I_0 Intensity in front of the object
μ Attenuation coefficient of the tissue
d Thickness of the object

When the vessels are filled with contrast medium (e.g. iodine), the absorption coefficient μ is replaced by μ_I according to the thickness of the vessel Δ:

$$I_F = I_0 \cdot e^{-[\mu(d-\Delta)+\mu_J \cdot \Delta]}. \tag{7.41}$$

I_F Intensity behind the object with contrast medium

Without transformation to a logarithmic intensity scale, the signal I_s in the subtraction image would be given by

$$\begin{aligned} I_s = I_F - I_M &= I_0 e^{-[\mu(d-\Delta)+\mu_j\Delta]} - I_0 e^{-\mu d} \\ &= I_0 e^{-\mu d - \Delta(\mu_j - \mu)} - I_0 e^{-\mu d} \end{aligned} \tag{7.42}$$

and thus would not only depend on the amount of contrast medium in the vessel (via μ_j Δ), but also on the input intensity and the total attenuation μd arising at the position in question.

By conversion to the logarithm (Fig. 7.125), before subtraction, however, one obtains

$$\begin{aligned} \log I_F - \log I_M &= \log I_0 - \mu d - \Delta(\mu_j - \mu) - \log I_0 + \mu d \\ &= -\Delta(\mu_j - \mu) \approx -\Delta \mu_j. \end{aligned} \tag{7.43}$$

As long as I_0 does not vary between mask and contrast images, this subtraction result is independent of the input intensity. It is also virtually independent

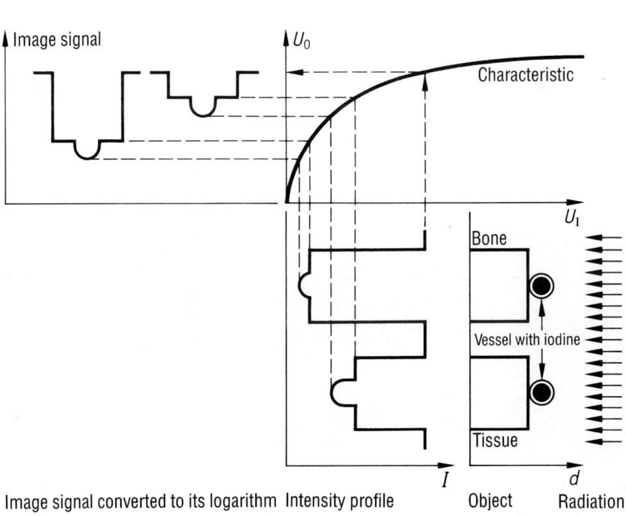

Fig. 7.125 Conversion of the image signal to its logarithm

of the superimposed body tissue as in the case of iodine contrast medium $\mu_j \gg \mu$. Thus a true representation of the amount of contrast medium is obtained.

Road-mapping

For selective catheterization, which has become more important because of interventional therapeutic methods, a fluoroscopic subtraction procedure called road-mapping is used. This procedure gives a continuous orientation aid concerning the position of the catheter in relation to the path of the vessel (Fig. 7.126).

Procedure for road-mapping:

In the vascular tree of interest a small quantity of contrast medium is injected. When the vessel has been filled to the maximum extent an image is stored in the memory, which serves as a mask for the rest of the procedure. While the catheter is being moved, this mask is continuously subtracted from the fluoroscopic image. In this way both the vascular image (path) and the advancing catheter (superimposed on the subtraction image) can be displayed.

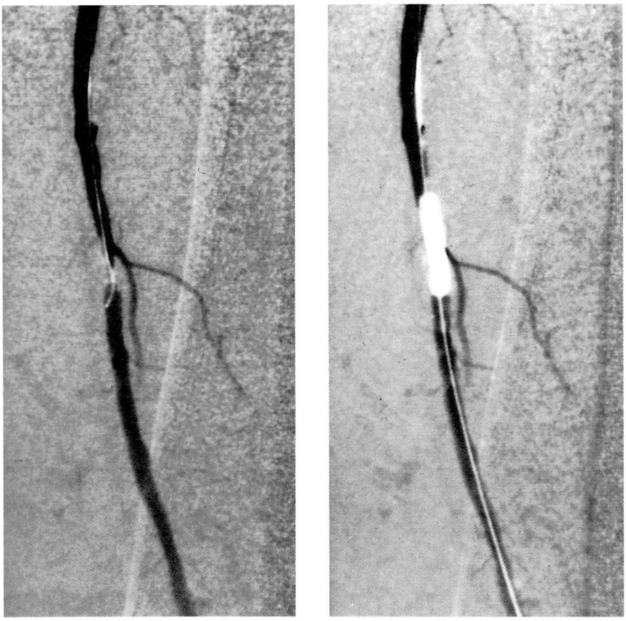

Fig. 7.126
Example illustrating the road-mapping technique. Left: image of vessel, right: guided catheter superimposed on the subtraction image

7.2.5 Dual energy imaging and hybrid subtraction

An x-ray image describes the locally variable attenuation of the radiation as it passes through the body. The degree of attenuation and thus the radiation intensity depends on the nature and thickness of the tissue. Each type of tissue is characterized by a linear attenuation coefficient μ, which depends on the energy. Table 7.7 shows some typical values. The radiation striking the patient is attenuated in accordance with the Lambert-Beer law:

$$I(x) = I_0 \, e^{-\mu x}. \tag{7.44}$$

I_0 Incident intensity
I Emerging intensity
μ Linear attenuation coefficient
x Thickness of object

This holds strictly only for an object made of uniform tissue and for monoenergetic radiation.

The linear attenuation coefficient can be written as the product of the mass attenuation coefficient μ/ϱ, which is characteristic of the tissue, and the local density $\varrho(s)$. The total attenuation is thus

$$I/I_0 = e^{-(\mu/\varrho)\int \varrho(s)\,ds}. \tag{7.45}$$

The x-ray tube delivers radiation over a wide spectrum $S(E)$. In the path of the radiation there are generally several types of tissue such as muscle, fat

Table 7.7
Linear attenuation coefficients of various body tissues. Based on Phelps et al. [7.80] and Mika and Reiss [7.81]

Energy (keV)	Attenuation coefficient μ (1/cm)		
	Fat	Muscle	Bone
30	0.272	0.390	1.750
40	0.216	0.278	0.930
50	0.193	0.235	0.631
60	0.180	0.213	0.493
80	0.165	0.189	0.375
100	0.155	0.176	0.324
150	0.138	0.155	0.268

and bone. The radiation intensity behind the object is

$$I = \int S(E)\, e^{-\sum_i (\mu/\varrho)_i(E) \int \varrho_i(s)\, ds}\, dE, \tag{7.46}$$

where $S(E)$ is the x-ray spectrum in front of the object. The summation is over the individual types of tissue and the integration is over the density along the beam and over the energy. An x-ray exposure yields an image of this integrated attenuation. The information contained in the energy dependence is not used. This is analogous to a black-and-white photograph, which only depicts shades of gray. The 'color' of the x radiation, i.e. the energy dependence, can yield information relevant to the diagnosis. An example of this can be found in the characterization of nodes in the case of a chest radiograph. With an x-ray or CT exposure, it often can not be determined with certainty whether increased attenuation values are due to diffuse calcification, i.e. to a higher mass attenuation coefficient, or to fibrosis, i.e. to an increase in the tissue density. If exposures are made at two different tube voltages, i.e. with different spectra, images can be reconstructed which only show bone and calcium or soft tissues. This procedure is known as dual energy imaging [7.82, 7.83].

Theoretical basis

In the energy range used in diagnostics, the attenuation of the x radiation is due primarily to the photoelectric effect and Compton scattering. The mass attenuation coefficient can then be written as follows:

$$(\mu/\varrho)(E) = a_p f_p(E) + a_c f_c(E), \tag{7.47}$$

where a_p and a_c are energy-independent material constants, while f_p and f_c express the energy dependence of the photoelectric and Compton effects respectively. The mass attenuation coefficient of any material may be represented as a linear combination of the two basis functions f_p and f_c. Instead of these functions, other linear independent functions can also be chosen as a new basis. One can, for instance, choose the attenuation coefficients of two sufficiently different materials. This results in:

$$(\mu/\varrho)(E) = a_1 (\mu/\varrho)_1 (E) + a_2 (\mu/\varrho)_2 (E). \tag{7.48}$$

The coefficients a_1 and a_2 are again characteristic of the material and are energy-independent. Any material may be represented as a linear combination of these two basis materials. As basis one can choose Plexiglas and aluminum or water (soft tissue) and calcium (bone).

X-ray systems essentially image the line integral $\int \mu(E,s)\,ds$ over the attenuation coefficients. This integral may be written as follows:

$$\int \mu(E,s)\,ds = (\mu/\varrho)_1(E)\,d_1 + (\mu/\varrho)_2(E)\,d_2. \tag{7.49}$$

$d_i = \int \varrho_i(s)\,ds$ area density of the basis material i
$\varrho_i(s)$ local density

Then one has

$$I(d_1, d_2) = \int S(E)\,e^{-\{(\mu/\varrho)_1(E)\,d_1 + (\mu/\varrho)_2(E)\,d_2\}}\,dE, \tag{7.50}$$

where $S(E)$ is the spectral distribution in front of the object. If one makes two exposures at different tube voltages, i.e. with different spectra, one has two non-linear integral equations with two unknowns d_1 and d_2:

$$I_l(d_1, d_2) = \int S_l(E)\,e^{-\{(\mu/\varrho)_1(E)\,d_1 + (\mu/\varrho)_2(E)\,d_2\}}\,dE, \tag{7.51}$$

$$I_h(d_1, d_2) = \int S_h(E)\,e^{-\{(\mu/\varrho)_1(E)\,d_1 + (\mu/\varrho)_2(E)\,d_2\}}\,dE, \tag{7.52}$$

The indices l and h refer to the low-energy (l) and the high-energy (h) spectrum respectively. The equations can be solved numerically with the aid of reference tables.

In this way material-selective images can be calculated which only display one of the basis materials such as a 'bone image' or a 'soft tissue image'.

Application in DSA: hybrid subtraction

In digital subtraction angiography (DSA), vessels are imaged by the temporal subtraction of two images, where an iodine contrast medium is injected into the vessel before the second exposure. The unchanged parts of the image are subtracted and what remains is the image of the iodine-filled vessel. Due to involuntary movements, such as swallowing or peristalsis of the intestine, artifacts arise. Dual energy imaging makes it possible to eliminate these artifacts, or at least to reduce them. The method (Fig. 7.127) consists of a combination of an energy subtraction and a temporal subtraction and is called hybrid subtraction [7.84 to 7.86]. Pairs of exposures are made at two different voltages and subsequently an 'empty image' (mask) and a 'contrast image' is calculated, which only shows bone or bone plus iodine respectively.

The temporal subtraction of the contrast image and the mask eliminates the bone. The hybrid subtraction image shows the vessel without artifacts. The time interval between the lower energy and the higher energy exposure should be as short as possible so that in this period virtually no movement takes

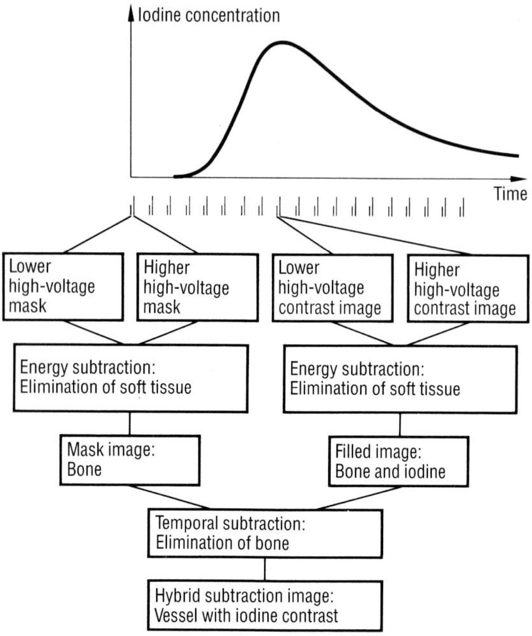

Fig. 7.127 Principle of hybrid subtraction

place. The minimum interval is given by the length of the x-ray pulse and the subsequent television scan. These times are below 100 ms and are sufficiently short for those areas where hybrid subtraction is used (carotid arteries, abdomen).

Fig. 7.128a shows an image of an abdomen phantom. In the path of the radiation, there is also an iodine line phantom and a phantom which simulates a bubble of intestinal gas. Fig. 7.128b shows the corresponding DSA image. The motion artifact shows up clearly. Fig. 7.128c shows the result of hybrid subtraction; the artifact has been eliminated, but at the expense of a distinctly worse signal-to-noise ratio. The clinical value of hybrid subtraction depends on how many nondiagnostic DSA studies due to soft tissue motion cannot be reduced by other methods such as compression.

Fig. 7.128
Hybrid subtraction of an artifact from a bubble of intestinal gas

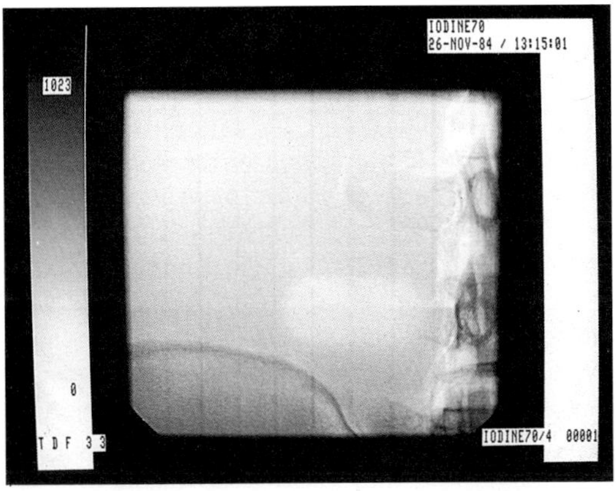

a) Abdomen phantom with iodine lines and air bubble

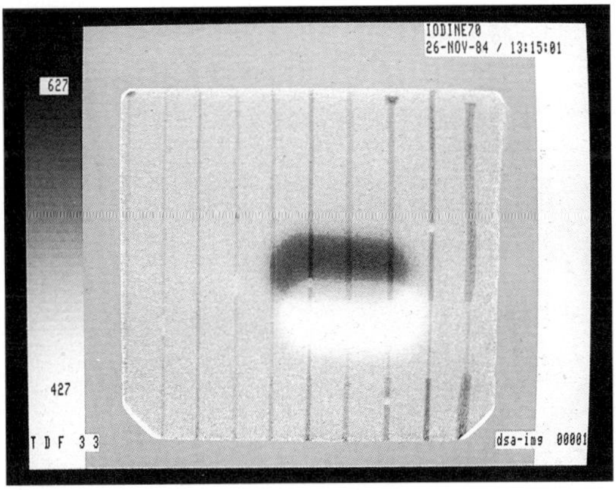

b) DSA image with motion artifact

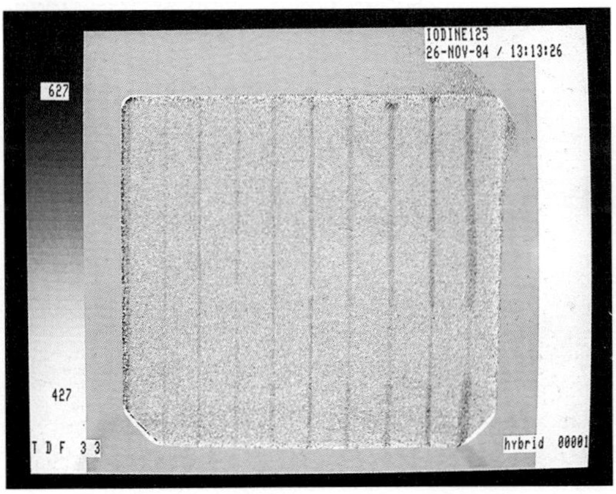

c) Hybrid subtraction

7.2.6 Digital multilayer tomography

In conventional film tomography a selected plane is imaged by a coupled opposite movement of the x-ray tube and the film during the exposure. Fig. 7.129 shows the basic principle of this method. Objects lying in the fulcrum plane P1 are imaged sharply because during the tomographic movement they are always projected onto the same position on the film. Contributions from neighboring planes are blurred by the movement which takes place during the exposure. In order to represent an anatomically interesting region sufficiently well, several exposures have to be made generally. This necessitates a correspondingly higher patient dose. Digital multilayer tomography makes it possible to reconstruct tomographic images in several planes from a single set of projection images taken at different angles during a tomographic exposure sequence [7.91 to 7.93]. The patient dose in tomosynthesis thus corresponds to the dose for a single conventional tomogram. The unshifted individual projections, when superimposed, result in a tomographic image of the plane defined by the imaging geometry. By shifting the individual exposures and subsequently superimposing them, as many parallel slices as desired can be reconstructed in principle. The

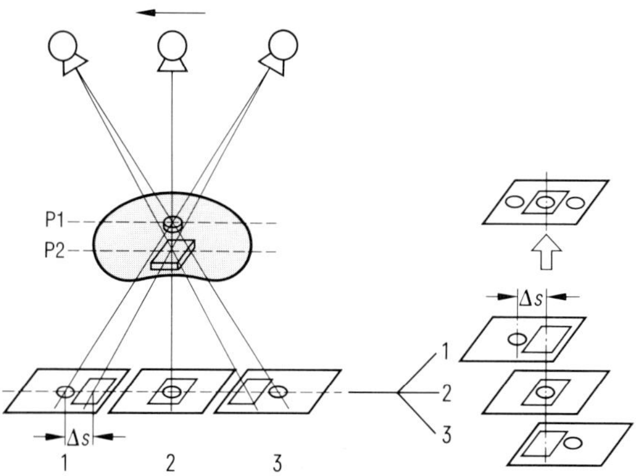

Fig. 7.129
Digital multilayer tomography (principle of reconstruction)
Superimposing the projections 1 to 3 yields a sharp image of the fulcrum plane P1. A tomogram of a parallel plane P2 can be reconstructed by shifting the individual projections before superimposition.

size and direction of each shift depends on the position of the x-ray tube and on the location of the layer to be reconstructed. Fig. 7.130 shows the geometrical relationships for linear digital multilayer tomography. The shift for each projection is given by Δs.

Digital image acquisition and processing systems such as those developed for digital subtraction angiography (DSA) can in principle be used for digital multilayer tomography. The image data are aquired with an image intensifier television chain, and subsequently digitized, stored, and processed in the DSA unit.

The aim of conventional tomography is to reduce contributions from objects outside the fulcrum plane by blurring these contributions through the tomographic movement. In digital multilayer tomography a further reduction of those contributions having low spatial frequencies can be achieved by processing the reconstructed image with a high-pass filter in the direction of the tomographic movement [7.94].

Fig. 7.131 a shows the reconstructed tomogram of a skull phantom. Reduction of the tomographic blurring using a high-pass filter is shown in Fig. 7.131 b.

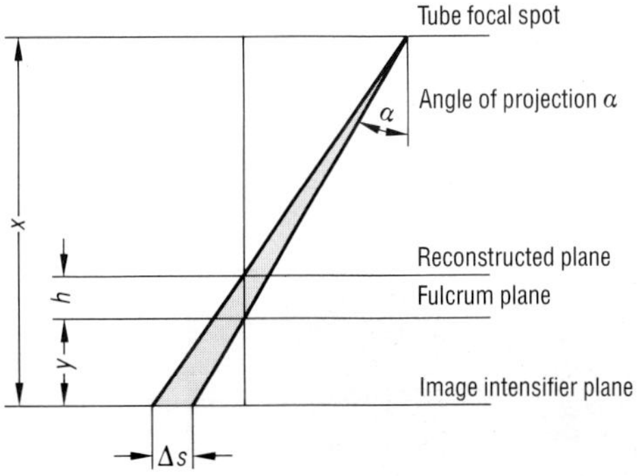

$$\Delta s = \frac{x \cdot h}{x - y - h} \cdot \tan \alpha$$

Fig. 7.130
Geometrical relationships in linear digital multilayer tomography.
Δs is the shift of the individual projection
as a function of the angle of projection α

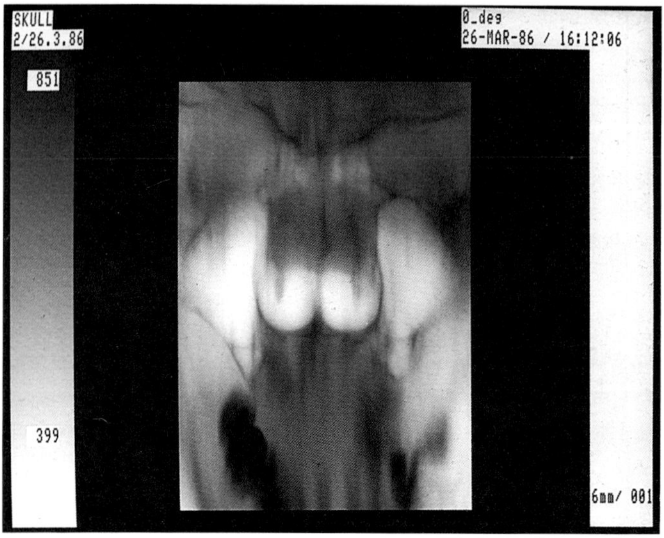

a) Tomogram of a skull phantom

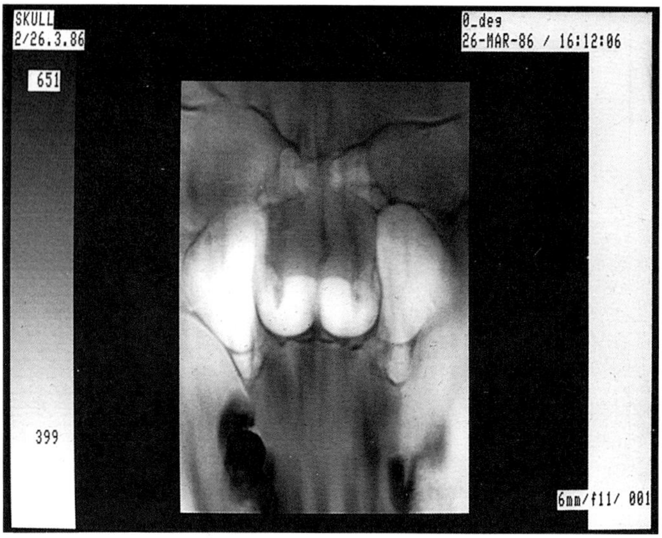

b) Reduction of linear blurring by high-pass filtering

Fig. 7.131 Linear digital multilayer tomography

7.2.7 Functional images

Information about the hemodynamic function cannot be obtained directly from a conventional x-ray image. It must therefore be derived by observing the dynamics of a sequence of images.

Digital image systems make it possible to determine hemodynamic quantities from a sequence of images [7.87 to 7.90]. Parameters are determined for each pixel and then represented as a gray scale or color coded image. The method is shown schematically in Fig. 7.132. For each pixel the temporal change of the DSA number, i.e. of the iodine contrast, is plotted in the form of a time-density curve. From these curves values such as the arrival time of the bolus, and the magnitude and time of the curve maximum can be determined. The aim is to describe the hemodynamics in a mathematical form. If such a mathematical description can be found with the aid of the parameters obtained, it is possible to make statements about the physiological function. Thus, for instance, the total area below the time-density curve is a relative measure for the local thickness of the vessels and hence for the blood volume. Even if the values obtained from the time-density curve are not sufficient for a complete mathematical description of the hemodynamics, the corresponding image can still be diagnostically relevant. Examples of this are the arrival time of the

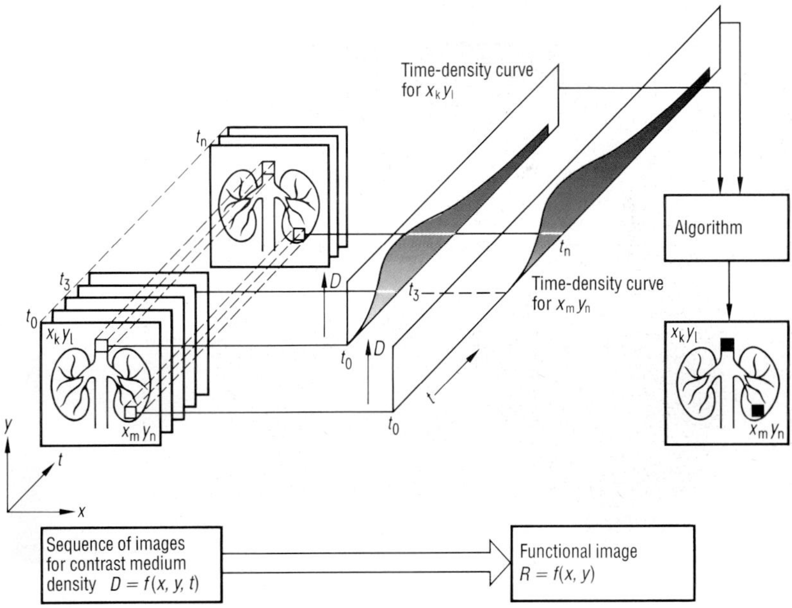

Fig. 7.132 Schematic representation for evaluation of the hemodynamic function

bolus, or the time of the bolus maximum. These two values only describe a limited part of the bolus dynamics, but can nevertheless indicate a delay in the filling process. However, this is not sufficient to enable an estimation of perfusion. There is no direct relationship between these parameters and physiological quantities.

Fig. 7.133 shows a functional image of a kidney in a graphically simplified form. The parameter is the bolus arrival time, early arrival times being coded with bright gray levels.

In the literature the terms parameter image and functional image are frequently used synonymously for the images described here.

In order to obtain genuine parameter images which describe physiological parameters in a quantitative way, we have to take into account effects of x-ray physics, such as beam hardening and radiation scattering.

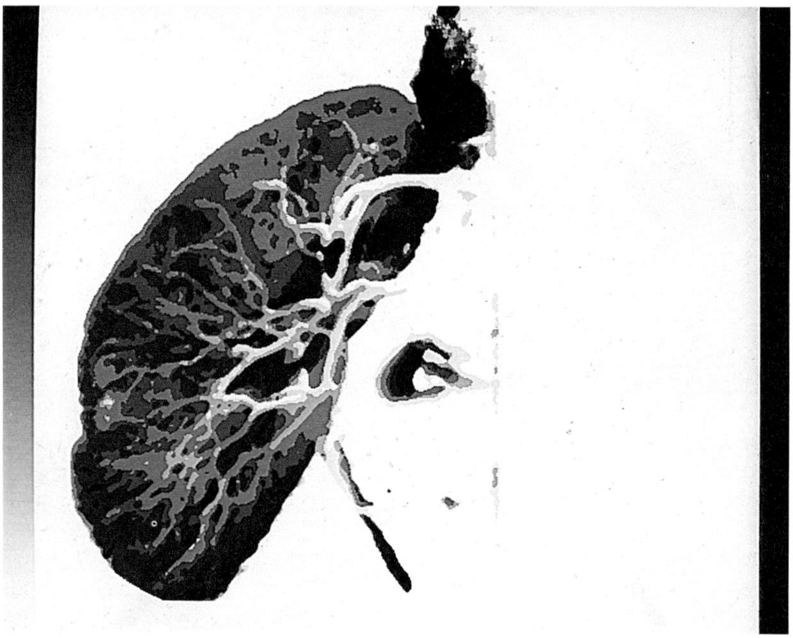

Fig. 7.133
Functional image of a kidney. The parameter displayed is the bolus arrival time

7.2.8 Image analysis

The information content of a radiological image may in principle be arranged in the form of a matrix. Morphology and function can be described qualitatively and quantitatively. Classical radiography primarily gives a qualitative representation of morphology. Digital radiography makes it possible to analyze images quantitatively with relatively little extra effort since the image data are already available in numerical form. Quantitative analysis is based on analyzing the pixel gray levels and their spatial and temporal relationships. The analysis of spatial data yields information about lengths, areas and volumes; using temporal data, organ movements, blood flow velocities and similar parameters may be determined. Although in each case the starting point is the gray level information of the pixels, a distinction is made between geometric and densitometric analysis.

Geometrical analysis

In this case pixel gray levels are only used to identify points, edges or surfaces. The analysis itself is based on distance and area measurements. Examples are the determination of the percent diameter narrowing of a blood vessel (degree of stenosis), and the calculation of the volume of the left heart ventricle with the area-length method.

In the numerical analysis one must take into account that every image generation system contains certain imaging errors. In the case of an image intensifier television system these are principally pincushion distortions. A pixel is shifted radially outwards, the shift being greater the further the pixel is away from the center. Measurements of distance therefore always contain systematic errors. The degree of distortion can be determined with a test image of a point grid. The differential distortion is expressed by $\{(\Delta R/\Delta R_0)-1\}\cdot 100\%$, where ΔR_0 is the distance between two points on the grid (typically 1 cm), and ΔR is the measured distance on the image matrix. For an x-ray image intensifier, the differential distortion increases from about 1% at a radius of 5 cm to about 15 to 30% (depending on the model) at the edge of the image. Corrections of distance and area measurements have to be performed according to the accuracy required and the degree of distortion, i.e. in a position-dependent way. To obtain relative values, as in the simplest form of stenosis determination, the measured values are generally not corrected. Measurements over a larger region of the image, e.g. when determining the ventricle volume, are affected by integral distortion. This is substantially smaller than differential distortion and can also often be ignored. When determining the volume of the left ventricle, the errors are about 5 ‰. This does not have to be corrected since the inaccuracy due to the underlying ventricular model is greater.

Densitometric analysis

The DSA signal is proportional to the iodine area density $\varrho_I d_I$ and hence, given a constant concentration ϱ_I of the contrast medium, proportional to the thickness of the vessel d_I. The sum of the DSA values over all the pixels of a region is therefore proportional to the volume. Following these simplifying assumptions, it would be possible to calculate the volume of the left ventricle from the DSA density values without making further assumptions about the shape of the ventricle. In practice, however, for accurate analysis, beam hardening, radiation scattering, and veiling glare in the image intensifier must be taken into account.

Beam hardening

Diagnostic x rays have a broad energy spectrum (see Fig. 3.6). When an x-ray beam passes through matter, the low-energy components are more strongly attenuated and the intensity spectrum is shifted to higher energies. On passing through a second material, this hardened radiation is attenuated less as the attenuation coefficient is now smaller. The x-ray absorption and hence the DSA number no longer depends only on the thickness of the material. The iodine signal of a blood vessel of constant thickness is reduced behind a bone and the iodine area density appears to become less. Beam hardening also takes place in the vessel or the heart ventricle itself. Densitometric errors due to beam hardening depend on the thickness of the tissue and the iodine concentration. In applications such as the determination of the ejection fraction of the left ventricle, the errors amount to a few percent and are small compared with the effects of radiation scattering.

Radiation scattering, veiling glare

The radiation emerging from the object $I(d)$ is composed of a primary radiation (P) and a scattered radiation (S) component:

$$I(d) = P + S. \tag{7.53}$$

In DSA one has for the filled image I_F

$$I_F(d, d_J) = I_0\, e^{-(\mu d + \mu_J d_J)} + S \tag{7.54}$$

and for the mask image I_M

$$I_M(d) = I_0\, e^{-(\mu d)} + S. \tag{7.55}$$

μ, d Attenuation coefficient, thickness of the object
μ_I, d_I Corresponding values of the vessel filled with iodine contrast medium

The DSA signal is

$$\ln I_F - \ln I_M = \ln\{I_0\, e^{-(\mu d + \mu_J d_J)} + S\} - \ln\{I_0\, e^{-(\mu d)} + S\}. \tag{7.56}$$

If the ratio S/P is small, one has approximately

$$\ln I_F - \ln I_M = (-\mu_J\, d_J)/(1 + S/P), \tag{7.57}$$

i.e. the subtraction signal is reduced by a factor $1/(1+S/P)$ and is therefore also dependent on the proportion of scattered radiation. The curves in Fig. 7.134 show this relationship. The range of the iodine area density extends up to about 200 mg/cm^2, corresponding to undiluted contrast medium in a blood vessel 5 mm in diameter. Even with a grid the proportion of scattered radiation can be around 20%. Thus, even for small and medium iodine surface densities there are signal reductions of about 10 to 20% [7.95].

A further source of scatter is the scattering of light in the image intensifier (veiling glare). The effect of x-ray scattering and veiling glare on densitometric analysis is considerably greater than the effect due to beam hardening. Radiation scattering cannot be calculated exactly and thus can only be numerically corrected in a very rough approximation. In a direct correction technique [7.96],

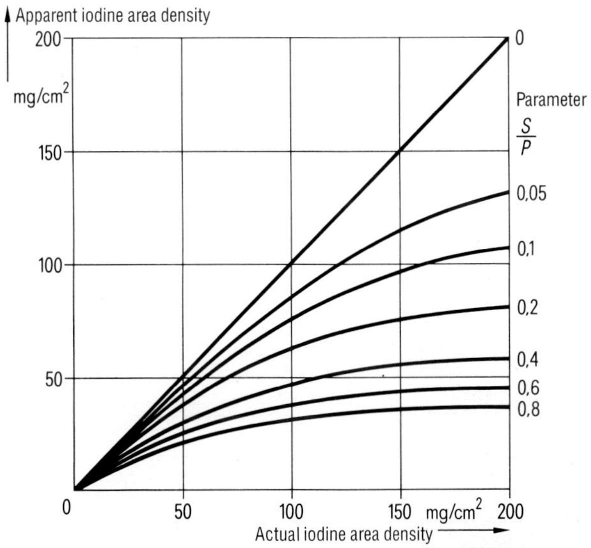

Fig. 7.134
Relationship between the actual and the 'apparent' iodine area density obtained in a density measurement neglecting radiation scattering

the suggestion is made to subtract the scattered radiation measured behind lead absorbers point-by point from the image signal. In spite of various attempts at finding solutions, however, a demonstrably useful and practicable correction technique has still to be found.

The accuracy of densitometric analysis is thus essentially determined by radiation scattering and it can therefore only be used to a limited extent for quantitative analysis in spite of its basic attractiveness. An important area of application is the determination of the degree of stenosis of blood vessels. Here both geometrical and densitometric techniques are applied. The analysis is based on a comparison of the narrowed section of the vessel with a 'normal' region. The two regions analyzed are relatively close to each other and thus the proportion of scattered radiation is roughly the same. This also holds for beam hardening insofar as it does not arise in the vessel itself. These effects therefore cancel in first approximation. The effect of pin cushion distortion is, however, generally corrected.

7.2.9 Multiformat cameras

Multiformat cameras, in short MFC, are used for photographic documentation of the television images made in medical diagnostics. Here the image information can be provided either as a video signal or in purely digital form, depending on the type of camera.

As film material, the following types of film are used: Polaroid films, dry sheet or paper films (in the case of low contrast range and resolution requirements) or large-format single-coated transparent films similar to those used in radiography.

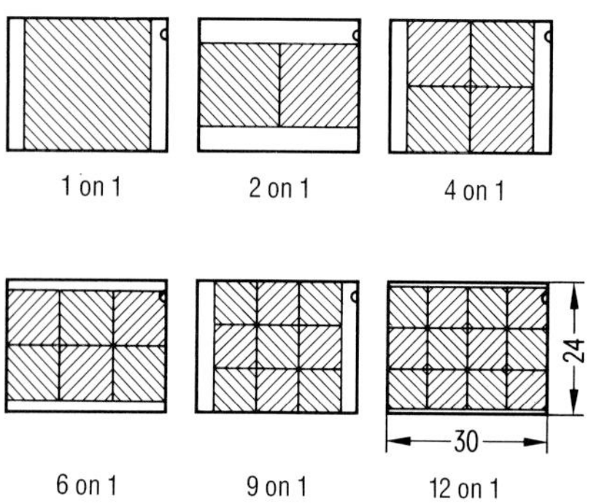

Fig. 7.135 Format subdivision of a film for multiformat cameras

A distinction is made between simple MFCs with a cassette system in which after each complete exposure of a film the cassette has to be taken out by hand by the user, and magazine cameras, which are capable of consecutively removing up to a hundred sheets of film from a supply magazine and automatically transporting them after exposure to a collecting magazine.

Depending on the type of examination and the requirements which must be met, MFCs give the user the possibility of exposing several images in fixed format subdivisions on one film. This ranges from the 1-format to as many as 84 images per film.

Some common format subdivisions are sketched in Fig. 7.135 using the example of a 24 cm × 30 cm film.

7.2.9.1 Cameras with a cathode ray tube

Apart from laser cameras, which will be gone into later in more detail, all multiformat cameras work on the same principle. The image of a high-resolution documentation monitor with a cathode ray tube (CRT) is deflected by mirrors (depending on the type of camera) and projected onto the film with the aid of a lens system (Fig. 7.136).

The image information must be supplied to the camera in the form of a video signal.

The lens system projects the monitor image onto that part of the film which is to be exposed at any particular moment. This can be done by means of several fixed lenses or a movable lens. The whole screen surface is available for each partial exposure of a subdivided film.

Between the exposures the beam current of the image tube is automatically switched off in order to prolong the life of the tube.

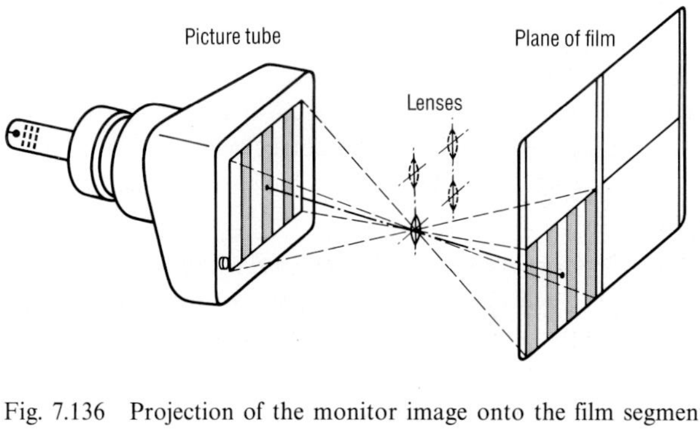

Fig. 7.136 Projection of the monitor image onto the film segment

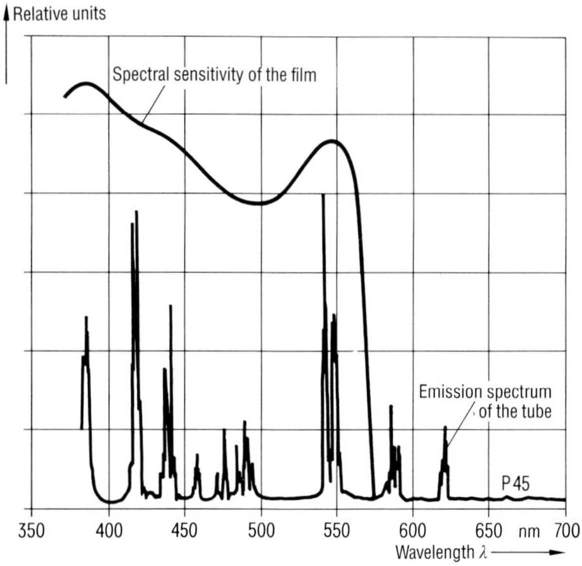

Fig. 7.137
Spectral emission of the cathode ray tube and spectral film sensitivity

The films used are so-called CRT films. These are negative cutfilms with a sensitivity which is matched to the light emitted by the luminescent substance (Fig. 7.137). As one is dealing with negative films, the documentation monitor has to perform an image inversion so that the film image has the same polarity as the image on the viewing monitor. As a rule, one can select either a positive or a negative image.

Documentation monitor

Because of the characteristics of the eye, irregularities on viewing monitors are covered up both by the line flicker and large-area flicker. Since the film, however, integrates several frames to achieve the correct exposure and since its average gradient is very steep, faults become visible on the images which are not normally perceptible.

Documentation monitors therefore constitue a special case within monitor technology. They must meet very high demands with respect to resolution, range of contrast, constancy of brightness, brightness distribution, line uniformity and image geometry as well as with respect to the transmision characteristics of the video amplifier and the picture tube.

The lines may deviate from each other by at most 3% from the theoretically required position. If this is not the case, a distracting line pairing effect becomes visible on the film. For a 625-line monitor and a real image height of 120 mm this implies a maximum permissible deviation of 2.9 μm.

Exposure regulation

In order to obtain a constant exposure result, i.e. a constant optical density of the film, without this being affected by the ageing of the picture tube or other components or by voltage and temperature drift, the brightness of the monitor has to be regulated.

The regulation system must be independent of the content of the image, however. The film image must correspond to the image on the viewing monitor. At the same time it is important that the image manipulations necessary for the diagnosis, such as changing the brightness or the contrast, are carried out centrally via the imaging system and not at the viewing monitor since a change in the image impression at the monitor has no effect on the video signal and therefore no effect on the film.

To regulate the monitor brightness one uses for example an optical clamping circuit (Fig. 7.138).

Outside the image matrix that is to be displayed, a light sensor (1) is attached to the cathode ray tube in such a way that it measures the actual brightness of the porch (2) of the video signal (which is independent of the image content). Via a regulation system (3) which feeds back to the grid of the picture tube, the brightness of the porch is kept constant at a preselected required value.

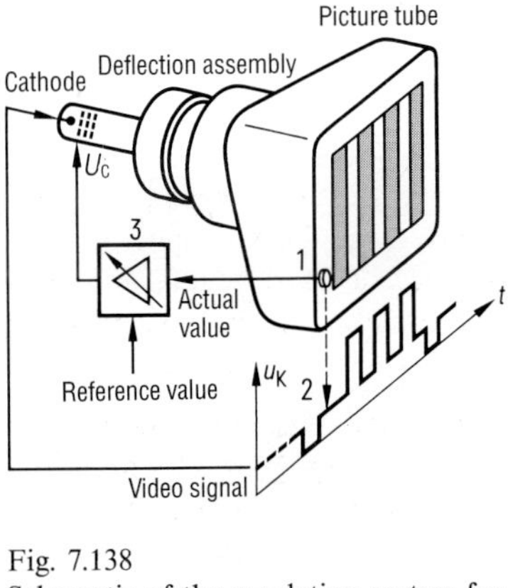

Fig. 7.138
Schematic of the regulation system for a cathode ray tube

Film characteristic, resulting gradation

The film characteristic of CRT films is very similar to that of conventional x-ray films (see Section 7.1.3.2).

The regulation system of the documentation monitor is set in such a way that even the smallest changes in the image signal close to the porch value are visible on the film as differences in optical density. To this end the film has to be pre-sensitized in such a way that even the porch value of the video signal produces an optical density of the film which is just above its base fog (Fig. 7.139).

The contrast and hence the amplification of the video signal must be set in such a way that the highest part of the image signal which can reasonably be expected comes to lie just within the upper range of the film characteristic so that no information is lost here in the black of the film.

The resulting gradation characteristic of the CRT and the film is not linear; it produces a distortion of the gray levels in an image. As can be seen in Fig. 7.139, the distortion consists of an increase in contrast in the middle gray level range and a reduction in contrast in the upper and lower range. In some applications this effect is positively desirable. The video signal is adjusted in such a way that the details relevant to the image lie in the middle gray level range, and the film therefore reproduces them with more contrast than the viewing monitor.

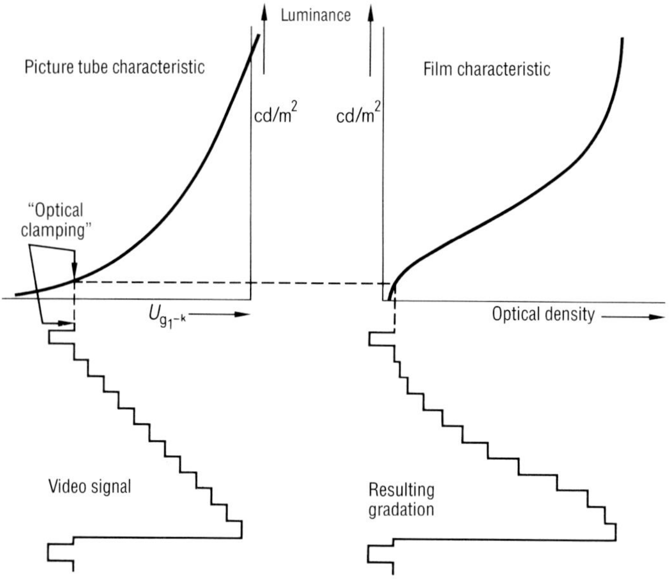

Fig. 7.139 The effect of the tube and film characteristic on the gradation

Should this effect not be desired, additional linearization measures have to be taken. This can be done by suitably distorting the gradation in advance on the documentation monitor or alternatively by means of so-called look-up tables in the imaging system.

Contrast and resolution

The profile of the electron beam and hence the luminance profile on the screen phosphor has approximately the form of a Gaussian function. Given sufficiently sharp focussing of the beam (high MTF), the spaces between the lines become visible on the film as bright lines; at these places, the film is not completely blackened. Because of the eye's mechanism for appraising surfaces, a loss of contrast occurs.

However, if the lines are defocussed or written close together in such a way that the image appears to be free of lines, the range of contrast is increased, but the image loses sharpness. Absence of lines in the image can be achieved by 'multi-interlacing'. In this process, after each full scan the vertical image position of the lattice on the picture tube is shifted by Δs, the film integrates the full scans thus shifted, and the total effect is that one obtains a line-free, high-contrast image, which, however, suffers a corresponding loss of sharpness.

The second way of generating a line-free image is provided by so-called line wobbling. Here a high-frequency deflection voltage moves the electron beam up and down, as it moves along each line, by half the distance between the lines, i.e. the electron beam is artificially broadened in the vertical direction.

7.2.9.2 Film processors for magazine cameras

The exposed films of a MFC are developed in conventional film processors. Here the films have to be taken out of the cassette or the magazine in a darkroom and introduced into the film processor. The developing process then takes place automatically; when the film is ready after about 90 s, it falls into a collecting chute.

This time-consuming processing of the film after exposure can be substantially shortened by adding a film transporting system between the MFC and the film processor. Instead of a collecting magazine, one now has a 'film feeder', which essentially consists of a kind of conveyor belt. After exposure the film is carried along this transporting system and automatically transported into the film processor (Fig. 7.140).

All the components of such a system are monitored by a central processor. They are connected up so as to exclude light and can be operated in daylight.

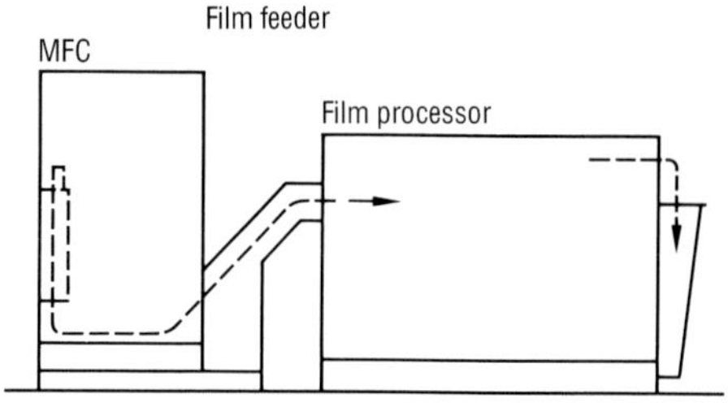

Fig. 7.140
Connection of a multiformat camera (MFC) to a film processor

To protect the film feeder and the MFC from the highly corrosive vapors from the developing baths, a permanent, slight positive pressure is produced in both of them by means of a ventilator.

7.2.9.3 Attachment of 35 mm and cine cameras

To make 35 mm negatives or slides, many MFCs give the option of attaching an SLR 35 mm camera. By automatically changing the path of the rays of light, e.g. by swivelling a mirror, the monitor image can be photographed by the 35 mm camera (Fig. 7.141). The shutter is then released by the electronics of the MFC and a winder takes care of the film transport.

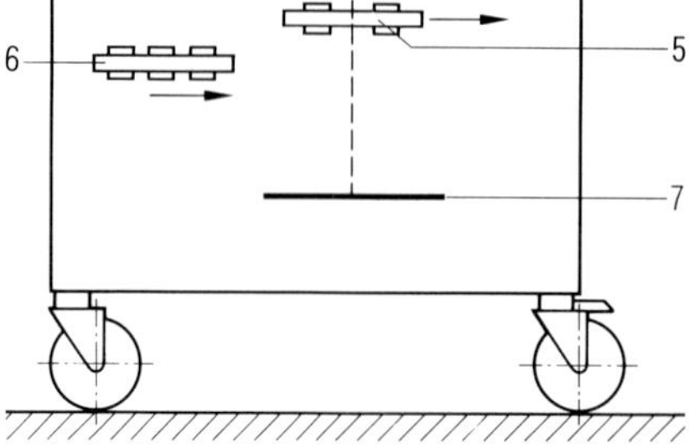

1 Monitor
2 Swivelling mirror
3 35 mm or cine camera
4, 5, 6 Lens system supports
7 Film stage (sheet film)

Fig. 7.141

Since 35 mm cameras do not, as a rule, have an electric film counter, the length of the film loaded must be known to the control system of the MFC. Some camera manufacturers offer special backs for their 35 mm cameras with which it is possible to load films with a length of up to 240 exposures. 35 mm films have proved their value as space-saving mass storage media and as presentation media at lectures and conferences.

In order to document dynamic processes as well, such as in angiocardiography, a cine camera with 35 mm film can be attached instead of a 35 mm camera. As opposed to a 35 mm camera, a cine camera has to be synchronized with the frame rate of the monitor. If this is not done, the changing of the image becomes visible as a black stripe slowly moving through the picture.

7.2.9.4 Multiformat cameras with laser

MFCs with a laser as writing system provide another possibility of documenting very-high-resolution images. Laser beams have some considerable advantages compared to electron beams which justify their use in very-high-resolution systems. The most outstanding of these is the high degree of focusability (low divergence) of the beam. The resolution of the system is determined solely by the diameter of the laser beam on the film and not, as is the case with the monitor, by the graininess of the screen phosphor and the MTF of the optical system as well.

Types of laser

The lasers which can be used are gas lasers with helium cadmium (blue), argon (blue) or helium neon (red or green), or semiconductor laser diodes (infrared, in short SC-IR diodes). The power needed is of the order of several 10 mW, depending on the efficiency of the lens system and the film.

SC-IR lasers have a number of advantages compared to gas lasers. They are relatively small and robust. The power of the laser is proportional to the current over a large range and can therefore be modulated easily.

The wavelength of SC-IR lasers requires the use of a special IR-film, however. Processing these films in conventional x-ray operation is not simple. They require a special kind of dark room illumination and they are heat-sensitive.

Amongst the gas lasers, helium-neon lasers are well-established. Compared to argon lasers they are cheaper and have a significantly longer life. With gas lasers it is possible to use the conventional documentation films which have been generally introduced.

Deflection and modulation

Leaving aside system-specific correction procedures, all laser cameras operate according to the same principle (Fig. 7.142). The intensity of the laser beam is modulated in SC lasers internally via the current, and in gas lasers by an external modulator (e.g. with the aid of polarization filters and acousto-optic couplers). Subsequently, the beam is diverged, deflected by rotating polygonal mirrors or galvanometer mirrors in the x-direction, and focussed on the film via a lens system. The movement in the y-direction is achieved either by advancing the film or by means of an additional mirror.

The attainable spot diameter d (Fig. 7.143) depends on the laser wavelength λ used, the beam diameter D and the focal length of the lens system f; D is inversely proportional to the spot diameter d.

Diverged beams can therefore be focussed to a smaller spot diameter than the direct beam:

$$d = k \frac{\lambda \cdot f}{D}. \tag{7.58}$$

The laser is driven in the basic transversal mode TEM_{00} (Fig. 7.144), i.e. the intensity I in the beam approximately obeys the relation

$$I = I_0 \, e^{\frac{-2r^2}{w^2}}. \tag{7.59}$$

I_0 Maximum intensity on the axis
w Beam radius

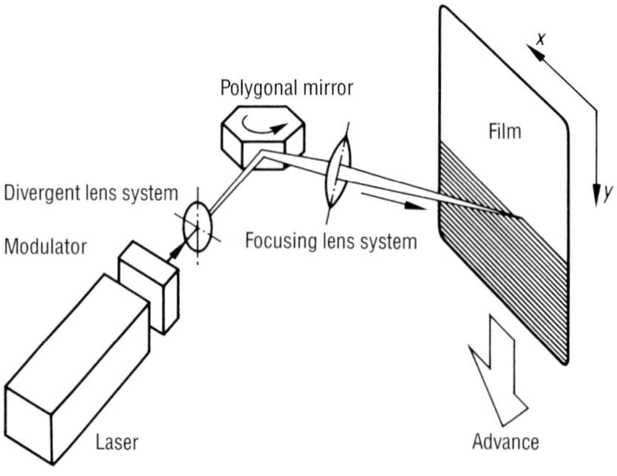

Fig. 7.142
Ray path
in a laser camera

The beam diameter $2w$ is defined here by the drop in intensity to $1/e^2$ times (i.e. 13.5% of) the peak value of a Gaussian curve.

The beam diameters and spot sizes so defined are about 65 to 80 μm for present-day systems and thus, for a film measuring 35 cm × 43 cm, make it possible to represent a 4096 × 5120 pixel matrix.

If one considers that, as in monitor photography, even a line error of 3% becomes visible and distracting, the laser beam has to be guided to an accuracy of ±1.3 μm. Consequently, the demands made with respect to accuracy in the lens system (e.g. flatness of the mirrors), the control system and the other mechanical components of the device are exceptionally high. Thus, for instance, any convection in the path of the laser beam must be avoided; the different refractive indices of air at different temperatures would lead to an unacceptable deflection of the beam.

The maximum scanning speed of the laser beam is given by the spectrum-dependent energy of the laser on the film required for the blackening of the film, and by the readout time of the digital image information. For a 4096 × 5120 matrix, one has exposure times of about 20 s.

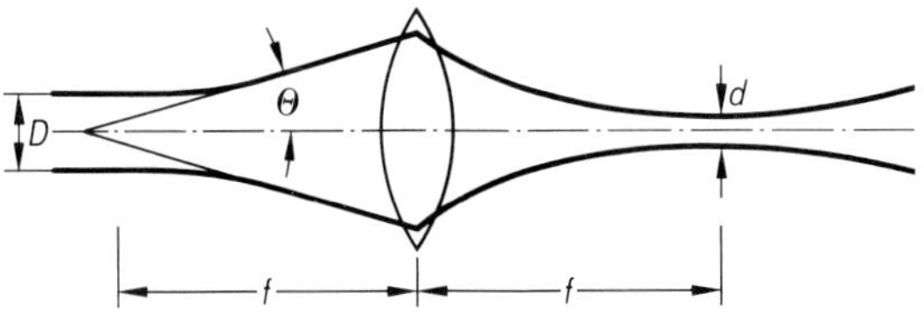

Fig. 7.143 Profile of a laser beam

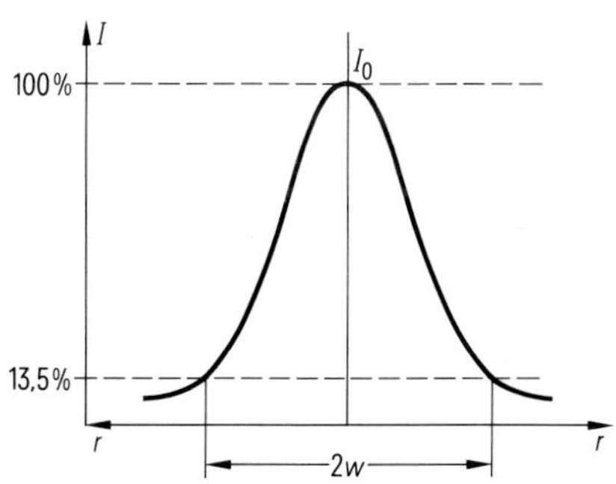

Fig. 7.144 Intensity distribution of a beam in the basic mode TEM_{00}

Camera interfaces

As a rule, laser cameras have a digital interface for the image information. The gray level for each individual pixel of the image matrix must be stored in a memory inside the camera before the film is exposed.

If the data matrix is smaller than the image matrix which can be displayed, e.g. if a 512 × 512 matrix is to be displayed in large format, i.e. with 4096 × 4096 pixels, the laser camera can fill in the missing pixels.

This can be done by a simple replication of pixels or by interpolation algorithms. In the first case the pixels are represented as clearly visible squares. Through interpolation an image can be produced which is completely free of grid lines.

One of the drawbacks of the laser camera arises from the limitation of the image matrix. In the case of format subdivisions where the sum of the data of the individual images exceeds the storage space of the camera or the matrix size of 4096 × 5120 which can be displayed, the image data are reduced. The consequence is loss of resolution in the individual images.

In a CRT system, where the format subdivision is carried out by optical means, there is no loss of resolution apart from the graininess of the film.

Documentation with lasers is not possible on 35 mm or cine film; the option of adding on a film transport system is, however, standard for all laser cameras.

7.3 X-ray systems for angiography and lithotripsy

The possibility of using x radiation for diagnostic purposes was recognized by Roentgen himself immediately after his epoch-making discovery: with the aid of the new type of rays he prepared images of hands and showed the resulting pictures to the public [7.97]. Since this first demonstration of their imaging properties, x-rays have been used in such a variety of ways for imaging purposes in medical diagnostics that even a moderately comprehensive survey of the areas of application and the corresponding examination equipment is not possible within the framework of this book. Instead our remarks must of necessity confine themselves to a few selected areas of application together with the relevant x-ray equipment, namely those areas which because of important technical improvements are of special interest at the present time:

universal angiography,
cardiac angiography,
digital subtraction angiography,
lithotripsy.

Here it should be particularly emphasized that to achieve the best examination results the individual components (as described in the previous sections with respect to their key features) must be integrated into a system which is adapted as well as possible from the medical and technical point of view to the requirements of the individual examination procedure. The essential components of such an optimized system are:

generator, tube assembly, collimators, secondary radiation grids,
image receptor,
image processing unit,
image display unit,
examination unit (arrangement of tube assembly, image receptor and unit for positioning the patient).

Further additional system components are e.g.

contrast medium injector,
ECG triggering device,
image storage device.

Before proceeding to a closer consideration of a few selected systems, the most important aspects which must be taken into account for the optimization of the system will be briefly surveyed below.

It goes almost without saying that the patient positioning unit must be designed in such a way that it allows the patient to lie down and be positioned without any complications in the most favorable way for the desired examination. Positioning the patient must be made as comfortable as possible so that attempts by the patient to change his position during the examination do not arise in the first place. At the same time the positioning unit must not impede the imaging of the body region to be examined; it must therefore be made out of material which is as homogeneous as possible with a low radiation attenuation capacity.

The examination unit must permit the most favorable directions of projection for the examination and at the same time be such that access to the patient is not restricted at all or only to an insignificant extent so that all the manipulations required in connection with the examination of the patient can be carried out without obstruction. This is extremely important both in the case of examinations of anesthetized patients and for examinations using vessel catheterization or similar invasive and interventional procedures, and naturally also facilitates medical intervention during the examination.

When selecting the image receiver components, it is of fundamental importance to decide upon the desired or required image techniques (fluoroscopy, indirect exposure techniques using medium format film, cine techniques, digital subtraction techniques, direct techniques) as well as the image field sizes and exposure frequencies required for the examination.

The spatial resolving power can only be varied to a limited extent. It depends on the one hand on the image receptor chosen and the image processing and reproduction systems connected to it, and on the other hand on the size of the focal spot and the imaging geometry (magnification of the object to be imaged) as well as on the movement of the object during the exposure time (or the integration time in the case of fluoroscopy). The focal spot size is in turn determined by the tube power needed, which depends in its turn on the minimum dose per image (or minimum dose rate in the case of fluoroscopy) which is necessary because of noise, on the most favorable value of the high voltage to be aimed for so as to achieve the optimum contrast for the object to be imaged, as well as on the exposure time which is still permissible for a given movement of the object, on the exposure frequency, and on the number of individual exposures (or the duration of fluoroscopy, as the case may be). The same parameters which determine the tube power also determine – albeit in a different way or with different weightings – the tube assembly power and the necessary generator data.

These relationships, which have merely been sketched here, make it clear that optimizing such a system is certainly not a trivial task, especially as there are yet more aspects to be taken into consideration. When using a secondary radiation grid, for instance, which is usually the case, one has to weigh up whether in a particular case (given the same grid design) it is better to use a grid with a higher grid ratio or a lower grid ratio. The grid with the higher ratio achieves a better suppression of the scattered radiation and therefore a better contrast as compared to the other grid (see section 7.1.2.5); nevertheless it may be that because of the available exposure time, the employment of the highly selective grid forces the use of a higher value for the voltage because of its lower total radiolucency, so that the primary radiation contrast is diminished with the overall result that there is no gain in contrast – and in certain circumstances possibly even a lower contrast.

A further aspect of optimization is the matching of the object and the receptor dynamics. In many situations when an exposure is being made the signal range in the relief pattern of the radiation behind the object will be broader than the range which can be processed by the image receptor. X-ray image intensifiers in particular exhibit loss of contrast in such cases even for signals which are well within the range covered by the image receptor. Matching of the dynamics can be achieved by the use of appropriate compensators, shaped filters or partially radiolucent diaphragms. These devices illustrate the fact that systems can only be fully exploited with the aid of small additional pieces of equipment which at first appear inessential.

Finally, operational aids and automatic operation systems which make a system manageable and efficient in its use are a decisive factor in the optimization of complex systems: a system which is extremely powerful from the technical point of view is diminished in value if its use is limited by the complexity of its operation.

7.3.1 Universal angiographic systems

Area of application

As their name implies, universal angiographic systems should be suitable for all angiographic examinations from head to toe. Also included in these are cardiac angiography and interventional techniques right up to PTCA (percutaneous transluminal cardangioplasty). While it is true that the use of special systems for cardiac angiography (see section 7.3.2) is becoming more and more established, setting up a special heart catheter laboratory in a clinic is only justified when the number of patients is sufficiently large.

Requirements

The universality of application necessitates an examination unit-patient positioning table combination which makes it possible to image every part of the body, and it may also be necessary to image different parts of the body one after another without changing the position of the patient (e.g. lower extremities and extracranial vessels). The different kinds of examination which are carried out with the aid of the system require different directions of projection: apart from the standard projections from the front to the back (a.p.), from the back to the front (p.a.) and from the side, complex oblique projections must be set up for cardiac angiography in particular in order to be able to image the individual vessels and sections of vessels so that they lie perpendicular to the direction of projection without distortion or superimposition (see subsection on requirements in 7.3.2). Some examinations (e.g. in the cranial region) require the use of magnification techniques for an accurate diagnosis.

In the different examination procedures which are carried out by a system for general angiography, various image recording procedures are used. Apart from the obligatory x-ray image intensifier television fluoroscopy, the following techniques are also employed: direct exposure series (e.g. in cranial angiography and angiography of the extremities), indirect exposure series on medium format film (e.g. in visceral angiography and angiography of the extremities) as well as image intensifier cine techniques (principally in cardiac angiography). It must also be possible to attach a DSA (digital subtraction angiography) unit if required.

Example of a system

As an example, a typical x-ray system for general angiography will be described below. The key components of this system are

the ANGIOSKOP D33 examination unit,
the KOORDINAT DII patient positioning table,
the OPTILIX 150/12/40/72C or
MEGALIX 125/15/40/82C x-ray tube assembly,
the POLYDOROS 80 generator (power 80 kW) or
POLYDOROS 100 (power 100 kW),
the PUCK UD cutfilm changer with a maximum of 4 images/s,
the high-resolution VIDEOMED H television system with a camera tube of the SATICON type,
the medium-format SIRCAM 106 camera with a maximum of 6 images/s,
the 35 mm ARRITECHNO cine camera with a maximum of 90 frames/s.

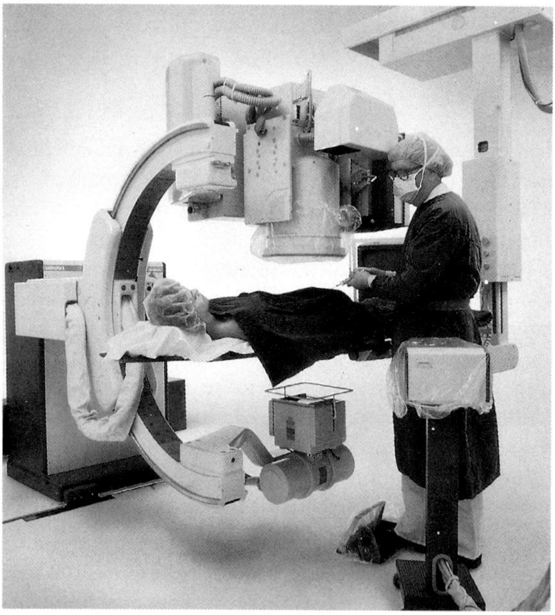

Fig. 7.145 ANGIOSKOP D33, examination unit for universal angiography, in combination with the KOORDINAT 3D II patient positioning table. The image receptor unit is in the fluoroscopy or indirect exposure position, the cutfilm changer has been rotated towards the feet.

Examination unit and patient positioning table

The examination unit (Fig. 7.145) is designed for isocentric operation, i.e. all the rotating or swivelling movements of the imaging system take place around a central point. If at the beginning of the examination the center of the object area of interest is positioned at this point by an appropriate horizontal and vertical adjustment of the positioning table, this object area will not move out of the image field if the direction of projection is changed at a later stage. In this way it is very much easier to make any changes in the direction of projection which may be necessary during the examination.

The principal components of the unit are as follows: the floor-mounted stand which can be moved by a motor parallel to the longitudinal direction of the positioning table. This carries an L-arm which can be rotated about a horizontal axis running perpendicular to the direction of movement of the stand. At the end of this arm there is a C-arm which can be rotated about an axis running perpendicular to the L-arm axis, and to which the tube assembly and the image receptor combination are attached. All the axes of movement and the central ray pass through a common point of intersection, the isocenter. The image receptor combination consists of the image intensifier with television camera and optionally attachable 100 mm cutfilm camera or 35 mm cine camera, as well as the cutfilm changer. The combination can be rotated around an axis in such a way that either the image intensifier (see Fig. 7.145) or the cutfilm changer (Fig. 7.146) is facing the tube assembly. Whilst the tube focal spot

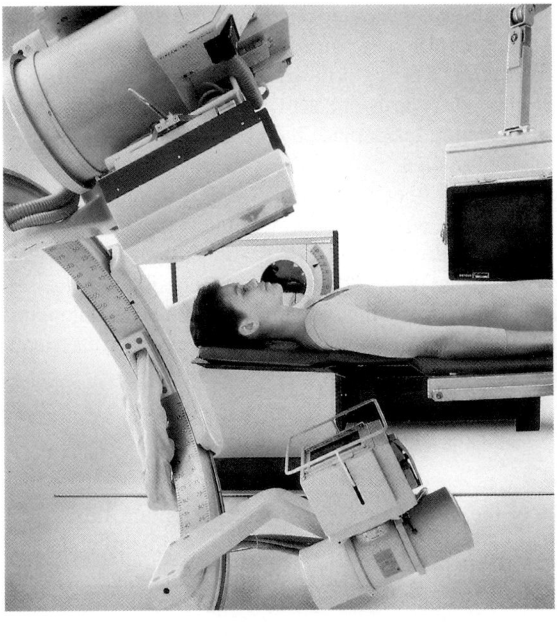

Fig. 7.146
ANGIOSKOP D33, examination unit for universal angiography, in combination with the KOORDINAT 3D II patient positioning table. The image receptor is in the direct exposure position, the x-ray image intensifier has been rotated out of the path of the radiation.

can be selected to have either a fixed or variable distance from the isocenter, the image receptor combination can be moved along the central ray in every version of the unit so that it is always possible to set the minimum object-image receptor distance or focal spot-image receptor distance. In this way the geometric magnification and the accompanying unsharpness, as well as the dose requirement, are kept as low as possible. The focal spot-image receptor distance is only set to the largest possible value when magnification techniques are used, which in any case employ a small focal spot.

Attaching the C-arm to an L-arm has the important advantage that the unit can easily be expanded to a biplane system (e.g. for biplane cranial angiography) by means of a second tube assembly attached in a movable way to a ceiling support and a receptor mounted in the same way or on a floor support.

The patient positioning table is made out of a carbon fiber board which only slightly attenuates the x radiation, and which is attached sideways to a ceiling support at the foot end. The raising movement of the table suspension is done by a motor, and lengthways and sideways movements are carried out easily by hand or else assisted by a motor. Since the table does not contain any obstacles anywhere in the patient region, it is not necessary to alter the patient's position when changing the field of examination. The ceiling suspension makes it possible for the examiner to get to any part of the table without obstruction. The unit and the table do not constrain him in any way e.g. with respect to the choice of the method of catheterization (following Sones via the artery in the arm or following Judkins via the artery in the leg).

The motor-powered maneuverability of the floor support in combination with a programming facility for stepping and for the cutfilm changer or medium-format camera makes angiography of the extremities particularly easy: whereas normally the patient table is moved towards the head end between the individual exposures, with this unit the stepping takes place by moving the support whilst the patient remains stationary. In this process the voltage for the exposure can, as usual, be lowered for the thinner regions of the object relative to the thicker ones. Moving the imaging system instead of moving the patient positioning table has two advantages: the danger associated with moving the patient when the catheter has been inserted is eliminated, as are possible feelings of fear and nervous starts of the patient caused by the movement. The new imaging technique has been made possible by the use of microprocessor control systems which ensure movement of the support free of jolts and vibrations.

The x-ray tube assembly

The x-ray tube assemblies of the above-mentioned systems contain tubes with compound anodes made out of rhenium-alloyed tungsten with molybdenum and graphite, which are distinguished by their particularly large heat storage capacity. Each of the tubes has three focal spots with the sizes 0.3/0.6/1.0 (to

DIN 6823/1) with a power of 12/40/70 kW (OPTILIX tube assemblies) or 15/40/80 kW (MEGALIX tube assemblies). Here the focal spot size of 0.3 is basically only used in cerebral magnification angiography. Its load capacity, which is determined by the focal spot size and is low in comparison with the other two focal spots, is more than sufficient for this examination especially since in magnification techniques one can dispense with the use of a secondary radiation grid in the cutfilm changer or in front of the image intensifier. The middle focal spot has been designed with respect to its size and load capacity so that it can be employed as a standard focal spot for the majority of applications. The large focal spot is essentially only used with corpulent patients for cine sequences. The tubes in both of the tube assemblies differ not only with respect to the load capacity of their focal spots but also in their heat storage capacity; whereas the tube in the OPTILIX tube assembly is able to store 450,000 J, the tube in the MEGALIX tube assembly can store more than twice as much, namely 1,000,000 J. The effect of this difference is noticed principally in the permissible duration of cine sequences, especially if the tube assembly has previously been subjected to a load arising from a fairly long fluoroscopy session at high power or from sequences taking place immediately before. This means that the MEGALIX tube assembly is definitely to be preferred if this application is to be the primary one.

The generator

The generators belonging to the series mentioned are high-frequency generators which are optimally matched to the tube assemblies employed with respect to their power specifications. The high voltage is produced in these generators from the power supply voltage, which has first been rectified, by a converter operating within a frequency range of a few kilohertz. Regulation of the converter permits a particularly high degree of reproducibility and accuracy of the high voltage values.

All the necessary automatic exposure control systems can be combined with each other: for dose rate regulation in the case of fluoroscopy various characteristics can be chosen, so that both fluoroscopy with the lowest possible skin dose (following the so-called anti-isowatt characteristic) is possible, as well as fluoroscopy with the best possible contrast: in the latter the automatic control system essentially first raises the fluoroscopy current with increasing object thickness and then, on reaching the highest permissible fluoroscopic power, changes over to increasing the voltage with the electric tube power held constant.

The amount of exposure in direct radiography can be controlled after preselection of the tube voltage by means of an automatic exposure timer with ionization chamber. Suitable automatic exposure timers are available for medium-format cameras and cine techniques, although in these cases the measuring signal is produced not via an ionization chamber, but by measuring the light in the telecentric ray path of the indirect exposure system.

In medium-format cameras and cine techniques the best tube voltage is automatically determined, set and displayed on the basis of the data from the preceding fluoroscopic examination and the selected exposure program.

Exposure in cine operation takes place with fixed, preprogrammed exposure times. Fine adjustments for each following image are made in accordance with the measured light signal via the current and the voltage. To avoid changes in the exposure during a sequence due to the contrast medium flowing into the image field, it is possible to maintain the exposure constant for the rest of the series at the values reached at a certain fixed, preselected point in time.

The image receptor

The cutfilm changer is constructed in such a way that it is able to function in an unrestricted way in any projection allowed by the unit. The frame speed is sufficient for all the examinations which come into consideration.

The image intensifier has an input screen made of cesium iodide and is therefore particularly suitable for examinations with iodine contrast mediums. The input field can be switched to three different values (33, 23 and 17 cm) and thus caters for all the requirements which arise in general angiography. The television system used is a high-resolution system with 1249 lines, which therefore exploits the resolution achieved with the image intensifier especially well. The use of a camera tube of the SATICON type which has a particularly small dark current allows a DSA system to be connected without difficulty.

Like the cutfilm changer, the medium-format camera, with its even higher frame speed, meets all the demands which arise. With its reduced dose requirement, it represents in many cases a real alternative to the cutfilm changer.

The cine camera is indispensible for angiocardiography for which as a rule frame rates of 25 to 50 frames per second are required. The maximum possible frame rate is 90 frames per second. This rate is essentially only used in pediatric cardiac angiography.

Image results

Since the following sections deal separately with the subjects of cardiac angiography and DSA, no image results for these areas will be shown here, but only examples which have been obtained using a medium-format camera and a cutfilm changer: Fig. 7.147 shows an image-intensifier exposure of a vascular occlusion of the femoral artery; Fig. 7.148 shows a direct exposure sequence of a bilateral leg arteriography made with a moving imaging system.

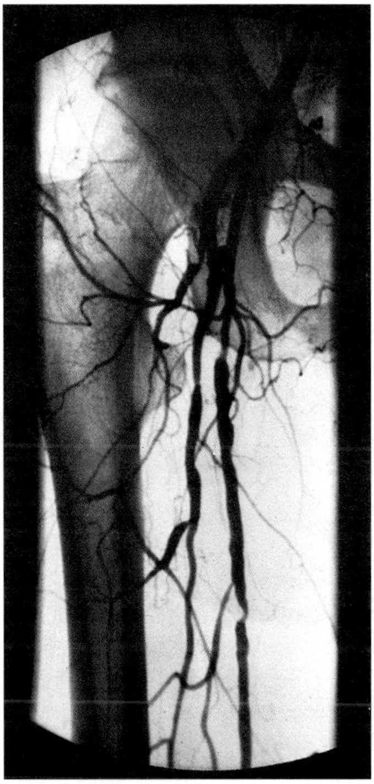

Fig. 7.147
Indirect exposure (100 mm exposure) of a femoral artery affected by multiple stenosis

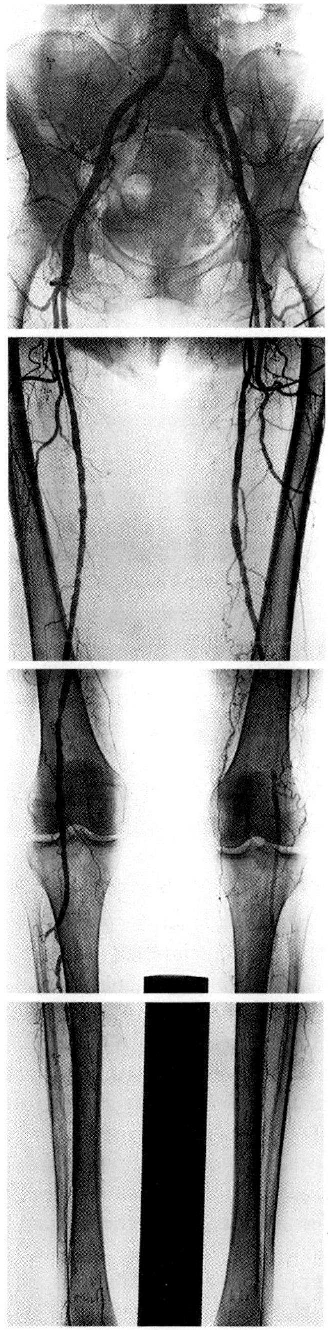

Fig. 7.148
Direct exposure sequence of a bilateral leg arteriography, taken by moving the imaging system while the patient remains stationary

7.3.2 Systems for cardiac angiography

Area of application

Systems for cardiac angiography are specially designed to display the ventricles, the cardiac valves and the heart vessels. To do this they must meet all the requirements of diagnostics as well as being able to support the relevant therapeutic operations which are possible using the methods of interventional cardiology. These operations include, for example, vascular dilatation with the aid of catheters according to Dotter or with the aid of balloon catheters according to Gruentzig, the widening of the cardiac valve cross-section with the aid of balloon catheters, thrombolysis by means of drugs applied directly at the site of the lesion via a catheter, and the recanalization of blocked coronary vessels by laser beams.

Requirements

Since the risk to the patient increases with the duration of the examination or the operation, any invasive examination of the heart or any possible therapeutic operation using interventional cardiology must be carried out in as short a time as possible – this is both in the interests of the patient as well as for economic reasons. Thus a system for these types of application should, if possible, permit simultaneous imaging in two different directions of projection (biplane operation), or else rapid changing between two directions of projection. In fluoroscopy, a biplane system makes orientation considerably simpler during positioning of the catheter, and when taking exposures it reduces the amount of contrast medium required and the length of time the catheter has to remain in the vessel, since with a single injection two directions of projection are recorded at once. At the same time, simultaneous biplane display simplifies the quantitative description or classification of the stenoses.

The coronary vessels meander across the curved surface of the heart and can therefore only be displayed without distortion from a single direction of projection if this is done section by section. For this reason, and in order to eliminate mutual superimpositions of individual vessels, several different projections are necessary for a complete examination of the coronary system. In these the central ray not only moves in a plane perpendicular to the longitudinal axis of the patient; it must also be rotated out of this plane by at least 30 degrees towards the head and towards the feet. The same flexibility is required when choosing the directions of projection for treating a stenosis, because for this the stenosis has to be imaged as orthographically as possible. Rapid setting up of the various projections to follow one another and optimization of the projections for treating a stenosis can only be achieved by using an isocentric system (see also section 7.3.1). All these degrees of freedom necessary for the direction of projection must not, however, hinder free access to the patient. In particular, the system must not impose any limitation on the examiner in the choice of the catheterization path.

Since the heart wall partly moves at high speed, exposure times must be around a few milliseconds to avoid motion blurring and image frequencies of up to 50 images/s must be attainable so that it is possible to carry out functional analyses of the hemodynamics and the movements of the heart valves and wall with sufficient spatial and temporal resolution.

In order to keep the time the catheter remains in the vessel as short as possible (particularly in the case of selective catheterization), it must be possible to quickly change from fluoroscopic to radiographic operation.

On top of all this, the actual imaging components of the system, namely the tube assembly, the x-ray image intensifier, the film cameras and the television systems, must of course ensure the best possible contrast with high geometric resolution in the image results.

Example of a system

The key components of the system which will be described below as an example are:

the BICOR, biplane examination unit,
the KOORDINAT 3D II patient positioning table,
two MEGALIX 125/40/82 C x-ray tube assemblies,
the PANDOROS 1200 A generator (biplane version),
two OPTILUX 27 HD-Triplex image intensifiers,
two VIDEOMED H high-resolution television systems with camera tubes of the SATICON type and
two 35 mm ARRITECHNO cine cameras with up to 150 frames/s.

Examination unit and patient positioning table
(The patient positioning table has already been described in Section 7.3.1)

The examination unit (Fig. 7.149) consists of two isocentric C-arm configurations, viz. the COROSKOP C floor-mounted stand and the COROSKOP L which is suspended from the ceiling. The C-arm of the COROSKOP C is mounted off-center in the same way as that of the ANGIOSKOP D33 (see section 7.3.1), so as to give the examiner the best possible access to the patient. The radius of the C-arm is chosen to be large enough for the imaging system still to be able to register the point of puncture in the arteria femoralis without any difficulty despite the floor stand being at the head end. The COROSKOP C permits the setting up of any desired projection including $\pm 45°$ cranio-caudal or caudo-cranial projections without changing the position of the patient.

In the COROSKOP L the C-arm is suspended centrally with the result that the tube assembly and the image intensifier can also be attached centrally to the C-arm. In this way one has a particularly slim C-arm arrangement which hardly hinders access to the patient at all. This makes it possible (e.g. for hygienic reasons) to already move the COROSKOP L from its space-saving parking position over the floor stand of the COROSKOP C to its exposure position while the preparations for the examination are taking place. In order to make this parking position possible, the tube mounting has been constructed in such a way that the tube can be swivelled through 180°. This possibility of swivelling the tube can be used as an extra means of facilitating access to the patient as long as the COROSKOP L is already in its exposure position but not yet

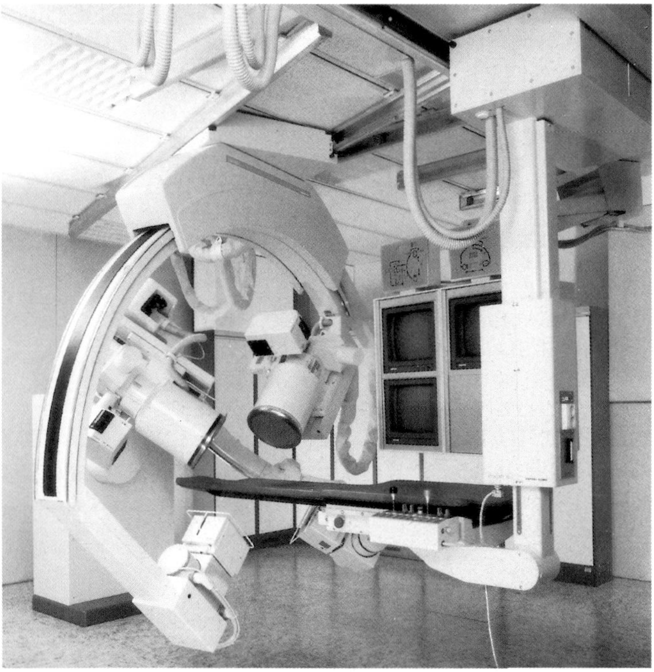

Fig. 7.149
BICOR, an examination unit for biplane cardiac angiography, in combination with the KOORDINAT 3D II patient positioning table. The COROSKOP C floor-mounted stand has a C-arm which is mounted off-center, to which the x-ray tube and the image receptor unit are also attached off-center. In the case of the ceiling-suspended support COROSKOP L, the x-ray tube and the image receptor unit are mounted centrally on the C-arm attached to it, which leads to an especially slim construction. The overall arrangement, together with the fact that the patient positioning table is secured at the ceiling and thus does not touch the floor, allows particularly easy access to the patient and very great freedom in the choice of the directions of projection.

in operation. With the COROSKOP L, the central ray can be rotated 120° to the left (LAO 120°) from the p.a. position. The angle range through which the C-arm can turn around the vertical axis is from 70° cranial to 70° caudal.

The directions of projection which can be realised with the two C-arm arrangements are well in excess of the demands of cardiac angiography.

To order to achieve an optimal imaging geometry, the image intensifier units can be moved along the central ray, as was the case with the ANGIOSKOP (see Section 7.3.1). It is especially advantageous with respect to the imaging geometry if instead of the 27 cm image intensifier one attaches a 17 cm image intensifier to the COROSKOP L, since then in certain circumstances it is possi-

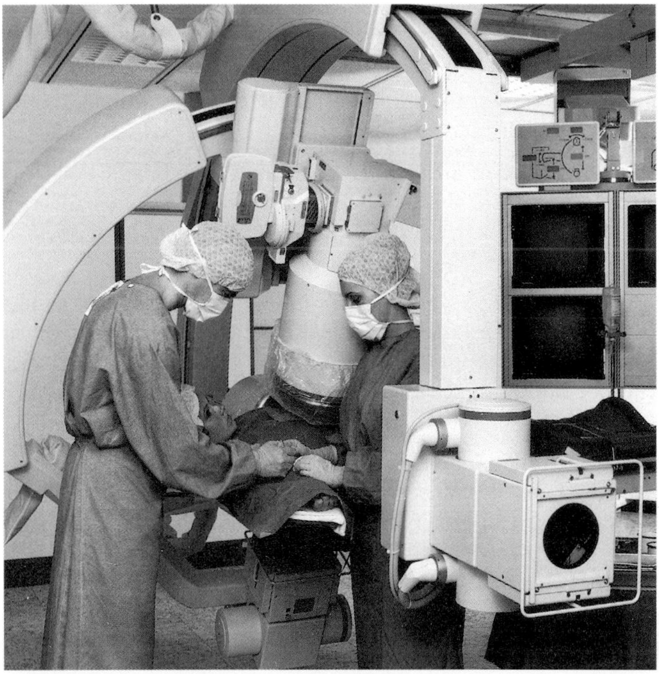

Fig. 7.150
BICOR, an examination unit for biplane cardiac angiography, in combination with the KOORDINAT 3D II patient positioning table. The x-ray tube attached to the COROSKOP L ceiling support has been rotated through 180° from its operating position thus facilitating access to the patient, especially so long as the relevant imaging system is not needed. With the tube in the position shown, the COROSKOP L can also be moved into its parking position over the floor stand of the other COROSKOP C imaging system. On the top of the ceiling-suspended monitor unit, large displays giving the angle of projection, in focus-image intensifier distance and the magnification factor of objects in the isocenter can clearly be seen.

ble to move the smaller image intensifier underneath the larger one. It is true that by doing this one sacrifices the equivalence of the two planes to some extent. The large number of projection possibilities means that the two planes are equivalent to such an extent that should one plane cease to function, the entire examination could, if necessary, be carried out with the remaining plane.

All movements of the unit are carried out with the aid of a motor, and controlled by the most modern microprocessor technology, which has numerous advantages for the user:

> Operation is simple and clear. The two C-arm units can either be moved separately or – irrespective of their starting position – synchronously in the same direction. Movements can be carried out at variable speeds, so that relatively large changes in position can be rapidly made and fine adjustments are possible. Automatic return of the COROSKOP L to its parking position from any other point can be brought about at the simple touch of a button.

As a particular aid to operation, an additional control system is available which enables the standard projections to be programmed.

If there is danger of a collision an automatic warning sounds and the speed of movement is reduced. If a collision actually takes place between different parts of the unit or between parts of the unit and the patient, movement is switched off by suitable sensors triggering before damage can occur.

The position signals from the various parts of the unit to the control system are also used to indicate by means of large digital displays the current values of certain variables for the isocenter, viz. the angle of projection, the distance between the focal spot and the image intensifier and the geometric magnification resulting from this taking into account the electronic magnification.

Finally, microprocessor technology also makes it easier to track down errors should a fault occur, since with the aid of the electronic diagnostic system the cause of the breakdown can usually be established immediately.

The tube assembly and the generator

The MEGALIX tube assembly which has already been described in section 7.3.1 is used in cardiac angiography in a version with only two focal spots. With its focal spots of 0.6 and 1.0 which have a high load capacity and its large heat capacity, the MEGALIX tube assembly has enough reserve power for any kind of cine-angiographic examination of the heart.

The tube assembly is provided with a motor-powered iris diaphragm which automatically restricts the x-ray beam to the image intensifier input field selected. Even narrower collimation can then be set by a remote control device.

If, in a projection, there are large differences in transparency between the heart and the neighboring lung region, these as a rule produce a deterioration in the image quality in the sense of a loss of contrast in the heart region. The causes of this are essentially an increased level of scattered radiation and the non-linear behavior of the image intensifier. Here a remedy is provided by a semitransparent diaphragm with a curved shape, the 'heart contour diaphragm', which is mounted in the diaphragm housing in such a way that it can be rotated about the central ray and shifted in a radial direction, and which, like the iris diaphragm, can be optimally adapted to the object to be imaged via a remote control device.

The PANDOROS 1200 A generator differs completely in its construction principle and also somewhat in its power specifications and properties from the POLYDOROS 80 or 100 high frequency generator, which was described in connection with the ANGIOSKOP D33 and which could also be perfectly well employed here. The PANDOROS 1200A is a generator which is regulated and switched on the secondary side, i.e. in this generator the power supply voltage is first transformed upwards and rectified, and the high voltage conducted to the x-ray tube via a suitable electronic regulator and switch. In this way switching times as low as 0.5 ms are possible, and the maximum frame rate of the camera of 150 frames/s is also managed by the generator without difficulty.

This generator too has suitable automatic control systems like the ones described above; however, in contrast to the POLYDOROS, it is possible in cine operation to change the automatically pre-set value of the high voltage manually before the beginning of the exposure sequence. Furthermore, here the exposure for each single image is controlled individually, and not determined from the data of the previous image for the subsequently following one.

A very important point as regards the image quality in biplane operation is the alternating exposure of the two planes. So that exposures in the two planes corresponding to each other reveal as far as possible the same state of the object, the exposure of the two planes for each pair of images takes place in close succession and not, for example, separated by exactly half an image period. If the two planes were to be exposed simultaneously, there would be a higher proportion of scattered radiation registered in both planes, which would of course reduce the contrast as a result. In addition, alternating operation gives a technical advantage as well: whilst two switching and regulating devices are required for the high voltage, only one high voltage generator is needed.

Image receptor

The image intensifiers recommended for purely cardiological use differ only in their formats, and not in their technology from the one described in 7.3.1.

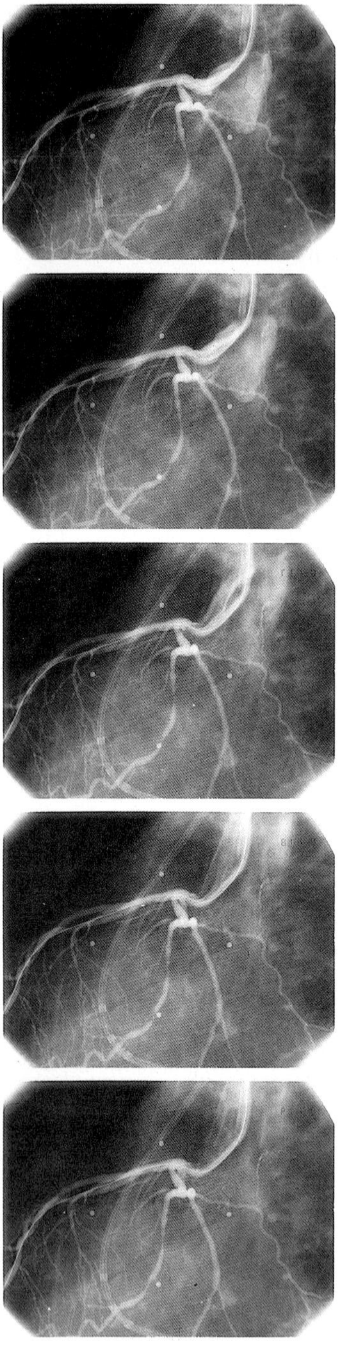

Fig. 7.151
Extract from a cine scene taken in the course of an cardiac angiographic examination.

The other components of the image intensifier unit have also already been dealt with there. It should be pointed out, however, that the television units as a rule are additionally equipped with video tape recorders so as to make it possible to store both fluoroscopic scenes and cine scenes, which are also received by the television camera via a semitransparent mirror in the light distributor of the image intensifier unit. This facility provides backup of the information, in particular if there should be faulty handling and processing of the cine film.

As a rule, the exposure of cine scenes is monitored by simultaneously viewing the television picture. Here there would be a distracting flicker for cine frame rates below the frame rate of the television. This flicker is suppressed by writing the video image corresponding to the single cine image into a suitable (digital) semiconductor memory from which it can be read out repeatedly at the television frequency until a new cine image is exposed. This technique is known as 'gap filling'.

Image results

An essential part of the diagnostic information in cine-angiography naturally resides in the reproduction of the dynamic processes in the heart which unfortunately cannot be shown as impressively in print as in cine projection. Nevertheless Fig. 7.151 shows some interesting details of an extract from a cine scene.

7.3.3 Systems for digital subtraction angiography (DSA)

Area of application

DSA is used today in practically all areas of angiography. For this reason DSA systems do not differ in their basic design from the corresponding angiographic systems, but merely have extra components for DSA.

The hope which was expressed when DSA was introduced that the procedure would largely make it possible to replace intra-arterial administration of contrast media by the less invasive intravenous method has not been fulfilled. Nevertheless, DSA allows one to work with smaller quantities of contrast medium when using intra-arterial application. The immediate display during the examination of the image results (which are always correctly exposed) leads to shorter examination times and permits decisions to be taken on the spot about how to proceed further in the examination. In this way DSA reduces the risk to the patient in many interventional radiological procedures or may even make the operation feasible in the first place [7.98].

Requirements

The requirements which a DSA system has to meet with respect to image intensifier format, image matrix size, image matrix depth, image acquisition, image storage, computing power, image processing, image analysis, overall control system and types of exposure operation, strongly depend in part on the medical application in question. Since the basic technical investment in such a system is extremely high, however, one does not design special systems for the individual types of examination, but instead uses various expansion levels of a powerful general design which are specially adapted to the particular task; the highest level of expansion is then also able to meet the demands of cardiac angiography.

A few of the key requirements of a system which can be used in all areas of application will be listed below:

The image matrix should contain at least 512 × 512 pixels. This value represents an acceptable compromise between on the one hand investment in storage and computational capacity, and on the other hand resolution and required dose per pixel. In combination with an image intensifier input format of 27/17/14 cm, this implies e.g. a limitation of the resolution to about 0.53/0.33/0.27 mm due to the matrix alone. Digitization of the video signal at the input of the DSA system should be carried out with a resolution of 10 bits. This means subdividing the input signal range into 1024 gray levels and thus meets the requirements with respect to the signal range and the signal-to-noise ratio of the image intensifier television picture even at high values for the dose or dose rate. The value of 10 bits can still be realised with an acceptable level of investment at the required measurement data rate of about 20 MHz.

Subtraction and display in real time must be possible both in continuous operation and in pulsed operation. For the purposes of cardiac angiography, an exposure frequency of at least 25 images/s at full resolution (512 × 512 matrix) is necessary; apart from this, the system should make it possible to operate cine and DSA simultaneously by means of a suitable synchronization system so that the information gained by using radiation can be exploited in the best way possible.

Since subtraction procedures can only eliminate the background perfectly if the position of the object in the path of the radiation does not change during the exposure series, the possibility must exist of ECG-controlled triggering of the exposure for those situations where the pulsation of vessels during exposure may falsify the result of the subtraction. Moreover it must be possible to establish a link between the individual images and the ECG.

In many applications, just like when using a cutfilm changer, it is necessary to change the exposure frequency (in certain circumstances, several times) during the exposure of a sequence in order to reduce both the patient's radiation exposure and the tube load, and to keep the number of images to be archived to a reasonable level.

Apart from subtraction, the most important image processing function which is required for practical use is the possibility of image integration. This is necessary both when taking the mask and the contrast image. Image integration achieves a reduction of noise in the subtraction image (admittedly sometimes with a simultaneous loss in temporal resolution) which facilitates the recognizability of weak contrasts, or actually makes it possible to recognize them at all.

As already mentioned, a usable subtraction result can only be expected if the mask and the contrast image are geometrically congruent. In practice this condition cannot always be met: depending on the exposure situation and the capacity of the patient to cooperate, voluntary or involuntary movement of the patient or of organs can occur during an exposure series in spite of careful preparation and execution of the examination. It should be possible to make retrospective corrections to deal with such movements, so that, should the results of subtraction be unsatisfactory as a consequence of inadequate geometric image congruence, another subtraction can be carried out with suitably shifted, stored originals.

A considerable computational capacity is necessary for data acquisition, image storage and subtraction which, as it is present in the system, can also be used for image analysis. Because of this there arises more or less automatically the demand for quantitative image analysis programs for those areas of application in which quantitative results form a key goal of the examination.

Finally, the last remaining requirement to be mentioned is the basic one for the greatest possible simplicity of operation of such a complex system. Here again part of the computing power can be used to good effect.

Example of a system

Apart from the components which serve the purpose of digital image processing and storage, DSA systems largely resemble conventional angiographic systems as already presented in sections 7.3.1 and 7.3.2. For this reason, essentially only the above-mentioned digital components and the overall control system will be dealt with here, using the example of the DIGITRON 3 VAC (Fig. 7.152).

This system fulfills the stated requirements. The block diagram in Fig. 7.153 shows the key component parts necessary for this purpose and their interaction. The system is capable of processing the video signals from up to three imaging entities, where by the concept 'imaging entity' is also meant a video tape storage system (SIRECORD) or a cine-video converter (CIPRO with attached television camera). After either logarithmic or linear amplification, according to what is chosen, the video signal arrives at the analog-digital converter, where it is converted into a digital signal 10 bits in depth at a sampling rate of 22.4 MHz when operating at 50 Hz or 18.5 MHz at 60 Hz. The digital measurement data

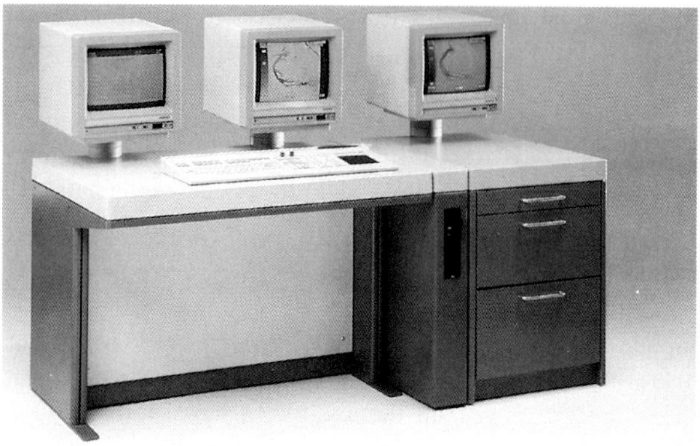

Fig. 7.152
Console of the DIGITRON 3 VAC. Behind the operating keyboard with its additional marking facility (on the right of the keyboard), e.g. for selecting areas of the image for analysis, there are three monitors: on the left the dialog monitor, in the middle the image monitor, and on the right an optionally available additional color monitor for image reproduction.

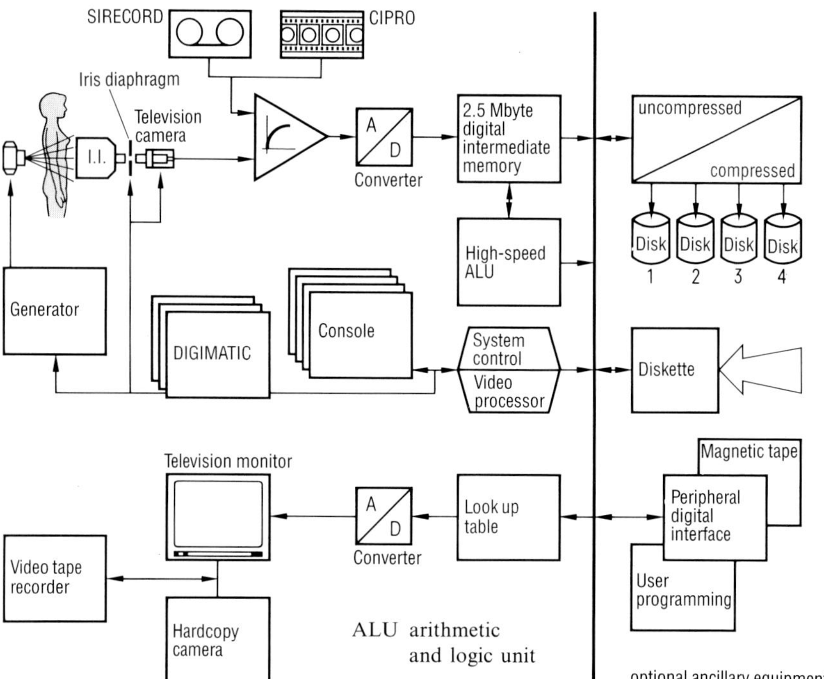

Fig. 7.153
Circuit diagram (overview) of the DIGITRON 3 VAC (see text for further details)

go into an intermediate memory with a capacity of 2.5 Mbyte. The latter is linked to an extremely fast arithmetic and logic unit (ALU) which is capable of carrying out the image subtraction and reproduction in real time.

In addition the images can be stored in a high-speed digital storage system with four disk drives. Operating at 50 or 60 Hz, this is capable of storing 3800 or 4400 image matrices respectively, consisting of 512×512 elements with a maximum frequency of 25 or 30 images/s respectively. The storage process is organized in such a way that only complete images are stored in the individual drives, which are employed cyclically one after the other.

Image processing is not only restricted to subtraction, integration, windowing and shifting of the image. In addition there exists amongst other things the possibility of moving subtraction with a fixed time interval between the mask and the 'contrast image'; likewise there exists the possibility of gray level inversion, image magnification, image filtration and the insertion of text anywhere in the image. Amongst the possibilities for quantitative image analysis, apart from the construction of time density curves for selected regions of interest (ROI) and density profiles together with the corresponding processing of the curves, one has, in particular, programs for stenosis quantification, flow analysis and heart function analysis. In addition the scientifically-oriented user can expand the program system with his own analysis programs.

The operation of the whole system is carried out with the aid of a menu program via the dialog station of the console. The generator, the television system and the iris diaphragm in the telecentric ray path between the x-ray image intensifier and the video camera are controlled by the DIGIMATIC exposure control unit.

The menu offers the user four different dose rate levels. The exposure parameters are selected automatically on the basis of the values of the previous fluoroscopic examination and the desired image frequency and number of images, so that no special test shots are needed. In this process the tube voltage is automatically set to the best possible value for displaying the iodine contrast medium used in the examinations. Fig. 7.154 illustrates diagramatically the setting of the exposure parameters and the function of the automatic exposure control system. All the exposure parameters are displayed before the start of data acquisition.

The exposure series can either be made in continuous operation or in pulsed operation; in the latter case the possibility exists both of using a constant pulse time and of switching off the single pulses individually in accordance with light measurement in the telecentric ray path of the receptor system (MEMOSPOT operation). The requirements with respect to parallel cine operation, ECG triggering or marking and variable exposure frequency are met. In simple fluoroscopy, the image memory can be used to hold the final fluoroscopic image (last image hold, LIH). Naturally the system allows the use of the road-mapping technique which is so important in interventional procedures [7.99]. Here one uses as a mask a contrast image of the vessel of interest which has been produced with a small amount of contrast medium and then subtracts this from the fluoroscopic image (without contrast medium), so that the vessel appears virtually isolated in the image. This subtraction image is superimposed on the image obtained during continuous fluoroscopy of the guide wire or catheter advancing in the vessel.

DSA image results occasionally suffer from the fact that the range of attenuation in the object is so large that in spite of logarithmic amplification of the signal, non-linearities occur which then cause inadequate subtraction results. Such cases can be remedied by the use of compensators (e.g. in the form of little bags of rice flour) or shaped filters. However, these are difficult to handle. For this reason a special wedge filter assembly (see Fig. 7.155) was created for DSA systems, which can be attached to the tube assembly in front of the usual multi-leaf collimator. This DSA filter contains in one of its planes a double wedge filter which can be freely rotated around the central ray and displaced sideways, in order for instance in angiography of the extremities to

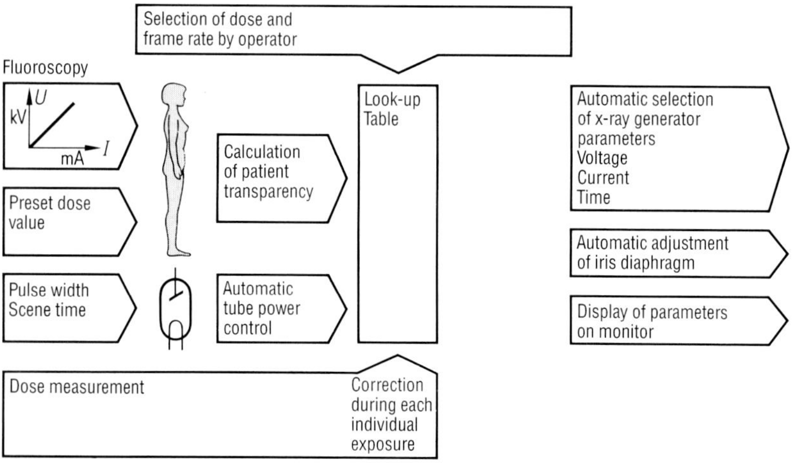

Fig. 7.154
Schematic diagram of the DIGIMATIC system interface and exposure control unit. After the image dose and image frequency have been selected by the operator, the DIGIMATIC automatically determines the optimum exposure parameters from the fluoroscopic data, sets these at the generator and also displays them on the monitor. The correct collimation value in the light-optical imaging system between the image intensifier output and the television camera tube is also selected automatically. Finally, the exposure is also automatically controlled during the radiographic series.

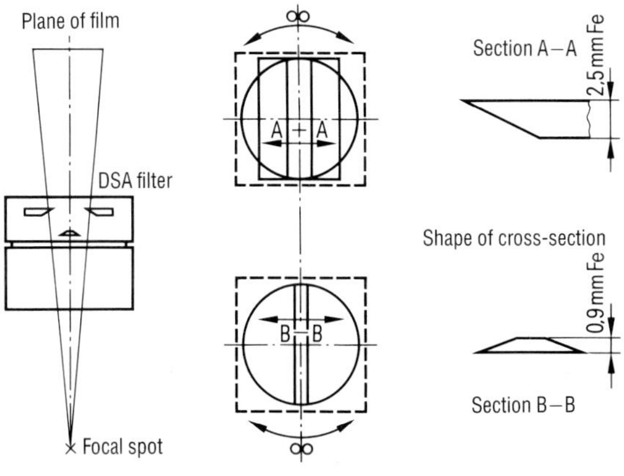

Fig. 7.155
Schematic view of a DSA filter. The device has two filter planes. Plane A consists of two wedge filters which can be displaced perpendicularly to their longitudinal direction in order to compensate for differences in object thickness at the edge of the body. Plane B contains a double wedge filter which can likewise be displaced perpendicularly to its longitudinal direction, which is intended in particular to eliminate direct radiation between the legs in leg arteriography. Both filter planes can be rotated around the central ray. All the movements are powered by a motor and under remote control.

attenuate the direct radiation in the region between the patient's legs. In the other plane there are two wedge filters which can be moved sideways independently of each other and rotated together around the central ray. These can be used for example at the edge of the body to harmonize the attenuation range. All filter movements are powered by a motor and under remote control.

For image documentation on film, two types of multiformat camera are available: MULTISPOT K with cassettes for two films each and MULTISPOT M with a supply and a collecting magazine for the film material. In addition, floppy disks and magnetic tapes can be used for digital image archival.

Image results

Figs. 7.156 a and b show levocardiograms on which quantitative analyses were carried out. Figs. 7.157 a and b show examples of images of coronary vessels.

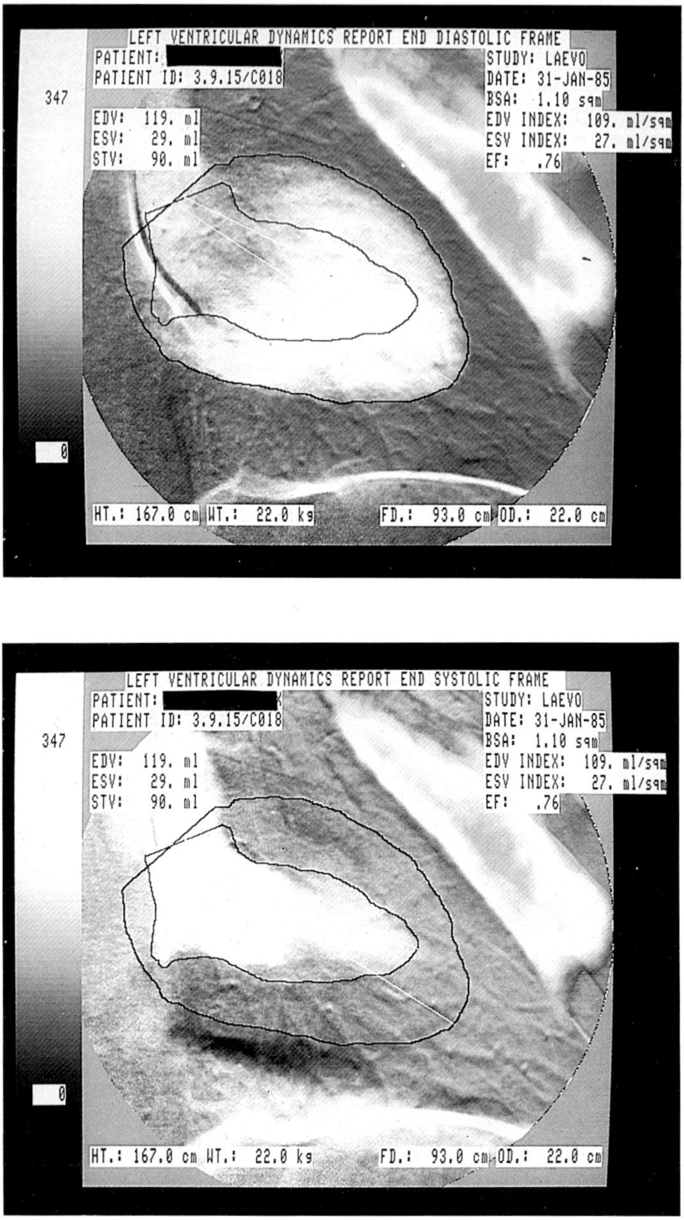

a)

b)

Fig. 7.156
Digital levocardiograms with analysis. Fig. a shows the left ventricle of the heart in the diastole, Fig. b in the systole.

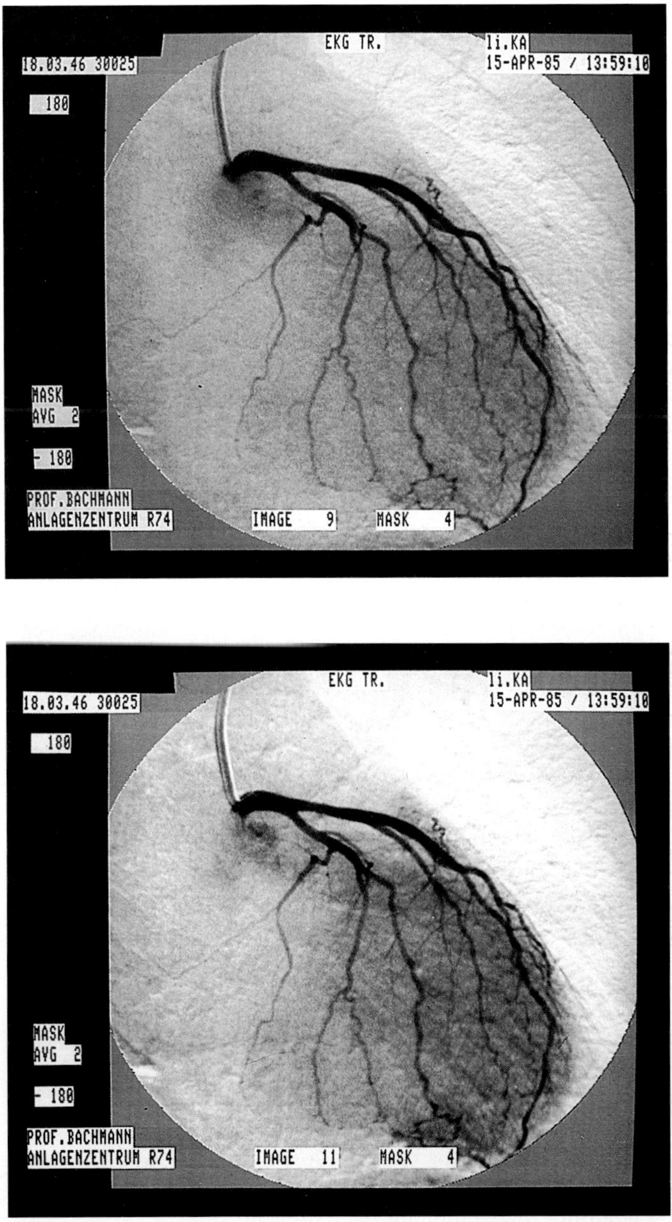

Fig. 7.157
Digital subtraction angiograms of coronary vessels. These image results were produced with the aid of ECG-controlled triggering of the exposure.

7.3.4 Systems for lithotripsy

Area of application

Lithotripsy systems are used in the treatment of stone disorders to fragment the stones by means of focused high-energy ultrasound pulses generated outside the body. While extracorporeal shock wave lithotripsy (ESWL) for the treatment of calculi of the urinary tract, particularly of kidney stones, can now be regarded as an established procedure, its application in other areas, e.g. for the treatment of gallstones, is still at the research stage. The rapid spread of the technique after it was first performed at the end of the seventies [7.100] is due to the fact that, as a rule, ESWL is considerably less stressful for the patient than lithothomy or the removal of the stone by percutaneous techniques, and moreover leads to a shortening of the patient's stay in hospital and a reduction in the cost of treatment.

Requirements

Whereas the systems described in the preceding sections 7.3.1 to 7.3.3 essentially serve diagnostic purposes and are used in the various invasive radiologial techniques mentioned as aids for the insertion of therapeutic instruments at the treatment site, lithotripsy systems also contain components which are exclusively used for treatment, viz. all those parts of the system which are intended for generating, guiding and focusing the shock waves and for 'coupling' them to the patient. The efficiency of the system is determined by the combination of the x-ray components needed for stone localization together with the shock wave components necessary for fragmenting the stone, as well as by the overall control system coordinating the two groups of components.

The x-ray system should be designed in such a way that it is not only suitable as a targeting aid for fragmenting stones, but also for urological examinations, for verifying findings and for checking and documenting the result of the treatment.

Apart from pure ESWL, a lithotripsy system should also make it possible to combine ESWL with e.g. percutaneous stone extraction, if this seems advisable or becomes necessary in a particular case. This requirement cannot be realized with the equipment design chosen for the first lithotripsy systems, where the patient is placed in a water bath for coupling to the shock waves. A system which dispenses with a water bath at the same time also has the advantage of needing a less laborious preparation for the treatment.

Lithotripsy systems with a water bath generate shock waves by means of an underwater spark gap; the spark gap is situated in one focus of an elliptical reflector, and the stone to be fragmented is brought into its other focus. This type of shock wave generation is characterized by strong wear on the electrodes of the source, which as a rule have to be changed at least after each treatment. This characteristic contradicts the basic requirement for a system that its operation should involve as little maintenance as possible.

In order to protect the tissue structures surrounding the stone, it is essential to make the ultrasonic energy in its concentrated form act as far as possible only on the stone. When treating kidney stones, because of the considerable displacement of the kidneys during breathing, this can only be realized if a suitable respiratory triggering of the localization and treatment system ensures that the calculus localization and the application of the shock waves occur at the same position of the object.

Example of a system

The LITHOSTAR lithotripsy system operates without a patient bath. The patient positioning table (Fig. 7.158) looks at the first glance like a normal urology examination table and can also be fitted with all the accessories necessary for urological x-ray examinations (Fig. 7.159). However, in the pedestal of the table there are two shock wave heads – one each for access from the left or right side of the body – which can be raised for the treatment after taking out the relevant parts of the table surface and brought into contact with the patient (Fig. 7.160), as well as two image intensifiers.

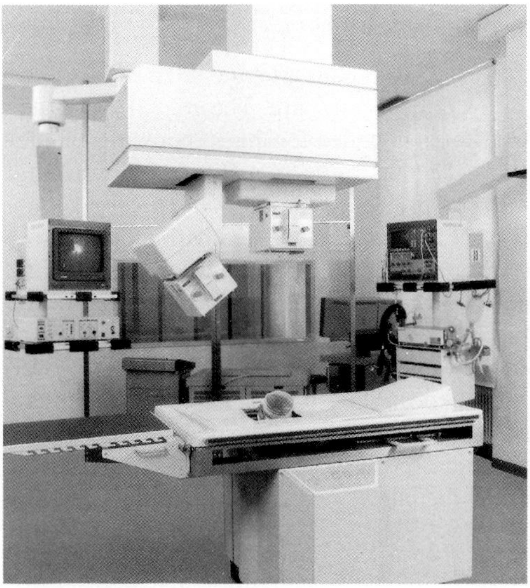

Fig. 7.158
LITHOSTAR, equipment for extracorporeal shock wave lithotripsy (ESWL). The ceiling-suspended mounting contains two single-tank x-ray tube assemblies. The associated image intensifiers and two shock wave heads for shattering stones are situated inside the table pedestal. The movable spotfilm device with moving grid can be seen in its parking position under the top of the table to the right.

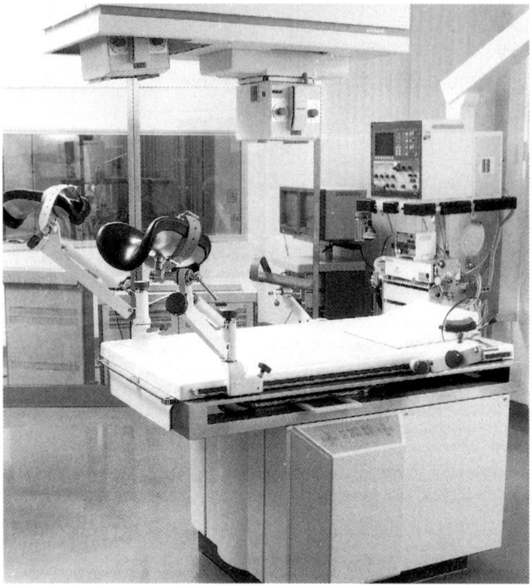

Fig. 7.159
Apart from its function as a therapy unit, the LITHOSTAR also meets all the requirements of a versatile urological examination apparatus and is equipped with all the necessary accessories for this purpose. The cassette-spotfilm device with moving grid is shown here in its recording position. The tube assembly for caudo-cranial projection has been put in its parking position inside the ceiling-suspended mounting so as to hinder access to the patient as little as possible. The second tube assembly can likewise be retracted into the ceiling-suspended mounting.

The x-ray unit consists of

a POLYPHOS 30 M high-frequency generator (power 30 kW),
two single-tank tube assemblies with motor-driven collimators,
two OPTILUX 17/12 HN image intensifiers,
two VIDEOMED N television systems
and a MEMOSKOP U/2 digital image memory.

The first x-ray tube assembly with its corresponding image intensifier is positioned in the vertical (a.p., antero-posterior) beam path. The second x-ray tube assembly/image intensifier combination is intended for fluoroscopy in a caudo-cranial projection at an angle of 45°. The a.p. projection shows the horizontal position of the stone, the caudo-cranial projection shows the vertical position. Fluoroscopy in both planes takes place with automatic collimation of the x-ray beam to the relevant image intensifier format and with automatic dose rate control. Apart from the two fluoroscopic units which are principally needed for localization of the stone, the apparatus also has a cassette device with a moving secondary radiation grid incorporated in the table. This can be moved easily from its park position into the exposure position when needed. For cassette radiographs the x-ray beam is automatically collimated to the cassette format used. In addition, an automatic exposure timer is built into the system in order to ensure correct exposure of the film.

The isocenter of the system is the point of intersection of the central beams of the two fluoroscopy configurations; the sound energy of the shock wave

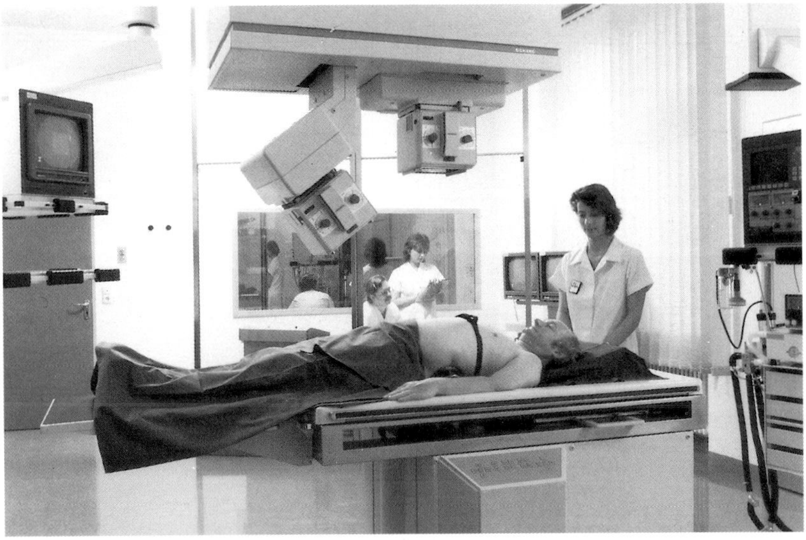

Fig. 7.160
LITHOSTAR with a patient. The raised shock wave head can clearly be seen below the left kidney region of the patient. Stretched around the patient's chest is the constraining tension band of the respiratory triggering device, which is used to trigger both the fluoroscopic pulses and the shock waves.

head selected is also focused on this point once it has been put in the treatment position (Fig. 7.161).

In order to fix the target for the shock wave treatment, the fluoroscopy pulses are under respiratory control so that the stone can be localized in a well-defined position. For especially strong noise suppression, the digital memory makes it possible to integrate from 2 up to 16 consecutive images. The option of windowing permits a further increase in contrast when stones or concrements with low contrast are being displayed. In this process a selected subregion of the brightness range of the stored image can be displayed over the whole luminance range of the monitor. The correct target position can be marked on both of the monitors by a superimposed cross. First of all the stone to be treated is brought to the target point on the monitor of the a.p. fluoroscopy unit by motor-driven excursion of the table in the two horizontal directions. Afterwards the corresponding adjustment on the other monitor is carried out by raising or lowering the table. In the horizontal plane, the stone naturally does not thereby move out of the target area again so that the targeting procedure is thus completed.

In the LITHOSTAR, shock waves are not produced with the aid of an underwater spark gap, but by means of an electromagnetic source using the principle

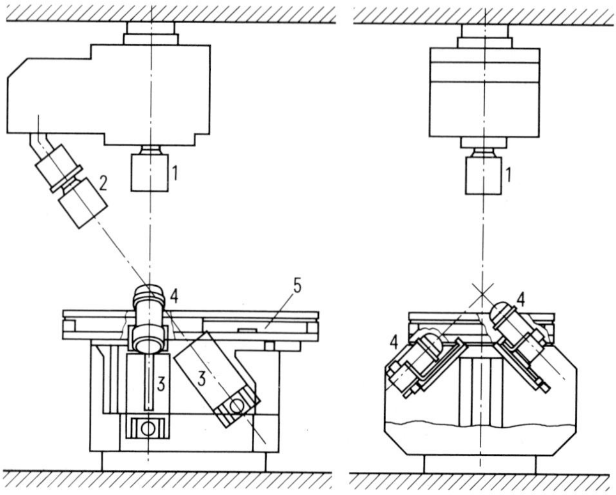

1 X-ray tube assembly plane 1 (a.p. projection)
2 X-ray tube assembly plane 2 (caudo-cranial 45°)
3 Image intensifier
4 Shock wave head
5 X-ray film cassette

Fig. 7.161
Isocenter of the LITHOSTAR. If a shock wave head is in the treatment position, its shock waves are focused on the point of intersection of the central rays of the two fluoroscopy systems. Thus the kidney stone to be shattered merely needs to be guided to this point of intersection by the fluoroscopy systems before the application of the shock waves

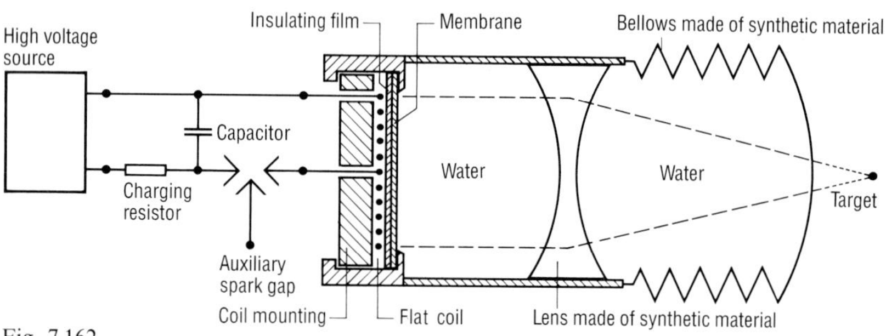

Fig. 7.162
Schematic of the shock wave generator with the LITHOSTAR shock wave head. The high voltage capacitor is discharged via a flat coil with only a few turns. The magnetic field thus induced generates eddy currents in a thin metallic membrane which is positioned so as to be insulated from the coil. The magnetic field of these currents is opposite to that of the coil and thus leads to a deflection of the membrane. Due to the high discharge current in the kA range this creates a very short, plane acoustic pulse with a large amplitude in the water-filled tube sealed by the membrane. The pulse is then focused onto a small region by means of a suitable acoustic lens made out of synthetic material. The free end of the tube is sealed by a soft bellows made of synthetic material which molds itself to the shape of the body and thus ensures that a sufficiently large entry area is available for the transmission of the sound energy into the body of the patient.

of the shock tube [7.101]. The relevant configuration is sketched in Fig. 7.162 following [7.102]. A tube filled with degassed water is sealed at one end by a plane acoustic source. This consists essentially of a high voltage capacitor, a suitable switch (e.g. an auxiliary spark gap), a flat coil with just a few turns and a very thin metallic membrane placed as near as possible in front of the coil, but electrically insulated from it. If in this configuration the capacitor is discharged via the coil, eddy currents are induced in the membrane by the magnetic field of the coil. The magnetic field of these currents is opposite to that of the coil and thus leads to a deflection of the membrane away from the coil. If the configuration is dimensioned in a suitable way, this process generates a very short, plane acoustic pulse with a large amplitude in the adjoining water. Due to transit time effects, the corresponding pressure wave becomes even steeper as it traverses the water-filled tube. The plane wave front is finally focused onto a point by an acoustic lens made out of a suitable synthetic material, which brings about another extreme increase in pressure. In clinical applications, one must then place the kidney stone (or whatever is to be treated) at this focal point. To make this possible, the free end of the water-filled tube is sealed by an elastic membrane made of synthetic material which can adapt itself to the shape of the body to a large extent. The acoustic coupling between the shock wave generator and the body of the patient is ensured by a specially developed 'gel disk', which should be placed between the synthetic bellows and the patient. The sound energy thus penetrates the body over a relatively large area, and the focal point lies deep inside the body, so that tissue damage is largely avoided.

The control system for generating the shock waves permits the choice of operating either of the two shock wave heads. The energy of the individual shock waves can be varied by changing the charging voltage of the high voltage capacitor. Both single shock wave pulses or sequences with a shock wave frequency of 100 per minute can be released, and the triggering can be controlled by respiration and/or by ECG. This method of shock wave release ensures a particularly effective use of the shock waves whilst causing as little damage as possible to the tissue surrounding the stone to be treated.

8 X-ray computed tomography

8.1 Equipment design

There are different types of requirements for a computer tomograph (CT). For example, although the main requirement for a skull image is the best contrast resolution, the exposure time being of minor importance, an image of the torso requires the shortest possible exposure time. Only then can one be certain that organ movements, respiration or peristalsis do not cause any interference in terms of image artifacts.

8.1.1 The CT system and its components

The components of a CT system are shown in the block diagram (Fig. 8.1). The operating console is the central communication unit for the user of the system. All equipment parameters and patient data are input here. The scan itself is initiated from here and here the reconstructed image is displayed on a monitor. A well designed operating concept is characterized by as few input

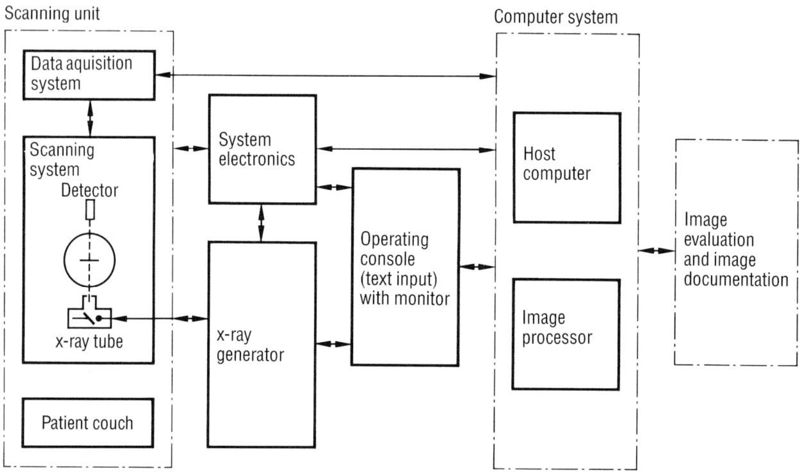

Fig. 8.1
Schematic diagram of a CT scanning system

procedures as possible which are as simple as possible. The computer system provides support to the operator and controls and monitors safety functions. The fastest possible imaging computer for image reconstruction forms the heart of the computer system. The scanning system with x-ray tube, diaphragm and detector as well as the electronics for processing the measurement data and the patient couch form the scanning unit. Here, the scanning system and the data aquisition system are housed in the scanning system, i.e. in the gantry. The x-ray generator, characterized by high output power and constancy of its output values, and also the system electronics are essential components of a CT system which, as the components for image evaluation and image documentation, are controlled by the computer system.

8.1.2 Scanning unit

Fig. 8.2 shows the scanning unit of a whole-body CT. The gantry can be tilted by +/−25°; the patient is moved into the measurement field on a couch. Seen from the outside, it is impossible to tell what is the operating principle of a CT scanner. The magnitude of the measurement field, the diameter of the measurement aperture and their accessibility from all sides determine the possible field of application.

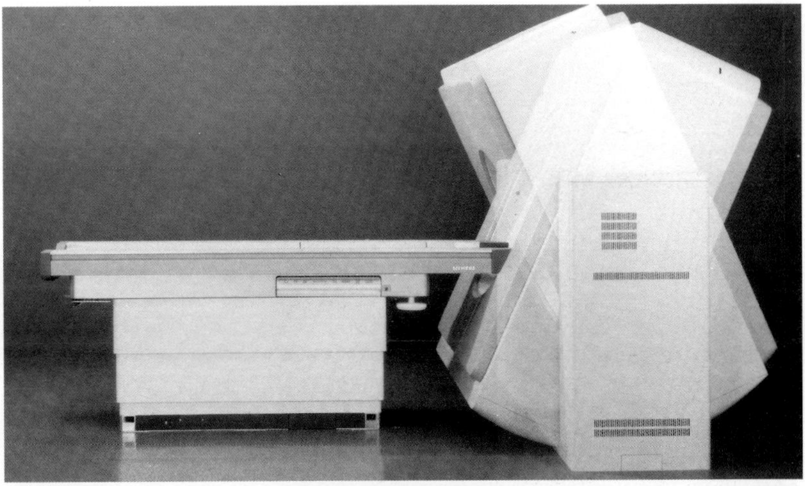

Fig. 8.2
The tilting gantry of a whole-body computer tomograph facilitates the measurement of coronary sections and allows the free projection of organs

8.1.2.1 Gantry

A parallel beam apparatus based on the translation-rotation principle requires alternating linear and rotational movements of the detector system, which is rigidly connected to the x-ray tube. It is understandable that, because of the relatively large mass, the exposure times have lower limits imposed on them. At present, measuring times as low as approximately 10 seconds can be achieved.

However, the most commonly used apparatus functions according to the fan-beam principle. Here, a distinction is made between scanning systems with detector and x-ray tube rotating with them and those with rotating x-ray tube and stationary detector ring. In installations with rotating x-ray tube-detector systems, several hundred radiation receivers are arranged on a circular arc opposite the x-ray tube with the focal spot as the center (Fig. 8.3). The large number of detector elements and scanning channels process a corresponding number of measured signals at the same time. This means that the scanning procedure is reduced to a single rotation movement, which allows short exposure times of less than one second for large scanning field diameters of, for example, 50 cm. Monitor detectors at the edge of the diaphragm system next to the x-ray tube constantly measure the unattenuated x-ray radiation outside the patient scanning field for normalization purposes. The x-ray tube is operated with constant radiation or in pulse mode. The demands made by the large number of scanning channels means that only the scanning of one slice per exposure is economically viable.

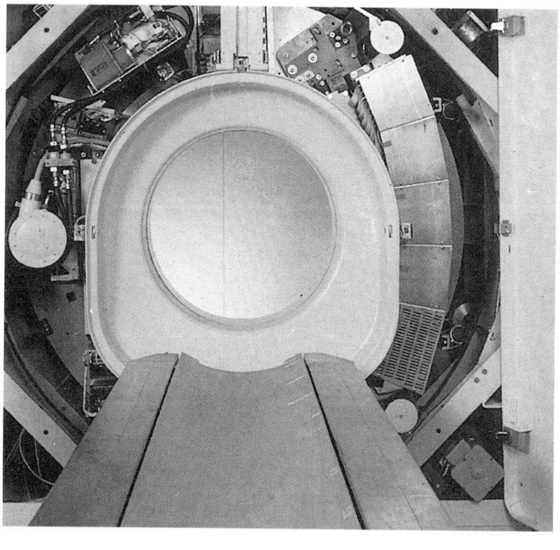

Fig. 8.3
Gantry unit
of the SOMATOM DR
fan-beam scanner,
with rotating detectors

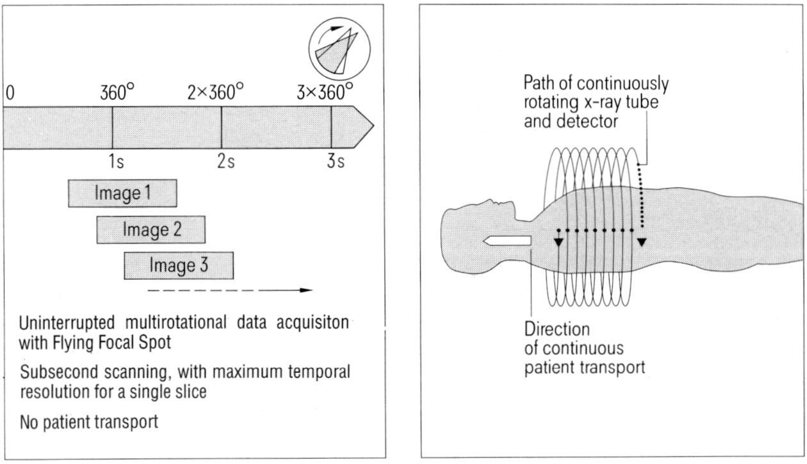

Fig. 8.4
Dynamic Multiscan with and without patient transport (Somatom Plus)

Very high demands are placed on the mechanical components. In these systems, the position of the "projection" must be known to a fraction of a degree and the positioning of the detector elements must be known to 0.01 mm. The short exposure times and interscan times enable a slice frequency of more than 10 slices per minute and thus make it possible to operate in "CT-angio" mode.

The latest generation of high-performance CT systems (SOMATOM PLUS) operates with continuous rotation of the radiation detector system and flying focal spot. This allows measurement times of less than 1 second and successive exposures without any breaks (Fig. 8.4). The continuous moving of the patient transport during this procedure allows the scan of a continuous volume of the body.

8.1.2.2 Patient positioning and slice positioning

The patient couches of these CT systems have adjustable height and can be adjusted to the height of the bed when it is necessary to transfer the patient. The patient on the couch is raised to the operating height and then moved into the exposure position. Tilting visors, a tilting gantry and automatic advance of the couch make it possible to provide a rapid and reproducible slice positioning. Fig. 8.5 shows an example of this.

The functions necessary for positioning the patient can be directly controlled from the couch, the gantry or remotely controlled from the central operating console.

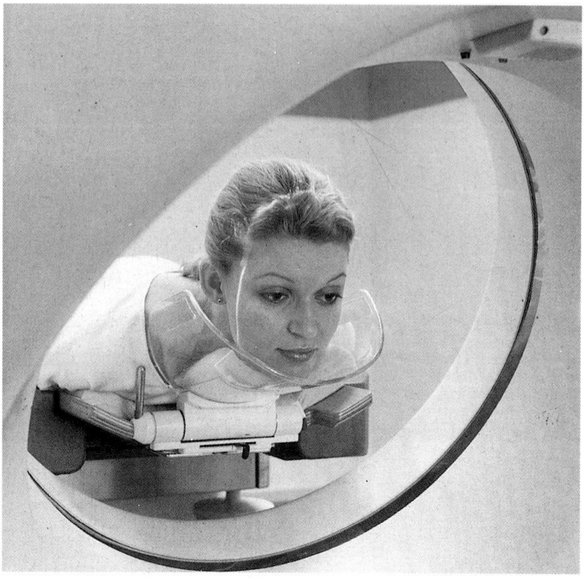

Fig. 8.5
Coronal section.
Prone position
of the patient
with inclined gantry

Localizer radiograph

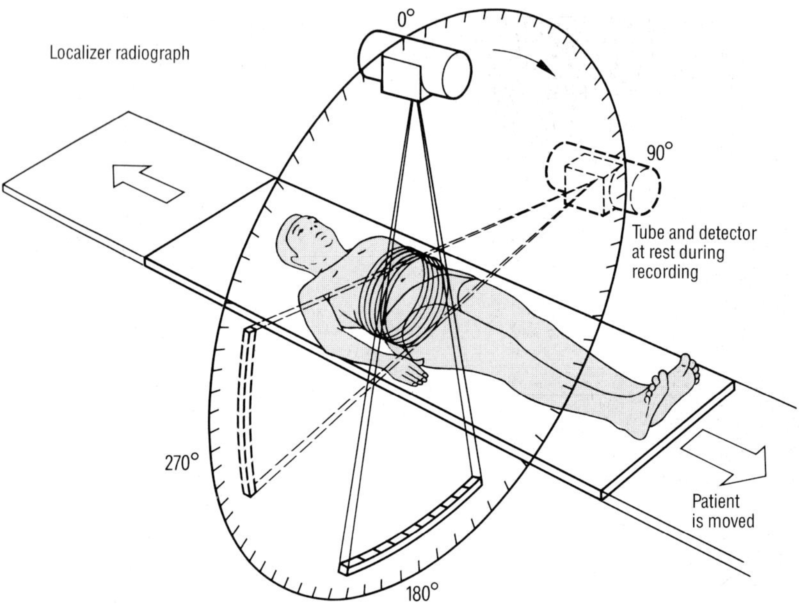

Fig. 8.6 Schematic diagram of a localizer radiograph (Topogram)

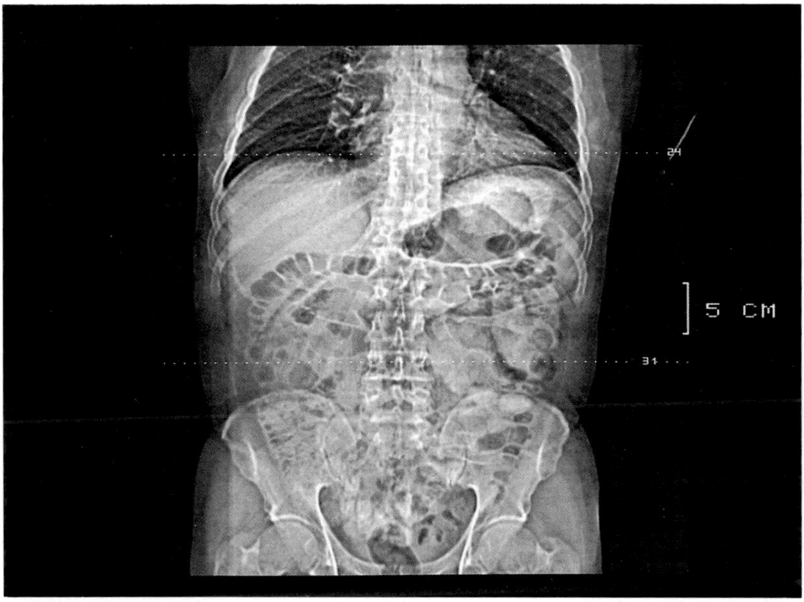

Fig. 8.7
Topogram to facilitate the localization of the examination area of the torso

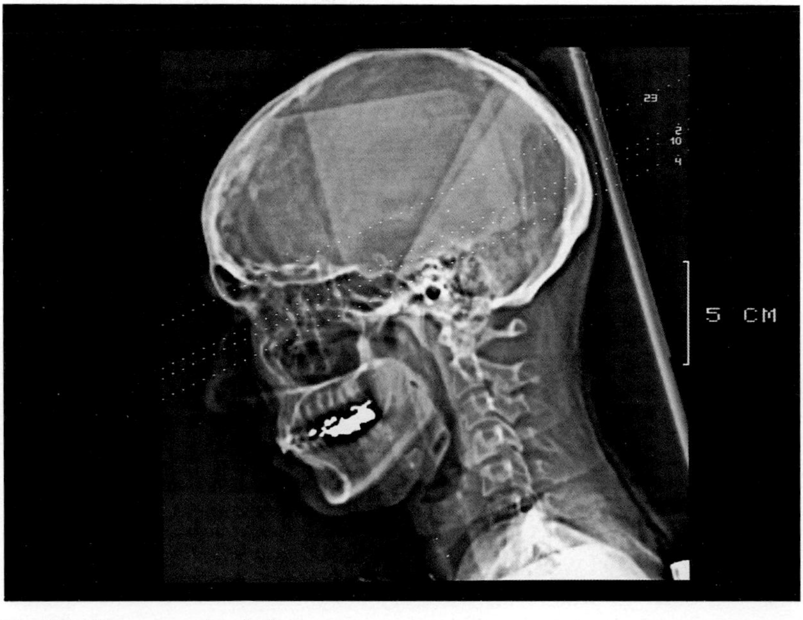

Fig. 8.8 Topogram of a skull

In addition, locating the correct slice can be considerably facilitated by means of a localizer radiograph (Topogram) (Fig. 8.6). With this imaging principle, the scanning system remains in a fixed position, e.g. x-ray tube above and detectors underneath the patient. The patient is then moved through the measurement aperture. The "line profiles" obtained in this way are combined by the computer to form an image and displayed on the monitor. The image produced in this way corresponds to a parallel projection in the forward movement direction of the patient and a central projection in the direction perpendicular to this. The dose applied for such an exposure is very low. The high density resolution and the possibility of displaying a good contrast area facilitate the slice definition. With the help of superimposed marks, the patient is automatically moved to the required exposure position (Figs. 8.7 and 8.8). This imaging mode can also be directly used for producing a diagnosis.

8.1.3 Scanning system

Corresponding to the block diagram (Fig. 8.1), the scanning system contains the x-ray tube with diaphragm system, the detectors with collimator and the electronics for processing the scanning data.

8.1.3.1 High-voltage generation and x-ray tube

In soft tissue diagnostics, as performed with computed tomography, the differences of the attenuation coefficients relative to the soft tissue structures to be differentiated are of the order of magnitude of percent or even per mil. The error limits for the measured values must have very narrow tolerances and so very high demands are placed on the necessary minimum number of x-ray quanta and their constancy per measured value because of quantum noise. In addition to this, it is necessary to maintain the spectrum of the emitted x-ray radiation as constant and reproducible as possible over the scan time, the exposure time or from pulse to pulse, because of the energy dependence of the attenuation coefficients. A fan-beam apparatus with rotating detectors may operate with pulsed radiation. In this case, imaging is carried out during continuous rotation of the imaging system at intervals of a few angle minutes per projection. The x-ray pulse duration for a five second system can only be a few milliseconds in order to avoid blurring effects.

A whole-body scanner such as the Somatom with its large measurement field and the large object thicknesses which this makes possible requires a slice energy of approximately 30 kWs and a pulse power of the x-ray tube of approximately 40 kW in order to achieve the necessary minimum number of x-ray quanta for an optical focal spot size of 1.6 mm $\times$ 1.6 mm. Only an oil-cooled rotary

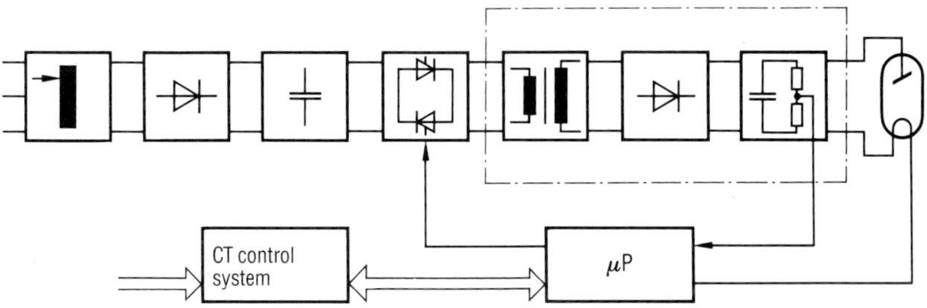

Fig. 8.9 Block diagram of a modern high-voltage generator

anode tube is suitable for this pulse mode. In order to be able to fully exploit the capabilities of a high-speed imaging system, the heat reservoir capacity of the anode must allow the scanning of more than 25 slices (in an uninterrupted sequence). The cooling time until the next series of slices should not significantly interfere with the examination procedure; this is achieved with high-performance oil-air cooling systems. X-ray tubes with a heat capacity up to 3.5 MHU are used.

In scanning systems with constant radiation, i.e. the x-ray tube continuously emits radiation during the entire exposure time, instead of a short x-ray pulse, a sampling frequency of the detectors as high as possible is used in order to again avoid blurring effects. A modern high-voltage generator (x-ray generator) with primary regulation by means of power level compensation and microprocessor control, such as the MIKROMATIC-CT, generates a stable x-ray voltage of 125 kV with a deviation of $<1\%$ (Fig. 8.9).

The whole-body scanner with continuous rotation uses high-voltage slip rings for transferring the x-ray voltage from the stationary part to the constantly rotating part of the gantry.

8.1.3.2 Measurement system

The detectors and the acquisition system for the scanning data form the measurement system, which converts the x-ray radiation attenuated by the object into a scanning signal suitable for computer input.

To date, three types of detector systems have been used in CT systems:

Scintillation crystals with photomultipliers
Scintillation crystals with photo-sensitive semiconductors
Rare gas ionization chambers

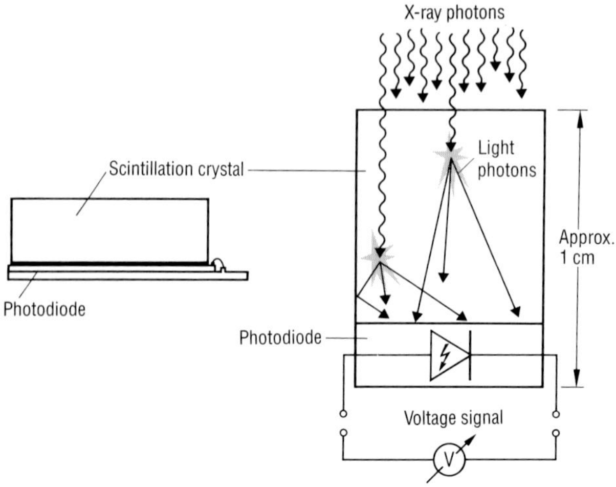

Fig. 8.10
Scintillation crystal with photo-sensitive semiconductor detector

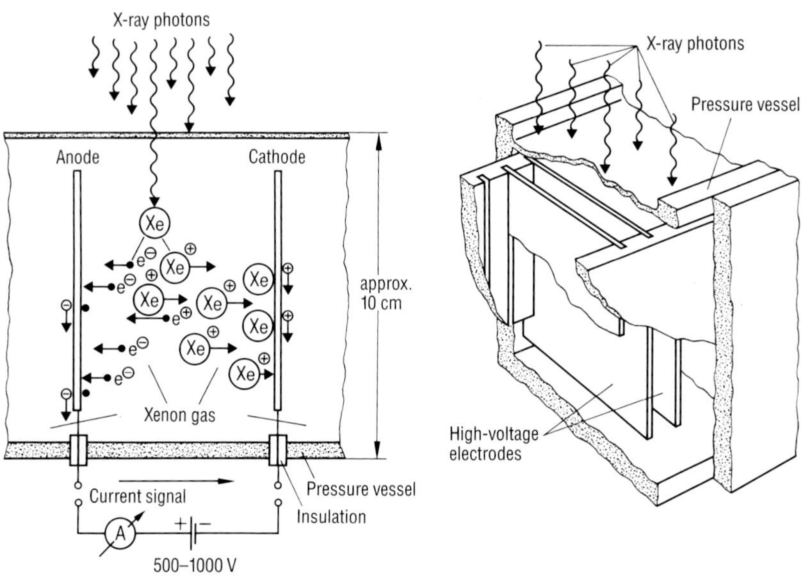

Fig. 8.11 Rare gas ionization chamber detector

Important criteria for the selection of the detector system are good absorption of the incident x-ray radiation and high efficiency in the conversion of the absorbed radiation energy to electrical signals. Naturally, the system must function in a monotonic and stable fashion and cover a large dynamic range. In this case, such crystals as cesium iodide (CsI) and bismuth germanate ($Bi_4Ge_3O_{12}$), with their very high quantum absorption, are more suitable than the rare gases (xenon). However, gas detectors can also be designed for very short decay times, an advantage for an extremely short scanning time. The largest electrical signal combined with a large signal-to-noise ratio for the followup electronics, is provided by the system photomultiplier crystal; however, it does not provide the high packing density of the crystal-semiconductor combination or ionization chambers. Figs. 8.10 and 8.11 show the structure and operation of the semiconductor and xenon detectors. In fan-beam equipment, it is important to position many detector elements as close as possible to each other. On the one hand, radiation losses must be kept as small as possible and, on the other hand, every effort is made to arrange as many elements per solid angle as possible in order to improve the spatial resolution of the system. As a result, the demands on the measurement electronics increase correspondingly, since every detector element must in general have its own measurement channel allocated to it (Fig. 8.12).

In the SOMATOM PLUS the effective number of measurement channels is effectively multiplied by means of rapid electromagnetic deflection of the focal spot of the x-ray tube during the rotation of the system, i.e. every projection is decomposed into several "viewing angles" and thus the resolution capacity of the equipment is increased.

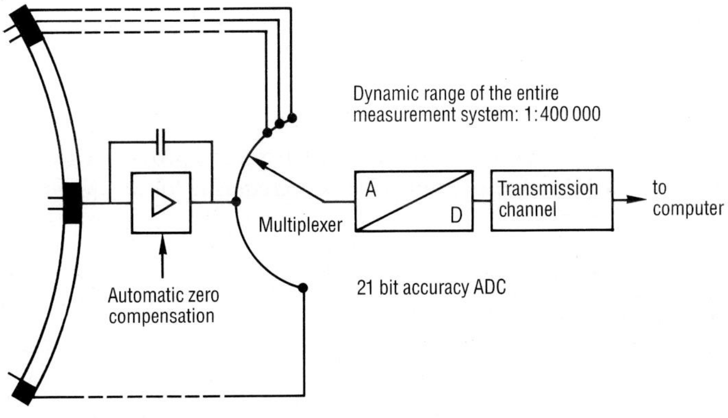

Fig. 8.12 Block diagram of a data acquisition system

The precision requirements of the measurement system follow from the permissible magnitude of the image errors. The point of departure is the radiation dose which can be applied for an image, restricted for a number of reasons, which generates minimum noise in the image. The noise of the measuring equipment must now be kept so small that it no longer makes any additional contribution to the noise in the image.

Thus, high demands are made on the analog amplifier, the integrator and the analog-digital converter, which provides correct computer conversion of the analog measurement values. In order to be able to convert the large signal value range of the analog scanning signal as generated in body images to a digital signal with the necessary high accuracy, converter systems with a resolution of more than 20 bits must be used.

A special technical challenge is noise-free data transmission with continuously rotating systems. Optical transmission systems or slip rings are used here which provide a transmission frequency of up to 200 Mbits/s.

8.1.3.3 Beam path

The beam path and collimating system of the fan-beam machine with rotating detectors can be seen in Fig. 8.13. The collimating system on the tube side is as close as possible to the patient and helps to limit the dose exposure to the necessary minimum for the patient. The lamellar collimator of a crystal detector arranged just above the detector elements and on the focal spot of the tube reduces the proportion of scattered radiation in the measured signal by a factor of approximately 10. This collimator must have an extremely high-precision construction; if the graduation is not equidistant or there is too great a mechanical tolerance, this would immediately affect the image and cause artifacts. Gas detectors are essentially self-collimating due to their electrodes being directed onto the focal spot.
In equipment with a stationary detector ring (ring detector equipment), the elements are directed to the isocenter of the scanning unit. A lamellar collimator therefore cannot be used. Other cylindrical or triangular constructions considerably reduce the radiation utilization.

Thus, only equipment with rotating radiation detector systems provides effective suppression of the scattered radiation, which is the prerequisite for the quantitative evaluation of a CT image.

8.1.3.4 Dose distribution

The dose distribution in the object imaged is quite different in CT systems from that in conventional equipment (Fig. 8.14) [8.1]. Whereas in a conventional x-ray unit, the dose continuously decreases in a ratio of approximately 1000:1

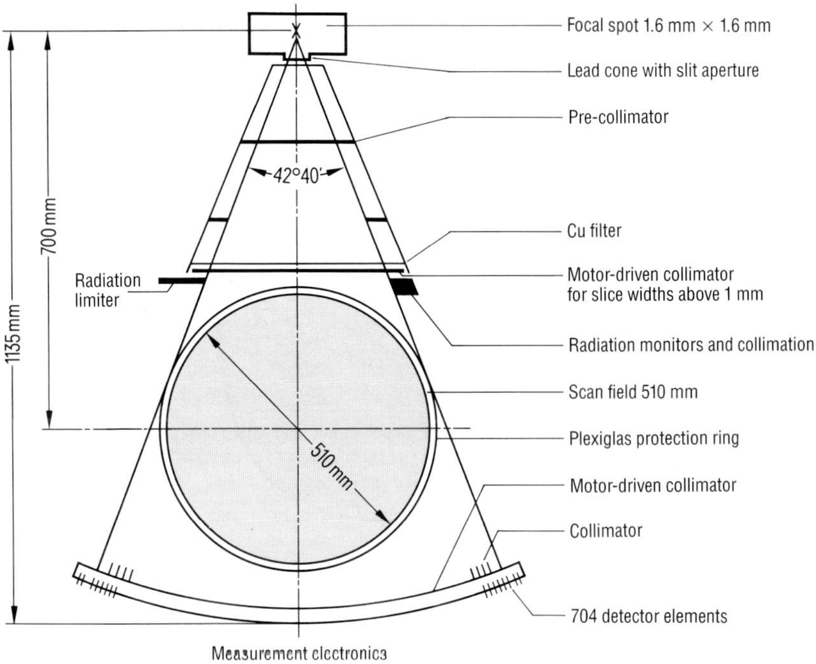

Fig. 8.13
Geometrical arrangement of x-ray tube, collimators and detector system (SOMATOM DRH)

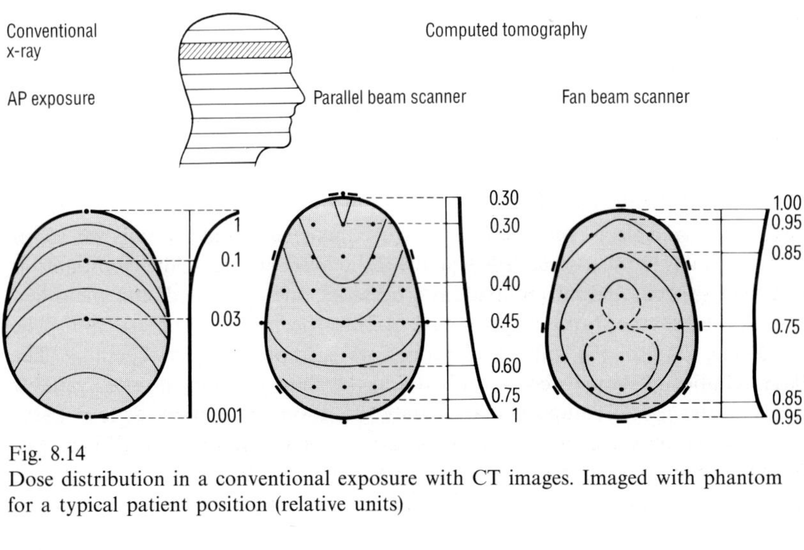

Fig. 8.14
Dose distribution in a conventional exposure with CT images. Imaged with phantom for a typical patient position (relative units)

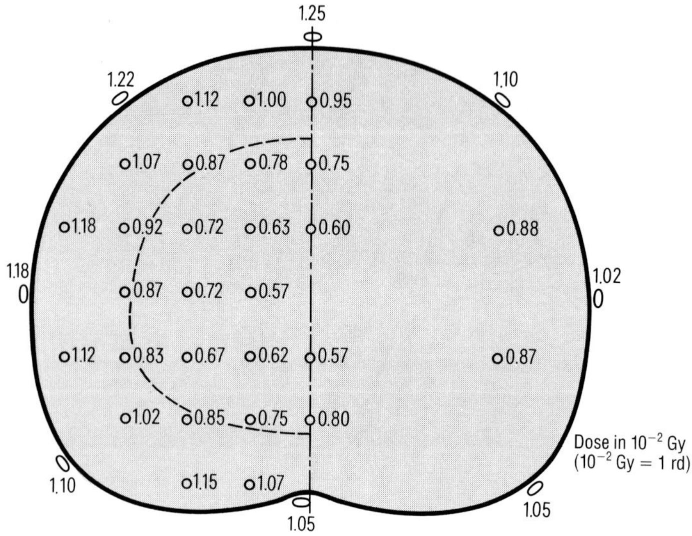

Fig. 8.15
Typical energy dose distribution of the center slice from seven adjacent slices in the liver-pancreas region measured with a fan-beam scanner with the Alderson phantom (disk 24)

going from the side of the body close to the tube to the side of the body far from the tube, in a fan-beam apparatus an almost uniform distribution is measured. The dose distribution in an image of the torso with a fan-beam apparatus can be seen in Fig. 8.15.

8.1.4 Computer system

The mathematical algorithm for CT equipment operating on the parallel or fan-beam principle is very well suited to concurrent image calculation. This is possible using the so-called pipeline principle. For this, the computer is regarded as separated into individual processors, one connected after the other. Each processor performs its own task during the image reconstruction. The processing time of the individual processors is approximately the same. The large number of steps to be performed and the short amount of time available preclude the use of computers commonly found on the market. Special hard-wired computers and chip processors are better suited to the problem. For example, with the SOMATOM it has been possible to make the processing time of a computational step of the same order of magnitude as the projection sequencing time, i.e. immediately on completion of the measurement process, the image is available in a calculated matrix of 512×512 elements (pixels) (Fig. 8.16) and can be displayed in a matrix of up to 1024×1024 elements.

Higher ordered control functions of the data processing system, such as equipment control, image display and image storage can be performed by an ordinary minicomputer (host computer). The system is equipped with floppy disk drives, magnetic tape and disk stores and also interactive terminals for inputting patient data, comments and control commands.

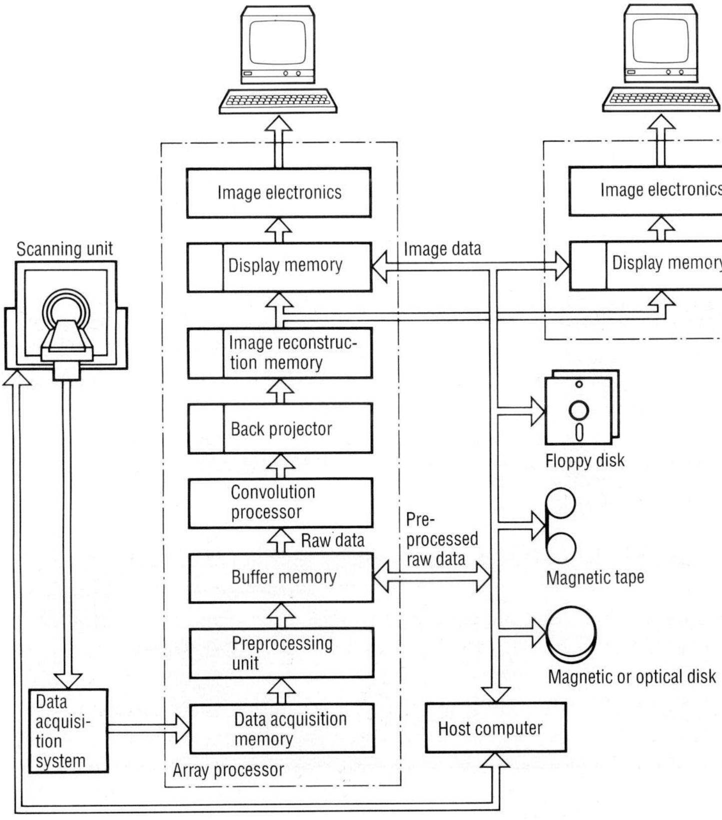

Fig. 8.16 Structure of the computer system

8.1.5 Operating concept

Routine functions such as the selection of scan parameters, exposure release, image recall and table feed are usually performed at an operating console (Fig. 8.17). A user-friendly system characterized by software-controlled dialog, menu-driven commands and only a few input elements to operate minimizes errors and provides a fast scanning sequence, thus ensuring a high patient throughput.

If the operating console is attached to its own image store, then after an image has been transferred to this store the computer is free for another scan and the observer can select the image representation which seems correct to him for diagnosis without any delay.

Every pixel of the calculated image is represented in the image memory by digital values. In order to display this information on the viewing monitor,

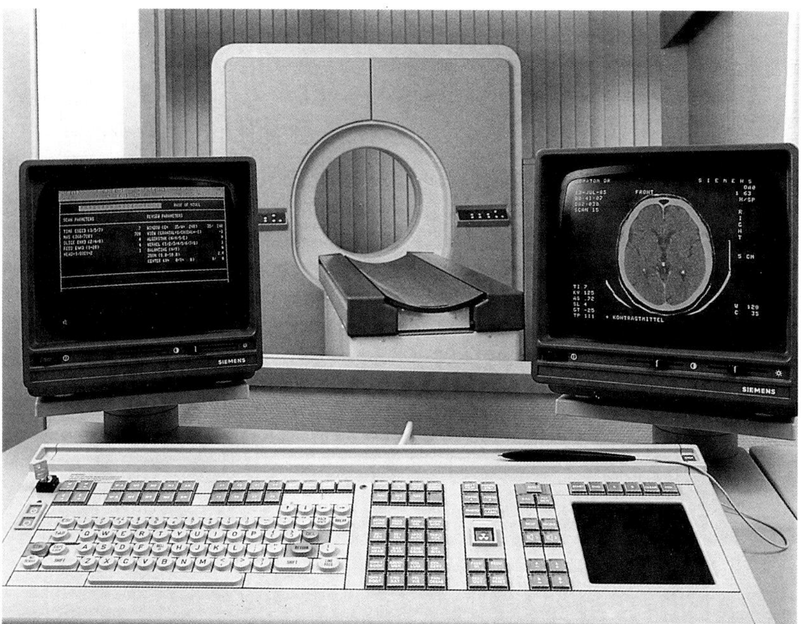

Fig. 8.17
One of the many functions of the CT system control console with the SOMATOM is to vary window position and width of the images displayed

it must be read out from the memory synchronously with the video sync signal. Every bit combination then has a signal amplitude allocated to it through a digital-analog converter, which in turn controls the brightness of the television image tube. Modern systems operate with high frame rates and more than 1200 lines per frame.

Of course, a computer-controlled operating concept is flexible enough that new scanning techniques and evaluation functions, as well as extensions and expansions to the CT system, can be implemented [8.2].

8.2 Image display, documentation and evaluation

8.2.1 Image display

For the morphological evaluation of a CT image, it is necessary to focus on the essential information for a given examination. The information inherent in the CT image lies in the absorption range between −1000 and approximately +3000 HU (Hounsfield Units, i.e. CT values). The absorption values of the CT image are therefore converted to gray levels and displayed on a viewing monitor. In an ideal case, the eye can distinguish approximately 100 brightness graduations in a television image, but under normal working conditions not much more than 30.

The user could thus never distinguish between the approximately 4000 values comprising the entire range of CT values. Furthermore, the observer is often only interested in a small section of the absorption range, e.g. the differentiation of gray and white brain matter, which only differ by approximately 10 CT values.

In order to display small absorption differences, so-called *image windowing* is therefore used. Here, only a part of the CT scale is selected and spread over all brightness values between black and white. Even small absorption differences inside the selected window are displayed as distinguishable gray tone differences, while all CT values below the window are displayed black and CT values above the window are displayed white.

Since the position and the width of the window can be varied at will, several different medical questions can be answered from the same CT image, depending on the window selected. Typical applications here are images in the heart-lung region and the optional display of soft tissue and bone structures.

If a linear gray scale is used for the display, this leads to a compression of the dark gray tones due to the distortion of the television tube characteristic. This favors differentiation between details, because, due to the physiology of the eye, gray tones can be more easily recognized in the dark parts of the image than gray tones in the bright parts of the image with the same differences in illumination density.

In order to improve the recognizability of the gray tone image, an additional distortion of the image is often also used in the form of look-up tables. Here, a fundamental distinction can be made between two applications:

▻ A distortion with the help of a look-up table *before* windowing can be used in order to spread out or compress specific CT-value ranges specific to an organ, e.g. in order to optically magnify the interval between the gray values of white and gray brain matter.

▻ A distortion with the help of a look-up table *after* windowing can be used in order to compensate for the effects of the blackening curve specific to the film when the CT image is recorded onto x-ray film.

In general, it can be said that apart from other factors such as dose, detector arrangement and reconstruction algorithm, considerable importance should be attached to the imaging system which, together with photographic documentation, represents the last component in the CT system imaging chain. Here, only a few key words will be mentioned, such as video bandwidth, modulation transfer function and flicker-free displays. Today, the dimensioning of the CT imaging system is normally based on display in a 512×512 matrix, where it is unimportant for the image system whether this display matrix has been directly calculated or has been produced by interpolation.

8.2.2 Image documentation and archiving

After the CT image has been displayed on the viewing monitor and a diagnosis has possibly been made, the question arises as to the documentation of the examination result and the archiving of the image material. These requirements take up a considerable proportion of the time spent in routine operations.

Depending on the nature of the CT image, image documentation and archiving can be divided into two methods:

▻ Photography: window position and width must be defined before exposure, all information outside the selected window is lost.
▻ Digital image storage: the entire information content of an image is kept; a specific image setting can be reproduced at any time or the image can be evaluated numerically based on latest findings.

For the foreseeable future, these two methods should be regarded as complementary and not competing.

8.2.2.1 Photography

Legally, the CT image should be regarded as an "image from an x-ray examination". This means that the law requires images to be safely stored for many years. Although the image in the form of a photographic document can clearly show the relevant information for the findings, the window selected may be completely unsuitable for other medical questions.

However, photographic documentation is certainly the most important type of long-term archiving at the present time. Multiformat cameras (see section 7.2.9) are available for this purpose. They allow to a large extent any subdivisions of the transparent film from large format to slides. Film magazines, which eliminate the need for frequent changing of the film cassettes, greatly simplify the operation of this equipment. A further step in the automation of photographic documentation is the direct connection between multiformat camera and developing machine with wet development in a 90 second process.

The software provides additional support functions for image documentation: image and patient data, evaluation results, as well as marker arrows and comments, can be superimposed. The layers examined can be marked in a Topogram for orientation. A characteristic which can be freely defined for the camera monitor enables the optimization of image results.

The digital camera, i.e. the so-called laser camer, only recently introduced to the market, represents a further advance in camera technology. With this type of camera, the image is not photographed from a monitor. Instead, the gray values of the pixels are transferred in digital form to the camera and directly control the exposure time for every individual pixel. The result is enhanced imaging accuracy and increased image dynamics. Today this type of camera is mainly used in upper class CT-systems. Special interfaces had to be developed for the CT scanning system to allow the digital transmission of images to the camera in a matter of seconds in order to provide the same operating speed as with conventional multiformat cameras.

8.2.2.2 Digital image storage

Digital image storage usually takes place onto magnetic tape or floppy disk (see section 7.2). However, this type of image storage has lost importance as a routine method of documentation with the increasing size of the matrix of the images. Even when coding procedures are used for reducing the redundance or when reduced matrix sizes are stored, the capacity of magnetic tape and in particular of floppy disks is inadequate or the costs per stored image are high. Further limiting factors, such as poor access to the images and limited lifetime of the data storage media – usually only a few years without resorting to exceptional measures – must also be considered.

However, this situation is considerably improved when another storage medium is used, the digital optical disk (see also section 7.2.2). With this data storage medium, the image information is burned in in digital form by means of a laser beam; it can then no longer be erased.

Optical disks provide a very high storage capacity (several thousand images per disk). This means low costs per image and in addition a long lifetime for the data storage medium. No special maintenance procedures are necessary for a period of at least 10 years.

Optical disks accommodated in so-called juke boxes, with direct access to a large number of disk cassettes, will in the future form the long-term archives of PACS systems.

PACS (Picture Archiving and Communication Systems) is the corner stone for a future x-ray department without film, in which all imaging systems are connected via fast data lines to a digital image archive from which the doctor can rapidly access every image in its original digital form.

8.2.3 Image evaluation

In recent years, certain evaluation procedures for CT images have emerged as useful aids for the doctor. However, none of the procedures can take away the doctor's responsibility in making his diagnosis. Only the tools are provided, to be used for answering certain diagnostic questions.

An image processing system is needed to perform the image evaluation. Usually one of the following three systems is used:

▻ The standard operating console of the CT system in departments with low numbers of patients, where imaging and evaluation can be carried out alternately;

▻ An additional evaluation console, connected to the computer system in the same way as the operating console and therefore allowing access to all peripheral image stores and to the image processor of the system;

▻ An independent evaluation console with its own computer, to which the images are either transferred by magnetic tape or floppy disk or to which they are directly transferred from the CT system by a data link.

The evaluation procedures themselves and the capabilities of the evaluation system can be roughly divided into two categories:

▻ *Subjective evaluation* procedures in which the doctor displays or prepares the images in a suitable form for making his diagnosis;

▻ *Objective evaluation* procedures in which the values of the image matrix are used directly for measurements or calculations and the results give information on the relevant diagnosis.

8.2.3.1 Subjective image evaluation procedures

These procedures include:

- Image display with suitable look-up tables
- Multi-window image display
- Multiple image displays
- Image subtraction
- Image filtering
- Image magnification
- Profile section
- Reconstruction of reformatted images
- 3-dimensional image display

Reference was made to image display with suitable look-up tables in section 8.2.1. A special case of a non-linear gray scale is the highlighting of density regions selected by the user. This makes it easier for him to find certain diagnostically relevant areas.

Image display with several windows makes it possible either to display a small density region with maximum contrast inside a body displayed with a large window or, in images with large differences in density, to display different regions with optimum contrast at the same time.

Multiple image displays make it possible to display several consecutive layers of an organ in order to produce a 3-dimensional impression.

A method often used for operational checks and contrast examinations is the comparison of two CT images. The difference can be seen after subtraction of the images. This method is limited by the spatial reproducibility of two images separated in time.

2-dimensional filtering of images is a well-known method for smoothing images or enhancing contours. In the first instance, image filtering is carried out by using a corresponding convolution kernel during image reconstruction. Subsequent image processing has usually only an additional cosmetic effect.

In order to improve the recognizability of an image detail, it can be enlarged with the help of image magnification. However, magnification does not produce any extra gain in information.

Small density differences can be more easily identified without selecting too narrow a window, which would increase the image noise, by using the profile section; the CT values are then plotted as a curve over the section of interest.

By suitable choice of the gray scale in displaying the section, even small density differences can be unambiguously differentiated.

One of the main advantages of a series of digitally processed transverse slice images, which together form a cube of CT values, is the possibility of reconstructing images with any orientation, i.e. reformatted images. Of special impor-

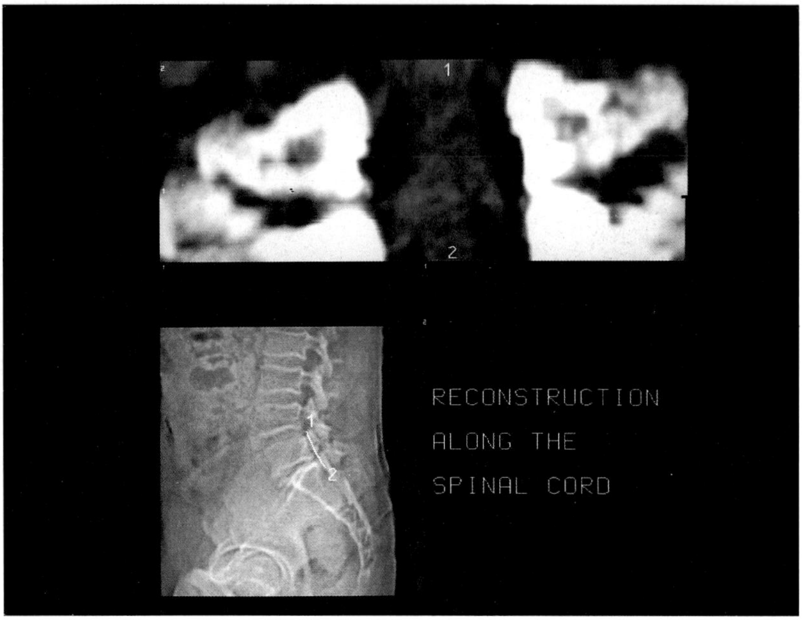

Fig. 8.18
Reconstruction of a curvilinear reformatted image

tance here are sections which are perpendicular to the original transverse sections and which thus give a quasi "technical" representation of the object of interest. In images of the skull and the spine, computer simulation of highly inclined positions of the scanning unit are also of great importance. Curved sections, e.g., along the spine, can also help in spinal examinations (Fig. 8.18). Even completely freely defined slice planes, e.g. through three marked points in different slices, are useful in the abdomen for certain diagnostic questions, although it is then often difficult to obtain a good spatial impression [8.3, 8.4].

The same cube of CT values can be used for calculating 3-dimensional images (Fig. 8.19). A special problem in the calculation of such images is the determination of the contours, which can only be automated at clearly defined boundaries, e.g. at the skin surface or at the edges of bones. The differentiation of soft tissue can still only be done manually and is therefore extremely time consuming.

However, the calculation of 3-dimensional images, e.g. in plastic surgery and in general in planning operations, is gaining in importance.

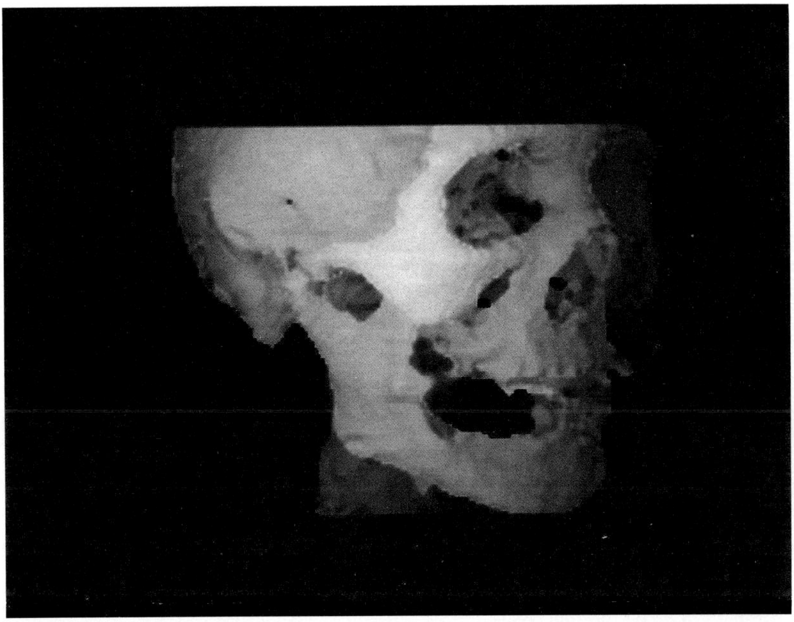

Fig. 8.19
Three-dimensional reconstruction of the cranial bone surface from a sequence of transverse CT images

8.2.3.2 Objective image evaluation procedures

These include:

- Distance and angle measurements
- Evaluation of area, volume and average density in regions of interest
- Symmetry comparison
- Histogram

The most important and the most frequently used evaluation function is the measurement of distances and angles in the image. Here, the fact that the CT design principle ensures perfect reproduction with no distortion is exploited.

Since the computational accuracy is limited by the pixel size and the accuracy with which the user sets a measurement point, it is recommended when measuring small objects to first magnify the corresponding image section.

There are many different ways of evaluating regions of interest (ROIs). The most important determinations are for the area, the volume or the average

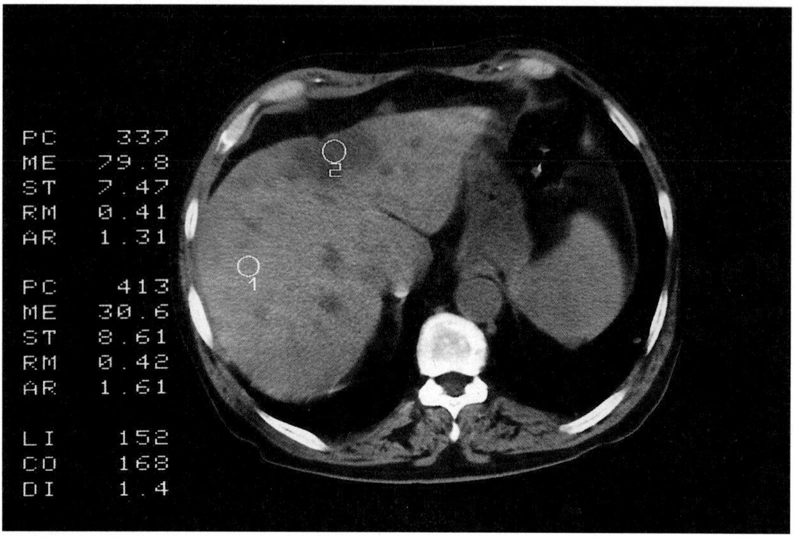

Fig. 8.20
Comparison of the average absorption values over two regions of interest

Region 1: 79.8 HU, normal tissue
Region 2: 30.6 HU, tumoral tissue

density of a region. Here, the ROI can itself be in the form of a point, a circle or any arbitrary shape (Fig. 8.20).

It is often necessary to compare two regions in the image with each other. A special case is that of symmetry comparison in the skull region, where the two regions to be compared are reflected about a selectable line of symmetry. In calculating the average density over an ROI, the standard deviation of the result is also usually calculated; this gives information on the variance of the density value. If one is interesterd in the exact distribution of the density values over the ROI, a histogram of the density values gives information on the internal composition of the ROI.

8.2.4 Applications

Special applications were already developed very early in CT. Some of these, e.g. dynamic computed tomography, have in the meantime become standard procedures. Other procedures are still under development or work in progress. Here, we will give a brief description of the most important special applications which are known today.

Evaluation of dynamic image series after contrast medium injection

CT scanners with short scanning times, high imaging frequencies and short delay times between image acquisitions make it possible to display fast physiological processes within a slice through the body. This permits the exact differentiation of lesions from the enhancement phase of a contrast bolus, e.g. in order to dispay vessel changes or the arterial and capillary phase in parenchymatous organs. Such a series of images is evaluated quantitatively by numerical determination of the density changes in the ROIs over time and displaying them in the form of curves (Fig. 8.21). Special programs are available to help in interpreting the density curves, e.g. for curve smoothing or calculating a gamma fit. Other possibilities of assessing the contrast dynamics are so-called parameter images or, often much more impressive, the display of the contrast medium enhancement by a sequence of images shown at real-time speeds on the image monitor [8.5, 8.6].

Evaluation of dynamic image series after xenon inhalation

In measurement of the brain blood flow by Dynamic CT, the patient inhales a mixture of stable xenon gas and oxygen or air over a period of several minutes. At the same time, CT images of selected layers of the brain are acquired. The time between the precontrast images and the corresponding contrast images is exactly measured together with the arterial xenon concentration. With the help of special programs, the regional cerebral blood flow and the xenon lambda coefficient (a tissue parameter which indicates the relative solubility of xenon) can be calculated from the measured data and the images. These values are displayed as so-called flow and lambda images (Fig. 8.22). Flow values are usually given in milliliters per 100 g brain tissue. Lambda values indicate the ratio of brain tissue to blood and are therefore dimensionless [8.7].

Evaluation of ECG-triggered cardiac images

ECG-triggered cardiac images can be obtained from a sequence of CT images in which the ECG information is plotted together with the scan data. In order to make the data acquisition more effective, the individual images are initiated at different times relative to the cardiac phase.

A program sorts the scan data for the desired cardiac phase and calculates the associated image. From a sequence of such images, the movement of the heart can be displayed in real time on the monitor [8.8].

CT image for biopsy and stereotaxy

The CT image can be used in a routine manner as the basis for biopsies and stereotactic interventions, because it provides a perfect 3-dimensional assign-

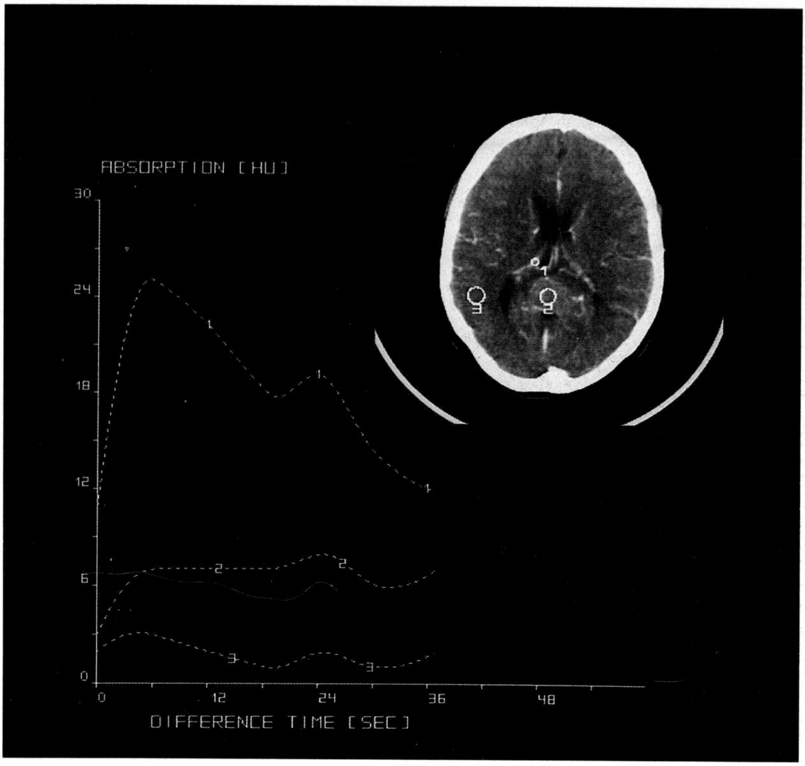

Fig. 8.21
Evaluation of the contrast medium distribution over time for different regions of the cranial slice displayed

Region 1: Vessel during contrast medium enhancement
Region 2: Tumor
Region 3: Normal tissue

ment of every pixel. It is particularly helpful when other methods, such as ultrasound or fluoroscopy, cannot display with sufficient precision the target volume or the structures endangered by the needle, lying between the incision point and the target volume. In these examinations, the patient is usually fixed in a stereotactic frame which defines a system of coordinates.

Programs can then be used to calculate the coordinates for the target apparatus after marking the incision and target points in the CT image [8.4].

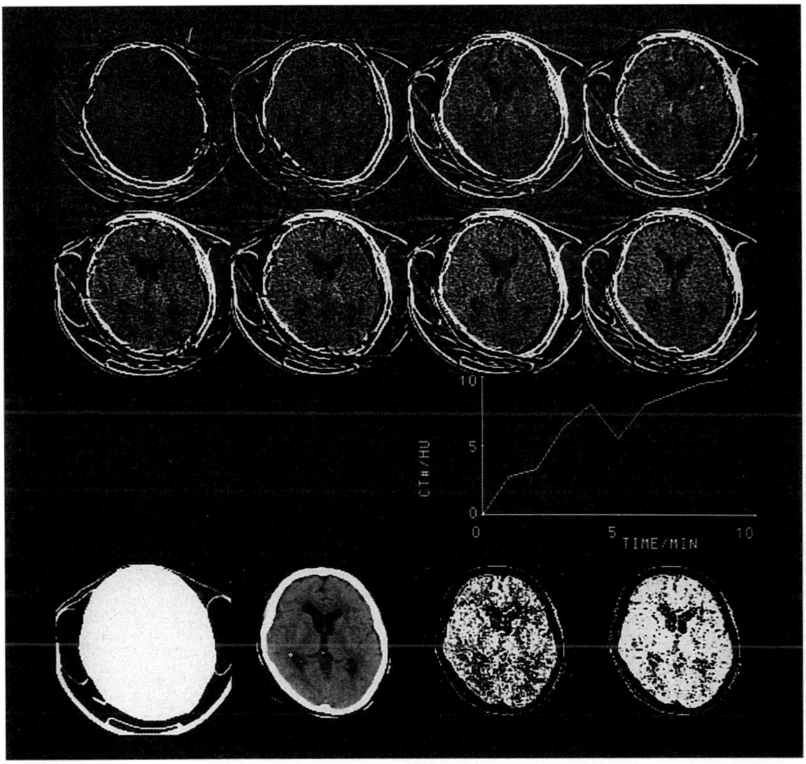

Fig. 8.22
Xenon contrast study. The top eight sections are subtraction images taken from a dynamic series. The bottom four figures show, from left to right: mask (scaled for higher accuracy and thus located outside the window), unsubtracted CT image, flow image and Lambda image. In between, diagram of contrast medium enhancement for a point marked in the CT image.

Generation of images from the dual energy method

CT images represent the linear attenuation coefficients for the volume elements of the imaged layer, but in no way are they images of the density as is usually asserted incorrectly. The linear attenuation coefficient is a product of the capacity for x-ray attenuation and the local density. If, for example, there is a lung node showing increased CT values in the image, then it is not certain whether

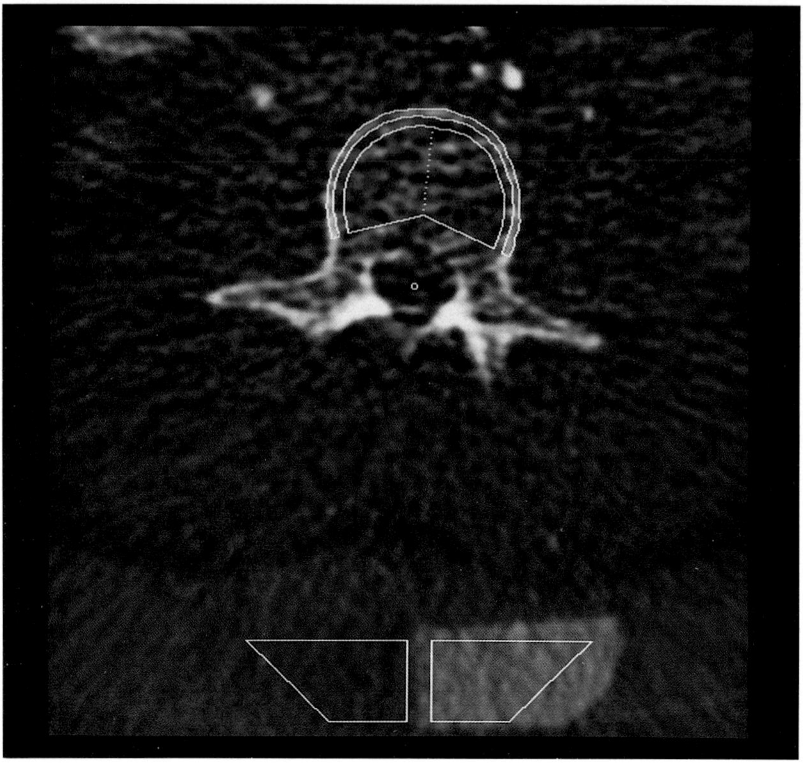

Fig. 8.23
Determination of bone mineral content. Here, the evaluation of a calcium density image from a dual energy measurement. Automatic contour finding for regions of interest (ROIs)

Top: cortical ROI, spongy ROI with symmetry axis, center of gravity of ROI through spinal cord

Below: reference materials for calcium equivalent (right) and water equivalent (not visible in the calcium density image)

the reason for this is diffuse calcification, i.e. elements with a higher atomic number, or a fibrosis, i.e. an increase in the density [8.9].

The image of a layer with two different spectra makes it possible to calculate images of the density distribution of specific materials with suitable programs instead of the usual CT images, e.g. so-called soft tissue images and bone images. Based on these, electron density images and so-called mono-energetic CT images can be reconstructed. The advantage of the latter is that artifacts caused by spectral hardening of the x-ray radiation are eliminated (e.g. the Hounsfield bars in the posterior cranial fossa).

Determination of the mineral calcium content in the vertebrae

In order to determine the mineral calcium content in vertebrae, the center of vertebrae L1 to L3 is imaged for each CT scan, with reference materials measured at the same time, e.g. embedded in the patient couch. With suitable software, the calcium content of the vertebra can be calculated in calcium equivalence units by means of ROI evaluation of the measured bone structures and the reference materials, assuming that computer assisted contour determination is available (Fig. 8.23) [8.7, 8.10].

The CT image in radiation therapy planning

The CT image directly provides important information for optimal radiation therapy planning. On the one hand, this involves information on the size and volume of a lesion and its topographical and anatomical relationship to neighboring structures and, on the other hand, information on the density of the structures which can be taken into account in the planning process.

The planning process results in the radiation plan and its local dose distribution, which can be directly superimposed on the CT image in the form of isodose curves.

9 Nuclear medical diagnostics

The function of nuclear medical diagnostics is to trace radioactive indicators in vivo and in vitro with the aim of obtaining information on transport, distribution, metabolic and clearance processes in the human body. Since a relatively small number of radioactive indicator atoms in the body is already sufficient to be able to identify them by external measurement, metabolic processes remain chemically unchanged. Such processes can therefore be observed in their natural state. However, it is necessary to measure the emitted radiation as proof of the indicator's presence with sufficient accuracy in order to have information on the concentration, dwell time and/or distribution in the measurement field.

The desire to image the distribution of a radioactive indicator in a region of interest is probably as old as nuclear medicine itself. The clinical diagnostician has always been visually biased; his desire to be able to gain a visual image of distribution states and transport mechanisms is urgent and understandable.

Unfortunately, nuclear medicine suffered for many years because of the question of functional measurement versus image; the high-speed functional measurement workstations did not provide any image and yet the imaging equipment was still too slow to yield additional functional information.

On the one hand, the lack of any image with the resulting lack of spatial selectivity made examinations difficult and this in turn meant that excellent opportunities for applying radioactive indicators in cardiology [9.1 to 9.4] were not part of established routines for many years. On the other hand, the inadequacy of earlier imaging equipment in terms of its temporal resolution led to an overemphasis of quasi-static scintigraphy, the end product of which, although it did provide a distribution pattern of the indicator, was only a single snapshot of a functional process.

The representation of the distribution of activity concentrations as an image over time

$$C_A = f(x, y, t)$$

opens up in the truest sense of the word new dimensions in nuclear medical diagnostics.

The synthesis of image and functional process which can be performed by modern instrumentation in the nuclear medicine department now puts the physician in the position of being able to fully exploit the diagnostic potential of his science.

9.1 Measurement technology

9.1.1 Structure and function of a radiation measurement channel

For the detection of gamma radiation the scintillation counter is used almost exclusively in most different designs (Fig. 9.1). The primary detector element is an optically highly transparent single crystal, usually consisting of sodium iodide, activated with traces of thallium. This emits light photons, the number emitted being proportional to the excitation energy on the average, excited by the absorption of energy-rich radiation. The resulting quanta make it possible to measure the event and its energy by means of optoelectronic and electronic devices.

The light quanta emitted by the crystal (scintillator) knock electrons out of the photocathode of a photomultiplier tube by means of the external photoeffect. The stream of electrons is amplified to a measurable signal by means of secondary electron emission at the dynodes of this high-vacuum tube [9.5]. The proportionality of the signal measured to the energy is ensured by the highly linear current amplification. Only due to statistical fluctuations in the generation of the light photons in the crystal, the limited efficiency of the light transfer to the photomultiplier and the fluctuating number of electrons released from

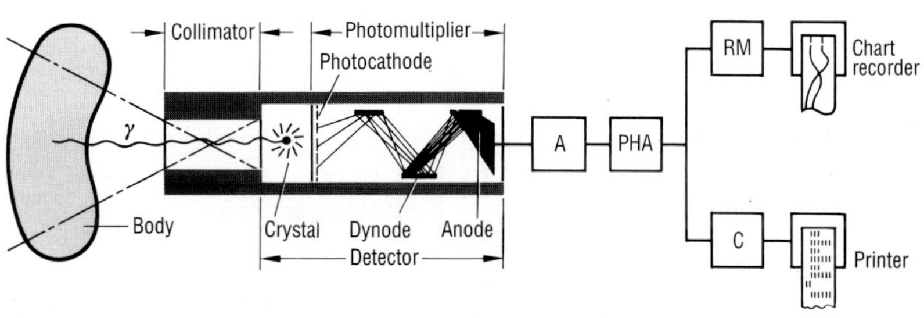

A amplifier
PHA pulse height analyzer
RM rate meter
C pulse counter

Fig. 9.1
Diagram of the radiation measurement channel of a scintillation counter

the photocathode per event, does the photoline (Eγ) in the energy spectrum experience a certain broadening (Fig. 9.2).

Fig. 9.3 shows a simple representation of all effects which contribute to the energy spectrum observed:

1. A gamma quantum reaches the detector unhindered and is completely absorbed in the crystal by a photo effect.
2. A gamma quantum is still fully absorbed in the crystal following Compton scattering. Since both these quanta give up all of their energy in the crystal, the amplitude of the measurement signal is on the average proportional to the energy. Such events account for the *photo peak* in the energy spectrum (see Fig. 9.2).
3. After Compton scattering and energy loss, a gamma quantum escapes from the crystal. The amplitude of the signal measured is proportional to the energy loss and not to the primary energy.
4. A gamma quantum is generated outside the measurement field (A–B) and is scattered inside the field, in the body. It only has a residual energy and is fully absorbed in the crystal. The signal measured is proportional to the residual energy; an incorrect point of origination (4′) is simulated.

The number of light quanta produced in the crystal is in cases three and four not proportional to the primary energy, which leads to smaller signal amplitudes. Such events account for the Compton continuum in the energy spectrum. The mixing of these effects in the radiation measurement leads to the typical energy spectrum shown in Fig. 9.2.

Since the events recorded in the Compton continuum partly originate outside the measurement field, they falsify the position-based measurement result and

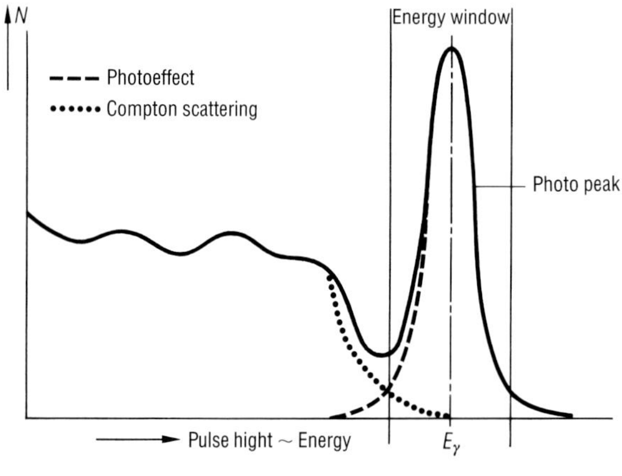

Fig. 9.2
Energy spectrum with energy window of the pulse height analyzer

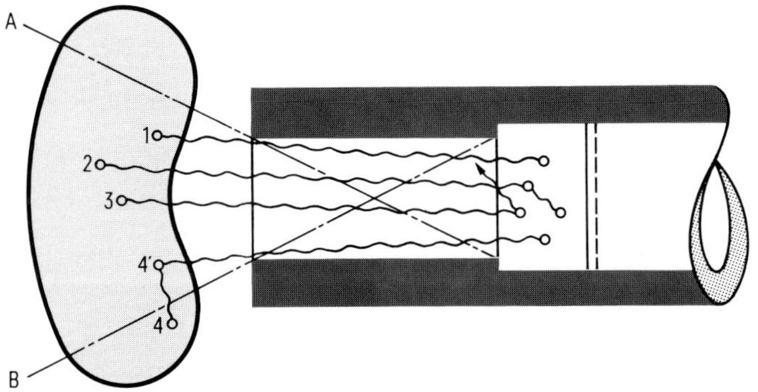

A, B limits of the measurement field

Fig. 9.3
General diagram of possible gamma radiation interactions for radiation measurement with the scintillation counter (1 to 4, see text)

must therefore be eliminated. This function is performed in the radiation measurement channel by the *pulse height analyzer* (see Fig. 9.1). It only allows pulses to pass for which the amplitude lies between two trigger thresholds connected in anticoincidence. This circuit generates an energy window which can be adapted in position and width according to the measurement required (see Fig. 9.2). In this way, only those events contribute to the measurement result for which the pulse amplitude is on the average proportional to the primary energy of the radionuclide which is used.

9.1.2 Effect of information density on the measured results

The way in which the measured result is obtained and its documentation depends on the type of measurement. For measurements with the collimated scintillation counter the evolution of the activity concentration over time is measured with constant position over the measurement field. It then follows that

$$C_A = f(t), \quad \text{because the coordinates } x \text{ and } y \text{ are fixed.}$$

Here, the relative activity concentration C_A is determined by the number of pulses N recorded during a measurement period t. If the activity concentration were to remain the same, it would be expected that a constant measurement period t_1 would always lead to the same measured result N_1. However, because of the spontaneous character of radioactive decay, this is not the case.

The average absolute error of such a single measurement is

$$\sigma_a = \pm\sqrt{N}, \tag{9.1}$$

which has the dimension of N. From this we obtain the average relative deviation,

$$\sigma_r = \pm\frac{\sqrt{N}}{N} = \pm\frac{1}{\sqrt{N}} \cdot 100\%. \tag{9.2}$$

It can be seen from this that, as the number N increases, the error becomes smaller and smaller [9.6, 9.7].

This is important not just for the measurement of the statistically distributed gamma photons, emitted but also applies to all information obtained on the basis of a single measurement of a number N of spontaneously generated information carriers.

The information density, that is the number N of the information carriers which can be processed in the available measurement time t, determines the exactness of the measurement.

9.2 The scanner, the first imaging unit in nuclear medicine

The advent of localization diagnostics in nuclear medicine came about with the description of the first automatic scanner (almost simultaneously by Cassen et al. [9.8] and Mayneord et al. [9.9] in 1951). The measurement principles used then are still applied today. The terms *scintigram* and *scintigraphy* coined at that time are also still common today for any type of image representation of the spatial distribution of a radionuclide.

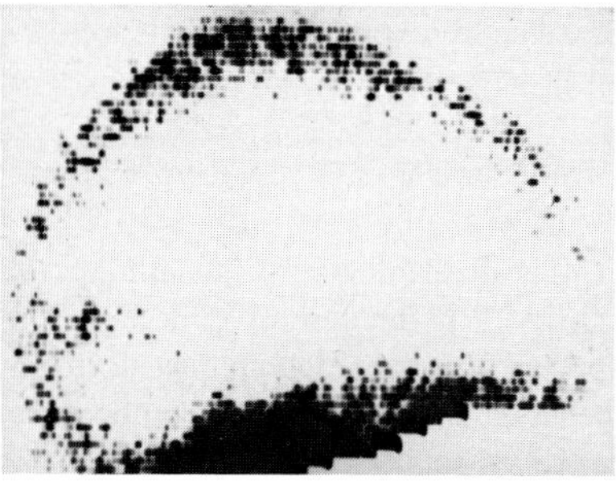

Fig. 9.4
Photoscintigraphic image of a skull

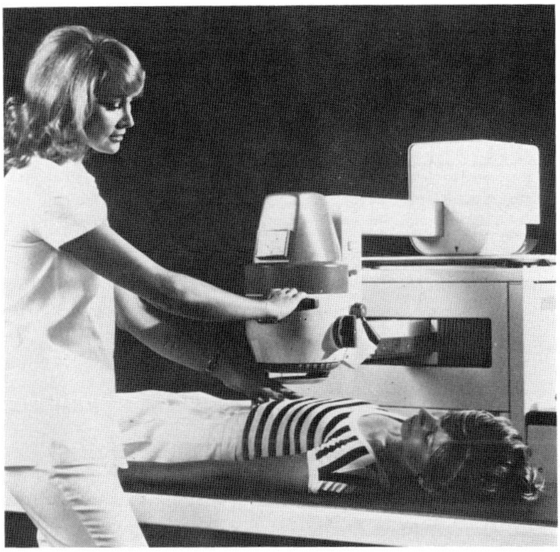

Fig. 9.5
Scintigraphy with the SCINTIMAT 2

In terms of its construction, the scanner is actually nothing more than a radiation measurement channel as described in section 9.1.1, with a moving detector and a collimator connected in front of it and a recording system operating synchronously with it. The detector is usually moved over the measurement field along a meandering path, which it scans line by line. The collimator in the scanner is designed so that it only covers a narrowly defined measurement field $\Delta x \, \Delta y$ within which the radiation reaching the detector is measured over a time t. The measured result $C_A = f(\Delta x, \Delta y, t)$ is assigned to the image element by a recording system as a blackening value in general proportional to $C_A(t)$.

Fig. 9.4 shows a photoscintigram and Fig. 9.5 the design of a scanner.

Today, scanners have been replaced by gamma cameras, because of the more meaningful diagnostic information which these provide. Scanners are therefore no longer manufactured, although a large number can still be found in use.

9.3 Gamma cameras

A gamma camera consists essentially of a large area collimator, which generates a radiation image, and a detector which converts this into the best possible image for documentation. In the past, different approaches were taken to develop such detectors [9.10 to 9.13], but only the camera developed by H.O. Anger [9.14] has made its mark on a large scale and, constantly undergoing improvements, has become the universal tool of the nuclear medical practitioner. Fig. 9.6 shows the measurement principle of an Anger gamma camera.

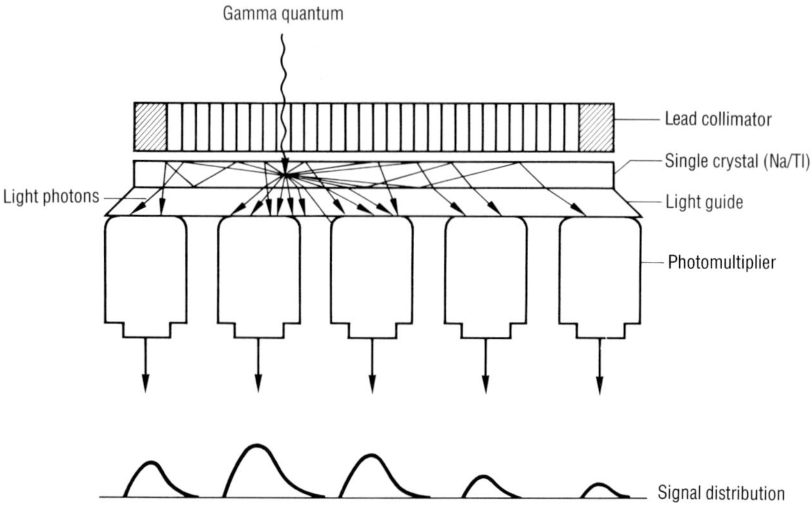

Fig. 9.6 Measurement princple of the Anger gamma camera

9.3.1 Design and operation of the Anger gamma camera

Collimator

Essentially, the collimator (Fig. 9.7) performs the task of dividing the entire measurement field $M(x, y, z)$ into a finite number of small individual fields $m(\Delta x, \Delta y, \Delta z)$ and imaging these onto the detector. Here, the size of these individual measurement fields in the object is a measure of the spatial resolution and the fraction of the total number of photons contributing to the image of this area element is a measure of the collimator sensitivity. Since these two criteria are of key importance for the quality of a scintigram, we will examine them in greater detail here.

Geometrical resolution

Following Anger [9.15], the radius R_c of the latent radiation image produced by imaging a point source at a distance Z from the collimator surface in the main absorption plane of the crystal is commonly taken as a measure of the geometrical resolution. From Fig. 9.7, we have

$$R_c = \frac{2r}{L}(L + Z + A). \qquad (9.3)$$

Since the septa between the individual collimator channels serve to insulate the channels from each other, they must have a finite thickness in order to prevent radiation penetration as far as possible. For this reason, the imaging of a point source is discontinuous and R_c should be regarded as a purely geometrical measure. The radius R' of the individual measurement field m of a collimator channel obeys the relationship

$$R' = \frac{r(L+2Z)}{L} \tag{9.4}$$

and is therefore proportional to the inter-measurement distance for the given collimator characteristics. It is therefore to be expected that the measured variables describing the spatial resolution performance of a gamma camera also satisfy this relationship, provided that the collimator is the determining element.

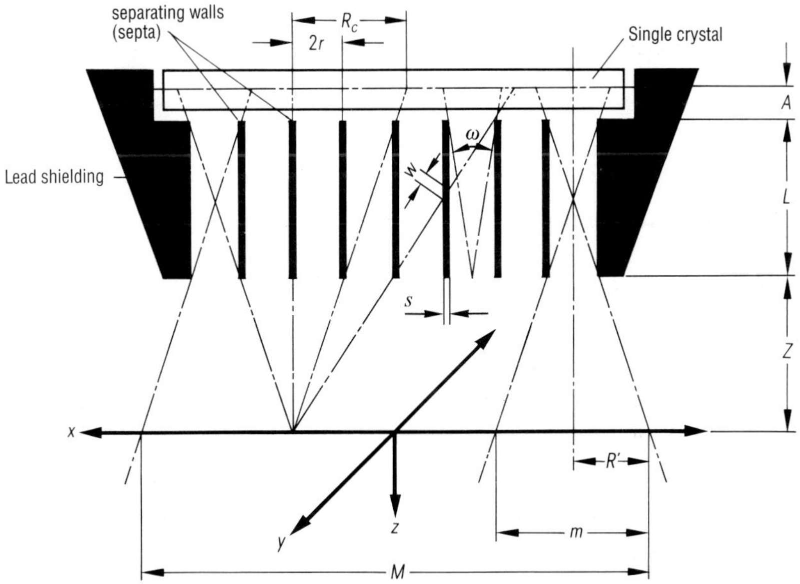

A	Distance	w	Path length in the septum
L	Collimator length	x, y, z	Spatial coordinates
Z	Object distance	ω	Solid angle
R_c	Blurring radius	M	Total field of view
$2r$	Channel diameter	m	Individual field of view
s	Septum thickness		

Fig. 9.7
Diagram of the parallel hole collimator for a gamma camera and the geometrical relationships

Until now, we have ignored the deterioration of the purely geometric values due to radiation penetrating the collimator septa at the edges with smaller path lengths and detected in the neighboring channel. According to Anger [9.15], this part of the radiation can be taken into account by introducing the so called effective length of the collimator in place of the geometric length. We then have

$$L_{eff} = L - 2\mu^{-1} \tag{9.5}$$

(e.g.: μ^{-1} for ^{99m}Tc (140 keV) $= 3.8 \cdot 10^{-2}$ cm in lead).

The blurring radius of the virtual image of a point source should therefore be taken as:

$$R_c = \frac{2r}{L_{eff}}(L_{eff} + Z + A). \tag{9.6}$$

Radiation components which magnify the blurring radius R_c are either accounted for by introducing the effective length L_{eff} or have to penetrate a septum along the minimum path length w (Fig. 9.7). Experimental investigations have shown that for $\leq 5\%$ penetration of a septum by radiation there is only an insignificant effect on the imaging properties of a camera collimator. From the attenuation formula

$$N = N_0 \, e^{-\mu w}. \tag{9.7}$$

w, for 95% absorption, is calculated as

$$w = \frac{-\ln 0.05}{\mu} = \frac{2.99}{\mu} \tag{9.8}$$

and the septum thickness s for $L \gg 2r$ as

$$s = \frac{120r}{\mu L - 3} \text{ mm}. \tag{9.9}$$

Sensitivity

Ignoring penetration of the septa by radiation, the sensitivity of a collimator only depends on its geometrical data. We therefore also speak of the geometrical efficiency. The geometrical efficiency of a collimator channel for a point source is in general

$$G_p = \frac{\omega(x, y, z)}{4\pi}, \tag{9.10}$$

where the solid angle $\omega(x, y, z)$ which is swept by the free path through the collimator channel is related to the full solid angle 4π. If we consider collimators which can be used in practice with satisfactory spatial resolution, the diameter $2r$ of the collimator channel is small compared to the collimator length L.

Then, to a good approximation, we have

$$\omega = \frac{\pi r^2}{L^2} \tag{9.11}$$

and for a point source at the collimator surface ($Z=0$)

$$G_p = \frac{r^2}{4L^2} \tag{9.12}$$

within the free area πr^2.

If we use a planar source which is always larger than the viewing field of the sum of all collimator channels, the geometrical area efficiency G_F is then calculated as

$$G_F = \frac{R'^2}{4(L+2Z)^2}. \tag{9.13}$$

It can be seen from this equation that the geometrical efficiency of the entire collimator for an area distribution is independent of distance, provided that its dimensions are $\geq M$ (see Fig. 9.). Equation (9.13) can therefore be transformed back to equation (9.12) and equation (9.12) is then used for calculating the geometrical efficiency from the collimator dimensions r and L. Here, we have not yet taken into account the fact that the part of the crystal area covered by the septa may not be used for integration over the area.

The final formula, which represents a good approximation for the geometrical efficiency of a parallel hole collimator with $d=2r$, taking into account the septum thickness s, is then

$$G = \frac{d^2}{16L^2} \cdot \left(\frac{d}{d+s}\right)^2. \tag{9.14}$$

This formula applies to collimators with round channels. However, by substituting the areas, it can be adapted to any shape of channel.

In order to allow for septum penetration, L_{eff} can be substituted into this equation as for equation (9.5).

If we examine equation (9.3), it can be seen that r and L depend on each other for a given resolution. It is clear from the dependence of the septum thickness on the ratio r/L in equation (9.9) that the construction of a collimator is an optimization problem for $L=f(r)$ and $s=f(L, r, E_\gamma)$ in terms of G_{max}. In this case, criteria such as avoiding the imaging of the septa and the collimator weight must also be taken into account.

Detector system

The radiation detector of the camera is a large-area highly transparent sodium iodide single crystal commonly 1/4 to 3/8″ (6.35 to 9.5 mm) thick. The measurement field diameters M lie between 250 and 500 mm or the measurement field is rectangular and up to 610 mm × 390 mm. As described in section 9.1, through the absorption of gamma photons the crystal produces a number of light quanta proportional to the gamma photon energy, for which the point of origin is calculated electronically. As follows from Fig. 9.6, the absorption position of every individual gamma photon is determined from the signal amplitudes of several photomultipliers arranged hexagonally (frequently 37, sometimes considerably more). The planar arrangement of the photomultipliers is shown in Fig. 9.8. The measurement field is divided up into a measurement coordinate system x, y. Since the determination of position is carried out independently for the x and the y coordinates, the localization mechanism can be regarded as 1-dimensional under simplified conditions.

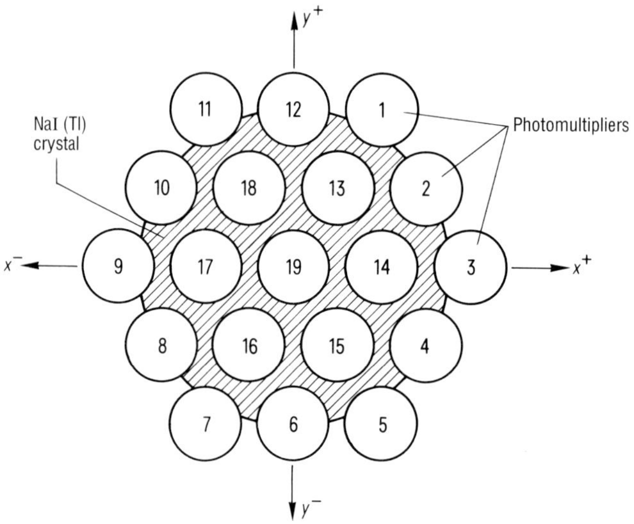

Fig. 9.8
Arrangement of the photomultipliers above the crystal (only 19 multipliers are shown here)

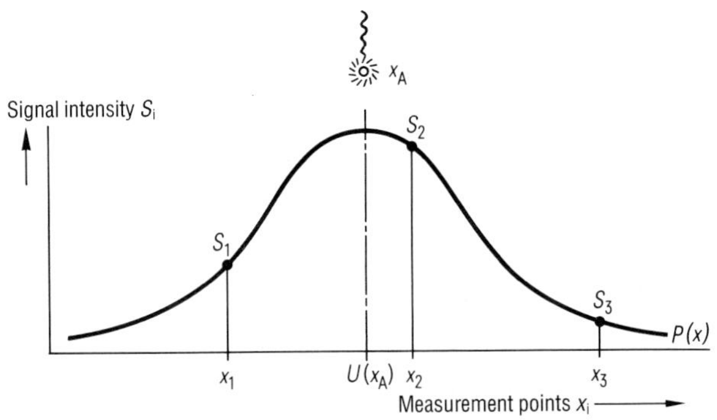

Fig. 9.9
Signal distribution $p(x)$ over the measurement points x_i generated by light photon emission from the absorption position x_A

Fig. 9.9 shows a typical signal distribution $p(x)$ here taken in the x-direction as obtained from the position of the point of absorption x_A relative to the system of measurement coordinates x_i. Here, the signal amplitudes S_i of the photomultipliers (e.g. S_1, S_2, S_3) are dependent on x_i and the shape of the light distribution. The center of gravity of the signal distribution, i.e. the localization signal $U(x_A)$, is calculated from the signals S_i at the measurement positions denoted by x_i as

$$U(x_A) = \frac{\sum_i x_i S_i}{\sum_i S_i} \tag{9.15}$$

and has the dimension of a length. Here, from the circuitry point of view, on the one hand all signals S_i are summed with the individual signals multiplied by the gain factor x_i determining the measurement position and, on the other hand, an unweighted sum is formed to determine the energy. This signal contributes to the determination of the localization signal, $U(x_A)$; however, it is also supplied to the pulse height analyzer, which generates an energy window (Fig. 9.2) and rejects events which do not belong to the photopeak. The localization in the y direction is carried out in a similar manner. The separately determined localization signals $U(x_A)$ and $U(y_A)$ deflect the blanked electron beam of an oscilloscope to the calculated image point position. If the amplitude of the associated energy signal satisfies the logical conditions of the pulse height analyzer, a pulse is generated which unblanks the oscilloscope for a period of approximately 10^{-6} s and produces a light point. The individual pixels produced in this way are summed over a measurement time t determined by the pulse number or a preselected time on a photographic medium and produce the image

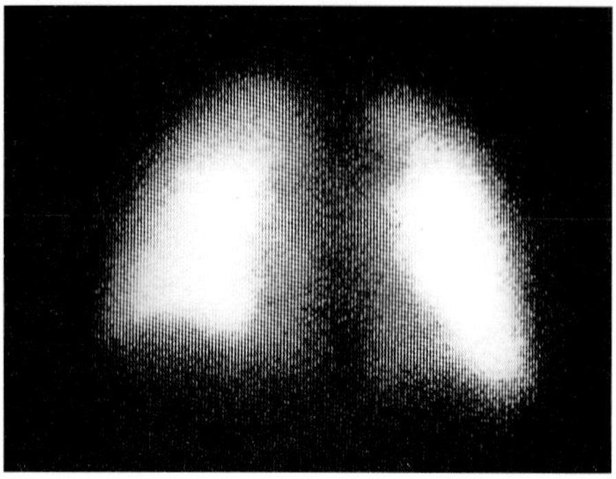

Fig. 9.10
Perfusion state of the lungs. Digital scintigram taken with the large-field camera

of the spatial distribution of the indicator $C_A(x, y, t)$. The enable signal of the pulse height analyzer can also initiate the transfer of the position coordinates to a computer system. In this case, the pixels are summed in the computer system's digital image memory to produce a scintigram. Fig. 9.10 shows a digitized lung perfusion scintigram produced with a large field camera.

Spatial resolution performance

If we consider the determination of the center of gravity $U(x_A)$ of the signal distribution $p(x)$ as a single measurement of statistically emitted information carriers, as described in section 9.1.2, then U must be subject to statistical fluctuations according to equation (9.1). The fluctuating variables are in this case the number of light photons l_i impinging upon the individual photomultipliers (PM) and the photoelectrons $N_i = q l_i$ released by them, where q describes the quantum yield of the photocathode. For modern photomultipliers, q should be set to approximately 0.3, from which it follows that the number n_i decisively influences the fluctuation width σ of the signals S_i from the multipliers. The statistical uncertainty of the signal U, resulting from the calculation of the center of gravity of a signal distribution in which the individual signals fluctuate independently of each other, approximately obeys a Gaussian distribution about the average value U for constant x and y according to the central limit theorem of probability theory [9.16].

The so-called inherent resolution performance of a camera detector (the resolution capacity of the detector alone) is today generally given by the full width at half maximum (FWHM) value of the line spread function. The FWHM of the fluctuation function about $\bar{U}$ corresponds to the FWHM of the point spread function in the 1-dimensional approximation. In the normalized Gaussian function

$$y = \mathrm{e}^{-\frac{x^2}{2\sigma^2}} \tag{9.16}$$

the FWHM is related to σ by

$$\mathrm{FHWM} = \sqrt{8 \ln 2} \cdot \sigma \tag{9.17}$$

This permits the calculation of the FWHM of this function from σ.

Assuming proportionality between the number of electrons n_i released in the cathode and the PM signal S_i, equation (9.15) can in general be written as

$$U = \frac{\sum_i x_i N_i}{\sum_i N_i} = \frac{\sum_i x_i N_i}{N_{el}}. \tag{9.18}$$

The fluctuating variable $N_i = q l_i$ depends on the fluctuation of L and l_i, i.e. on the total number of the light photons generated per γ photon absorption and their transmission to the individual PMs and on the fluctuation of q, the quantum efficiency of the PM cathode. If the energy resolution is sufficiently good, the standard deviation of $U(x_A)$ can be calculated according to [9.16] through the law of error propagation to give

$$\sigma^2 = \frac{\sigma_{p^2}}{\bar{N}_{el}} \tag{9.19}$$

and the half width value

$$\mathrm{HWB} = 2.35 \cdot \frac{\sigma_p}{\sqrt{\bar{N}_{el}}}. \tag{9.20}$$

In this way it can be shown that σ and therefore also the half width value of the point spread function is only dependent on the number $\bar{N}_{el}$ of electrons (information carriers) contributing on the average to the imaging and the deviation σ_p of the signal distribution $p(x)$ according to Fig. 9.9, which in turn is closely related to the light distribution over the plane of the PM. However, this approach only accounts for the effect of the interaction of detector and localization system on the resolution for optimal design of the electronics and does not allow for the lack of sharpness already generated in the crystal due to Compton scattering and subsequent photoabsorption, described in [9.15, 9.17, 9.18]. The typical value for the FWHM of the inherent line spread function presently lies between 3.5 and 5 mm for a large field camera. Fig. 9.11 shows the inherent imaging of a lead strip test phantom.

The modulation transfer function (MTF) has been introduced as a measure for assessing the quality of an imaging system. For the camera, the MTF is

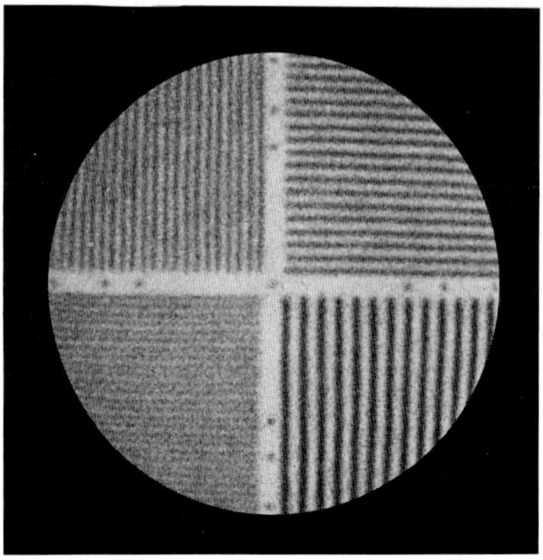

Fig. 9.11
Image of a lead strip test phantom for visual assessment of the inherent spatial resolution of a gamma camera. The spatial resolution in the quadrants with the finest grid patterns is 3 mm

generally calculated by a Fourier transformation from the line spread function $L(x, Z)$ at a distance Z of the source from the collimator according to

$$\mathrm{MTF}(v, Z)=\frac{\sum_{i=1}^{m} L(x_i, Z)\cos 2\pi v x_i}{\sum_{i=1}^{m} L(x_i, Z)} \tag{9.21}$$

$(x_i = i-1)$ [9.19]. Fig. 9.12 shows the MTF of a large-field camera with a high-resolution collimator for a distance of the line source to the collimator $Z = 100$ mm.

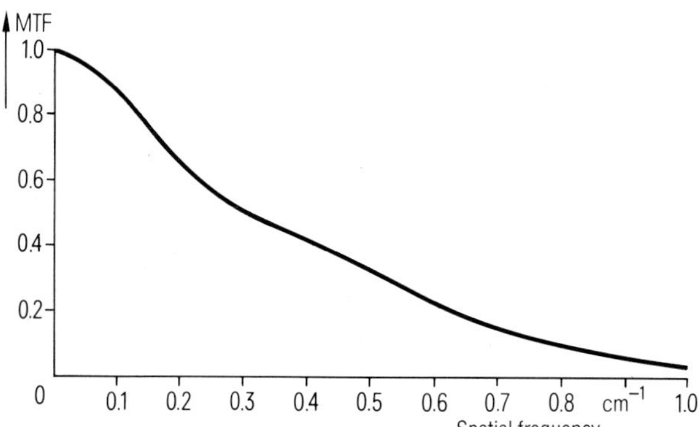

Fig. 9.12
Modulation transfer function (MTF) of a gamma camera with high-resolution collimator. Distance Z of the line source from the collimator 100 mm. Measurement in a scattering medium (water)

Homogeneity and linearity

In attempting to improve the resolution performance of the camera, there is a risk of impairing the linearity and homogeneity of the camera image. If the light distribution is narrowed down, which according to equation (9.20) is the most effective way for improving the resolution without change of the given measuring grid, $\bar{N}_{el}$ depends more strongly on position; this means that the position of the spectrum in the pulse height analyzer is also subject to position fluctuations. In this way, the sensitivity of the detector can become dependent on position and so the image becomes inhomogeneous [9.18, 9.20]. Furthermore, the linearity $U(x, y)$ is disturbed by position-dependent fluctuating sums, such as non-linear compression of the positioning at the edge of the measurement field (edge packing), which produces disturbing inhomogeneities. Many approaches have been made in an attempt to avoid these disadvantages, some optically by clever coupling of the PM to the crystal, some electronically by digital correction of the energy and position signals (ZLC). In the meantime, it is possible to reduce the inhomogeneity to $\pm 5\%$ with maximum resolution.

The prerequisites for such effective quality improvements are long-term and short-term stability of the system. Simultaneous monitoring and guarantee of this stability in the DIGITRAC camera (Fig. 9.13) provide a good example of advanced camera technology.

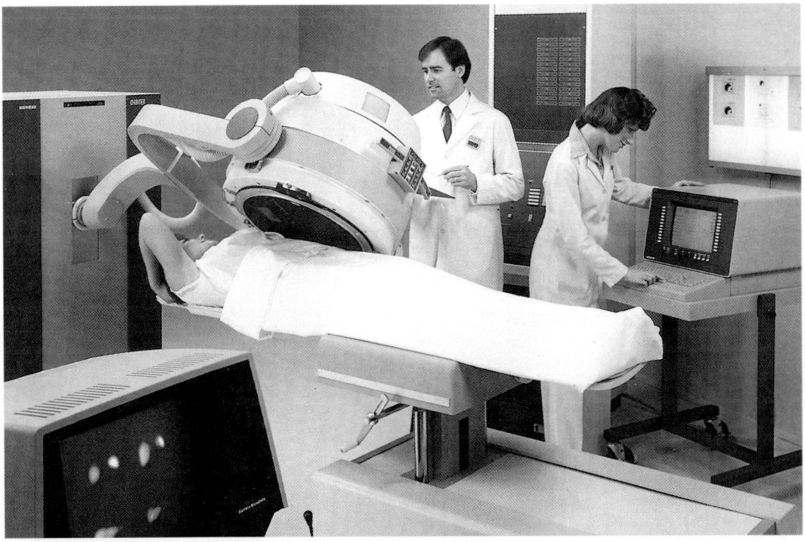

Fig. 9.13
ORBITER 7500 DIGITRAC gamma camera with MicroDELTA nuclear medicine computer system

Image stability for high count rates

The measurement of radioactive radiation requires event-based information processing because of the energy discrimination. A finite processing time is therefore necessary to identify and characterize an event.

In the gamma camera, the necessary processing time is of course longer due to the additional task of exact localization. In general, this means that the counting rate which can be processed is more severely limited. However, for high counting rates an impairment of the resolution or even a complete disintegration of the image is already observed below this limit in the camera [9.21]. This effect is due to the fact that two or more events are separated by too small an interval, so that they mutually interfere in the localization. Due to the finite decay time of the light emitted from the scintillator ($\tau = 2.5 \cdot 10^{-7}$ s), especially at high counting rates pileup of the pulses can occur. This may result in the detection of scattering events which are normally not seen due to energy discrimination; that is, in the detection of events having false position information which are still accepted by the pulse height analyzer. For high counting rates, false localization and counting losses are produced in this way. Intensive studies [9.22 to 9.24] have been able to explain these effects and their causes

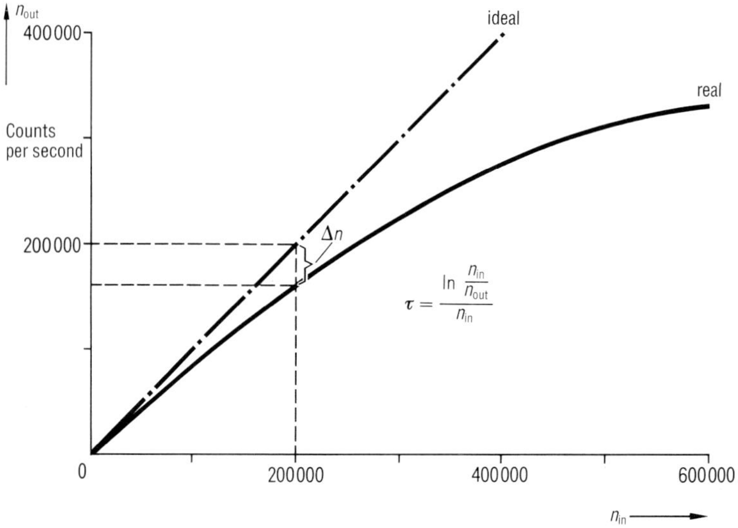

Δn Counting loss
τ Camera dead time
n_{in} Number of incident photons
n_{out} Number of measured events

Fig. 9.14
Counting rate behavior of an Anger camera (example). Relationship between dead time and counting loss

and, as one result, for a few years the Anger cameras have largely kept up with the increased demands on nuclear medicine for fast functional diagnostics in terms of image stability at high counting rates through the use of the most advanced electronic components and circuits, although the counting loss is still an unsatisfactorily solved problem because here technology is confronted with physically imposed limits (Fig. 9.14).

The Anger gamma camera is the "universal instrument" of the nuclear practitioner, because it fulfills the most important requirement of nuclear diagnostics: to make functional processes in the human body visible and measurable.

9.4 Scintigraphic data processing

Due to the large amount of information acquired, scintigraphic functional diagnostics requires storage of this information for subsequent selective evaluation. Already at the beginning of the sixties, digital magnetic tapes and a little later the first minicomputers were therefore used to solve these problems. With the progressive integration of digital components and the fall of the initial hardware costs, it is possible today to design scintigraphic data processing systems in which both software and hardware are tailored to the demands of functional camera scintigraphy.

Large-scale image and data memories are in step with the good resolution capability of modern cameras. Large and fast image memories ensure that high event processing rates and amounts of data are not limited by the data processing system. The marking of regions of interest (ROI) makes it possible to generate selective function curves, even with a time resolution of <50 ms, e.g. in cardiac function diagnostics [9.25].

The specialized software can be preprogrammed to automatically control such functional studies and to take over their evaluation. Sophisticated image processing and the reconstruction of tomographic slices are today standard in nuclear medicine routine diagnostics.

9.5 Emission computed tomography (ECT)

The first successful attempts at transverse tomography in nuclear medicine were made by D. Kuhl in 1963 [9.26]. The goal was to image a selected, isolated volume without the contrast-reducing information of the total volume by proper slice separation. Already in 1968, i.e. 4 years before the advent of x-ray computed tomography, the same author used a digital computer for image reconstruction [9.27]. In the wake of the tempestuous development of x-ray computed tomography (CT), ECT in recent years has experienced an equally rapid upsurge.

It has become an integral part of nuclear medicine imaging diagnostics and is constantly undergoing further development in terms of methodology and technology.

Complementing CT and magnetic resonance imaging, ECT provides slice images of the organ and tissue function, regional blood flow and regional metabolism with maximum sensitivity. It therefore plays an important role in imaging diagnostics. Two completely different techniques led to true tomography with radioisotopes:

1. ECT with gamma photon emitting (single photon emitting) isotopes: **S**ingle **P**hoton **E**mission **C**omputed **T**omography or SPECT
2. ECT with positron emitting isotopes: **P**ositron **E**mission **T**omography or PET.

9.5.1 SPECT

In general, a rotating gamma camera measurement head based on the Anger principle is used for SPECT. According to the so-called translate-rotate principle, the tomographic data is collected and reconstructed to the slice image in a manner similar to CT. By suitable measurement head suspension, today almost all modern gamma cameras are capable of being rotated and therefore performing SPECT (see Fig. 9.13). Sensitivity and resolution can be optimized for special tomographic tasks. The development of new radio-labelled drugs has considerably enhanced the value of the procedure.

9.5.2 PET

The measurement principle of tomography with positron emitters is based on the phenomenon of annihilation radiation. Fig. 9.15 shows a simplified diagram of the measurement principle for PET. The incorporated radioisotope emits a positron, which after a short distance through the tissue combines with an electron. Both particles are annihilated and two gamma photons are produced with an energy corresponding to the energy equivalent of the electron mass, 511 keV. Their directions differ by exactly 180°, so that the two trajectories describe a straight line. If the two photons arrive at two detectors at the same time (coincidence measurement), the measurement system assigns the event to the line joining the two detectors. Since only the line is known and not the position of generation on this line, the result of the measurement of many such events is called a line integral, as in CT. Thus, by corresponding coincidence concatenation, the slice can also be reconstructed as with a CT scanner with fan-beam geometry. Fig. 9.16 shows an investigation of the circulation and metabolic processes in the brain with the positron emission tomograph, ECAT.

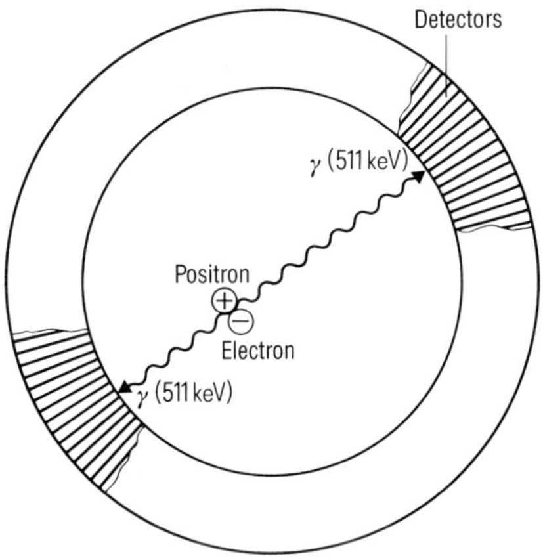

Fig. 9.15
Simplified diagram of tomography with positron emitters (PET)

For PET, the elements belonging to the human body – carbon, nitrogen and oxygen, represented by their positron emitting isotopes ^{11}C, ^{13}N and ^{15}O – can be used for radioactive labelling. Even the fluorine isotope ^{18}F has gained considerable importance in the labelling of e.g. glucose. Since the amounts of labelled substrate can be extremely minute, the metabolic processes to be measured remain undisturbed.

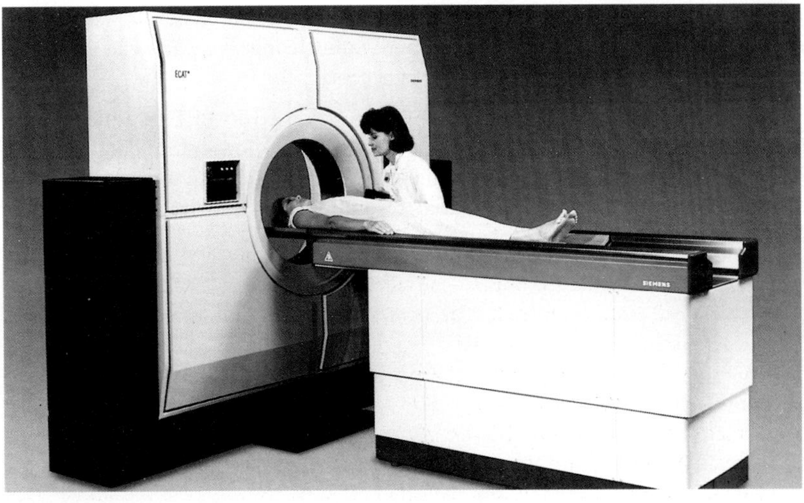

Fig. 9.16
Positron emission tomograph (ECAT) for circulatory and metabolic measurements

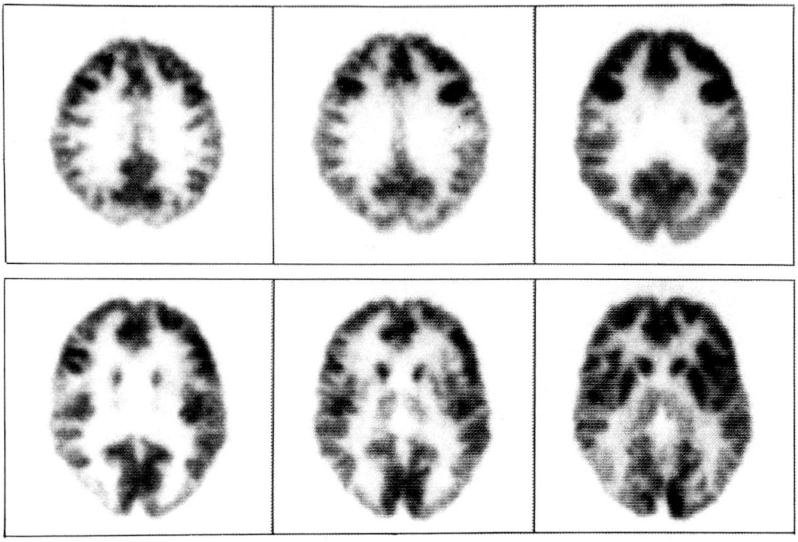

Fig. 9.17
^{18}F desoxyglucose distribution in six layers of the brain (with permission of M.E. Phelps, Ph.D., UCLA School of Medicine, University of California, Los Angeles)

Because of the short half lives of these isotopes – of the order of minutes – they have to be produced in the immediate vicinity of the PET camera. For this, small, highly automated production units have been developed, consisting of self-shielded mini cyclotrons and radiochemistry. They can generate sufficiently high activities of the isotopes necessary for PET.

Since, by contrast with SPECT, no collimator is used in PET, the unit which limits the resolution and sensitivity in SPECT is no longer present. The ^{18}F desoxyglucose distribution in the brain (Fig. 9.17), taken with a modern ECAT scanner, shows how good the spatial resolution can be with high-sensitivity PET. The spatial resolution is better than 5 mm.

10 Magnetic resonance imaging

10.1 System Overview

A magnetic resonance imaging (MRI) system is similar to the type of processor-controlled Fourier NMR Spectrometer (NMR = Nuclear Magnetic Resonance) used routinely today in analytical chemistry for the determination of molecular structure. In addition to standard NMR components an MRI system has gradient field coils and the appropriate pulsed power supply for the spatial encoding of the magnetic resonance signal (MR signal), as well as monitors for image display. The system is also adapted to the size of a normal patient, and the control program is structured to meet imaging requirements.

Figure 10.1 shows the basic arrangement and interaction of the components of an MRI system. Important aspects of the construction and specifications for these components will be discussed in more detail in the following sections: Magnet with Shim Coil and Gradient Coil System, RF System, System Control and Patient Table, on which the patient – reclining on a cradle-shaped support – can be moved into the gantry of the scanning system.

The main magnet system (1) generates a magnetic field constant in time, in order to polarize the nuclei of the atoms of the patient's body. The necessary spatial homogeneity within the measurement volume is guaranteed by the shim coils (2) in the magnet bore and by iron plates mounted both inside and outside when necessary. The cylindrical gradient coil (3) is placed concentrically in the opening. It consists of three sets of windings, which generate a linear gradient field in the direction of the Cartesian coordinates (see Fig. 10.2) proportional to the superimposed current. Inside the gradient coil there is a radio-frequency (RF) coil or RF resonator (antenna, 4). The purpose of this antenna is to transform the RF pulse generated by a power transmitter into an alternating magnetic field to excite the spins in the tissue being examined. This antenna then picks up the alternating field generated by the excited spins and converts it into a voltage which is forwarded to the receiver.

After the pulse sequence controller has been supplied with appropriate control programs, it runs the measurement sequence for the most part independently of the system processor. It assures the correct timing of the gradients via digital-to-analog (DAC, 9) converters and an RF pulse with defined phase and amplitude via a modulator. The time base is the synthesizer which functions as a central clock. The control processor generates the conversion pulse for the analog-to-digital (ADC, 8) converters, which translate the low frequency demodulated MR signals into digital numbers which can be utilized by a computer.

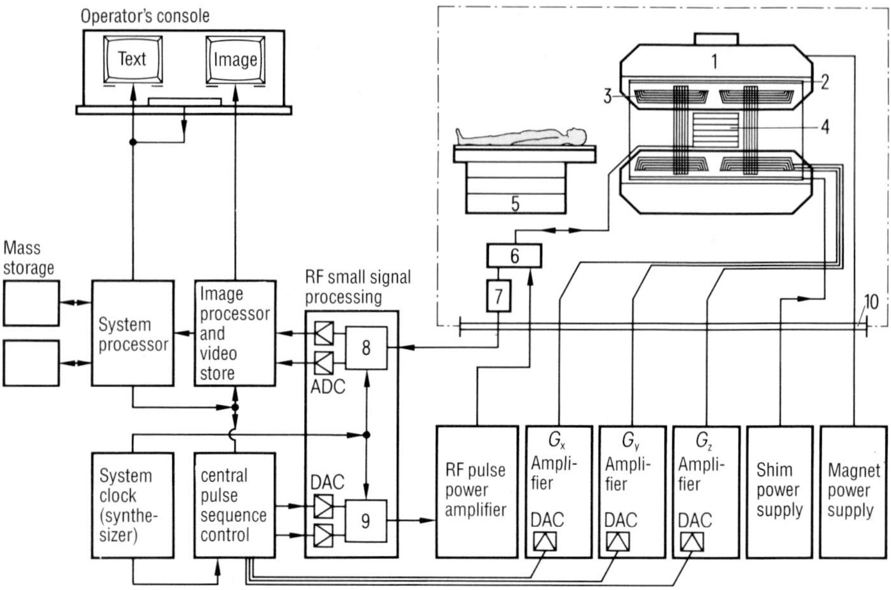

1 Magnet with cryo tank and cryogenic shielding
2 Shim coil system
3 Gradient coil system
4 RF resonator (antenna)
5 Patient table
6 Transmit-receive switch
7 Preamplifier
8 Quadrature demodulator with two low-frequency low-pass filters and ADC
9 SSB modulator with two DACs
10 RF-proof leadthroughs

Fig. 10.1 Schematic wiring diagram of an MRI scanning system

Fig. 10.2
Coordinate system (Cartesian and spherical coordinates) of the gradient coils; definition of field polarity

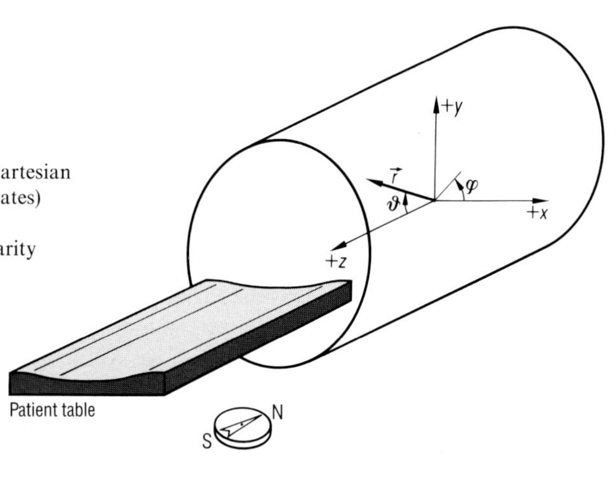

Measurement data are fed directly into the programmable image processor, which reconstructs them as image data immediately after data acquisition. Image data are copied to the video memory of the control console monitor.

The host computer manages the measurement data, image data and control programs. The video terminal serves as the interface between the host computer and the user.

10.2 System components

10.2.1 Magnet

Criteria for the selection of field strength

As has been shown in Section 5.1.8 the signal-to-noise-ratio (SNR) increases linearly with the main magnetic field B_0 (assuming a scanning object which generates RF losses, as is the case with a patient). This fact could lead to the assumption that the quality of an MRI system, expressed as the attainable SNR per volume element (and per square root of the invested measurement time), increases without limit with an increase in field strength. There are several practical and physical reasons, however, for not increasing the field strength to any arbitrary value, especially for systems used primarily for hydrogen imaging [10.1]. As will be discussed, the selection of field strength also has an important effect on the gradient and RF systems.

Considerations in regard to the technical implementation of these components are governing factors in the selection of field strength.

Those factors which must be taken into consideration are summarized in Table 10.1.

Chemical shift

The chemical shift is the main characteristic employed in NMR spectroscopy. The resonant frequency of the MR signal shifts slightly depending upon the type of chemical bond in which the nucleus of the material being examined occurs. This is caused by the diamagnetic shielding effect which the electron cloud within the molecule has on the nucleus and which is proportional to the main field B_0.

Due to their concentration in the human body, the hydrogen nuclei of free water (H_2O) and in aliphatic bonds (fat, $-CH_2-$) comprise essentially all protons visible in the MR image. Their relative resonance frequency difference δ is approximately 3 ppm, i.e. about 130 Hz at a field strength of 1 Tesla (T) (42.6 MHz). As explained in Section 5.2.3, spatial information is encoded in frequencies during readout in field gradients. Since the nuclei do not differentiate

Table 10.1 Factors to consider in selecting the field strength for ^{1}H MRI

Cause	Effect
Chemical shift	Image shift between fatty and aqueous tissue
Constant field inhomogeneity	Distortion
RF penetration characteristics (skin effect)	Inhomogeneity of intensity
RF losses	Patient warming
Field-dependent T_1 time	Change of contrast-to-noise ratio
Fringe field	Attraction of ferromagnetic objects, interference with cardiac pacemakers and other equipment

between outer and molecular fields, the result is a spatial shift between fat and water in the image (Fig. 10.3):

$$\delta x = \delta B_0 / G_x. \tag{10.1}$$

δx Spatial shift caused by chemical shift
G_x Readout gradient

In order to prevent spatial shifts from becoming too large, one must increase the readout gradient and therefore also the sampling bandwidth. Since noise

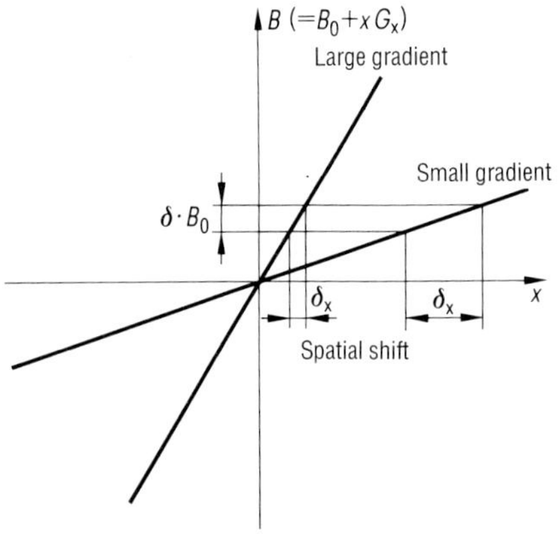

Fig. 10.3
Fat/water shifts as a function of the field gradient

increases with the square root of the bandwidth, however, a significant amount of the improvement in the SNR will be lost.

The same applies to selective slice excitation, i.e. the fat slice position is shifted with respect to the water slice position:

$$\delta z = \delta B_0 / G_z. \tag{10.2}$$

This requires an increase in the selection gradient G_z in proportion to the field. If the slice thickness, Δz, remains constant, the pulse bandwidth will increase, since:

$$\Delta\omega_p = \Delta z \gamma G_z. \tag{10.3}$$

As the bandwidth increases, the pulse duration becomes shorter, so that a higher RF field amplitude peak or pulse power becomes necessary.

Inhomogeneity of the constant magnetic field

The constant field inhomogeneity has an effect similar to a chemical shift. A field changed in relation to the nominal field strength by external influences acts on the nuclei. The result is a spatially-dependent dislocation of volume elements in the direction of the readout or slice selection gradients, which is calculated analogously to equation 10.1 and 10.2 by replacing the "chemical shift" with the relative field inhomogeneity.

$$\delta = (B(x, y, z) - B_0)/B_0. \tag{10.4}$$

Since magnetic field inhomogeneities cannot be reduced at will, owing to the magnet's construction, undesirable distortions must be reduced by increasing the gradient strengths with the field strength. An additional undesirable effect is caused by the inhomogeneity of the field across a volume element. This results in a dispersion of the phases of the nuclear magnetization (T_2^* effect) and, therefore, in a signal loss.

Irregularities in the macroscopic magnetic susceptibility of the subject can also cause local distortions, which increase with field strength at constant gradient strength.

RF power loss in the subject under study

According to the Maxwell equations, there is always a proportional electric field linked to a given time derivative of the magnetic field [10.2].

$$\vec{\nabla} \times \vec{E} = \frac{\partial \vec{B}}{\partial t} \quad \text{or} \quad \oint \vec{E}\, d\vec{r} = \int_F \frac{\partial \vec{B}}{\partial t}\, d\vec{F}. \tag{10.5}$$

The electric field induces eddy currents with a current density of $\vec{j}$ in a conductive material. When B_1 is sine-shaped the eddy currents increase linearly with the frequency ω_0 due to the proportionality between E and $\frac{\partial B}{\partial t}$.

Disregarding the losses in the RF coil (resonator) and the minimal frequency dependence of the conductivity in the subject, the transmit power P required to generate a given B_1 field strength increases as the square of the nuclear resonance frequency, because:

$$P = \int_V \vec{j}\vec{E}\,\mathrm{d}V = \int_V \sigma E^2\,\mathrm{d}V. \tag{10.6}$$

Thus

$$P \sim \omega_0^2. \tag{10.7}$$

This increase in required RF power must be multiplied by the increase resulting from the pulse bandwidth, as shown in Equation (10.3). The RF output warms the patient like a diathermy unit. Since a patient's thermoregulation system may not be functioning properly, the regulatory agencies of some countries have established relatively low specific absorption rates (SAR) (the permissible levels of absorbed RF power per unit of body weight). The Food and Drug Administration in the USA, for example, recognizes the ANSI guidelines of 0.4 W/kg. Fig. 10.4 shows the experimentally determined pulse output per B_1^2 field for an average patient during transmission using a whole-body antenna as a function of the field strength, B_0. Coil loss is subtracted using the following equation:

$$P_{\text{sample}} = P_{\text{input}} - P_{\text{coil}} = P_{\text{input}}\left(1 - \frac{Q_1}{Q_0}\right). \tag{10.8}$$

$$Q_1/Q_0 = \text{Loaded/unloaded } Q$$

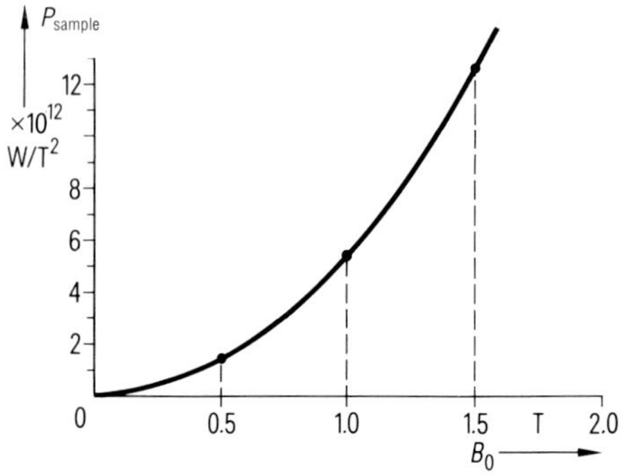

Fig. 10.4
Pulse power, P_{sample}, required per B_1 field squared for a given field strength B_0. (B_1 field – circular component – for a linearly polarized resonator; average patient weight approx. 70 kg)

There are limitations for the sequence repetition time at fields of 1.5 Tesla or greater for spin-echo sequences with two 180° pulses of approximately 1 ms duration. In this case, the sequence repetition time is no longer limited by the capabilities of the measurement system, but by the SAR.

RF penetration characteristics

The eddy currents induced by the RF field themselves generate an opposing field which weakens the applied RF field. This so-called skin effect [10.3] causes a spatially inhomogeneous excitation of the nuclear spins. RF field penetration decreases as the frequency, or conductivity, increases. At frequencies higher than approximately 40 MHz, shading of varying degrees, depending on the shape of the body being examined, may become visible.

Field dependence of the T_1 relaxation

The increase in the T_1 relaxation time with an increase in field strength [10.4] causes the relative saturation of the nuclear magnetization to increase with the field strength when the repetition time, T_r, remains constant. Consequently the increase in the SNR is less than proportional to the field strength, B_0 (Fig. 10.5).

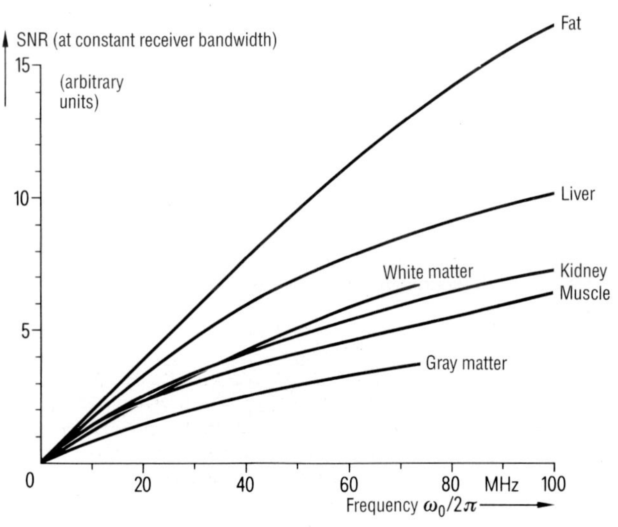

Fig. 10.5
Increase in the SNR with field strength, taking into consideration the dependence of the T_1 relaxation time on the field strength B_0 for a constant repetition time T_r

Safety considerations

It is obvious that the operation of large magnets with high field strengths is not possible without considering safety problems. The stored field energy increases with the square of the field strength. It must be possible to dissipate this energy quickly in an emergency (quench for superconducting magnets).

Large fields exert a substantial force on ferromagnetic objects, such as oxygen tanks, fire extinguishers, transport machinery or tools inadvertently brought near the magnet. If these objects are magnetically saturated – whether this occurs depends strongly on the material, shape and orientation of the object – the forces increase linearly with the fringe field. For unsaturated objects, the increase in the force is quadratic. In order to avoid accidents, ferromagnetic objects must be kept at a safe distance from the magnetic resonance equipment.

Patients with cardiac pacemakers or other electronic implants may not enter an area having a fringe field strength greater than 0.5 mT without medical supervision. The so-called pacemaker zone becomes larger with increasing field strength. Table 10.2 shows the distance of the 0.5 mT line from magnets of the same size, but for field strengths of 0.5 to 2.0 T.

Installation problems

There are several types of medical equipment in a physician's practice which are sensitive to static magnetic fields (see Table 10.3) and which cannot be set up in close proximity to a magnetic resonance scanning system. The selected field strength therefore has a direct effect on the amount of space required for an MR system and thus on installation costs, including any system shielding which might be necessary.

A consideration of the above mentioned points makes clear that there is no well defined optimum for field strength in an MR system. Along with the desire for high image quality and short exposure times, there is the important question of expenditure for the system itself and its operation. As will be shown in greater detail later in this chapter, the technological requirements increase at

Table 10.2
Safe distance for cardiac pacemaker wearers (for magnets having a 1.05 m bore and a length of 2.30 m without shielding)

B_0	0.5 mT line (radial)	0.5 mT line (axial)
0.5 T	6.5 m	8.3 m
1.0 T	8.2 m	10.5 m
1.5 T	9.4 m	12.0 m
2.0 T	10.3 m	13.1 m

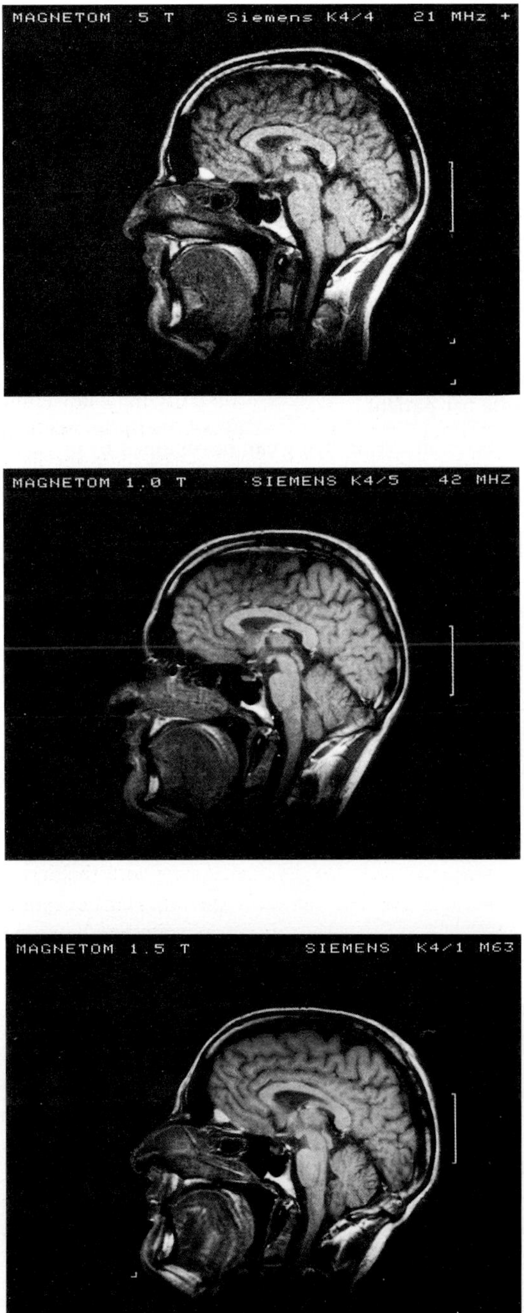

Fig. 10.6
Comparison of magnetic resonance image quality of cranial images at field strengths of

a) 0.5 T

b) 1.0 T

c) 1.5 T

Magnetic disks or tapes	3 mT
Video monitors with shielding or correction	3 mT
Video monitors (monochromatic)	1 mT
Cardiac pacemakers	0.5 mT
X-ray units	0.2 mT
Image intensifiers	50 μT
Photomultipliers	50 μT
Earth's magnetic field for comparison	50 μT

Table 10.3
Sensitivity of different systems to (static) magnetic fields

field strengths above 1 T without a corresponding increase in image quality or decrease in examination time per patient.

Since spatial and contrast resolution in MR imaging can be obtained by increasing the measurement time, systems with relatively low field strengths can be useful if purchase and operation costs are low enough to compensate for reduced patient throughput.

Figure 10.6 shows three cranial images taken at three different field strengths, but with otherwise identical parameters, including the bandwidth per pixel. The image quality (SNR) is clearly better from 0.5 T to 1.0 T, but the improvement is not as striking from 1.0 T to 1.5 T.

It should be noted that magnetic resonance imaging or spectroscopy on a living subject with nuclei other than hydrogen (sodium, phosphorus or fluorine, for example) is, for reasons of sensitivity, nearly impossible at field strengths of less than 1.5 T.

Types of magnets

Permanent magnets, resistive electromagnets and superconducting magnets are all used in analytical magnetic resonance spectroscopy as well as in medical magnetic resonance imaging. Either the air-core or the iron yoke construction is used for resistive electromagnets. Figure 10.7 shows the construction of several types of magnets. Table 10.4 summarizes the characteristics of the various types. The most important will be discussed further in the following.

In addition to field strength, other particularly important characteristics in magnetic resonance imaging are field stability, especially short-term stability ranging from milliseconds to several seconds, and the degree of homogeneity which can be achieved by shimming procedures within the measurement volume, which is almost always spherical in shape and which should be at least 40 cm, or preferably 50 cm, in diameter.

Field strength

The attainable field strength in the effective volume of a permanent magnet is determined by the required field energy produced there in relation to the energy stored in the permanent magnetic material. In consideration of the relatively large air gaps involved, such a magnet then requires either an extremely large amount of fairly inexpensive material or a smaller amount of very expensive material having a high magnetic remanence. The limitation in resistive magnets, on the other hand, is caused by the required electrical power. In both cases the maximum field strength is approximately 0.3 T.

Superconducting magnets with an inner bore of approximately 1 m can be constructed with field strengths of up to 4 T. Its limits are defined by the fact that current carrying capacity decreases as the field of the superconductor increases and also by the forces generated.

Homogeneity

A large homogeneous image volume requires a correspondingly large main magnetic coil, i.e. a large permanent magnet. Since power requirements in a typical clinical installation should not exceed 100 kW, more volume in a resistive magnet can only be achieved by sacrificing field strength. The homogeneous volume in superconductive magnets can be influenced by the length of the magnet and can therefore be adapted to requirements relatively easily.

Field stability

The Fourier MRI procedure requires an extremely stable main magnetic field over time in order to generate images free of artifacts. The reason for this

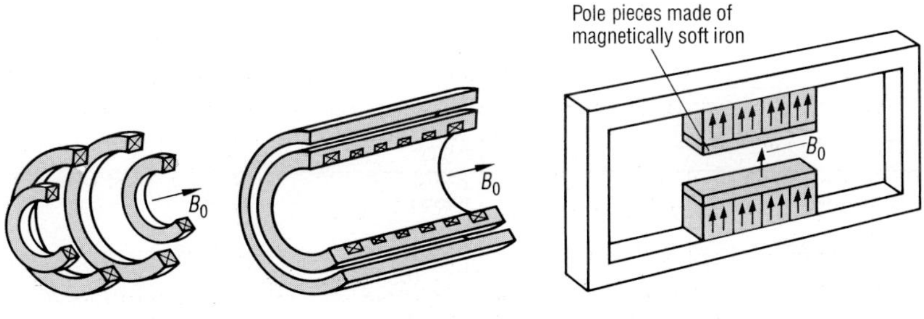

a) resistive magnet (air coil)   b) superconducting magnet   c) permanent magnet (yoke type)

Fig. 10.7 Construction of various types of magnets

Table 10.4
Comparison of magnet types for MRI Systems

	Superconductor	Resistive	Permanent Magnet
1. Technical characteristics			
Field strength	very high field possible (to 4 T)	relatively small to 0.3 T	to 0.3 T
Effective volume and typical homogenity	large 15 ppm/50 cm dia.	sufficient 40 ppm/40 cm diam.	sufficient 40 ppm/40 cm diam.
Field stability	very good	moderate, dependent upon power supply 0.3 to 1 ppm	very good
Shielding of external interfering fields	significant	extensive shielding with iron yoke; no shielding without iron yoke	good shielding
Eddy currents due to pulsed gradients	Extensive compensating measures needed	very limited (feedback to power supply)	very limited anisotropic
Field orientation	Z	Z (or Y)	Y
Fringe field	very large	small (due to small B_0)	negligible
Emergency shutdown	relatively slow due to quench	can be shut down immediately (small L/R)	cannot be shut down
Dimensions	large: 1.8 m diam. × 2 m	average: 1.5 m diam. × 1.6 m	very large: 4.2 m × 2.5 m × 2.3 m
Mass	average: 6 t	relatively low: 2 t	very large (yoke type) 80 t
2. Costs			
Initial price	high	low	high
Energy usage	none	very high to 100 kW ($\sim B_0^2$)	none
Cooling	Cryogens 0.5 l liquid helium per hour	large amount of cooling water needed	none

is that the spatial information is encoded in the phase of the signal generated by the volume elements to be imaged. Simulations show that phase errors as small as approximately 3° can generate visible artifacts. In the simplest of MR experiments, the FID, the phase errors $\Delta\varphi$ caused by time varying field shifts, $\Delta B_0(t)$, accumulate up to the read-out time, t, to:

$$\Delta\varphi=\gamma\int_0^t \Delta B_0(t')\,dt' \tag{10.9}$$

$t=0$ represents the time of the excitation pulse. The equation for a spin echo experiment is as follows:

$$\Delta\varphi=\gamma\left[\int_{T_e/2}^{t} \Delta B_0(t')\,dt'-\int_0^{T_e/2} \Delta B_0(t')\,dt'\right] \tag{10.10}$$

where $T_e/2$ is the time between the 90° and 180° pulse. The phase error, $\Delta\varphi$ can be calculated for a sinusoidal field modulation of frequency ω_b and phase φ_b. Other time characteristics can be described as a Fourier synthesis of sinusoidal modulations. For:

$$\Delta B_0(t)=\Delta B_0\sin(\omega_b t+\varphi_b) \tag{10.11}$$

the following expression results:

$$\Delta\varphi=-\frac{1}{\omega_b}\gamma\Delta B_0[\cos(\omega_b t+\varphi_b)-\cos\varphi_b]. \tag{10.12}$$

At very low $\omega_b\left(\omega_b\ll\frac{\pi}{t}\right)$ and an unfavorable phase angle, $\varphi_b=\frac{\pi}{2}$, the following relation applies:

$$\Delta\varphi(t)\approx\gamma\Delta B_0 t. \tag{10.13}$$

Otherwise, the phase error decreases as the reciprocal of the interfering frequency:

$$\Delta\varphi_{max}\leq\frac{1}{\omega_b}\gamma\Delta B_0. \tag{10.14}$$

At $t=5$ ms, for example, this gives: $\Delta B_0<0.04$ μT. The amplitude of a 60 Hz ripple field should be less than 0.06 μT. These requirements demand a current stability of less than 0.2 ppm, a condition technically difficult to achieve for a resistive magnet. In contrast, superconducting magnets, which are short-circuit operated, and permanent magnets are absolutely stable with respect to measurement time for an MR image. Superconducting magnets also shield very effectively against external interfering fields. Experience shows that an external interference field strength of up to 0.6 μT can be tolerated for the above frequency range without affecting image quality.

A consideration of all the advantages and disadvantages, including those pertaining to image quality and operating costs, leads to the conclusion that superconducting magnets are to be preferred for magnetic resonance imaging. All major manufacturers therefore employ this type of magnet almost exclusively.

Superconducting magnets

The following is a discussion of the technical considerations important to the construction and operation of large superconducting (SC) magnets in magnetic resonance imaging. For further information on construction of the magnets, the physics of superconductivity and producing the extremely low temperatures required refer to the relevant publications [10.5].

The characteristic parameters of an SC magnet are the maximum possible field strength, field homogeneity across a given volume generally spherical in shape and the consumption rates for cryogens, especially liquid helium, which is relatively expensive.

Field strength and homogeneity

The current carrying capacity of the wire material must be taken into consideration when constructing a magnet. It must be superconductive at the temperature of liquid helium, i.e. the critical temperature at which the wire in a magnetic field becomes resistive must be appreciably higher than 4.2 K, the boiling temperature of helium at atmospheric pressure. A suitable material is a multifilament wire composed of 30 niobium-titanium strands of 0.1 mm diameter, each of which, for reasons of stability, is embedded in a copper matrix having a diameter of approximately 2 mm. Such a wire can carry currents of up to 500 A. The desired field strength determines the number of windings on a core of pre-determined length. A 2 T magnet comprises wire lengths of approximately 60 km and has an average radius of 650 mm. The winding is divided into 6 subcoils and the number of windings on each is calculated so that the field is optimally homogeneous at the central spherical volume of 50 cm diameter. Without external interference or assembly tolerances, which are unavoidable, such a field coil would exhibit an inhomogeneity of less than 5 ppm within a spherical volume of 50 cm diameter. In practice, this figure is only approximately 100 ppm, even in environments which are nearly free of iron, so that additional shimming procedures are required (see section on shimming).

Cryostat

The required thermal insulation for the coils can be calculated using the allowable rate of evaporation, (V/t), the surface area of the helium tank, $F(\approx 26\ \mathrm{m}^2)$, the specific evaporation energy, $E_M = 21$ kWs/kg and the density, $\varrho_{He} = 0.1$ kg/l of helium as follows:

$$R_T = \frac{\Delta T \cdot F}{\frac{V}{t} \cdot E_M \cdot \varrho_{He}}. \tag{10.15}$$

If an evaporation rate of less than 0.5 l/h is required for the liquid helium, the surface-specific thermal resistance must be $R_T > 2 \cdot 10^4\ \mathrm{Km^2/W}$. Figure 10.8 shows a cross section of the cryostat for a superconducting magnet. The figure illustrates the individual measures taken to insure such low heat transfer.

Care must be taken to prevent convection, as well any kind of thermal radiation, from penetrating to the helium tank, which contains the steel cylinder with the superconducting coils. The latter is accomplished by a radiation shield and superinsulating foil and the former by evacuating the entire magnet container to high vacuum. The components of a cryostat are suspended within each other on thin, extremely strong, fiberglass-reinforced plastic rods with low thermal conductivity. At the top of the cryostat there is a so-called service

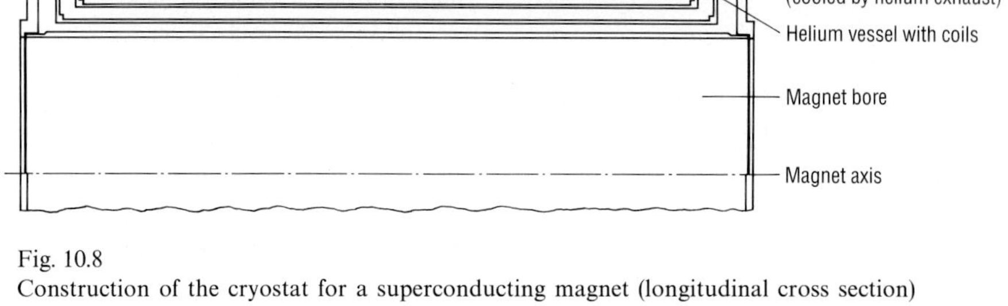

Fig. 10.8
Construction of the cryostat for a superconducting magnet (longitudinal cross section)

turret with openings to allow cryogens (N_2 and He) to be refilled and for the attachment of power cables. The evaporation of cryogens can be reduced to a reasonable level through using shield cooling machines (so-called refrigerators).

Loading and quenching

When the magnetic coil has been properly cooled and has reached the temperature of the helium it becomes superconductive and the field can be ramped up by connecting the coil to a power supply. This is illustrated in the circuit diagram shown in Fig. 10.9. In the quiescent state, switch S_L is at helium temperature and therefore represents the ideal short circuit. An electrical heater is used to warm S_L above the critical temperature, at which it takes on the resistance R_S, i.e. poorly conductive in comparison to the SC coil; the current superimposed by the magnet PSU begins to flow through the field coil. The rate of increase is determined by the voltage (U) generated by the power supply and the inductance of the magnet:

$$U = L\frac{dI}{dt}. \tag{10.16}$$

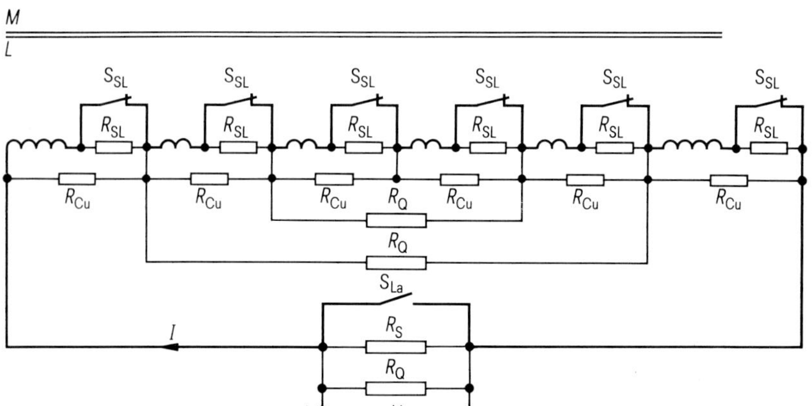

M Inductive coupling between the coils

L Winding inductance

S_{SL} Switch closed during SC state

S_{LA} SL switch (open during ramping)

R_{SL} Distributed ohmic resistance of the SC

R_{Cu} Distributed ohmic resistance of the copper matrix

R_Q Quench protection resistors

R_S SL switch resistor S_{La} – open

Fig. 10.9 Equivalent circuit diagram of an SC magnet with six coils

When the preselected current level or field has been established, the current regulator decreases the voltage to zero and S_L is closed by switching the heater off. The power supply system may then be removed; recharging is not necessary.

Controlled discharging of the stored field energy (for a 2T magnet with an inner bore of 1 m approximately 7 MWs) is performed by reversing the energizing procedure, i.e. the power supply superimposes the current that was set before the S_L switch is opened. A negative voltage is then applied until the current is reduced to zero.

A quench is understood to be the loss of superconductivity, either spontaneous or through external influences. In case of emergency, electrical heating elements increase the temperature of the coil windings beyond the critical point, thus precipitating a quench. Otherwise a quench is most often caused by negligence or the improper handling of the magnet, e.g. allowing the liquid helium level to drop too low.

The rate of current reduction is determined by the resistivity in the resistive zone of each coil winding, as well as their self inductance and mutual inductance. Since the resistive state spreads through the wire at finite speed, the values of these resistors are time dependent. In order to limit voltages, the so-called quench protection resistors are connected in parallel to the windings, giving the induced current a low resistance alternate path (see Fig. 10.9).

The total field energy is converted to heat in both the resistors and coils, which causes the liquid helium to boil off. A quench, especially at high field strength, is therefore highly undesirable and very expensive. In addition, the helium containers and the vacuum tank are subjected to great mechanical stress, due to the increase in pressure and eddy currents during a quench.

Fringe field shielding

If the space available for the installation of an MR system is limited, it is necessary to provide adequate shielding from the magnet's fringe field. Only ferromagnetic materials are suitable as shielding for static magnetic fields.

One differentiates between room shielding, such as iron plates in the walls of the examination room [10.6], and shielding mounted directly on the magnet, so-called self-shielding.

A considerable mass of iron is necessary for effective shielding, because the efficiency of the shielding is lost if the levels of magnetization rise above saturation inductance levels. One may assume that the same iron mass is required for comparable shielding effects in either room or self-shielding; although the thickness of the shielding material required is less at greater distances from the magnet, the total surface area to be shielded is larger. Highly permeable materials, such as Permalloy, are not suitable since they do not exhibit high saturation inductance and are too expensive.

Shielding measures have a substantial effect on the field homogeneity of the measurement volume. The tighter and more eccentric the distribution of ferromagnetic material is, the more difficult it is to compensate for field distortions. Room shielding is generally dependent on conditions in the building and is seldom positioned symmetrically around the magnet. Self-shielding, on the other hand, is highly symmetrical and provides for minimal fringe fields relatively close to the magnet. The major disadvantage of self-shielding is the loading capacity required of the floor at the installation site. Figure 10.10 shows a 1 Tesla magnet in a 21 t self-shield. In comparison to an unshielded magnet (see Table 10.2) the 0.5 mT limit lies at 4.3 m in the radial and at 6.5 m in the axial direction.

Instead of complete shielding, it is sometimes sufficient to use a single iron plate as partial shielding in order to shield an adjoining room, for example, from the pacemaker control area.

Recently, so called actively shielded magnets have been developed. In these magnets the fringe field is reduced via an opposing, external, current-carrying winding. The active shield is integrated into the cryostat; this increases the size and cost of such a magnet considerably. Such magnets are constructed so that the dipole field (decreasing with the cube of the distance) is almost fully suppressed and only a quadrupole field (decreasing with the fifth power of the distance) remains. The advantage of an actively shielded SC magnet is its relatively low total weight compared with an iron-shielded magnet for the same fringe field distribution.

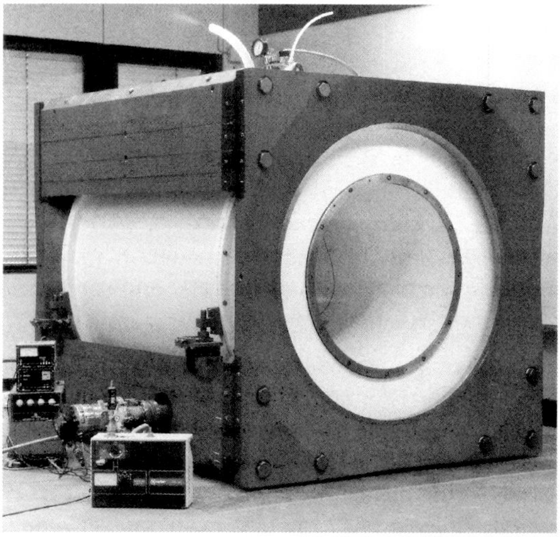

Fig. 10.10
1 T magnet with a
21 ton self shield

Shimming

Shimming is the elimination of constant field inhomogeneities originating from environmental influences and manufacturing imperfections.

The following technique is generally adopted: The field is measured using an MR probe on the surface of the spherical homogeneity volume, with expansion of the field according to spherical harmonics, followed by the determination of the expansion coefficients from measurement data and setting the corresponding currents for the shim coils, for which the windings are configured in such a manner that each generates a correction field closely approximating one expansion coefficient. Shimming is also possible by lining the bore surface or the external surface of the magnet with a suitable combination of iron plates.

Expansion by spherical harmonics

The characteristics of the magnetic field can be described by the Laplace equation:

$$\vec{\nabla}^2 \cdot (B_x, B_y, B_z) = 0. \tag{10.17}$$

As long as the field is sufficiently homogeneous, the field magnitude most important for the magnetic resonance frequency is equal to the field component $B_z = B_0$. The following spherical harmonic expansion is a solution of the Laplace equation in spherical coordinates, taking the center of the magnet as the origin:

$$B_0(r, \vartheta, \varphi) = \sum_{n=0}^{N} \sum_{m=0}^{M \leq N} \frac{r^n}{R^n} P_n^m(\cos \vartheta)[A_n^m \cos m\varphi + B_n^m \sin m\varphi]. \tag{10.18}$$

The coordinate system is illustrated in Fig. 10.2. The functions P_n^m are designated associated Legendre polynomials of the nth degree and mth order [10.7]. The coefficients A_n^m and B_n^m comprise the so-called spectrum of the spherical harmonic expansion. They are expressed either as absolute field units (in T) or as relative field deviations $(B(\vec{r}) - B_0/B_0$ (in ppm), each normalized to the radius R. The purpose of the spherical harmonics expansion is the evaluation of the spectrum from the field measurements across the surface of the sphere with radius R (analysis). Using the coefficients, the reverse is also possible; that is, calculation of the field at any point within the sphere (synthesis).

A simple interpretation of the expansion in spherical harmonics is possible for the special case of $m = 0$:

$$B_0(r, \vartheta) = \sum_{n=0}^{N} \frac{r^n}{R^n} P_n(\cos \vartheta)\, A_n^0. \tag{10.19}$$

On the surface of the sphere the field is not dependent upon the angle φ. The coefficients A_n^0 are also called zonal terms, while terms in which m is not equal to 0 are called tesseral terms. The P_n functions are Legendre polynomials of the nth degree. P_0 is the constant 1, so that the A_0^0 coefficient can be interpreted as the strength of the constant field without any perturbations and all other terms as perturbations. P_1 describes a linear change in the field in the z direction. A_1^0 is then the z gradient. The tesseral coefficients A_1^1 and B_1^1 correspond to the linear gradients in the x and y directions.

The factors $(r/R)^n$ show that for small radii substantial field perturbations are generated only by terms of low degree, while perturbations of higher degree are only effective at the edges of the spherical volume. The magnitudes of the coefficients decrease with increasing degree. For this reason, the expansion can be terminated beyond a certain degree.

Measurement and determination of shim coefficients

In order to calculate the spectral term of the nth degree and the mth order from measurement values, the field must be measured to $n+1$ circles parallel to the xy plane at $2m$ points. The sampling points are equidistant in ϑ and φ, i.e. the distances from the circles to the origin are on the order of $R \cos \varphi$. Field measurement is performed by using a small MR probe attached to a positioning gear, which allows the coordinates $r = R \sin \vartheta$ and $z = R \cos \vartheta$ to be adjusted. The field spectrum is calculated from the values acquired at the points of measurement.

Shimming with correction coils

Current-carrying windings are arranged on a cylindrical tube inside the magnet bore. The windings are configured so that the field of each partial winding corresponds exactly to one coefficient of the spherical harmonics expansion. Figure 10.11 shows the arrangement of the twelve windings for the terms which are usually compensated electrically. The cylindrical windings correspond to the zonal and saddle-shaped configuration of the tesseral coefficients. The higher the degree and order, the more complex and less effective the coil set becomes. The orthogonality of the spherical harmonics expansion corresponds to coil sets which are almost completely decoupled both from the SC coil and from each other. The linear gradients may not be activated on the shim coil, since they couple strongly with the pulsed gradients. They can therefore be eliminated and are compensated by offset currents from the pulsed gradient coil. The winding geometry of the coils determines the (non-linear) gradients generated per current unit. This value can also be determined experimentally: The spectrum of the magnet without shimming current and with a defined current level applied to one coil set is determined as described. The difference calculated from the two coefficient spectra should, ideally, have only one coefficient. This coefficient divided by the current results in the calibration factor for the corresponding shim coil. If all the factors are known, the magnet can be shimmed by setting the coil currents via a precision power supply.

Shimming with iron

One can also compensate for field inhomogeneity by mounting iron plates in the magnet bore or on the outside of the cryostat [10.8]. For each standard plate position one can determine, either by calculation or experiment, the field spectrum generated. The field spectra, of course, do not contain only one coefficient. It is practical that each position be located on a fixed grid. At such high field strengths, the iron plates are fully saturated, so that n number of plates will cause n times as much interference. Through varying the linear combi-

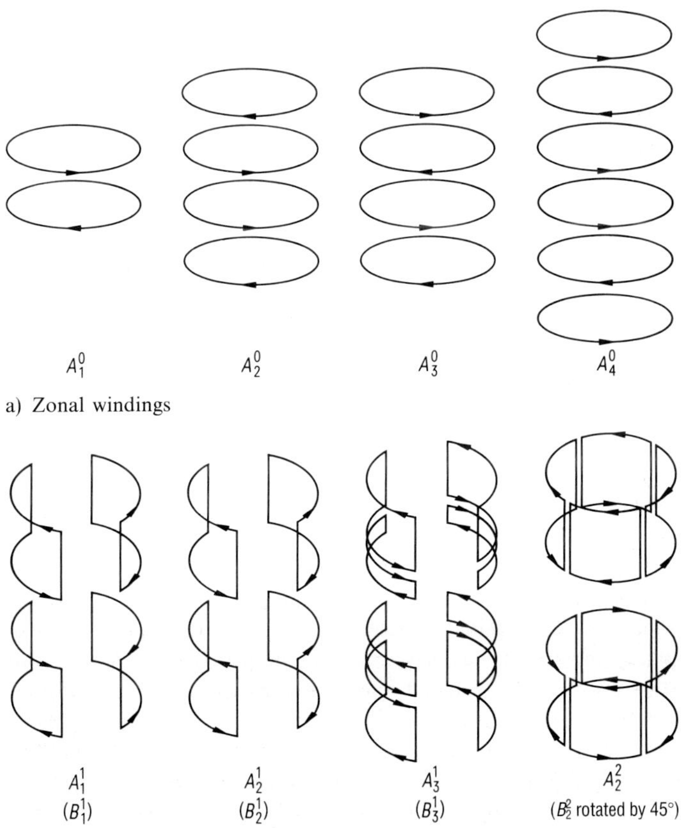

Fig. 10.11 Schematic drawing of shim coil windings

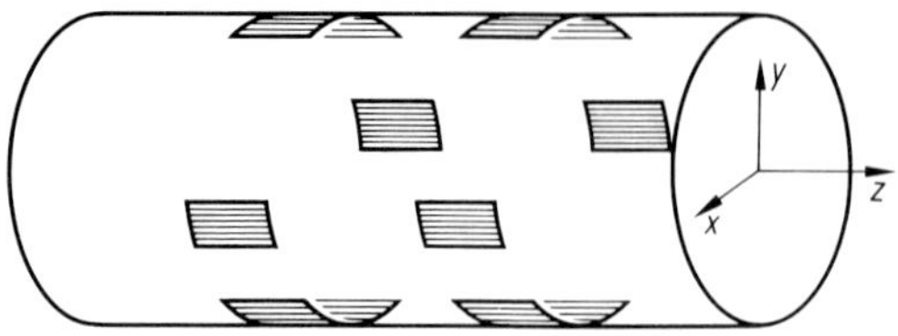

Fig. 10.12
Positioning of iron plates (passive shim) of the A_4^4 Term

nation of the different spectra corresponding to the various positions of the iron plates, one can establish a plate geometry that will compensate for the inhomogeneity of the magnet. This procedure can also be used with a magnet that is already electrically pre-shimmed.

Shimming with iron has the great advantage that the number of possible degrees of freedom, and therefore the degree and the order of the shimmable terms, is substantially higher than with electric shimming coils. A typical example is the compensation of the A_4^4 term, which is reasonably large in magnets with self-shielding (see Fig. 10.10) and which can be eliminated with passive shimming (Fig. 10.12). An added advantage is the reduced power consumption. When one dispenses with electrical shimming, the complex coils and the precision shim current regulator are eliminated and, along with them, a potential source of field instability. The main disadvantages of iron plate shimming: Retrofitting is extensive and time consuming. For spectroscopic application, this means that an additional correction coil system is usually necessary. Additionally, the iron mass per position is quantized and cannot be negative. These restrictions must be taken into consideration when writing a program for positioning the iron plates.

10.2.2 Gradient system

Criteria for required gradient field strength

As in the discussion of optimal field strength, the question arises here regarding the extent to which the maximum available gradient strengths influence attainable image quality. Here, too, the answer is not immediately obvious, since the dependencies which must be taken into consideration are quite complex. Since expenditures for a gradient system increase considerably with the maximum obtainable gradient strength and technological limits are quickly reached, practical compromises must be found here as well. The major parameters of immediate interest are the contrast/noise ratio ($\Delta S/N$) and the desired spatial resolution. $\Delta S/N$ at a constant spatial resolution is dependent only on the length of the pulse sequence time intervals [10.9]. If these are set for an optimal S/N ratio, the gradients necessary for a certain spatial resolution are defined.

Pulse sequence time intervals

Since the design of a pulse sequence can be very flexible and there is a great range of variation in contrast which is influenced by the relaxation times T_1 and T_2 and the spin density of the subject, the optimization procedure can only be achieved through the use of several examples. The T_2 relaxation time plays an essential role.

The MR image contrast between two adjacent materials excited by 90° pulses can be approximately described by the following proportionality (see section 5.2.4):

$$\Delta S \sim \varrho' e^{-T_e/T_2'}(1-e^{-T_r/T_1'}) - \varrho'' e^{-T_e/T_2''}(1-e^{-T_r/T_1''}) \tag{10.20}$$

T_e represents the time between excitation and readout of the MR signal (echo time) and T_r the repetition time of the pulse sequence. Prerequisite to the approximation are short pulse (T_r) and sampling (T_s) and echo (T_e) times, respectively ($T_e \ll T_1$, $T_p \ll T_2$, $T_s \ll T_2$) and a long repetition time ($T_r \gg T_2$) in comparison to the relaxation times. Image noise (N), on the other hand, is inversely proportional to the square root of T_s:

$$N \sim 1/\sqrt{T_s}. \tag{10.21}$$

The relationship between T_e and T_s is dependent upon the form of the pulse sequence. For spin-echo sequences capable of probing multiple slices (often

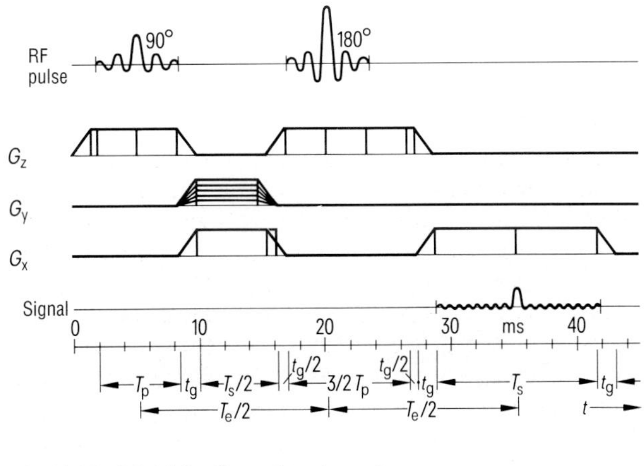

Fig. 10.13 Multiple slice spin-echo pulse sequence

used in practice) having one selective 90° and 180° pulse of the same length T_p (Fig. 10.13), T_e is:

$$T_e = T_s + 2\,T_p + 3\,t_g \tag{10.22}$$

(t_g is the rise and fall time of the gradients, which must be less than $T_s/2$), so that the noise is given by:

$$N \sim 1/\sqrt{T_e - 2\,T_p - 3\,t_g}. \tag{10.23}$$

Using the above formulas (10.20 and 10.23) ΔS/N can then be calculated as a function of T_e for various pairs of materials. Figure 10.14 illustrates a few examples; tissue parameters are taken from the literature [10.10].

It can be seen from the graph that the ΔS/N maximum lies at a rather long readout time and, consequently, at long echo times in relation to T_2. If the pulse time (or the sum $2\,T_p + 3\,t_g$) is added as an additional parameter, this results in ΔS/N curves such as those in Fig. 10.15. Shortening the quasi-parasitic T_p and t_g times yields a substantial improvement in MR image contrast.

There are additional limiting factors to be considered in the selection of sequence times:

On the one hand, due to the shifts between fat and water portions in the MR image and the constant field inhomogeneity, it is impractical to select

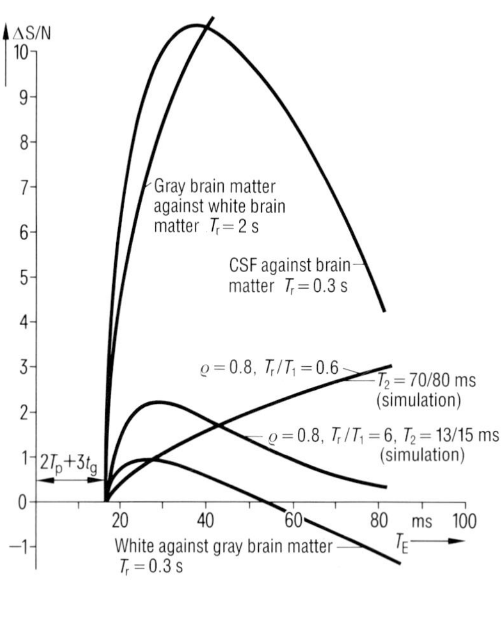

Fig. 10.14 Contrast/noise ratio as a function of echo time for gray and white brain matter at different pulse times

too small a receiving bandwidth, and therefore a T_s time which is too long. An acceptable compromise is to allow a fat/water shift equal to the pixel size, Δx.

Because

$$\delta x = \delta B_0 / G_x \quad \text{and} \quad \Delta x = \frac{2\pi}{\gamma G_x T_s} \tag{10.24}$$

the following is true for the data acquisition interval with $\delta x = \Delta x$:

$$T_s = \frac{2\pi}{\delta \gamma B_0}. \tag{10.25}$$

For a constant field strength of 1 T the readout interval is approximately 7.8 ms.

Another factor preventing an arbitrary decrease in pulse time is the fact that such a decrease causes a quadratic increase in the peak pulse power and therefore (if the pulse repetition rate is constant) a linear increase in power dissipation in the patient. As a compromise between the conflicting requirements of a short T_p, limited RF output and the sharpness of the slice profile, an (effective) pulse band width, $\Delta\omega_p/2\pi$, of approximately 0.8 kHz is chosen for the selective 90° pulse. In general a weighted sinc-pulse (see Section 5.2.2) with a length of at least twice the reciprocal bandwidth is used. This results in pulse lengths

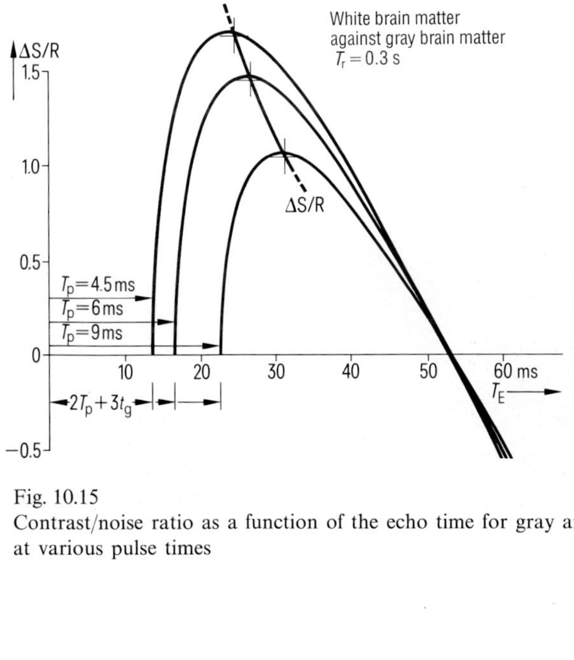

Fig. 10.15
Contrast/noise ratio as a function of the echo time for gray and white brain matter at various pulse times

of at least 2.5 ms. After the pulse sequence time intervals have been determined, the necessary gradients are calculated from the desired spatial resolution in readout, phase encoding and slice select direction as follows:

$$\Delta x = \frac{2\pi}{\gamma G_x T_s}, \quad \Delta y = \frac{2\pi}{\gamma G_y T_s}, \quad \Delta z = \frac{\Delta\omega_p}{\gamma G_z}. \tag{10.26}$$

At a minimum slice thickness of 3 mm or a pixel size of 0.5 mm, a maximum gradient of approximately 6 mT/m is required for a 1 T constant field under the above conditions. If the condition $\delta x = \Delta x$ is to be maintained at higher field strengths, or if even finer spatial resolution is desired, correspondingly larger field gradients are required.

Several of the special imaging procedures, such as flow refocussing, can also be implemented only when relatively high gradient field strengths are available.

Gradient coil

In principle the gradient coil set exhibits the same design as the shim coils of the first order. The dimensions of the winding, however, are adapted to the different requirements, namely high gradients and short switching times. High efficiency precludes the coil set's large linearity volume and free choice of diameter. The required number of ampere turns per gradient increases, taking into account the eddy currents generated in the cryo-shield, by the 4th or 5th

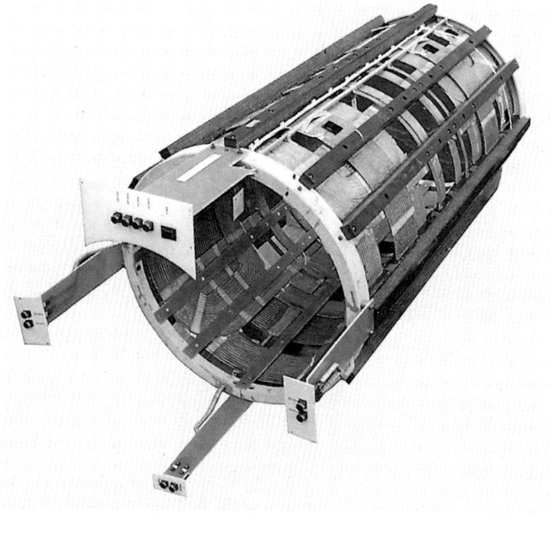

Fig. 10.16
Gradient coil system with 72 cm diameter for 6 mT/m at 100 A

power of the coil radius. A coil with a large number of windings requires less current. Such a coil shows, however, considerably more inductance and requires a correspondingly high voltage to switch the gradient fields in as short a time as possible. Figure 10.16 shows a gradient coil system having a 72 cm diameter, which generates a field of approximately 6 mT/m at 100 A.

Pulsed gradient power supply

The function of the gradient power supply is to generate current pulses of the correct amplitude and duration which correspond to the commands programmed in the pulse sequence controller. The currents required, including eddy current compensation (see section on effects of eddy currents), are 120 to 150 A. Since the gradient switching times are detrimental to the pulse sequence and should therefore be kept as short as possible, current increase rates of 150 kA/s are necessary. The inductive load requires a correspondingly high output voltage. Powerful amplifiers are required for this function alone. In addition, the power supply must be extremely precise and function with little ripple or noise. As described in Section 5.2.3, the gradient strength as a function of time directly determines the location of the sampled point in the spatial frequency domain (k space). The sampling error is the integrated time function of the gradient amplitude error from one sampling point to another. The sampling error, δk, is easily calculated for a sinusoidal gradient ripple of amplitude δG_{b}. Any other modulation can be expanded into a sum of sinusoidal modulations. The greatest sampling error occurs when the phase 0 or π coincides with the sampling time. It is then:

$$\begin{aligned}\delta k &= \delta G_{\mathrm{b}}\,\gamma \int_0^{\Delta t_{\mathrm{s}}} \sin \omega_3\, t'\,\mathrm{d}t' \\ &= 2\delta G_{\mathrm{b}}\,\gamma \int_0^{\Delta t_{\mathrm{s}}/2} \cos \omega_{\mathrm{b}}\, t'\,\mathrm{d}t' \\ &= \frac{2}{\omega_{\mathrm{b}}}\,\delta G_{\mathrm{b}}\,\gamma \sin \frac{1}{2}\,\omega_{\mathrm{b}}\,\Delta t_{\mathrm{s}}. \end{aligned} \tag{10.27}$$

One can see that the sampling error disappears regardless of the phase when the ripple frequency is a multiple of the sampling frequency. Figure 10.17 shows the frequency-dependent limit curve for the permissible relative gradient interference amplitudes for each sampling error relative to the sampling interval. Simulations show that this should be less than 1% for incoherent and 0.2% for coherent (with respect to the sampling interval, Δk) gradient modulations and that these levels may not be exceeded if visible artifacts are to be avoided. This applies to the readout gradients as well as to the phase encoding gradients, as can be seen from the equivalence of $\Delta t_{\mathrm{s}} \cdot G_{\mathrm{x}}$ and $\Delta G_{\mathrm{y}} \cdot T_{\mathrm{s}}/2$.

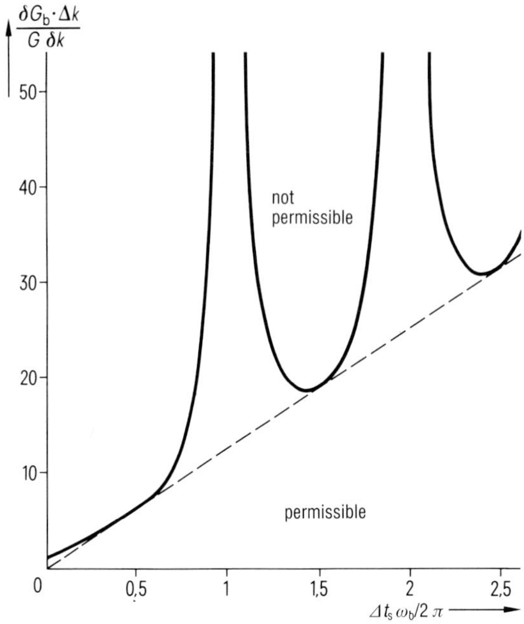

Fig. 10.17
Permissible gradient field ripple as a function of the ripple frequency

The reciprocal time between the RF pulses can be designated as the lowest ripple frequency that must be considered, since slower periodic interferences across a sampling line for all practical purposes cause a constant shift in the k space, for which

$$\frac{\delta G}{\Delta G} \leq \frac{\delta k}{\Delta k}. \tag{10.28}$$

Here, $\Delta G = G/N$, with an image matrix size of N is required. This is identical to the necessary reproducibility for the gradient amplitude.

For a field of view of 50 cm and a readout time of 8 ms, ΔG has the value 12 µT/m. For incoherent, low-frequency fluctuations of the gradient strength, 0.12 µT/m or 20 ppm of the maximum gradient strength of 6 mT/m or of the coil current is permissible.

For slice positions which do not pass through the center of the magnet, an instable gradient field has the same effect as a fluctuation of the constant field:

$$\delta B_0(t) = z\,\delta G_z(t). \tag{10.29}$$

The limits for this were formulated in Section 10.2.1.

As expected the resulting stability requirements are comparable to those discussed above.

Current amplifiers having a linear final stage or a switch-mode final stage operating at a relatively high frequency are used to comply with the required output specifications (Fig. 10.18). The gradient pulse, which is in digital form, is converted to an appropriate voltage pulse via a digital-to-analog converter (DAC). This pulse is predistorted using a high-pass filter which, in general, comprises multiple time constants in order to compensate for the field pulse distortion due to the cryo-shield eddy currents (see next section). The driver amplifier and the final stage follow, both powered by a high output bi-polar DC power supply. All the components in the amplifier chain must meet the stringent requirements mentioned above.

The regulator circuitry is particularly critical, since it is essential that this is not prone to oscillations, despite the required level of precision and a large bandwidth (≈ 1 kHz). It must be able to stabilize oscillating counter-EMF voltages resulting from the mechanical vibrations of the gradient coil in the constant field, as well as ripple caused by the DC power supply. The fundamental difference between linear amplifiers and switching amplifiers lies in the control over the final stage: The linear amplifier is directly driven by the analog signal, whereas a so-called modulator is connected just prior to the final stage of the switched amplifier. The modulator converts the control voltage into a rapid series of rectangular switching pulses having a pulse duty factor proportional to the desired output current. The current flows through the gradient coils via diodes during the "off" phase and falls off with the time constant, L/R. The frequency of the pulse signal must be significantly higher than R/L, in order that the current ripple remain sufficiently small. In addition, higher frequency ripple causes less interference.

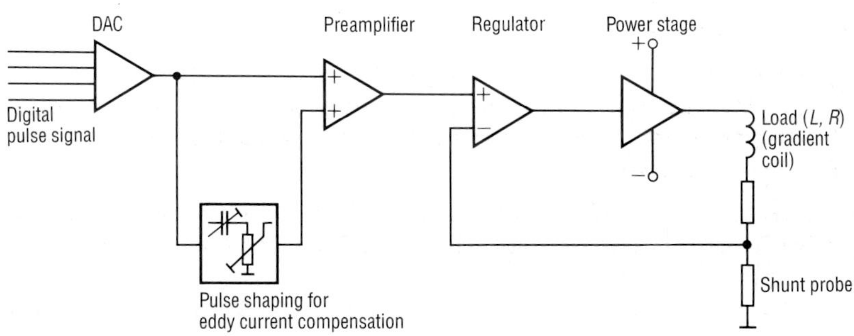

Fig. 10.18 Block circuit diagram of a gradient amplifier

The switching amplifier has several advantages over the linear final stage that make its use worth the extra technological effort. The power dissipation of the final stage, and therefore energy usage and cooling effort, is significantly lower. In the linear final stage the full supply voltage is present between the collector and the emitter of the output transistors after the gradient coil has been excited to the programmed current level; with the switching amplifier there is only the saturation voltage. The power supply in this case needs to supply power to compensate for losses in the coil and the cables only. As can be seen in Fig. 10.13, the excitation and de-energization of the gradient field is accomplished in exactly defined time periods. The power transistors in a linear controller must withstand a high counter-EMF voltage at high currents during the fall time. Diodes cannot take over the induced voltage in this case, because this would lead to current-dependent switching times. The effective switching times of the output transistors in a switching amplifier, on the other hand, are only about 1 μs. Inductive voltages can be handled by diodes, since transients are irrelevant in relation to the effective current through the gradient coil. This technology therefore allows for substantially more compact and powerful amplifiers.

Eddy current effects

Since the tradient coils are surrounded concentrically by the cryostat, as shown in Fig. 10.1, the magnetic flux in the cryoshields changes when the coil current is changed. This leads to the formation of eddy currents which counteract the field changes according to Lenz's law, as demonstrated for the *Z*-gradient in Fig. 10.19. Since the eddy current distribution, especially in the radial direction, differs from the coil current distribution, the spatial dependence of the eddy current field is different from that of the coil field. This must be taken into consideration when calculating the design of the coil, in order to avoid dynamic gradient non-linearity. Eddy currents increase with increasing coil current. As soon as the coil current has reached a constant value, the eddy current begins to decay. This can be closely approximated using an exponential function with

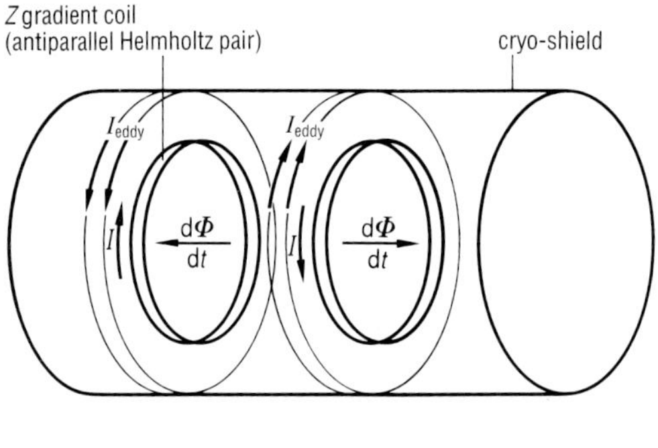

Fig. 10.19
Eddy currents generated by a pulsed gradient field

a time constant determined by the conductivity and the effective inductance of the cryo-shield. As the field penetrates through the first shield, eddy currents are induced in the outer shield and possibly in the superconducting coil itself. This leads to a complex distribution of eddy currents, in turn resulting in a gradient counter-field. For the rise times of approximately 1 ms considered here, the initial strength of the eddy current (and therefore the weakening effect on the field) is determined solely by the geometry of the coils and the innermost shield, i.e. by their inductive coupling. For the most part, only the ratio of diameters has to be taken into consideration, while the conductivity of the shield is practically irrelevant.

The gradient field increases as the eddy currents decay (Fig. 10.20a) and also changes in regard to its spatial dependence. This dynamic change in field distribution, which can be as much as a few percent of the eddy current field, cannot be compensated for by a modification of the current pulse form. This means that the conductivity of the innermost shield of the cryostat should be relatively high, so that the eddy current time constants are significantly longer than the length of the gradient pulses normally used. Such a time/space dependency of the gradient field makes it impossible to reconstruct an image exactly from the measurement data with the help of a Fourier transformation and can lead to image degradation. In addition, good conductivity reduces heat generation in the shield and prevents the boil-off rate for the nitrogen and helium from rising.

In addition to spatial changes in the field, the eddy current field has the same effect on the gradient pulse sequence as a low-pass filter. The inclusion of an adjustable high-pass filter in the gradient amplifier distorts the shape of the pulse in such a way that the desired gradient pulse shape is re-established (see Fig. 10.0b).

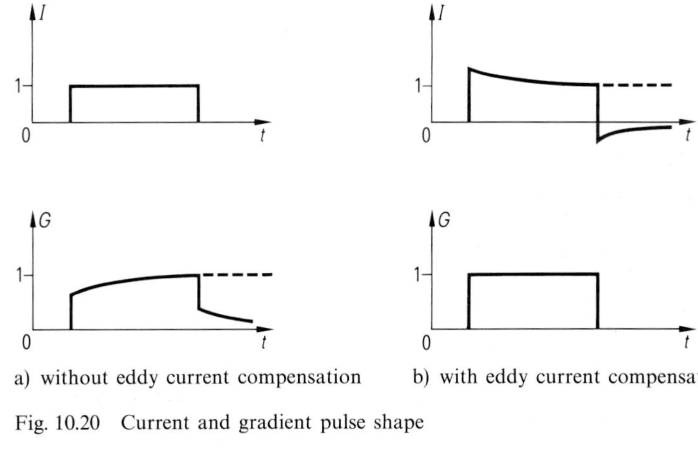

a) without eddy current compensation b) with eddy current compensation

Fig. 10.20 Current and gradient pulse shape

There are several aspects to the importance of exact eddy current compensation. A short discussion of the most important of these follows.

Equidistant sampling points in the spatial frequency domain (k space)

The same considerations apply here as were presented for the specifications of gradient amplifier stability. It follows at once from

$$k=\gamma\int_{0}^{t} G(t')\,\mathrm{d}t' \quad \text{or} \quad \Delta k=\gamma\int_{t_s}^{t+\Delta t_s} G(t')\,\mathrm{d}t' \tag{10.30}$$

that the gradient must be constant during the readout of the MR signal in equidistant time steps, Δt_s, so that the spatial frequency domain is evenly sampled. The same applies to the slice selection method with frequency selective excitation pulses in the gradient field.

Refocussing in selection Gradients

As explained in section 5.2.2, a gradient pulse of appropriate length and amplitude must make up for the phase dispersion of nuclear magnetization in the slice direction after an excitation pulse. Improper refocussing across the slice leads to signal loss, since only magnetization parallel to the direction of magnetization at the center of the slice contributes constructively to the signal. This is illustrated in Fig. 10.21.

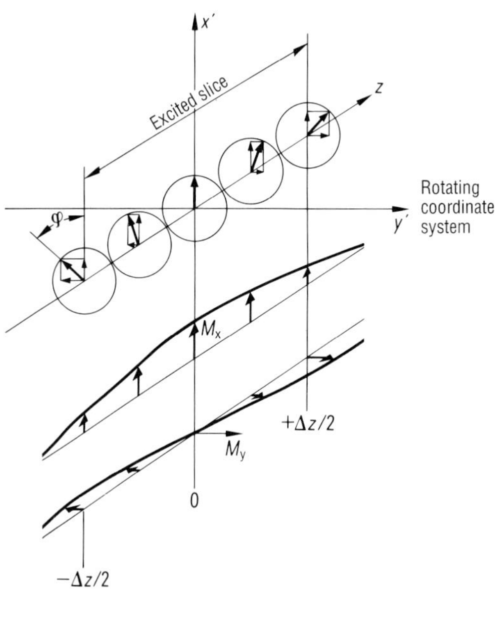

Fig. 10.21
Phase dispersion of magnetization across the slice due to incomplete refocussing

The phase angle in the slice direction is:

$$\varphi(z) = z\gamma \int G_z(t)\,\mathrm{d}t = z\Delta k_z. \tag{10.31}$$

Integration limits for a pulse sequence without a 180° pulse extend from the center of an excitation pulse to the readout interval. This also applies to spin echoes, but the time integrals before and after the center of the 180° pulse must be added together with opposite signs. Since the expression for the signal across the slice behaves as $\cos\varphi(z)$, the relative signal loss as a function of Δk_z is:

$$\frac{S}{S_{\max}} = \frac{2}{\Delta z} \int_0^{\Delta z/2} \cos \Delta k_z z\,\mathrm{d}z = \mathrm{sinc}(\tfrac{1}{2}\Delta z \Delta k_z). \tag{10.32}$$

Since the pulse sequence programs are written independently of the system, with the length of the refocussing gradient pulse just equal to 0.5 T_p (apart from a small correction for the rise time, t_g) (Fig. 10.13), a trapezoidal gradient pulse form must be assured via correct eddy current adjustment. This is necessary to achieve $\Delta k_z = 0$, i.e. an optimal signal/noise ratio.

It should be mentioned that the potential problems caused by eddy currents can be eliminated, at least partially, by so-called active shielding; that is, an external, opposed winding similar to the shielding of the fringe field for a magnet [10.11]. In principle, the active shield is a second set of gradient coils mounted concentrically on a cylinder of a larger radius. The windings are connected in series electrically opposite to the direction of their corresponding field windings. Their dimensions are such that flux changes at the cryo-shield (and as a result the eddy currents) during current changes are kept to a minimum. At the same time the useful gradient amplitude is reduced, since the shield coil field is superimposed on the field of the inner coil. The size and weight of this configuration are also disadvantages. Ohmic loss is disproportionately high, because the necessary degree of efficiency can only be obtained by raising the number of ampere turns and because the power dissipation of the shield winding must also be taken into account.

10.2.3 RF system

Transmit and receive system

The RF electronics of an MR system are designed to generate the pulsed RF output required to excite magnetic resonance and to prepare the signals picked up by the antenna for the image processor. The signal paths are illustrated in Fig. 10.22.

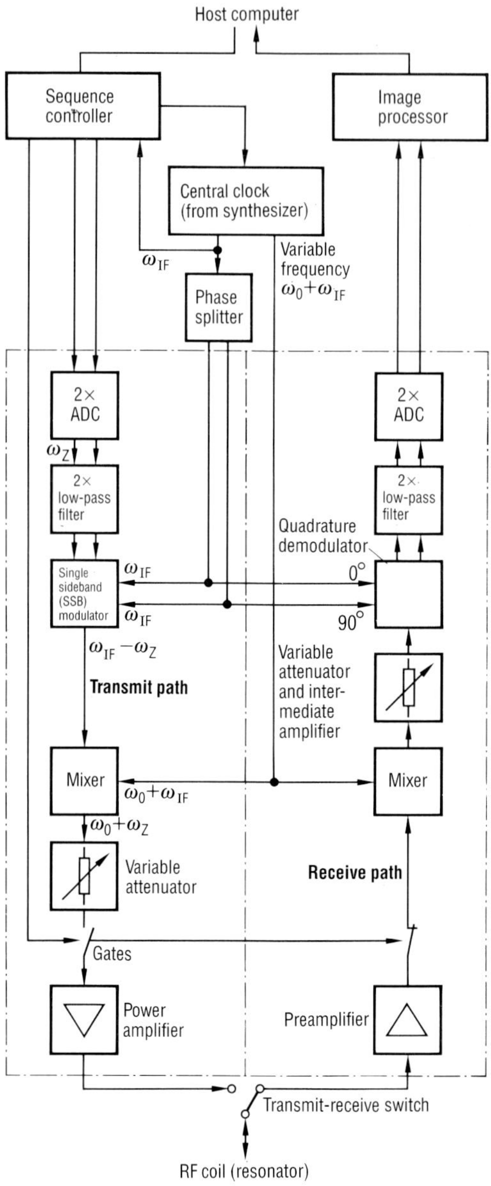

Fig. 10.22
Circuit diagram of the RF System

Transmit path

The RF pulses required for magnetic resonance are supplied digitally as a series of complex numbers by the sequence controller. The magnitude of a complex numerical value represents the momentary amplitude and the phase determines the direction of the B_1 field in the rotating frame. The series of complex numbers is converted to low-frequency voltage pulses by two digital-to-analog converters (DACs). The bandwidth and the length of the programmed pulse form are determined by the sample clock and the number of data points. The signals are fed into the modulator via two low-pass filters, which suppress the undesirable harmonics caused by the digital generation of the pulse.

Modulator

The function of the modulator corresponds to the transformation from the rotating frame to the laboratory frame. It multiplies the complex pulse form (the low frequency signal), $\mathcal{F}(t)$, by the complex carrier signal, $e^{i\omega_0 t}$ (Fig. 10.23 a). The real part of the product appears at the output of the modulator:

$$\mathrm{Re}[\mathcal{F}(t)\,e^{i\omega_0 t}] = \mathrm{Re}[\mathcal{F}(t)]\cos\omega_0 t - \mathrm{Im}[\mathcal{F}(t)]\sin\omega_0 t. \qquad (10.33)$$

If the low-frequency signal is:

$$\cos(\omega_z t + \varphi) + i\sin(\omega_z t + \varphi) = e^{i(\omega_z t + \varphi)},$$

the output signal is:

$$\mathrm{Re}[e^{i(\omega_0 t + \omega_z t + \varphi)}] = \cos[\omega_0 t + \omega_z t + \varphi).$$

By introducing the factor $e^{i(\omega_z t + \varphi)}$ into the low-frequency pulse signal, the frequency and phase of the high frequency excitation pulse can be shifted as

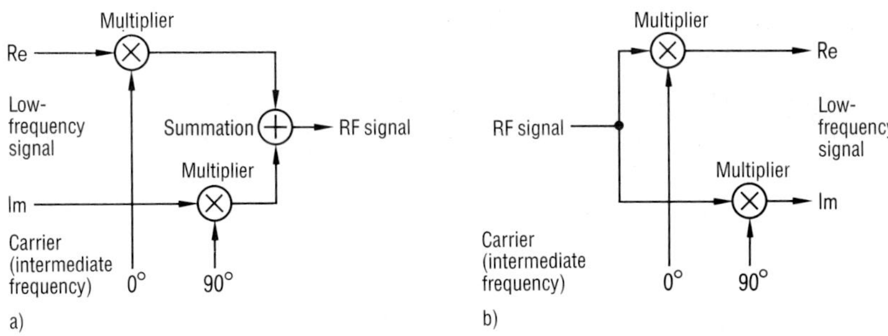

Fig. 10.23 Single sideband modulator (a) and quadrature demodulator (b)

desired. When feeding the modulator with $e^{i\omega_z t}$ only one frequency, $\omega_0+\omega_z$, appears at the output. Since the carrier frequency, ω_0, as well as the mirror frequency, $\omega_0-\omega_z$, are suppressed, the configuration is referred to as a single side-band modulator (SSB) [10.12].

Programming a frequency offset is a simple method of achieving a shift, z, of the slice excited with the help of a selective pulse while the gradient, G_z, is switched on:

$$z=\omega_z/(\gamma G_z). \tag{10.34}$$

The modulator is composed of a pair of ring mixers, supplied with the carrier signals shifted in phase by 0° or 90°. The most important characteristics are the linearity (i.e., the absence of spurious signals and harmonics), which determines the fidelity of the pulse shape, and the suppression of carrier and unwanted sideband signals. Insufficient suppression of undesirable frequencies results in magnetic resonance excitation at locations other than the slice selected and therefore leads to artifacts. A constant DC voltage on the low-frequency side generates a carrier signal at the modulator output. A signal from the unwanted sideband is generated if the two ring mixers are not precisely balanced or when the carrier signals are not shifted in phase by exactly 90°.

A single sideband modulator possessing good side-band suppression and carrier attenuation is best realized at sufficiently narrow frequency ranges. An intermediate frequency is used as a carrier, so that it is not necessary to have a different modulator for each type of nucleus or each variation in field strength. The mixer, coupled at the output side of the modulator, generates the pulse signal at a center frequency, ω_0, for the corresponding MR frequency. Transmission output is regulated for the differing B_1 field strength requirements using adjustable, variable attenuators. A gate circuit inhibits the transmit path while the system is in the receive mode. This prevents the noise and the carrier signal generated by the modulator from reaching the receiver circuitry via the power stage and interfering with the weak MR signal.

RF power transmitter

The RF final stage must amplify the pulse so that a (rotating) B_1 field is generated in the subject surrounded by the resonator. This field must fulfill the following requirements:

$$B_1=\frac{\alpha}{\gamma t_p} \tag{10.35}$$

α = Flip angle of magnetization
t_p = effective time for the B_1 field

If the RF field is linearly polarized, twice the B_1 amplitude is required for the same flip angle. Power is required because there are losses in the object being measured, as well as in the resonator and its connecting lines. For a cylinder with its axis parallel to the constant field and therefore perpendicular to the B_1 field, the power required to generate a given B_1 field can be approximated as follows:

$$P_{\text{sample}} = \frac{\pi}{512}\,\omega_0^2\,\sigma B_1^2\left[D^4 l + \tfrac{4}{3} D^2 l^3\right]. \tag{10.36}$$

If one assumes the following values, for example: Cylinder dimensions: $D = l = 40$ cm, conductivity $\sigma = 0.5/\Omega$m (equivalent to a physiological saline solution), flip angle = 180° with an effective time of $t_p = 1.0$ ms, thus resulting in a linearly oscillating field $B_1 = 23.5\,\mu$T and a center frequency $\omega_0 = 2\pi \cdot 42.576$ MHz, then P_{sample} is approximately 2.8 kW. Under experimental conditions using a patient of average weight (approximately 80 kg), 1.3 kW of power can be measured at the input of the antenna. As was determined by the measurement of loaded and unloaded Q, (Eq. 10.8 in Sect. 10.2.1) approximately 20% of this is lost in the resonator. Only slightly more than 1 kW will therefore be absorbed by the patient; the cylindrical model is therefore too pessimistic. This can be explained by the inhomogeneity of conductivity and the shape of the human body. The cables and components of the transmit/receive switch attenuate the RF output by approximately 1 dB. The final stage, therefore, must be able to provide 2 kW of pulse power. The final stage at 42 MHz is designed for 8 kW, so that shorter pulses are possible and so that there is some reserve power to compensate for the greater degree of attenuation caused by heavier patients. The 63 MHz final stage is designed for a pulse output of 15 kW to allow for the rise in loss, proportional to ω_0^2, within the measured object.

The average available output power may be considerably lower than the above. Output power is basically governed by local regulations for medical equipment and by how much the patient's safety will be affected by the specific rate of absorption. Thermal dimensioning and the power supply for the final stage are designed for the continuous output power needs, while the energy for a high-output pulse or series of pulses is taken from a buffer storage device, such as a capacitor battery, which is recharged during off times. Figure 10.24 shows the operating range of the transmitter between the pulse period and the continuous output power limits. The pulse duty factor and pulse output are approximately inversely proportional to one another over the operating range. The position of this range in the diagram marks the storage capacity.

Power amplifiers with these characteristics are equipped with tubes, since these are less sensitive to short-term overloads and are less expensive. The output circuit is tuned to the resonance frequency and is simultaneously the primary

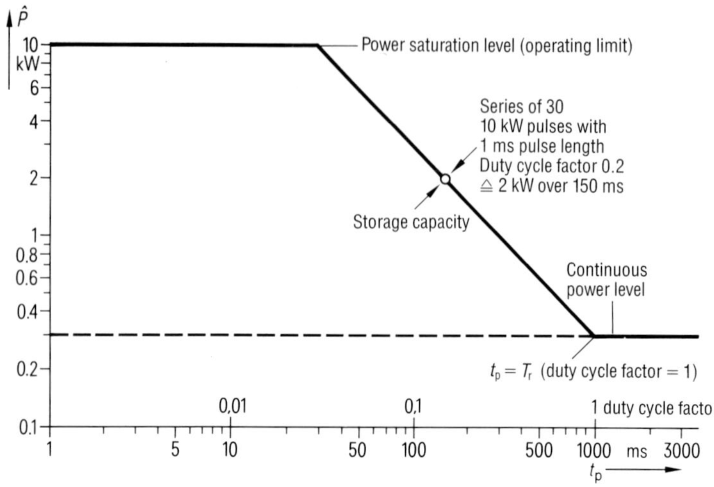

Fig. 10.24 Effective operating range of the pulsed RF final stage

side of the output transformer, which matches the final stage to the line impedance. Final stages are biased as Class C, i.e. without quiescent current when no input signals are present, as well as in the pulsed Class A (quiescent current equal to half of the maximum current during the transmit phase). The Class-C mode is characterized by an efficiency of nearly 1, but the RF output voltage is not proportional to the input voltage. This can be compensated for by pre-distorting the amplitude of the pulse shape, $|\mathscr{F}(t)|$. When using pulsed Class A operation, the power supply must generate power independently of the RF amplitude during the entire transmit phase; i.e., the amount of power dissipated is relatively high, especially for amplitude-modulated pulses. On the other hand, amplitude correction (pre-distorting) may not be necessary. The gain during the receive intervals for both modes is minimal, so that noise from the modulator, mixer and driver amplifier is largely suppressed.

Receive path

The receiving channel is shown in the right half of Figure 10.22. The MR signals are received by the receiver coil and then amplified to a sufficient level by the preamplifier, so that line attenuation and input noise from the following stage is negligible. The frequencies received from the coil are approximately the nuclear resonance frequency, ω_0. This band of frequencies is then translated by the mixer to an intermediate frequency range, so that a standard attenuator/demodulator assembly can be used regardless of the type of nucleus or the constant field strength.

Demodulator

The function of the demodulator is complementary to that of the modulator, namely the transformation of the laboratory coordinate system into the coordinate system that rotates with ω_0. The input voltage represents the transverse magnetization as

$$M_x \cos \omega_0 t + M_y \sin \omega_0 t, \tag{10.37}$$

where

$$M_x + iM_y = M_\perp \, e^{i(\omega_0 t + \varphi)}$$

and

$M_\perp$ = Magnitude of magnetization
φ = Phase of magnetization.

The demodulator multiplies (see Fig. 10.23b) the complex carrier signal by the input signal as follows:

$$\begin{aligned}(M_x \cos \omega_0 t + M_y \sin \omega_0 t) \cos \omega_0 t &= \tfrac{1}{2} M_x + \tfrac{1}{2} M_x \cos 2\omega_0 t - \\ &\quad - \tfrac{1}{2} M_y \sin 2\omega_0 t \\ (M_x \cos \omega_0 t + M_y \sin \omega_0 t) \sin \omega_0 t &= \tfrac{1}{2} M_y - \tfrac{1}{2} M_x \sin 2\omega_0 t + \\ &\quad + \tfrac{1}{2} M_y \cos 2\omega_0 t. \end{aligned} \tag{10.38}$$

With the exception of terms having twice the carrier frequency, signals representing the M_x and M_y components of the nuclear magnetization reach both outputs. This type of circuit is called a quadrature demodulator. Since it can distinguish between frequencies greater and smaller than ω_0 (upper and lower side bands) the output bandwidth is half of the input bandwidth. This improves the signal-to-noise ratio by $\sqrt{2}$ in comparison to simple phase-sensitive rectifiers [10.13], which can represent only one component (M_x or M_y). In addition, only half the conversion rate is necessary for the analog-to-digital conversion. On the other hand, there must be two of each of the components following the demodulator. Output signals are transmitted through a pair of low-pass filters which cut off all frequencies exceeding half the sampling frequency (the Nyquist frequency). The two ADCs then convert these into a sequence of complex numbers suitable for processing by computer.

The frequency responses and the phases of the ring mixers, filters and ADCs must be in exactly equal pairs, and the two carrier signals for the quadrature demodulator must be shifted by exactly 90°. If these conditions are not met, the result will be artifacts, such as mirror images, corresponding to the incomplete separation of the upper and lower side bands.

Signal levels

In order to specify the necessary total gain and dynamic range; i.e., the operating limit divided by the noise level, the expected signal-to-noise ratio and input voltage at the preamplifier must be known. Prognoses, however, as discussed in the section on pulse output, are only valid within limits, because the human body can not be described by a simple mathematical model. It is also not possible to calculate coil characteristics exactly. One must rely on the results of empirical studies. If the antenna impedance is always matched to the actual line impedance, R_L (50 Ω), via tunable circuits, the noise voltage at the input of the preamplifier (input impedance Z_i) is always the same, regardless of the coil load.

$$U_N = \frac{|Z_i|}{R_L + |Z_i|} \left(4kTR_L \frac{\Delta\omega_s}{2\pi} \cdot 10^{F/10\,\mathrm{dB}}\right)^{1/2}, \tag{10.39}$$

where F is the noise figure of the preamplifier in dB.

The total gain of the receive channel is given by the gain of the individual components minus the attenuation values of both the attenuator and the cables. The antenna and preamplifier noise, which is dependent upon the input bandwidth $\Delta\omega_s = \pi/\Delta t_s$, should be sufficiently higher than the frequency-independent ADC quantization noise. For the smallest commonly used bandwidth the gain must be greater than:

$$\frac{U_0}{U_i} > \frac{1}{\sqrt{12}} \frac{U_{LSB}}{U_N} \tag{10.40}$$

(see level plan, Fig. 10.25).

The amplitude of a useful signal depends largely on the type of MR experiment performed, especially on the volume excited. Several typical results for $\omega_0/2\pi = 63$ MHz are shown in Fig. 10.25. The dynamic range of the MR signal is substantially higher than 100 dB, especially for non-selective excitation. This means that the S/N gain resulting from the excitation of a large volume (e.g., for three-dimensional imaging) cannot be fully realized in any case with conventional 16-bit ADCs. It is then obvious that the dynamic range of all the components in the receive branch should not be smaller than that of the ADC. The adaptability of the preamplifier as well as the variable attenuation elements in the intermediate amplifier also allow the processing of high input signals, such as found when dealing with thick slices and non-selective excitation. This can be performed without overloading the ADC or the output of the preamplifier.

Transmit/receive switch

The transmit/receive switch is the link between the RF resonator and the RF pulse transmitter or the preamplifier. It must enable the path from the transmitter to the antenna during the RF pulse and at the same time protect the sensitive preamplifier from the high pulse power. In the receive mode the weak MR signal must reach the preamplifier with as little attenuation as possible, and the noise of the final stage must be excluded from the antenna circuit. Figure 10.26 shows a simplified wiring diagram of the switch, which automatically toggles between transmit and receive without additional control circuitry. The anti-parallel pair of diodes in the transmit cable does not conduct during the receive mode and prevents noise generated by the power section from reaching the preamplifier, as well as preventing the MR signal from disappearing in the transmitter. In the transmit mode, the voltages are high enough to switch on the diodes, so that the power reaches the antenna (resonator) with practically no loss. The pair of diodes at the preamplifier input also conducts. The $\lambda/4$ cable connected in front of the diodes transforms the short circuit to a high impedance at the input of the antenna. In the receive mode, the impedance

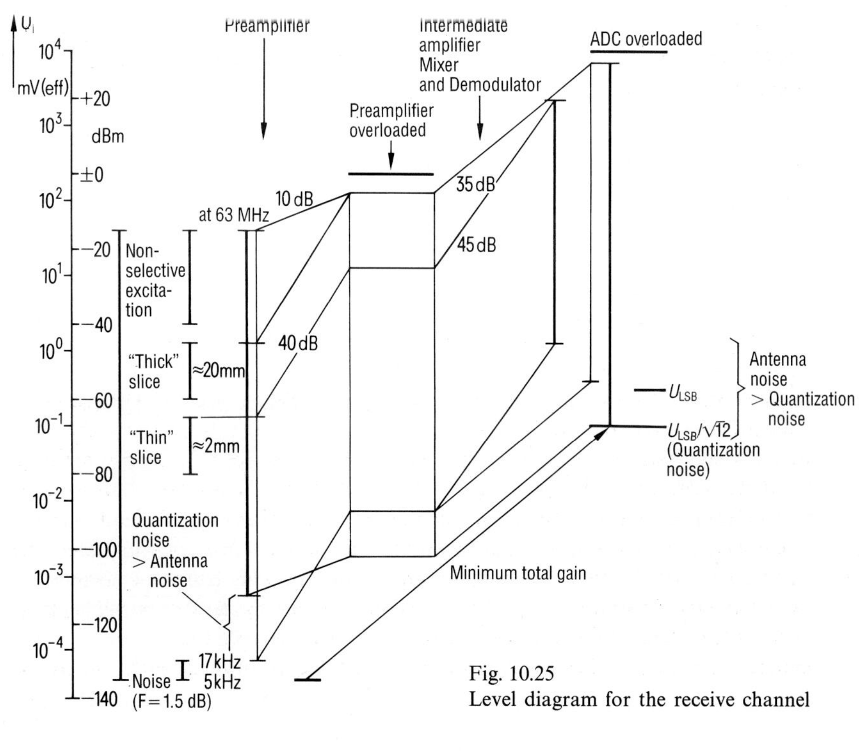

Fig. 10.25
Level diagram for the receive channel

of the diodes is high and the signal reaches the preamplifier virtually unattenuated via the $\lambda/4$ line. The circuit contains other adjustable components which neutralize the diode capacitance.

Phase noise

Section 2.1 mentions the importance of the phase stability in MR signals for the generation of artifact-free images when using the Fourier method. It therefore follows that all phase fluctuations generated by all the RF components together must remain significantly under the critical 3° limit. This is especially true for the frequency synthesizer, which serves as the system clock.

Coils and resonators

Coils and resonators, generally called antennas, generate the alternating magnetic field for magnetic resonance excitation and receive the field emitted by the precessing nuclear moment. They therefore comprise the component of the MR system directly interacting with the object to be measured.

In connection with the discussion of the signal-to-noise ratio of the magnetic resonance experiment presented in Section 5.1.8, the most important properties of antennas were described. These are the distribution function of the B_1 field resulting from the current in relation to the sample geometry and the coil quality factor, Q.

Antenna characteristics

The peak output voltage $\hat{U}$ from a coil characterized by a field-current distribution $\vec{B}_\mathrm{i}(\vec{r})$ over a sample with precessing nuclear magnetization is:

$$\hat{U} = \omega_0 \int_{V_\mathrm{sample}} \vec{M}\vec{B}_\mathrm{i}\,\mathrm{d}V. \tag{10.41}$$

The resulting received output power (short circuit at the coil outputs) is then:

$$P = \tfrac{1}{2}\hat{U}^2/R. \tag{10.42}$$

A maximum of only half the output is available when the coil has been matched to subsequent components; e.g., using the matching circuitry illustrated in Figs. 10.26, 10.27 or 10.33 (impedance transformers). This fact is of no importance, however, for the following discussion (see equivalent circuit diagram 10.27). Important is that the useful signal output amplitude increases with matching the spatial coil field distribution to the distribution of the magnetization and falls with the resistive loss. The term "matching" is to be understood

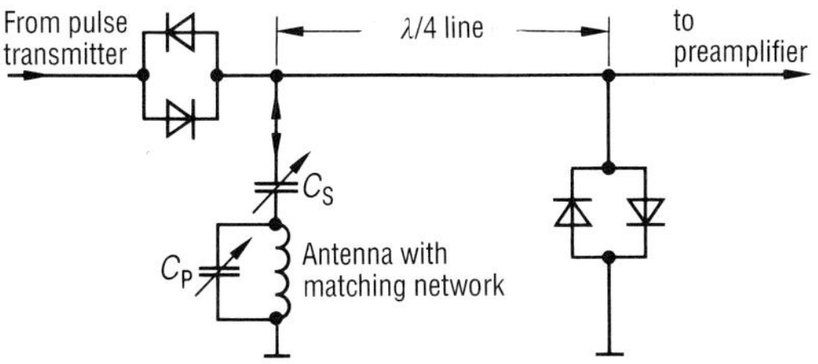

Fig. 10.26
Simplified circuit diagram of transmit-receive switch

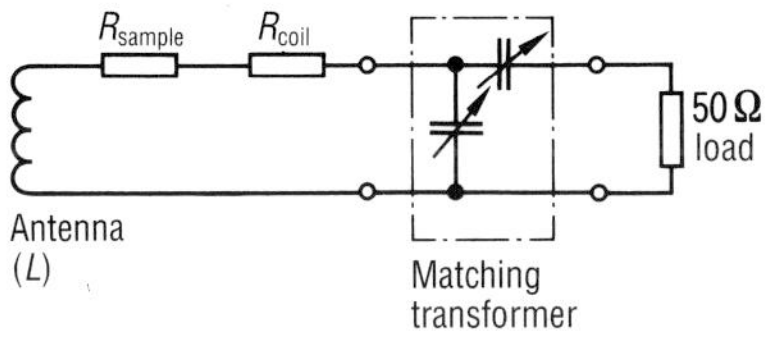

Fig. 10.27
Equivalent circuit diagram of a transmit-receive coil (antenna) with loss

in a very general manner; i.e., not only that the probe volume should correspond to the sensitive volume of the antenna, but that the vectors $\vec{M}$ and $\vec{B}_i$ should be parallel. It then follows that an antenna whose B_1 field is perpendicular to B_0 and is circularly polarized should be, theoretically, superior to any other configuration, because the nuclear magnetization precesses about the B_0 direction. Loss due to resistance is simultaneously the source of undesirable noise. It can be divided into the resistance induced by the sample and that caused by the coil:

$$R = R_{sample} + R_{coil}. \tag{10.43}$$

The loss in useful signal caused by the subject to be measuremend and the noise it generates is unavoidable. An expression for R_{sample} can be found in Section 5.1.8. R_{coil}, on the other hand, can be optimized:

$$R_{coil} = \frac{\omega_0 \int_{V_{coil}} B_i^2 \, dV}{2\mu_0 Q_0}. \tag{10.44}$$

With the definition of the filling factor η:

$$\eta = \int_{V_{sample}} B_i^2 \, dV \Big/ \int_{V_{coil}} B_i^2 \, dV \tag{10.45}$$

i.e., the fraction of the field energy penetrating the sample in relation to the total field energy produced, it follows that:

$$R_{\text{coil}} = \frac{\omega_0 \int\limits_{V_{\text{sample}}} B_1^2 \, dV}{2\mu_0 \, \eta \, Q_0}. \tag{10.46}$$

Coil losses therefore increase with frequency and sample volume and decrease with the unloaded Q_0 and the filling factor. In summary, the following characteristics are required for an optimized MR antenna:

1. The field distribution should be homogeneous across the measurement volume to assure spatially uniform nuclear resonance excitation.
2. The filling factor should be large.
3. The direction of polarization should be perpendicular to the constant field and (if possible) circular.
4. Energy losses should be minimal compared to the losses induced by the subject to be measured; i.e., the unloaded Q_0 should be high.

Characteristics 1 and 2 may occasionally conflict in medical practice, namely when a portion of the body which cannot be surrounded by a coil is to be imaged. For these cases so-called surface coils are used; i.e. the homogeneity of the B_1 field (in general, only in the receive mode) is sacrificed in favor of a large filling factor in order to achieve the largest possible $\Delta S/N$. In turn, this can be traded off against adequate spatial resolution.

Antennas with homogeneous field distribution

Coils and resonators (antennas) must surround the subject to be measured in order to generate a homogeneous B_1 field within the subject. A suitable configuration would be a solenoid arranged coaxially with the axis of the body. Since B_1 and B_0 must be perpendicular to one another, this type of coil configuration can be used only with yoke or resistive magnets (see Sect. 10.2.1 and Fig. 10.7). In addition, the resonance frequency of a solenoid having a diameter corresponding to the size of a human body is substantially lower (due to unavoidable parasitic capacitance) than the MR frequency normally used. It is necessary to find cylindrical structures, which at high frequencies generate a homogeneous field polarized in the direction perpendicular to the axis of the magnet. A sufficiently long tube, subjected to a constant current distribution $J(\varphi)$

$$J(\varphi) = \hat{J} \sin \varphi, \tag{10.47}$$

as shown in Figs. 10.28a and b, will generate the desired field distribution [10.14].

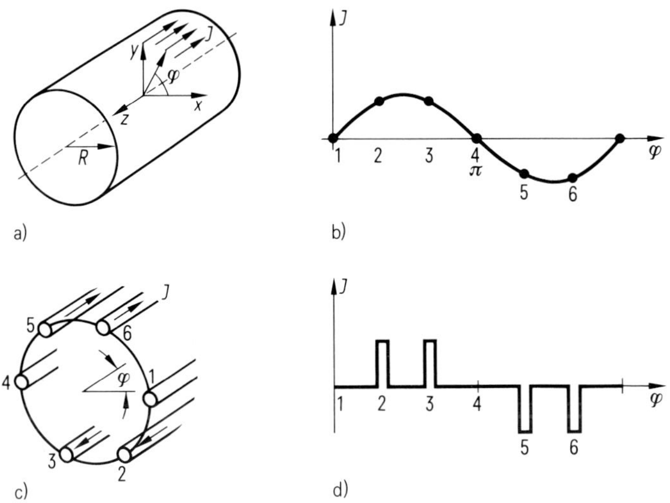

Fig. 10.28 RF Antenna with homogeneous B_1 field

a) Hollow tube with current density distribution in longitudinal direction
b) Ideal current distribution
c) Resonant conductors arranged as a discrete hollow tube
d) Current distribution in a discrete hollow tube for a nearly homogeneous B_1 field

Implementing this current distribution is not a simple matter. The current density can be approximated for several angles with discrete conductor paths (Figs. 10.28c and d). The conductors at $\varphi=0$ and 2π may be eliminated, since they do not carry any current. If the wire rods are connected in the manner shown in Fig. 10.29, the result is a so-called saddle coil, which can be used in situations when the frequency is not too high or the diameter not too large (up to 30 cm at approximately 25 MHz).

At higher frequencies and larger diameters (whole-body antennas) the length of the conductors is no longer short compared to the RF wave length, so

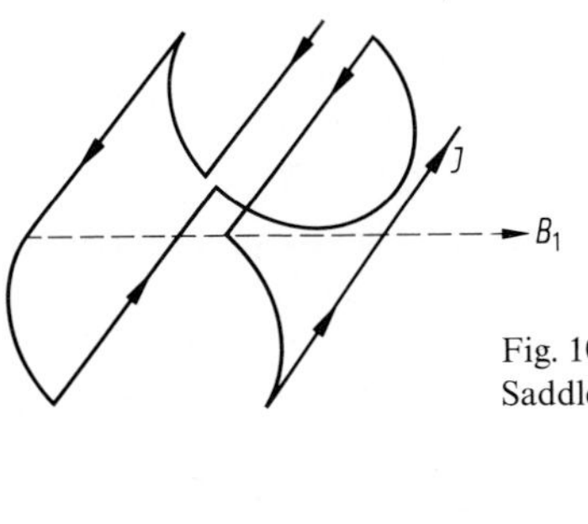

Fig. 10.29
Saddle coil for low frequencies or small coil dimensions

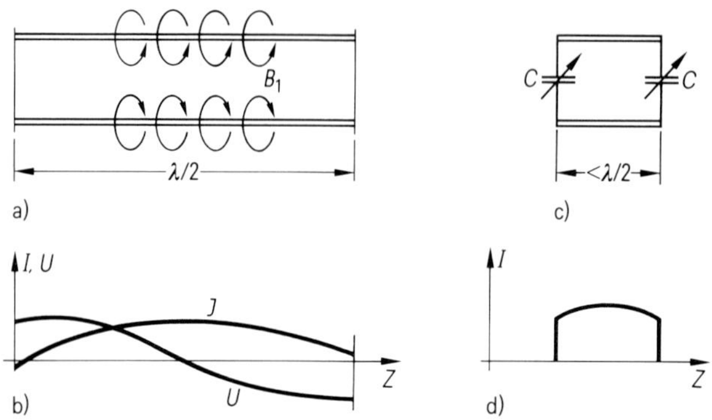

Fig. 10.30 λ/2 (half wavelength) resonator (antenna)

a) Conductor configuration
b) Current distribution
c) Shortening the conductors by applying a capacitive load to the ends
d) Current distribution with shortened conductors

that the desired current distribution can no longer be achieved with a saddle coil. Here the λ/2 resonator principle (see Fig. 10.30) becomes of interest. If a wave having the length $\lambda = 2\pi c/\omega_0$ (where c is the velocity of wave propagation) is generated on a double conductor (Fig. 10.30a) and the conductor is λ/2 long, a resonance or standing wave is produced which has a current distribution as shown in Fig. 10.30b, resulting in the corresponding B_1 field distribution. The circuit can be shortened symmetrically by adding capacitances, so that a nearly uniform current distribution arises in the longitudinal direction (Fig. 10.30c, d). Such resonant conductors can be configured as a hollow tube, as shown in Fig. 10.28d. A cross section of such a configuration is shown in Figure 10.31. The sections of the conductors are composed of rods having adjustable capacitors connected between the antenna and ground (exterior shielding). This λ/2 resonator [10.15] can be used as a transmit/receive antenna for whole-body magnetic resonance imaging up to 63 MHz.

Aldermann and Grant have developed a variation of this principle (Fig. 10.32) [10.16]. It is used primarily for head-imaging antennas, since the structure is open on two sides and is therefore more pleasant for the patient. The symmetrization to ground potential is accomplished via two inner rings.

A circularly polarized B_1 field can be generated with the above antennas by joining pairs of resonators attached coaxially, but at a 90° angle to one another. These partial systems are driven during the transmit mode via a power divider and a phase shifter in such a way that a high-frequency rotating field is generated

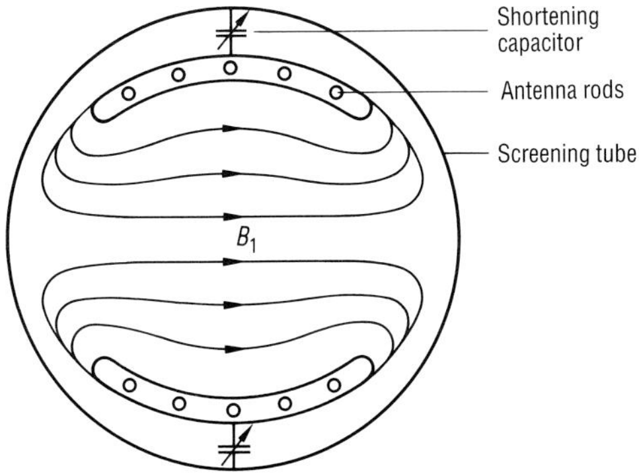

Fig. 10.31
Cross section of a whole-body antenna using the conductor resonance principle (suitable for high frequencies)

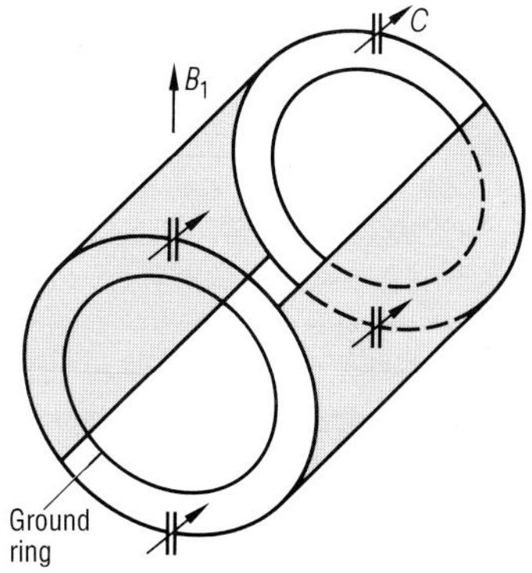

Fig. 10.32
Aldermann-Grant variation of the conductor resonance principle

in the antenna. In the opposite direction, the voltages induced in the resonators by the precessing magnetization, shifted by 90°, are transmitted to the preamplifier via a summation network. This configuration requires only half the RF output to generate a rotating B_1 field and results in a signal-to-noise ratio [10.17] improved by a factor of the square root of two if the Q of the antenna under load conditions (loaded by the subject to be measured) corresponds to that of a comparable linearly polarized configuration. Since a cross section of the human body is more elliptical in shape, the advantages of circular polarization cannot be fully realized in practice.

Surface coils

As the name indicates, these coils are used for imaging organs located close to the surface of the patient's body. They are placed on the patient directly over the position at which the organ is located. The coil must be oriented so that the B_1 field is perpendicular to B_0. In the simplest case, the coil comprises

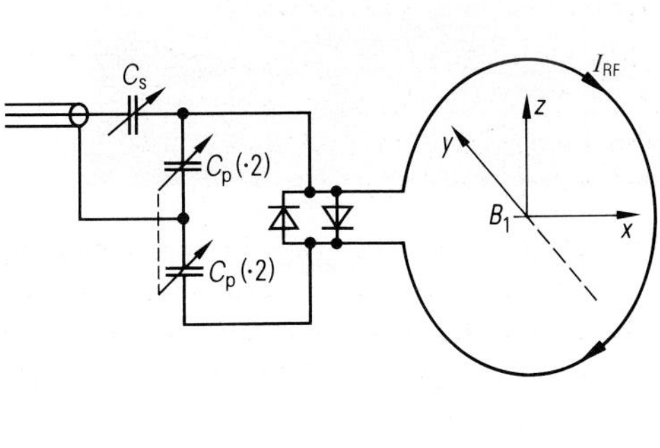

Fig. 10.33
Surface coil with symmetrical matching network

a single wire ring which is tuned to resonance at ω_0 via variable capacitors (Fig. 10.33). The field distribution of a current-carrying circular loop with radius r is described along the y axis of the coil by the following equation:

$$B_i(y) = \frac{\mu_0 r^2}{2(r^2 + y^2)^{3/2}}. \qquad (10.48)$$

The sensitivity along the coil axis and also the remaining field about the wire loop decreases rapidly with increasing distance between the subject and the coil plane. Experience shows that the effective penetration depth is approximately equal to the radius of the coil. In addition, B_i decreases as the radius increases. Depending upon the imaging objective, it is possible in general terms to trade sensitivity for the magnitude of the useful volume by varying the dimensions of the coil. The configuration of the coil windings can also be adapted to the surface of the human body. Surface coils are generally used only to receive MR signals, because of the inhomogeneity of the field distribution. Whole-body resonators are used for uniform excitation. The surface coil may not oscillate

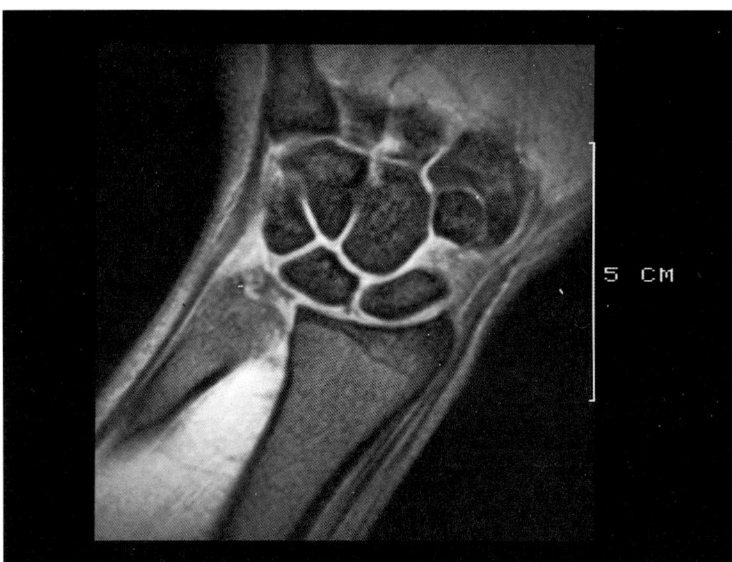

Fig. 10.34
High-resolution MR image of a wrist with carpal bones and ulna, taken with a surface coil
(pixel size: 0.5 mm, $T_r = 0.65$ s, $T_E = 10$ ms, slice thickness: 4 mm, measurement time: 2.5 min, field strength: 1.5 T)

during the transmit phase, since the distribution of the transmitter field would then be distorted. Complete decoupling through the appropriate orientation of the surface coil to the direction of polarization of the transmission antenna is not usually possible. Decoupling is therefore forced via the detuning diodes illustrated in Fig. 10.33; these diodes are switched into the conductive state by the induced voltage.

Figure 10.34 shows the high resolution in MR images which can be obtained using surface coils.

RF-shielded room

Effective antenna shielding against RF interference is essential, because of the extreme sensitivity of the receiving system to high-frequency fields. Antenna sensitivity, self-shielding capacity (a function of the length and diameter of the antenna resonator) and estimates of the intensity of possible RF interference (e.g., short-wave broadcasting stations) must all be included in the calculation of the required attenuation factor.

Experience has shown that the shielding factor must be greater than 100 dB to prevent interference from a 5 kW single-frequency transmitter at a distance of 10 km. In order to obtain such shielding the receiving antenna must be inside a metal housing, which is, for all practical purposes, completely closed. An extension of the shielding tube [10.18] in which the antenna is located, a practice seen occasionally, can only be effective in areas completely free of interference and when using low frequencies. Since high-frequency magnetic fields can hardly penetrate conductive material due to the skin effect, electrostatic shielding of a thickness of several times the skin depth is sufficient (e.g., 0.5 mm copper foil). Gaps in the shielding are to be avoided if possible. If necessary, however, the linear dimensions of such gaps must be clearly smaller than those of the wavelength corresponding to the MR frequency. Doors must be constructed so that they are RF-proof when closed. In general, the entire field generation system, i.e. the magnet, shim, gradient and RF coils and the patient table must all be set up inside the shielded room (see Fig. 10.1). This means that all the cables for these components must be routed through appropriately dimensioned suppression filters. Otherwise these cables, which are excellent antennas for high-frequency interference, would conduct RF noise into the shielded room.

If even these extensive measures are insufficient (in the case of a high-powered short-wave transmitter in the area), the constant field must be changed to provide for sufficient distance between the frequency band used for MR imaging and that of the interference.

10.2.4 System control

Processor systems for examination sequence, monitoring and image reconstruction

Alongside the central system computer, for which the tasks were already listed in Sect. 10.1, the MAGNETOM MRI system, for example, includes a number of additional processors, which control the pulse sequence, reconstruct images from raw data and initiate, as well as monitor, the correct functioning of all essential system components. This decentralization of computer tasks frees the system computer in particular from those operations which depend critically on time. In view of the significance of such a structuring for MR imaging, the function of the pulse sequence control will be dealt with in greater detail in the following. The image processor and also the image display units correspond to the system employed in x-ray computed tomography. The tasks assigned to the other control processors (Table 10.5) are comparatively trivial.

Table 10.5 Tasks of the monitoring processors

Function	Implemented in function module					
	Table	RF antenna control	RF power amplifier	RF small signal part	gradient amplifier	shim current power supply
Remote control on/off switch	×	×	×	×	×	×
Special switch-on procedure			×		×	
Self-testing routine	×	×	×	×	×	×
Electrical overloading			×		×	×
Thermal overloading (cooling)			×		×	×
Special functions	Table lift, table positioning, light localizer	Antenna switching, automatic tuning	Frequency and power range switching	Attenuator and gain switching, synthesizer frequency	None	Shim currents

Pulse sequence control

Fig. 10.35 shows a schematic diagram of the pulse sequence control. The procedure to be executed is present before the beginning of the measurement in the form of control words in the control memory. The bit pattern transferred from here by means of a control logic to the control word register determines what takes place in the corresponding time slice: this may be a gradient pulse, an RF pulse, a data acquisition interval, a delay time or several such events simultaneously. The control word only initiates the functions programmed, which are then executed independently under the control of programmed trigger pulse generators; that is, according to their clock speeds, the data present in the pulse shape memories are transmitted to the DACs or the MR signals are sampled. The image processor receives the measured data directly from the two ADCs and processes them to image data. The pulse data must, just as for the control word sequence before beginning the measurement, already be present in the memories. The same applies for the trigger pulse programs used to determine the time scale for the individual parts of the sequence. The

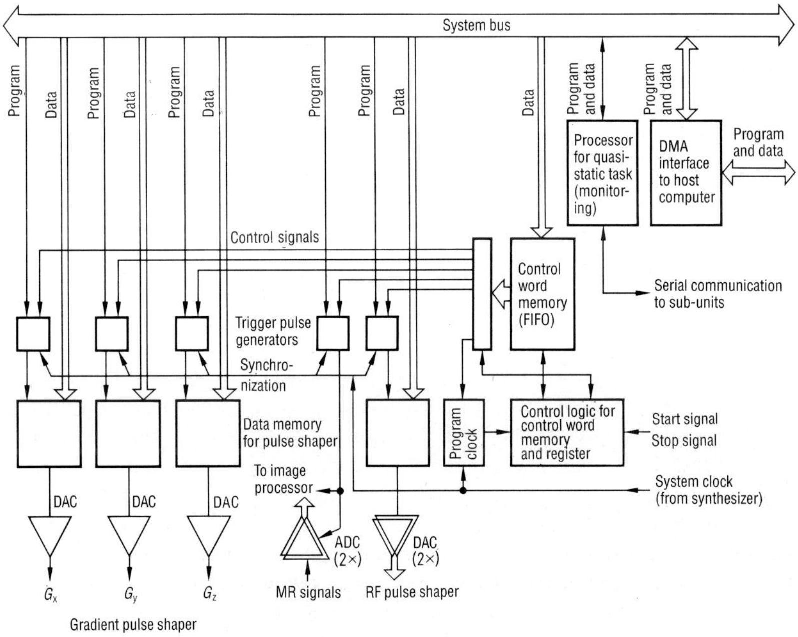

Fig. 10.35 Schematic diagram of pulse sequence control

entire sequence is synchronized from the frequency synthesizer, which serves as the system clock.

This control structure has the property that a control operation; that is, reading and decoding a control word, must only be initiated for each sequence function block and not for each change of an output value. The control word memory can therefore be relatively small. By comparison, the pulse shape data memories are generously dimensioned in order to support long pulse sequences comprising several different pulses.

The pulse sequence control is integrated into a microcomputer system, for which Fig. 10.35 shows only the general data flow path (system bus).

The system computer is connected via an interface with direct memory access (DMA) to the control and supplies the machine language program for the pulse sequence selected, in the form of data which the microprocessor makes available to the appropriate memories.

In the event of insufficient memory capacity, the microprocessor can load data from the backup buffer memories during the measurement process.

Operating program

In an imaging system which performs both measurement sequences and image reconstruction by means of digital computers, the operating program is of particular importance. Moreover, in normal operation the operating program represents the interface through which the user initiates measuring system functions and retrieves results – usually, images (Fig. 10.36).

The particular properties of the imaging process also clearly affect the software design. By contrast, for example, with x-ray computed tomography, MR imaging as a measuring process is relatively slow. The acquisition of a complete raw data file generally requires several minutes. A necessary consequence of this is that the delay time to accommodate other functions, such as image callup and manipulation, must be filled out. The operating system must therefore be able to perform several tasks quasi-simultaneously. This so-called time sharing capability is in conflict with the requirement of real-time operation during measurement. In spite of the long duration of measurement, there is a high rate of data flow: over the course of a single measurement, data for entire series of images can be acquired. This means that the program must be capable of managing large data files and rapidly accessing certain images. Finally, it must also be mentioned for magnetic resonance tomography that the possibilities for variations in the measuring procedure are greater and depend less on the system configuration than for any other modality. A high-capability dialog system for inputting the parameters of measurement is essential in order to be able to take full advantage of the potential which MRI offers.

The generation of the NUMARIS (Nuclear Magnetic Resonance Imaging Program) operating program for the MAGNETOM takes these points into account. It is able to run on a system computer (DEC-VAX) with the VMS Multitask operating system, which supports the requirement of performing several tasks simultaneously. The general structure of the operating program is shown in Fig. 10.37. According to the task at hand, the function blocks will differ.

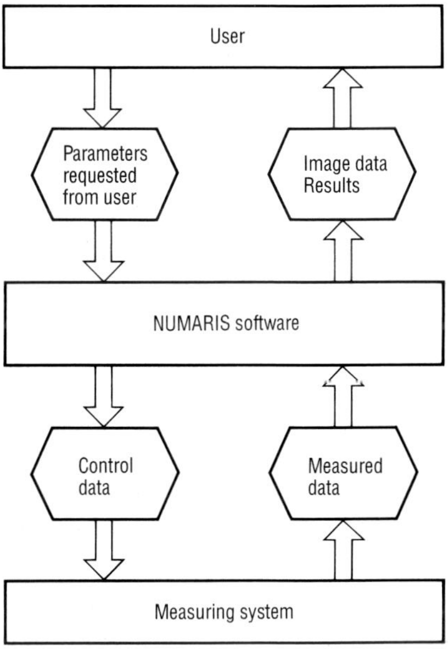

Fig. 10.36
Operating program as interface between user and measuring system

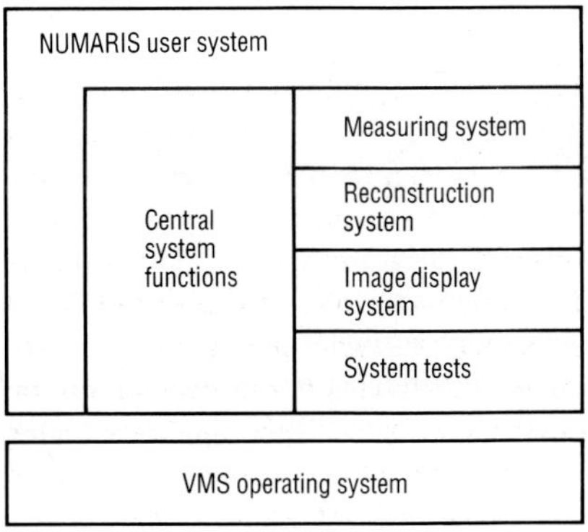

Fig. 10.37
General structure of the NUMARIS operating program

Central system functions:

To these belong process generation (the concept process will be defined more precisely in the following), communication between processes; that is, the transfer of information between processes which depend on each other, coordination of system components, processing of inputs through the operator's keyboard, interpretation of commands and function key codes and the management of the monitor terminal; that is, the assignment of display area to the various processes.

Measuring system:

This comprises the coupling of the system computer to the measurement sequence control, the modification of measurement parameters and the related generation of pulse programs, implementation of settings required and recognition of system status.

Reconstruction system:

This includes the functions of coupling the system computer to the image processor, acquiring measured data, image reconstruction and intermediate storage of measured data and image data files.

Image display system:

To this belong the coupling of the system computer to the image output units, control of image output and presentation (windowing), image evaluation routines, graphics and graphics inputs, and the management of patient and image data (file management).

System test:

This function block is provided for servicing purposes and includes the test routines for all digital components, as well as for adjustments and functional checkouts required in connection with the system installation and optimization.

At the basis of the operating program is the VMS operating system, with functions supporting NUMARIS, in particular during the dynamic assignment of host computer capacity (to take best advantage of the central processing unit and available memory) for processes, as well as for the management of peripheral mass storage devices.

The concept "process" [10.19] means the execution of a task, as well as the provision of the operating means required for performance of the task: computer capacity and programs. Within a process, only a single program can run at any one time, from which it follows that tasks which must be performed simultaneously must be assigned to different processes. A typical time-sharing application, for example, would be the creation of text data files for several users at different video terminals at the same time. For each user, a process is started, in the framework of which the (same) editor program can run. In this case, the processes would be fully independent of one another. However, in the NUMARIS operating program, the processes form a single system, since they are more or less dependent on each other; that is, they must continuously exchange data and messages among each other. Furthermore, they make use of a common terminal. It would not be meaningful and would only complicate operation if each process had to be operated from a separate input unit.

Distribution of operating functions in processes

Fig. 10.38 shows, in simplified form, the system of processes, their communications paths and the MR system components which they serve. The total number of processes implemented is greater than the number of function blocks described, because interrelated tasks (for example, an adjustment; i.e., specific measurements followed by the immediate calculation of results and control reactions) are combined within a single process and certain partial functions must be able to run together with others from the same block. So far as one or more operator consoles are additionally installed for evaluation tasks on the system, the given processes can be activated several times using identical program segments. The processes communicate with each other through the exchange of messages deposited in so-called mailboxes. The receiving process reads the messages entered and reacts accordingly.

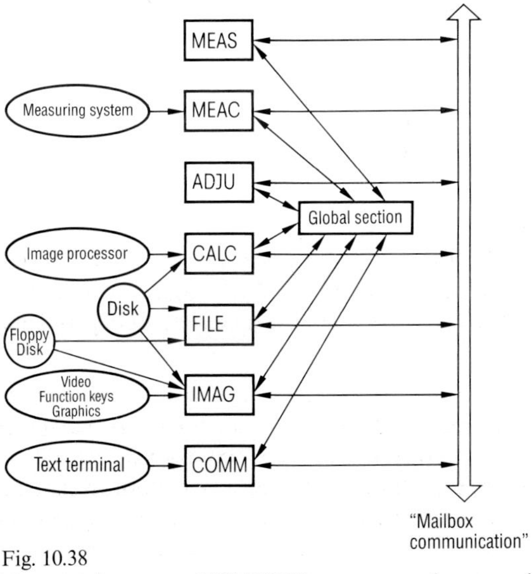

Fig. 10.38
The most important NUMARIS processes and communications paths

Table 10.6 Functions of the important NUMARIS processes

Process name	Process function
COMM[1]	Text terminal management, command input, assignment of text monitor screen into status, error and confirmation message fields and corresponding processor assignment
MEAS	Generation, modification and display of measurement programs (pulse sequences)
MEAC	Transfer of measurement programs to measurement sequence control
ADJU	Measurement programs for subject-dependent system calibration
CALC	Transfer of reconstruction algorithms and measured data or image data files to and from image processor
FILE[1]	Management of peripheral mass storage devices (patient, image and measured data)
IMAG[1]	Image presentation (video memory control), image manipulation, graphics input and output, management of function keys

[1] These processes can run twice in the system when a 2nd satellite console (2nd control console for separate image evaluation) is present.

The processes also obtain information from the common memories (global sections), in which system data of general use, such as system configuration, results of adjustments or conditions of measurement, are entered. Processes not performing a task are switched off in order to relieve the central processing unit of the host computer.

The functions of the NUMARIS processes illustrated in Fig. 10.38 are summarized in Table 10.6.

10.3 Imaging techniques

10.3.1 Subject-dependent system calibrations

After the patient has been positioned, the parameters influenced by the the subject to be measured must be calibrated before the measurement can be started. Calibration procedures for an MR examination are performed as follows:

1. Patient positioning
2. Matching of resonator/coils
3. Setting the MR center frequency
4. Pulse amplitude calibration
5. Selection of measurement parameters (or pulse sequence)
6. Setting the receiver gain
7. Starting the measurement
8. Image reconstruction and image retrieval

Steps 2–4 must be repeated only when the patient has been repositioned. The selection of measurement parameters (step 5) may be performed earlier in this sequence.

Antenna adjustment

The transmit/receive coil impedance, which is dependent on the size and position of the patient, must first be matched to the impedance of the transmission line. With the help of a fully automatic control system the capacitors of the matching network (Fig. 10.27) are set so that there is practically no reflection of the RF power fed into the antenna.

After the desired measurement parameters have been selected, the required procedures described in the following are normally performed automatically by the system.

Setting the center frequency

The next step is the determination of the magnetic resonance frequency. This would seem to be a superfluous step when dealing with the stability of superconducting magnets, but the frequency will change by tens of Hz from patient to patient due to varying susceptibility. A variation in resonance, as shown in Eq. (10.1), would cause a noticeable shift in the image, corresponding to the gradient strength employed. The resonance frequency can be determined by a simple MR experiment, namely the excitation and readout of an FID (free induction decay). The synthesizer is then readjusted accordingly.

Adjustment of pulse amplitude

Since the degree of efficiency of the transmission antenna, expressed in generated B_1 field per square root of the RF power input, is strongly dependent on the subject under examination, the pulse amplitude must be adjusted. This determines the RF output necessary to tip the nuclear magnetization by an angle α by using a pulse of length t_p. A practical method makes use of the following relationship between transverse magnetization $M_\perp$, which is proportional to the nuclear resonance signal apart from a constant phase factor, and the B_1 amplitude (Fig. 10.39):

$$M_\perp = M_0 \sin(\gamma t_p B_1). \tag{10.49}$$

The first zero passage of the MR signal directly after the RF pulse is sought by increasing the pulse amplitude in a series of FID excitations (Fig. 10.39a), first in larger steps and then in fine steps. The first signal minimum corresponds to a nutation angle of 180°.

Using the pulse length t_p and the amplitude determined during calibration, the scale factor of any other pulse shape of known effective length can be computed.

Receiver gain

The last step in the calibration process is the adjustment of receiver gain with respect to the maximum MR signal occurring during imaging. The importance of this adjustment is discussed in section 10.2.3. The same pulse sequence is used for the measurement as for the following imaging, except for the fact that the phase encoding gradient is not switched on, because the MR signal is at its maximum in this case. For this reason, with few exceptions – such as the size of the field of view, the pulse sequence parameters must be selected prior to this step.

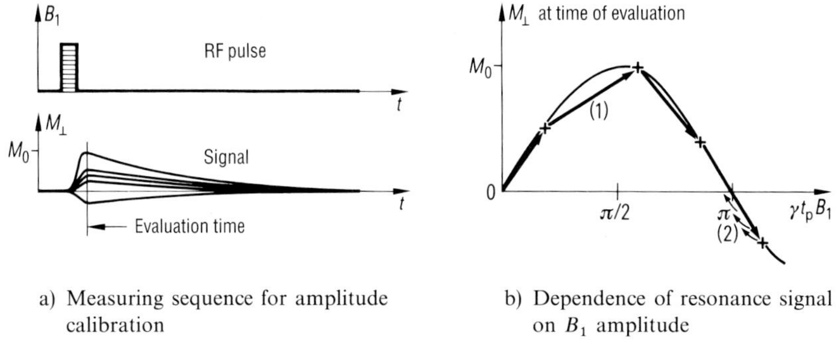

a) Measuring sequence for amplitude calibration

b) Dependence of resonance signal on B_1 amplitude

Fig. 10.39
Pulse amplitude calibration procedure. The condition $\gamma t_p B_1 = \pi$ is first attained in coarse steps (1) up to the sign reversal of $M_\perp$ and then in fine steps (2) up to the signal minimum

If no overload has occurred, the resulting measurement data can be used to calculate the amplifier settings necessary for proper modulation of the receiving components. If this is not the case, the calibration measurement must be repeated using reduced gain.

10.3.2 Spin-echo pulse sequences

Due to its relative insensitivity to inhomogeneities in the static constant field and to other imprecisions of the measuring system and also because of the easily characterized dependence of the resulting image contrast on the parameters echo time, T_e, and pulse repetition time, T_r, the spin-echo sequence remains the most widely used pulse sequence for MR imaging:

$$S \sim \varrho \, e^{-T_e/T_2}(1-e^{-T_r/T_1}). \qquad (10.50)$$

$$T_e \ll T_1$$

$$T_2 \ll T_r.$$

The underlying principle is described in section 5.2.3, while the form for the individual parts of the sequence was discussed in connection with the gradient strength (see Sect. 10.2.2). In the following, a few variations will be dealt with. Multiple-echo imaging for the production of a series of images with different T_2 weighting and the problems resulting will also be discussed.

Sequences with one spin-echo

The pulse sequence is again illustrated schematically in Fig. 10.40a, without taking the gradient switching times into account. Fig. 10.40b shows the path

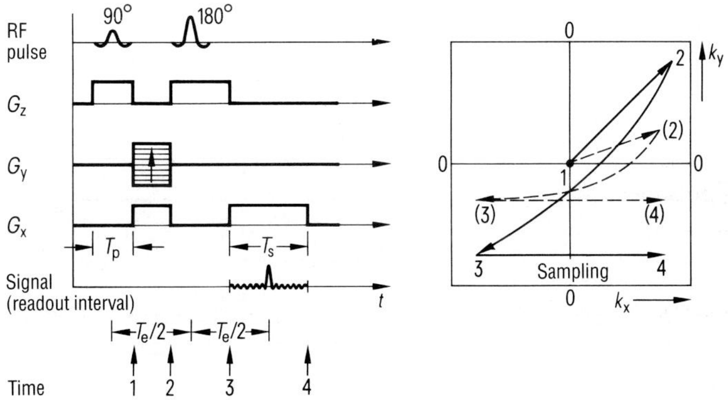

a) Pulse sequence b) Sampling in k space

Fig. 10.40 Simple spin-echo pulse sequence

over which the plane of spatial frequencies, represented by the measured MR signals, runs. In the following, this plane is referred to as the k plane, or in the three-dimensional extension, as the k space:

$$k_x = \gamma G_x t_x; \quad k_y = \gamma G_y t_y. \tag{10.51}$$

For each 90° – 180° pulse pair; that is, for each repetition interval T_r, a Fourier projection is acquired through changing the strength of the phase encoding gradient, G_y, in equidistant steps and stored in the measured data matrix, until all four quadrants are fully occupied. The reconstruction to an MR image then takes place through the Fourier transform following and the modulus values are then calculated in order to eliminate phase factors of the form $e^{i\varphi(x,y)}$. This is permissible, because the imaginary part of the object function vanishes for the symmetric sampling of four quadrants [10.20]. The phase factors are essentially the result of incomplete diagonalization of the measured data in the k matrix, particularly in the readout direction, due to the generally non-ideal gradient pulse shape. The entire spatial information is already contained in two quadrants, so that the measurement can be terminated after the acquisition of one half of the k plane. The other half is then filled with zeroes. From the complex result of the reconstruction, it is then necessary to extract the real part; due to the determination of phase factors required for this task, this process is generally problematic [10.21]. Halving the time of measurement is of course only possible at the expense of accepting a decrease in the signal-to-noise ratio by a factor of at least $\sqrt{2}$.

For the sequencing of gradient pulses there are various possibilities, as Fig. 10.41 illustrates: thus, the refocussing of the selection gradient can be placed before the 180° pulse (a) or the preparation period; that is, defocussing in the readout

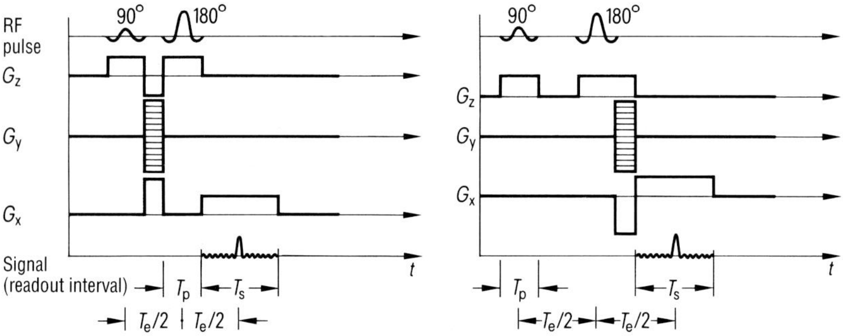

a) Refocussing before the 180° pulse   b) Defocussing following the 180° pulse

Fig. 10.41 Variations of the spin-echo sequence

direction and phase encoding, can follow upon the 180° pulse (b). The first variation permits a shorter echo time, T_e, provided that there is sufficient reserve in the gradient strength and switching time and that $T_p < T_s$. The second variation has the advantage that the phase encoding is also effective with respect to the signals induced by the 180° pulse, referred to in the following as the residual FID. As a result of its finite pulse length, the 180° pulse cannot bring about even an approximately homogeneous inversion of the magnetization, $M = (M_x, M_y, M_z)$, over the entire slice thickness. Furthermore, the B_1 inhomogeneity and the finite pulse calibration error also give rise to deviations from the ideal case. Since the buildup of M_z with the time constant T_1 already becomes noticeable within the time $T_e/2$, the 180° pulse can cause measurable transverse magnetization. If the phase encoding for these signal components is missing (as for the sequence in Figs. 10.40a and 10.41a), a disturbance in the form of a streak artifact is seen in the middle of the image field, in the direction of the readout gradient (x).

Through the alternation of the sign for the 180° pulse with every second Fourier projection, it is nevertheless possible to shift this streak to the edge of the image field, where it no longer represents a disturbance, but not to eliminate it altogether. The periodic alternation of signs modulates the residual FID with the highest frequency which can be represented in the sampling grid in y. This corresponds to the outermost lying position in the y direction. Still better is to alternate the 90° pulses and to take into account the changes in sign of the spin echo during image reconstruction. This also eliminates any offset error of the ADC, which would otherwise be reconstructed to a point in the middle of the image.

The variation depicted in Fig. 10.41b therefore appears less attractive for single echo sequences.

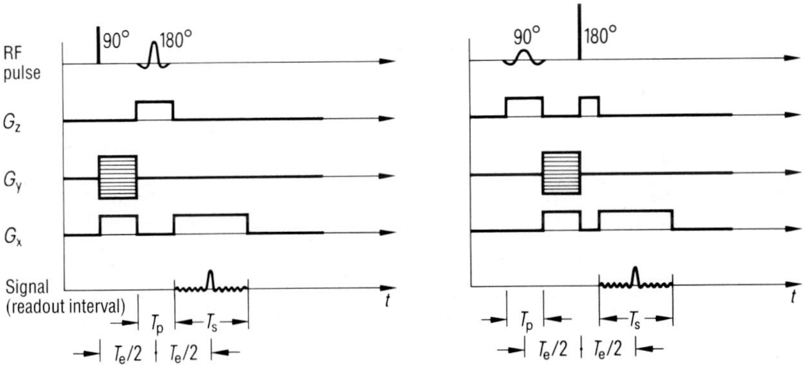

a) 90° pulse (nonselective) b) 180° pulse (nonselective)

Fig. 10.42 Variations of the spin-echo sequence with a nonselective RF pulse

In the interest of shortening, the echo time, one of the two RF pulses can be made nonselective: either the 90° pulse in Fig. 10.42a or the 180° pulse in Fig. 10.42b. But with this the multislice capability is lost. The version with the nonselective 90° pulse is preferable, because there is no switching process for G_z or the – mostly very intense – residual FID, which is excited from the nonselective 180° pulse acting over the entire object. The minimum T_e time possible is then reduced by T_p.

These represent the most important variations of the spin-echo pulse sequence.

In summary, the most important rules for designing such a sequence are as follows:

1. Symmetry rule: The time integrals of the gradient pulse from the middle of the 90° pulse to the middle of the 180° pulse should agree with those from the middle of the 180° pulse to the middle of the readout interval. This is equivalent to occurring at the same point in time as the spin-echo maximum, with and without gradient pulses, and brings about a complete refocussing of the phase dispersion resulting from field inhomogeneities and the chemical shift. This condition remains satisfied once a pulse sequence has been optimized for different gradient strengths when the gradient switching time is constant instead of the switching speed.

2. With the RF pulse, only one (generally constant) gradient field may act; otherwise, a rotation of the slice normals will take place in the direction of the gradient vector sum.

3. During readout, only a constant gradient field may be switched on; otherwise, a rotated or distorted image will result.

4. Pulse time and pulse bandwidth: The pulse bandwidth, $\Delta\omega_p$, together with G_z, determines the slice thickness and the necessary RF power. The slice profile sharpness is essentially a function of the product $\Delta\omega_p \, T_p$.

5. Readout time: Together with G_x and G_y, this determines the pixel size, the relative distortion due to field inhomogeneities and the chemical shift, and the signal-to-noise ratio.

Multiecho sequences

The single-echo pulse sequence can be extended through the addition of further – to maintain the multislice capability, preferably selective 180° pulses and readout intervals (Fig. 10.43a) – to a multiecho sequence. Fig. 10.43b shows the associated sampling path in the k plane. As can be seen, the phase reversal through the 180° pulse causes the spatial frequency matrix, and thus the image matrix for each even echo, to be the mirror image of the odd echoes about $y=0$. The reconstructed images are, according to Eq. (10.50), increasingly T_2-weighted with increasing echo number. Examples of this can be seen in Section 5.2.4, Fig. 5.22. In practice, however, such a simple extension does not function satisfactorily; that is, interference from mirror images and superimposed structures, with the formation of wave patterns, and streak artifacts occur. The cause, as for the residual FID, is to be found in the unavoidable incompleteness of the 180° pulse. Within a pulse sequence, as soon as more than one further RF pulse with a nutation angle not equal to 180° follows an excitation pulse, along with the desired echo for the T_2 determination for each readout interval spurious echos and stimulated echos also appear [10.22]. A detailed account of these rather complex relationships is not possible in this context. A descriptive explanation for the spurious echos is the following: each RF pulse in the sequence can form an excitation pulse or refocussing pair with each following pulse, just as for the normal single-echo sequence. The intensity of these spurious echos depends on the values of both relaxation times and also on the deviation of the pulse angle from its theoretical value (90° or 180°). The number of spurious echos increases strongly with the number of RF pulses, since each echo can in turn be refocussed through the following pulses. After only the second 180° pulse, two spurious echos can already appear with the second echo.

The origin of stimulated echos can be visualized as follows: the second RF pulse folds a part of the magnetization, dephased due to constant field inhomogeneities (the inhomogeneities introduced intentionally through the spatially coding gradients also belong to these), into the xz or yz plane of the coordinate system, which rotates with ω_0. As a result of T_2 relaxation and field inhomogeneities, this part loses its phase coherence in the transverse (xy) direction, so that after a certain time the magnetization executes a conically shaped precession, at an angle corresponding to the dephasing which has occurred up to the second RF pulse. This means that, except for the part which – as a result

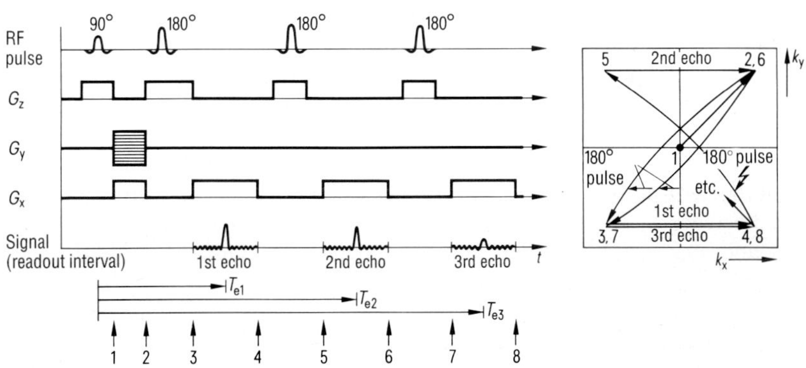

a) Pulse sequence

b) Sampling in k space

Fig. 10.43
Multiecho sequence. Even and odd echos belong to the corresponding Fourier projection

of T_1 relaxation – vanishes into M_z; the magnetization "remembers" the phase angle. The third RF pulse then folds the magnetization again, at least partially, into the xy plane, where it is refocussed and forms the stimulated echo. For the purposes of imaging technology, this can be summarized in the form a rule of thumb:

The stimulated echo generated by three RF pulses does not "see" the effect of the static fields over the time between the second and third RF pulses.

Stimulated echos are generated from any three non-180° RF pulse series; through further pulses, they can form new ordinary echos and spurious echos. In view of this, it appears questionable whether it is possible at all to obtain meaningful multiecho images from this utter confusion of echos, spurious echos and stimulated echos, together with the residual FID.

Fortunately, for the greatest part of the undesirable echos, for even the simplest multiecho sequence, as shown in Figure 10.43, no phase encoding of the spatial dimension y takes place, nor is the refocussing condition in the slice (z) direction or the readout (x) direction satisfied. All signal components not subject to the phase encoding give rise to a streak artifact, corresponding to object extension in the x direction. As for the single-echo sequence, this can be displaced to the edge of the image through alternating the signs of the 90° pulse.

The occurrence of mirror images is explained most easily with the aid of the rule developed above: this says that the stimulated echo signal (STE) does not take part in the mirror imaging of a point, caused by the (second) 180° pulse. In [10.23], without introducing the concept of an STE, the intensity of the mirror image for the second echo is given quantitatively as a function of the pulse angle error. It can be largely eliminated through addition (even echos) or subtraction (odd echos) of the signals from every two measurements for each Fourier projection, which differ only by a 90° phase shift of the 180° pulse (PHAPS sequence). However, this requires – among other things – that the normal spin echo appear at the same time as the STE. Otherwise, through the superposition of images arising from the partial signals, wave patterns will result in accordance with the known rules of Fourier transformations [10.20]. Their occurrence at the same moment in time is guaranteed by satisfying a symmetry rule, which – its meaning extended to the STE and the second echo – can be derived from the rule given for the creation of single-echo sequences: the difference of the time integrals of the readout gradients (G_x) before the first and after the second 180° pulse up to the echo must be equal to their sum minus the G_x integral between the two pulses. Such a pulse sequence can be programmed easily, as long as the G_x pulses are in the ideal trapezoid shape. Nevertheless, the smallest deviations – such as due to insufficient eddy current compensation – are already problematic.

One possibility, related to the PHAPS sequence, should be mentioned without further explanation: the suppression of the mirror image-generating STE at least for the echos of order not equal to $4n+2 (n=0, 1, 2, \ldots)$. This makes the twofold measurement of each Fourier projection unnecessary. Each two 180° refocussing pulses following each other in this sequence are rotated by 90° in their phase. The method is also sensitive to minute inaccuracies of the refocussing and defocussing gradients.

Owing to these difficulties, other variations of the multiecho sequence have also been developed. One of these makes a virtue of violating the symmetry rule mentioned earlier. The duration of the readout gradient is set so that the interfering signals occur outside the readout interval. Alternatively, or in addition, the slice selection gradient is extended by the third and further 180° pulses in such a way that the undesired echos are defocussed and no longer contribute to the image [10.25]. Figure 10.44 shows such a pulse sequence. Since the number of interfering echos for which the refocussing condition must be violated increases with the number of RF pulses, the required time integrals of the gradients around the 180° pulse become increasingly large with increasing echo number. This means that the application of this strategy is practically limited to sequences of no more than about four echos.

It must be mentioned that a completely exact T_2 determination is not possible with any of the methods described. Either, according to the distribution of the flip angle for nuclear magnetization over the slice, a more or less definite admixture of T_1 values, i.e. the time constants describing the STE relaxation, is always present in the image signal or the signal is reduced due to incomplete refocussing.

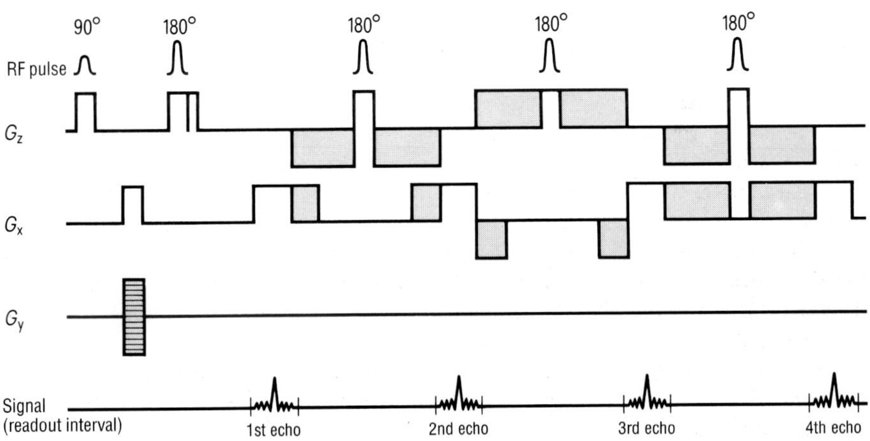

Figure 10.44
Multiecho sequence with dephasing and displacement of undesirable spurious echos (gray areas of the gradient pulse)

10.3.3 Fast MR imaging methods

The production of an MR image of sufficient spatial resolution and with an acceptable field of view with the spin-echo sequences described requires a few minutes; that is, at least the repetition time, T_r, times the number of Fourier projections, N.

Particularly for examinations of the thorax and abdomen, with their unavoidable involuntary movements, it is essential that the time of measurement be shortened. Two main methods are known today for achieving this goal. One of these is to reduce T_r as far as possible and so – through appropriate structuring of the sequence – to optimize the measurable transverse magnetization and thus the signal. The other possibility is, within the T_r interval; that is, beginning with a 90° excitation pulse, to acquire as many measurement points from the k matrix as possible at once.

Sequences with extremely short T_r times

Through a reduction of the pulse repetition time to below 0.3 s, the necessary conditions cited for using Eq. (10.50) are no longer satisfied sufficiently. Beginning with the formula of Ernst and Anderson [10.26] for equilibrium magnetization induced by periodic excitation with RF pulses of nutation angle α, for $T_2 \ll T_r$ the relation

$$M_L = M_0 \frac{(1-e^{-T_r/T_1}) \sin\alpha}{1-\cos\alpha\, e^{-T_r/T_1}} e^{-T_e/T_2} \text{ results.} \tag{10.52}$$

As a result of the inadequacies described in Section 10.3.2, the refocussing of the magnetization with a 180° pulse leads to unpredictable complications

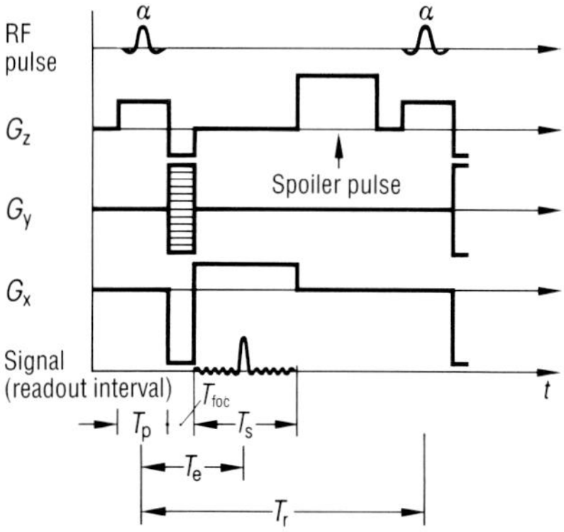

Fig. 10.45
FLASH sequence

with the method. The generation of the echo signal therefore follows without a 180° pulse through gradient polarity reversal in the slice and readout directions. The resulting MR signal is therefore known as the gradient echo. Figure 10.45 illustrates such a pulse sequence. Because of the missing 180° pulse, the minimum possible echo time is considerably shorter than for the spin-echo sequence. However, a dephasing of the spins due to B_0 field inhomogeneities and the chemical shift is not compensated. The signal intensity is then really dependent on T_2^* (see Section 5.1.5) and not on T_2. Since the transverse magnetization at the end of the readout interval, especially with extremely short T_r times ($T_e \leq 2T_r < T_2$), is generally still of a significant magnitude, a so-called spoiler pulse; that is, a gradient pulse having a large $t \cdot G_z$ product, is appended to the sequence in order to disperse the magnetization in the direction of the slice as completely as possible. This is done to at least satisfy the condition $T_2^* \ll T_r$.

As follows from Eq. (10.52), the signal intensity for this pulse sequence depends, in addition to its time data in relation to the relaxation times, on the nutation angle of the excitation pulse as well. One therefore has an additional parameter available, with which the signal-to-noise ratio or the image contrast can be optimally adjusted. The relation between the magnetization in equilibrium, determining the signal strength, and the ratio T_r/T_1 is shown in Fig. 10.46 for a few pulse angles. The pulse angle for the maximum signal is:

$$\alpha = \arccos(e^{-T_r/T_1}). \tag{10.53}$$

This means that, for long spin-lattice relaxation times (compared with the time T_r) weak RF pulses yield the largest – relative – signal. Following a suggestion

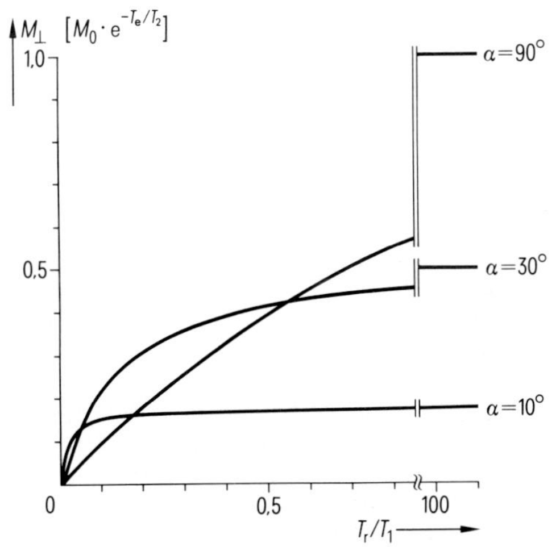

Fig. 10.46
MR signal for the FLASH sequence as a function of T_r/T_1 for different pulse angles, α (note that for relatively short repetition times, T_r, small pulse angles, α, yield a greater signal than large angles)

in [10.27], this sequence is given the name FLASH (Fast Low Angle SHot), because, for the short T_r times, the T_1 times of body tissue needed for an optimal signal-to-noise ratio require a pulse angle much smaller than 90° (usually 20–60°). The minimum total time of measurement is about 10 s for 256 Fourier projections.

Another possibility to obtain a relatively high equilibrium level transverse magnetization, in spite of very short pulse repetition times, is to bring about a complete rephasing of the spin in the RF pulses. Instead of the spoiler pulse of the gradient-echo sequence, refocussing gradient pulses occur in both the readout and also the phase encoding and selection directions, as can be seen in Fig. 10.47. The RF pulses alternate in sign. For signal behavior, the following equation [10.28], taken from Ernst and Anderson [10.26] and making use of the approximation $e^{-T_r/T_1}=1-T_r/T_1$ with $T_1 \gg T_r$ (and similarly for T_2) is generally given. This is the equation of Steady State Free Precession (SSFP):

$$M_\perp = M_0 \frac{\sin\alpha}{1+T_1/T_2+(1-T_1/T_2)\cos\alpha}. \tag{10.54}$$

In practice, though, it is found that for a non-homogeneous field the dynamic equilibrium described is not distributed uniformly over the object of measurement; this can lead to very disturbing image artifacts. A better result is achieved when the pulse sequence shown in Fig. 10.47 is modified by removing the gradient pulses marked in gray. Such a sequence is known by the name FISP (Fast Imaging with Steady Precession). Here, only the phase encoding is compensated. Otherwise, this sequence differs from the FLASH sequence only through the missing spoiler pulse. The image signal, which is a function of T_1, T_2 and α, behaves qualitatively in a way similar to that described by Eq. (10.54): object regions with $T_1=T_2$, such as aqueous body fluids, are imaged bright, in particular when $\alpha=90°$. The exact signal behavior can be derived from the equations given in [10.26] through averaging of the magnetization as a function of the angle of precession, α, over a volume element [10.29].

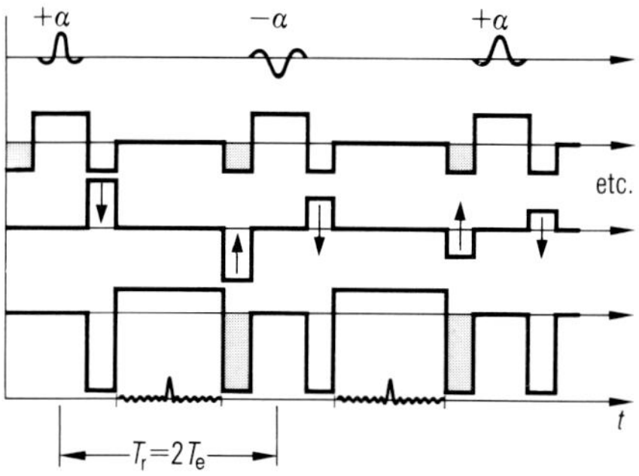

Fig. 10.47
SSFP pulse sequence.
The FISP sequence is obtained by omitting the gradient pulses (shown in gray)

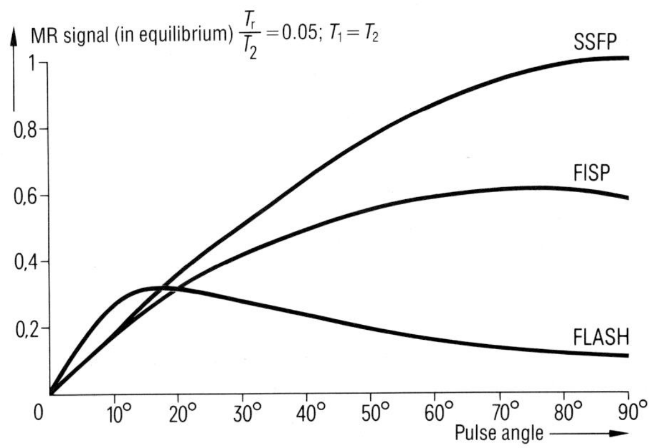

Fig. 10.48
FISP signal as a function of the pulse angle, α, compared with FLASH and SSFP signals
(Source: Dr. Oppelt)

Figure 10.48 gives the FISP signal as a function of α, calculated in this way, in comparison with FLASH and SSFP.

Thanks to their fast repetition rates, both methods permit the use of three-dimensional sampling with a high spatial resolution over an acceptable time of measurement: for example, 128 × 256 × 256 data acquisitions in about 13 min. For this, the slice gradient, G_z, is switched in stepwise – for each Fourier plane acquired – for phase encoding of the third dimension. Figure 10.49 shows sagittal head scans from three-dimensional data files measured with FLASH and with FISP sequences. In the FISP image (a) the "low viscosity" regions (edema about the solid tumor and liquor) are clearly brighter, whereas the FLASH image (b) shows approximately the contrast behavior of a T_1-weighted spin-echo image, with its typical demarcation between gray and white brain matter. Impressive is the outstanding signal-to-noise ratio, in spite of very small volume elements.

Echoplanar methods

The basic idea, which accounts for designating those methods described below "echoplanar imaging" [10.30], consists of the following: after a single selective RF excitation to produce a series of spin echos or gradient echos in the readout gradient (G_x), the different lines in the k plane are ordered with the help of a suitable modulation of the phase encoding gradient (G_y). The readout of the echo sequence must be completed within a time, the order of magnitude of which does not exceed T_2 or T_2^*: the decay of the transverse magnetization causes, in addition to a signal loss, a weighting of the Fourier projections in accordance with the order of their acquisition, so that an undesirable anisotropic change in the modulation transfer function would then result in the phase encoding direction. Figure 10.50a shows the echoplanar pulse

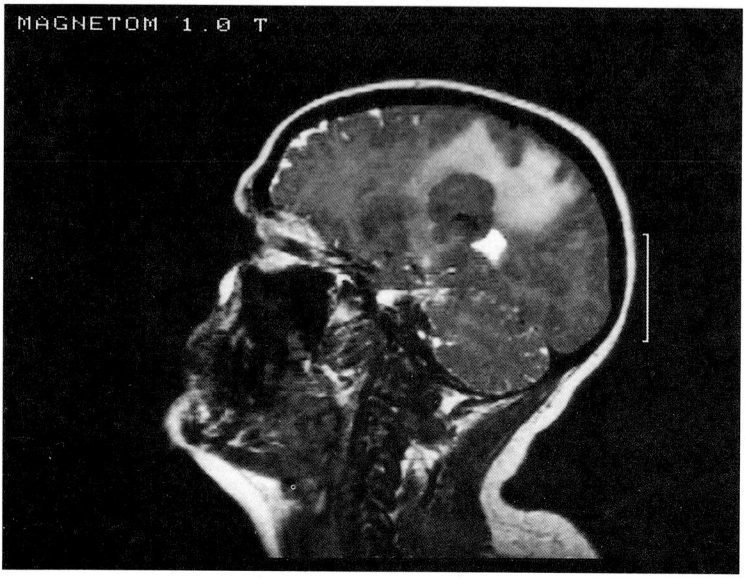

a)

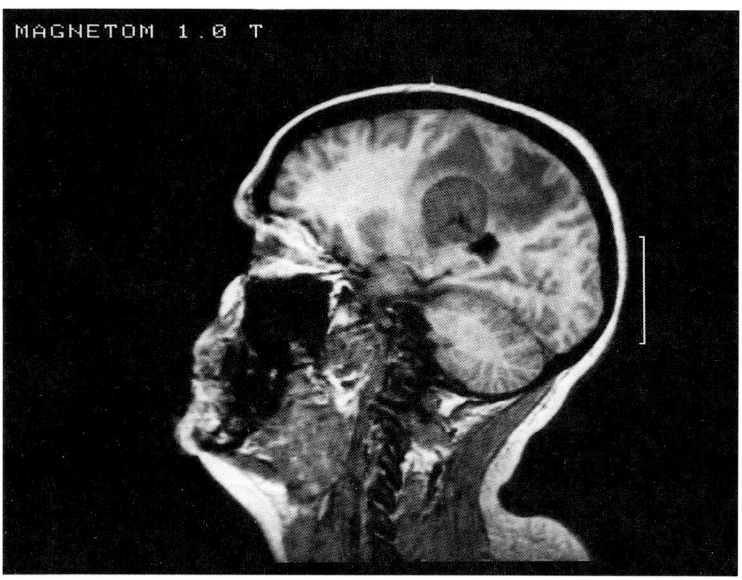

b)

Fig. 10.49
Sagittal head scan from a FISP image (a), showing bright low-viscosity regions, and from a FLASH image (b), with typical delineation of gray and white brain matter

sequence described in [10.30] in a slightly modified form. The needle-shaped G_y pulses in the switching intervals give rise to the meandering passes through the spatial frequency matrix (Fig. 10.30 b), so that the sampling points are made to occur equidistantly. Every other time function of the x or y gradient (among others, a sine-shaped G_x modulation and/or a constant G_y have been proposed) fundamentally leads to a non-uniform occupation of the k plane for sampling equidistantly in time. For the image reconstruction a Fourier transformation is then no longer sufficient, and it becomes necessary to make use of either interpolative matrix regeneration or more general integral transformations. If the requirements placed on the field of view or the spatial resolution are not too demanding, it is possible to sample the spatial frequency half-space with one "shot". In accordance with Eq. (10.26), for a pixel size of 5 mm and a pulse flat top length of 1 ms, a gradient strength of 4.7 mT/m is necessary. For a gradient polarity reversal time of 1 ms, about 70 ms would be necessary for the acquisition of measurement data for an image of 64 × 64 pixels. If one wishes, however, to obtain the level of resolution and pixel number known from spin-echo sequences, the demands on the gradient system rapidly overstep the limits imposed by technological feasibility. This is particularly true for the switching times, which act parasitically. This is the main reason why the echo-planar method has, in practice, not become established in MRI, even though – for the optimum choice of T_e or T_s relative to T_2 – it is the equal of the spin-echo method in terms of the signal-to-noise ratio per square root of the total data acquisition time ($N \cdot T_s$).

The technical problems just described can be avoided if, for each excitation pulse, only a few Fourier projections are acquired at the same time. These

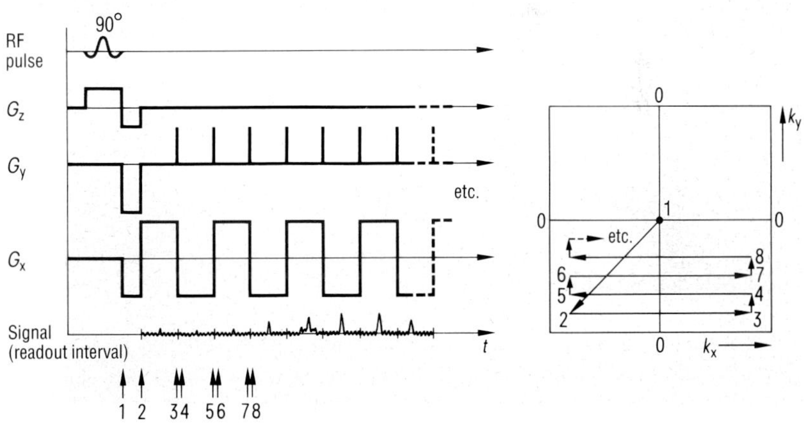

a) Pulse sequence

b) Sampling path in k space

Fig. 10.50 Echoplanar pulse sequence

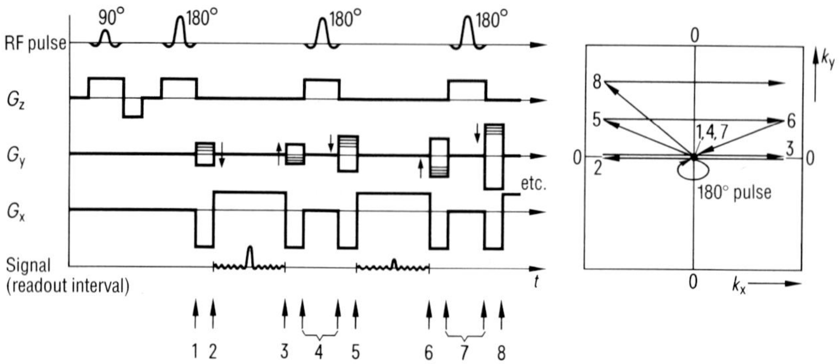

a) Pulse sequence b) Sampling path

Fig. 10.51
Modified echoplanar pulse sequence for a small number of Fourier projections with 180° pulses

so-called hybrid methods reduce the minimum time of measurement and the number of echo signals acquired over each T_r interval. Under certain conditions, 180° pulses can again be introduced to generate echos [10.31], so that a refocussing of the constant field inhomogeneities takes place. Figure 10.51 shows such a pulse sequence and its sampling path in the k plane. A phase encoding performed periodically at the echo position would not be suitable, because this would cause a repeating amplitude modulation of the form e^{-nT_e/T_2}, corresponding to each Fourier line, for each excitation pulse. The reconstructed image would then show a multiply imaged object. The phase encoding of each echo must be performed in such a way as to define a monotonic relationship between the T_2 weighting and the spatial frequency.

In addition to the examples of echoplanar methods described here, there are also other variations [10.32]; however, their description would go beyond the framework of our present discussion.

10.3.4 MR angiography

Apart from T_1, T_2 and the spin density, ϱ, magnetic resonance tomography also offers the possibility of using the velocity of the excited spins as an imaging parameter (see section 5.2.5). This opens the way to a fully new and medically significant field, namely the non-invasive presentation of vascular structures, known as MR angiography. This method, which has already proven itself through a series of clinical studies, will now be presented in detail.

Principle

Equation (10.50) characterizes the signal from a normal spin-echo sequence. We assume that the excited spins do not undergo motion relative to the magnetic field gradient. If this is not the case, then the MR signal will deviate more or less from that given by Eq. (10.50). Motion artifacts or flow artifacts will also occur [10.33], which complicate the interpretation of the MR image or – especially for high flow velocities – prevent evaluation altogether. In order to understand the change in signal intensity with nonstationary spins, it is necessary to examine the development of the phase for the transverse magnetization over time within a volume element. In its general form, this is given by:

$$\varphi(t)=\gamma\int_0^t \vec{G}(t')\,\vec{r}(t')\,\mathrm{d}t'. \tag{10.55}$$

Here, $\vec{G}$ is the magnetic field gradient vector and $\vec{r}$ the – usually – time-dependent position vector. For motion in the direction of a gradient, it then follows that:

$$\varphi(t)=\gamma\int_0^t G_x(t')\,x(t')\,\mathrm{d}t'. \tag{10.56}$$

Expanding $x(t)$ in a Taylor series,

$$x(t)=x_0+\frac{\mathrm{d}x}{\mathrm{d}t}(t-t_0)+\tfrac{1}{2}\frac{\mathrm{d}^2x}{\mathrm{d}t^2}(t-t_0)^2+\ \ldots, \tag{10.57}$$

it is then possible to represent Eq. (10.56) in the following form:

$$\varphi(t)=\varphi_0(t)+\varphi_v(t)+\varphi_\mathrm{b}(t), \tag{10.58}$$

where

$$\varphi_0(t)=\gamma x_0\int_0^t G_x(t')\,\mathrm{d}t',$$

$$\varphi_v(t)=\gamma v\int_0^t G(t')\,t'\,\mathrm{d}t$$

and

$$\varphi_\mathrm{a}(t)=\tfrac{1}{2}\gamma_\mathrm{a}\int_0^t G(t')\,t^2\,\mathrm{d}t',$$

in which the point t_0 can be set to zero without any limitations and the first and second spatial derivatives correspond to the velocity, v, and the acceleration, a, respectively. The first term, $\varphi_0(t)$, in Eq. (10.58), describes the dependence of the phase on the spin position x_0. The maximum phase coherence occurs at a zero of the time integral over G_x. This is the case at the time at which the spin echo appears. The other terms give rise, through motion at constant velocity and accelerated motion of the spin during the measurement, to additional phase contributions.

As an example, if we examine a uniform motion (that is, with $a=0$) in the direction of the readout gradient, G_x, the dashed line drawn in Fig. 10.52 represents the time dependence of the phase, $\varphi_v(t)$. This behavior describes a typical spin-echo sequence, such as shown in Fig. 10.40. At the time of appearance of the spin echo, T_e, the magnitude of φ_v is proportional to the velocity, v. For a material all parts of which move with the same velocity through the volume of measurement, this simply means that an additional phase factor occurs in the reconstructed image; the modulus image therefore remains unaffected by any motion. In general, however, other imaging conditions apply: the slice thickness is larger than the blood vessel diameter, and the velocity vector is parallel to the slice. The assumed laminar flow profile then gives different phase angles for the transverse magnetization at the time of the spin echo's occurrence. The MR signal for a pixel within the volume element arises through the superposition of all magnetization vectors. For a sufficiently large velocity, all phase angles between 0 and 2π would be present, and the resulting MR signal would then vanish due to destructive interference. The vessel, with blood flowing through it, is then seen with a lower intensity than the surrounding stationary tissue. These conditions can be described formally through the inclusion of an additional factor, $f(\Delta v)$, in Eq. (10.50):

$$S=\varrho f(\Delta v)\,\mathrm{e}^{-T_e/T_2}(1-\mathrm{e}^{-T_r/T_1}), \tag{10.59}$$

where $f(\Delta v)$ is a function of the velocity distribution within the volume element from which the pixel is taken. In a specific case, $f(\Delta v)$ must be determined from the particular velocity distribution and the sequence employed.

A simple method shows us how to keep the magnitude of the additional phase term, φ_v, in Eq. (10.58) small. In accordance with Fig. 10.53 two negative gradients, arranged symmetrically about the 180° pulse, are added on to the sequence [10.34]. Due to their symmetrical positioning, the time dependence of the phase, $\varphi_0(t)$, remains unchanged during the readout interval; this means that the MR signal for stationary spins also remains unchanged. The time dependence of the phase for uniformly moving spins is indicated in Fig. 10.52 by the unbroken line. It can be seen that, for suitable dimensioning of the gradient pulses (in terms of duration and amplitude), the phase, φ_v, passes through zero at the time of the spin echo's occurrence – independently of the velocity.

For the case of laminar flow, all magnetization vectors then point in the same direction. This implies constructive interference and the maximum value for the resulting MR signal. This so-called flow-rephasing, or bipolar, sequence (Fig. 10.53) consequently represents the vessel as a bright structure. The normal spin-echo sequence, by contrast, is a flow-dephasing sequence, since the moving spins are not rephased at the time of occurrence of the spin echo. A simple method for the production of a pure vessel image can be derived from the fact that the MR signal remains unchanged for stationary spins: two MR images are acquired, the first by means of a flow-rephasing, bipolar sequence, and the second by means of a normal, flow-dephasing sequence. The remaining parameters of measurement, T_e and T_r, are unchanged. Following this, a subtraction is performed between the two MR images in order to eliminate all stationary image parts: the resulting image is then composed only of spins undergoing uniform motion.

The inclusion of further gradient pulses permits compensating for higher-order phase terms of the motion, such as acceleration. As a rule, though, the echo time must be lengthened in order to provide room to accommodate additional gradient pulses. The dimensioning of flow-rephasing, bipolar sequences takes

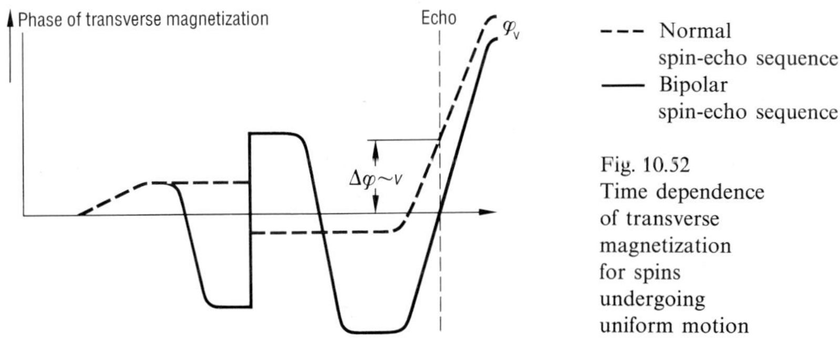

Fig. 10.52
Time dependence of transverse magnetization for spins undergoing uniform motion

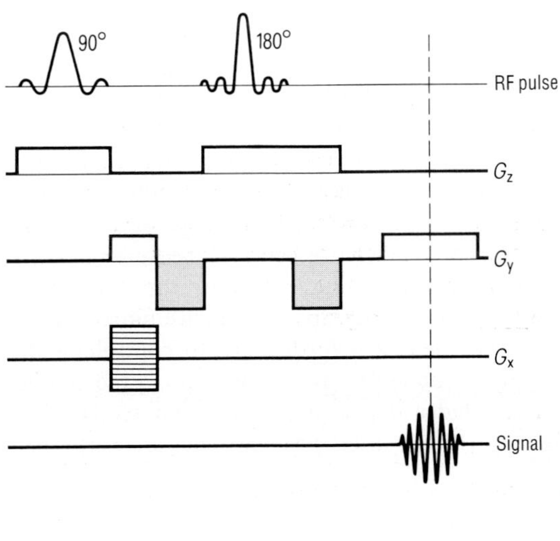

Fig. 10.53
Schematic representation of a bipolar spin-echo sequence

place as follows: beginning with a normal spin-echo sequence, the two additional gradient pulses are chosen to be of such duration and amplitude that the phase term, φ_v, present in Eq. (10.59) vanishes at the time of occurrence of the spin echo; that is,

$$\int_0^{T_e} G_x(t')\, t' \mathrm{d}t' = 0. \tag{10.60}$$

If one still wishes to compensate for acceleration effects, it is then necessary that the phase term φ_a vanish as well, so that

$$\int_0^{T_e} G_x(t')\, t'^2 \mathrm{d}t' = 0. \tag{10.61}$$

For spin-echo sequences, the integration runs up to $T_e/2$ (the midpoint of the 180° pulse) with a positive integrand and, from this point to T_e (that is, from the midpoint of the 180° pulse to the echo), with a negative integrand, analogously to Eq. (10.10) in section 10.2.1.

Based on Eq. (10.60) and (10.61), it is possible to determine the gradient pulses needed for "motion refocussing". At the same time, these pulses must lie within the technical possibilities of the given gradient system (see section 10.2.2). In order to obtain short echo times in the range from 20 to 30 ms, it is necessary to choose short pulse lengths and correspondingly large amplitudes.

Clinical studies

In order to be able to follow vascular structures over a larger region, slice thicknesses between 30 and 60 mm are required. In general, this leads to low contrast between arteries and stationary tissue. In order to improve the recognizability of vascular structures, use of the subtraction procedure already mentioned – according to which a flow-rephased and a flow-dephased image are measured and the stationary part of the image subtracted out – is recommended. Nevertheless, the flow-rephasing technique only functions well under the assumption of uniform motion. Spins accelerated during the pulse sequence cannot be optimally rephased. It is known that this is the case for an arterial vascular system in which there is a large difference between the flow velocities between the diastole and the systole. The measurements are therefore ECG-triggered, so that the same velocity relationships apply for each Fourier projection. The position of the trigger in time is a further aid to controlling the contrast between vascular structures and stationary tissue. During the systole, the arterial velocities are so large that a dephasing results from acceleration, and the arteries then appear dark. In all, three measurements are performed (Figs. 10.54a to c):

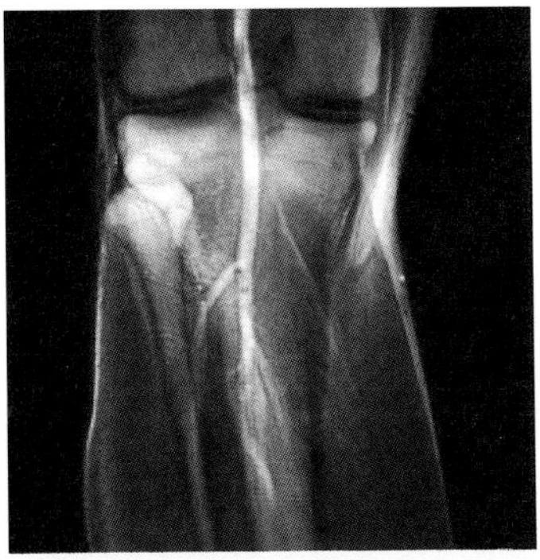

a) Flow-rephased, diastole:
arteries bright, veins bright

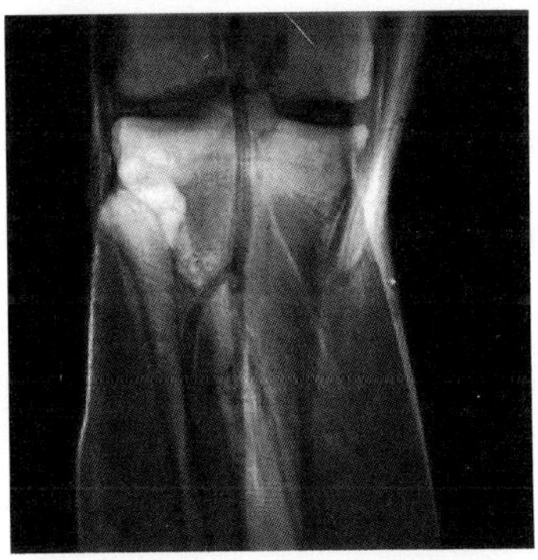

b) Flow-rephased, systole:
arteries dark, veins bright

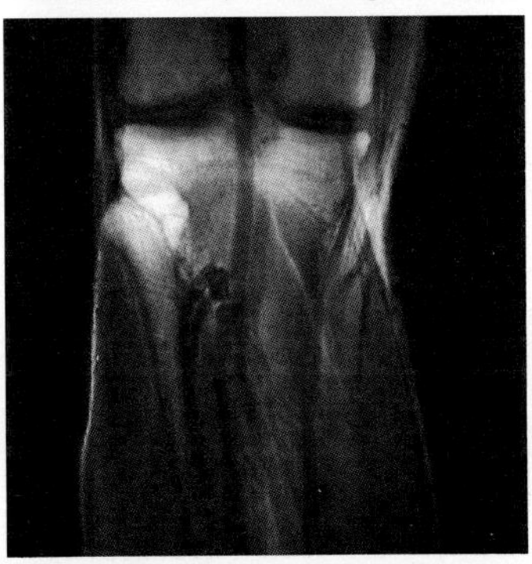

c) Flow-dephased, diastole:
arteries dark, veins dark

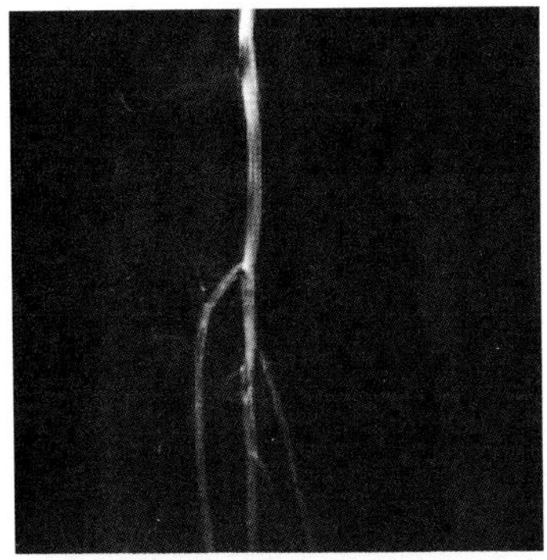

d) Arterial image
(difference of a and b)

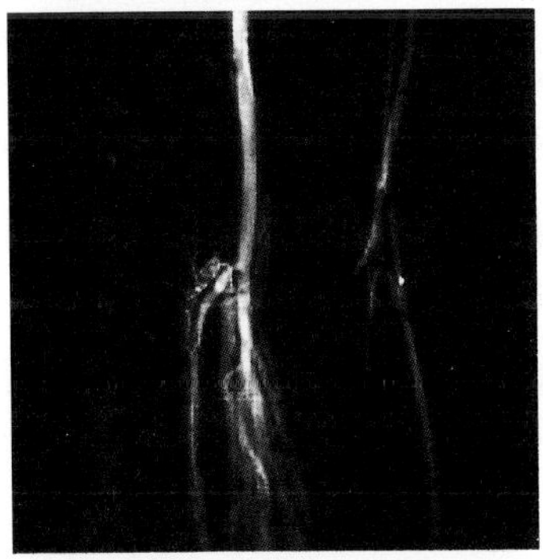

e) Arterial and venous image
(difference of a and c)

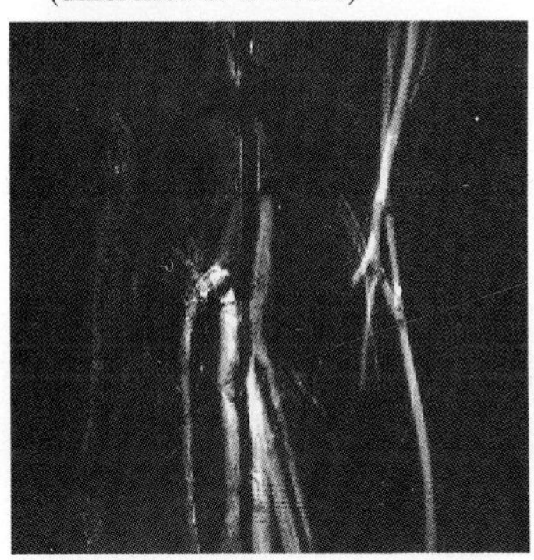

f) Venous image
(difference of d and e)

Fig. 10.54
ECG-triggered images (a to c) and subtraction images (d to f) of a part of the tibia for a healthy test subject: echo time 56 ms, slice thickness 34 mm, pixel size 0.8 mm, time measured approx. 4 min per image

a) flow-rephased, diastole (arteries: bright, veins: bright)
b) flow-rephased, systole (arteries: dark, veins: bright)
c) flow-dephased, diastole (arteries: dark, veins: dark)

The intensity of stationary tissue is the same for all three sequences. Figures 10.54a to c show for example these three images for a part of the tibia below the knee of a healthy test subject. The echo time was 56 ms, the slice thickness 34 mm and the pixel size 0.8 mm. The time of measurement for each image was 256 heart beats; that is, about four minutes. From these images, subtraction images were produced (Figures 10.54d to f), namely

d) the difference between a) and b): arterial image
e) the difference between a) and c): arterial and venous image
f) the difference between d) and e): venous image.

The individual images reproduce the anatomical details very faithfully. In particular, the bifurcation of the arteria poplitea into three tibial trunk arteries can be seen clearly.

The method of MR vascular presentation introduced here demonstrates that, in the field of angiography, MRI is capable of producing images very bit as good as those taken from conventional x-ray angiography or digital subtraction angiography (DSA).

11 Sonography

The development of ultrasound equipment started in the fifties with equipment for examining the skull and heart. Stimulated by sonar and radar technology, these developments culminated in 2-dimensional ultrasound examination of the abdominal organs and thyroid glands, obstetric examinations and sectional displays of the heart. Today, combination units using several scanning methods and satisfying all diagnostic requirements are widespread. The choice and consideration of subjects treated is limited by the scope of this book. Reference is made to the literature for a more detailed treatment (see page 609).

11.1 Scanning methods

11.1.1 Echo pulse technique

Almost all ultrasound methods used today in medical diagnostics are based on the echo pulse technique (Fig. 11.1): a transmitter excites a piezoelectric transducer to a short-lived damped oscillation. This is propagated in the medi-

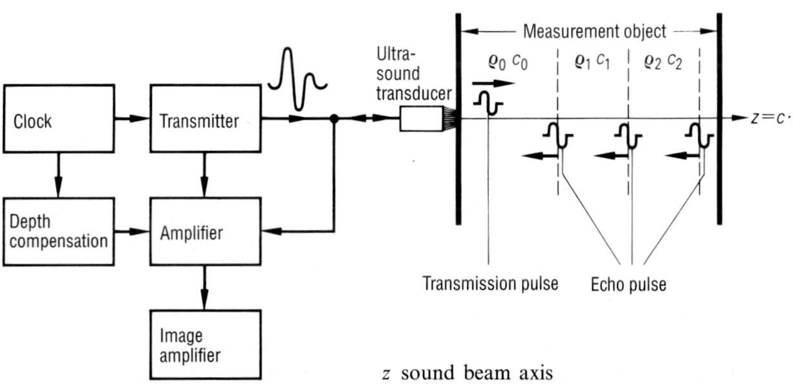

Fig. 11.1
Diagram illustrating the principle of the echo pulse method

z sound beam axis

Average values for soft biological tissue:

Velocity of sound c	1 540 m/s
Acoustical impedance $Z=\varrho c$	$1.5\cdot 10^6$ Pa s/m
Wavelength λ at 3.5 MHz	0.44 mm

um with the velocity of sound, c. Acoustically effective boundary surfaces and structures in the medium are characterized by changes in the acoustic impedance, Z, which is the product of the density ϱ and the velocity of sound c:

$$Z = \varrho c.$$

For soft human tissue, the average velocity of sound is 1540 m/s. Every change in impedance along the axis of the ultrasound beam z causes some of the incident ultrasound intensity to be reflected and return as an echo to the transducer.

The ultrasound transducer, as a first approximation, acts as a piston oscillating forwards and backwards, which alternately compresses and expands the coupled medium. The changes in density produced in this way are propagated in liquids as well as in soft biological tissue as longitudinal waves. The wavelength λ, the ultrasound frequency f and the velocity of sound c are related by the well known formula:

$$c = \lambda f.$$

The ratio of the reflected to the incident intensity at a boundary surface is the reflection factor, r. For vertical incidence, r is a function of the impedances in front of and behind the boundary surface. The transmission factor, d, is defined in a similar manner as the ratio of the intensity passing through the boundary surface to the incident intensity.

The impedance differences between different soft types of tissue are very small; the values for the reflection factor, r, in the human body are only a few per mil. Therefore, a large number of echoes are obtained along the axis of the beam, which can be received in a time sequence t proportional to the distance z of the point of origin of the echo from the transducer, and can be displayed as pixels.

For sonography, it is of special importance that ultrasound is almost totally reflected at the tissue-air boundary layer and approximately 50% reflected at the tissue-bone boundary layer. Therefore, access to certain body organs is restricted. Thus, the heart can be irradiated through the "acoustic window" which is produced by the intercostal space between the sternum and the left lung lobes.

A basic distinction must be made between mirror and diffuse reflection. Mirror reflection occurs at boundary surfaces which are large compared to the wavelength. This applies, for example, to the surfaces of the internal organs and large vessels. The incident sound beam is reflected by diffuse scattering at objects which are small compared to the wavelength. The echoes returning from such scattering centers are considerably weaker. However, they are carriers of important information on the condition of the tissue inside the organ. Of importance here is an effect known from laser technology which is called "speckle". This is understood as the echo pattern from scattering regions which do not correspond to the direct imaging of the scattering centers. These patterns are generated by interference caused by the coherence of the ultrasound waves [11.10].

Because of the fine structure of the surface, diffuse scattering also occurs at large organ surfaces in addition to mirror reflection. This makes it possible to display non-vertical surfaces in the ultrasound image. On the other hand, it is also found that oblique organ boundaries are imaged more and more weakly.

The ultrasound pulse passing through the body is subject to attenuation by absorption, partial reflection and scattering in the tissue, as well as field dilution in the ultrasound beam. The attenuation is taken into account by the equipment through depth compensation, i.e. by a runtime-dependent, user-defined echo amplification control.

The absorption increases exponentially in the tissue with the traversed path, but also increases exponentially with frequency (equation 6.26). This restricts the penetration depth of the ultrasound pulse. For the ultrasound intensities which are used today, the choice of the ultrasound frequency is a compromise between penetration depth and image resolution.

It should be pointed out here that until now no harmful effect has been observed for the intensities used in ultrasound diagnostics (see section 6.4) [11.19, 11.20].

11.1.2 Ultrasound field, axial and lateral resolution

The quality of ultrasound images is influenced by various parameters. Physically, the image quality is limited by the resolution which can be achieved. This is understood as the minimum distance between objects in millimeters for which these can still be distinguished in the ultrasound image. The limit of the resolution which can be achieved is given by the wavelength, λ; at 3.5 MHz it is approximately 0.44 mm. However, such values are not obtained in practice.

A distinction is made between the axial resolution, Δz, which is the resolution in the direction of the sound beam axis, and the lateral resolution, Δx, in the plane vertical to the sound beam axis. The axial resolution is only determined by the duration of the ultrasound pulse and, with present day equipment and technology, it is less than a millimeter and therefore close to the physical resolution limit of a wavelength (at 3.5 MHz). The field distribution in the ultrasound beam has the effect that equally good resolution values are not obtained in the lateral direction. The lateral resolution, Δx, is of the order of a few millimeters and depends on the geometrical shape of the transducer, the ultrasound frequency and the axial distance.

Fig. 11.2 shows the definition of the lateral resolution. If an ultrasound transducer is moved along the x axis, i.e. vertically to the radiation axis z, the two bell-shaped curves on the right-hand side of the image are obtained as echo signals from two neighboring point objects as a result of the 3-dimensional shape of the ultrasound cone. The lateral resolution, Δx, is the minimum distance between two objects which can still be distinguished from each other. Δx is defined as the -6 dB width or half width value of the echo signal from a point object.

The lateral resolution directly reflects the outgoing sound radiation characteristic of the ultrasound transducer, which will be discussed in detail below because of its special importance for image quality [11.7, 11.8, 11.9].

According to Huygens' principle, every point on the surface of an ultrasound transducer can be regarded as the starting point for an elementary spherical wave. Interference of the elementary waves produces a 3-dimensional sound field, which is defined by the characteristic near field and far field properties.

Fig. 11.3 shows an ultrasound field of a 2-dimensional spherical ultrasound transducer. The center of the transducer is at the coordinate origin and has a radius a. The lateral distance from the axis is based on this radius and the axial distance is normalized to the ratio a^2/λ. The figure shows curves of constant sound pressure drop compared to the maximum pressure arising in every plane vertical to the axis. In the echo pulse method, the ultrasound fields from the transmitting and receiving transducers are superimposed. If they are both identical, the characteristic shown in Fig. 11.3 should be multiplied by itself. Then the ultrasound cone, which is bounded by the two -3 dB curves, corresponds to the definition of the lateral resolution given in Fig. 11.2: for every axial distance, the value for Δx can be read off from the diameter of the -3 dB cone in Fig. 11.3 for a given transducer radius and given wavelength.

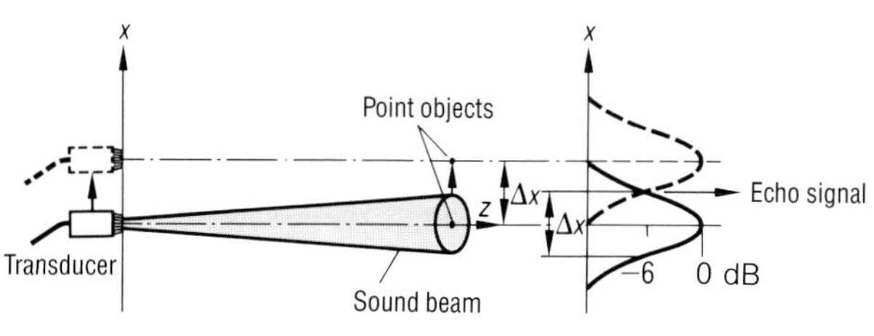

Fig. 11.2
Definition of the lateral resolution: Δx is the -6 dB width of the echo signal from a point object. Two point objects with a lateral separation of at least Δx can be distinguished

If, in what follows, we only consider this -3 dB lobe, some typical properties can be read off from Fig. 11.3. The sound field is characterized by the near field in the range of axial distances $< a^2/\lambda$ and by the far field for axial distances $> a^2/\lambda$.

In the vicinity of the near field, the -3 dB lobe is wide and so the resolution is unfavorable. In addition there are also interference effects here which can lead to ambiguities in the ultrasound image. Between the near field and the far field is the so-called focus region, which confines the sound lobe to yield

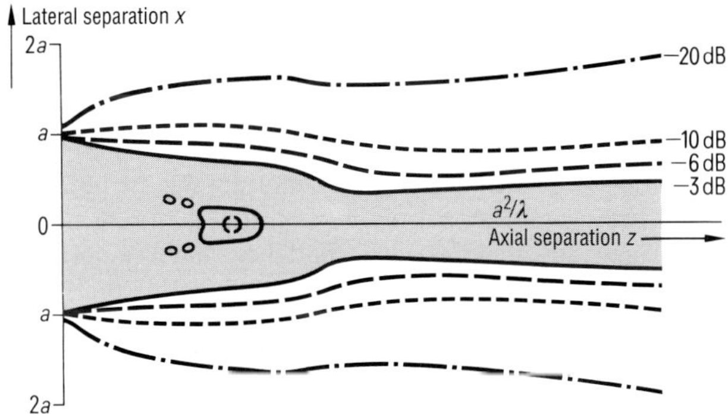

Fig. 11.3
Ultrasound field of a flat circular ultrasound transducer of radius a with pulse excitation. The figure shows curves of constant pressure drop compared to the maximum pressure occurring in every plane perpendicular to the axis

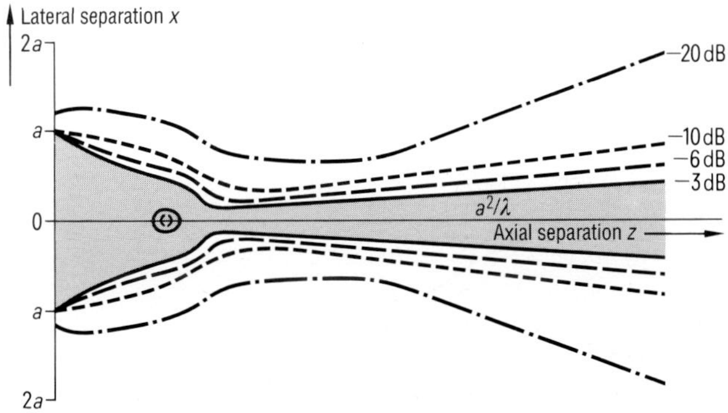

Fig. 11.4
Ultrasound field of a spherically curved circular transducer with radius *a*. The figure shows curves of constant pressure drop compared to the maximum pressure in every plane perpendicular to the axis

the best lateral resolution. The circular flat transducer generates this confinement at a distance of $z=0.75\,a^2/\lambda$. In the vicinity of the far field, the ultrasound lobe is wider and proportional to the transducer distance so that the resolution is worse.

For a flat circular transducer, the lateral resolution at the focus is approximately one third of the transducer diameter, 2a. For a transducer with radius $a=7.5$ mm, the lateral focus resolution is approximately 5 mm. The near field length, N, for a frequency of 3.5 MHz is $N=0.75\,a^2/\lambda=9.6$ cm. The focus resolution is improved by reducing the transducer diameter, but the focal length, a^2/λ, is smaller at the same time and the aperture angle of the ultrasound beam larger in the far field. On the other hand, the focal distance can be influenced by a suitable choice of the frequency or wavelength.

The ultrasound field of a transducer can be considerably changed if instead of a flat surface (Fig. 11.3) a spherically curved surface is chosen or an acoustic lens is placed in front of the flat transducer. Fig. 11.4 shows the example of an ultrasound field for a transducer with a radius of curvature $R=1.1$ normalized to the distance a^2/λ. Such a transducer is usually called a focussing transducer. The focussing measures act in such a way that they shift the position of optimum resolution in the direction of smaller distances and at the same time increase the sharpness of focus, i.e. the lateral resolution in the focus region. This becomes clear when Figs. 11.3 and 11.4 are compared. A transducer with radius $a=7.5$ mm and a radius of curvature of $1.1\,a^2/\lambda=10.5$ cm generates a focal resolution of approximately 1.5 mm for a focal distance of 5 cm at 3.5 MHz.

However, there are limits to this type of extra focussing, as shown in Fig. 11.5. In this figure, the -3 dB lobes of transducers with different radii of curva-

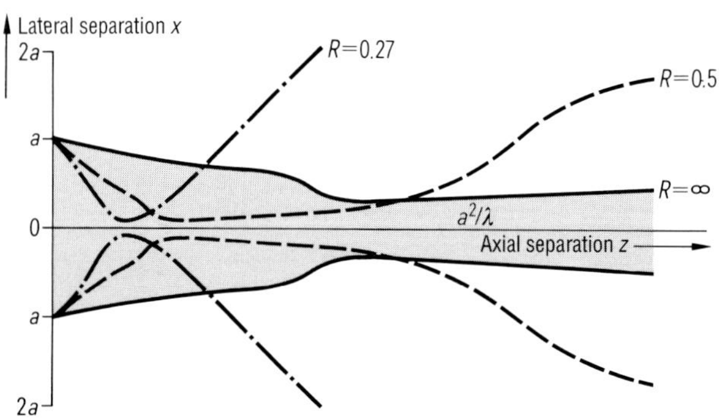

Fig. 11.5
-3 dB ultrasound lobes of spherically curved circular transducers with radius a for different normalized radii of curvature, R. The figure shows curves of constant pressure drop compared to the maximum pressure occurring in every plane perpendicular to the axis

ture are compared. As the radius of curvature becomes smaller, i.e. with increasing strength of focussing, the focal distance becomes shorter and shorter and the focal resolution better and better. However, at the same time the acuity depth becomes smaller and smaller. In other words, the far field resolution becomes more and more unfavorable. The sound lobe for $R \to \infty$ is in this representation identical to the -3 dB lobe for the non-curved transducer in Fig. 11.3.

The above discussion shows how the lateral resolution, apart from the axial distance and the ultrasound frequency, depends on the geometrical parameters: transducer radius and radius of curvature.

Unfortunately, these parameters can not be used independently of each other for optimizing the resolution behavior. The choice of the suitable ultrasound transducer with fixed focussing is a compromise which has to be made in each case, depending on the medical objectives.

11.1.3 Imaging methods

In ultrasound technology, the high-speed real time method has gained acceptance today. Other displays are also offered by modern equipment, as will be explained below.

A mode (A for amplitude modulation) is obtained with a transducer fixed in position on the body surface (Fig. 11.6). The amplitude of the echo signals

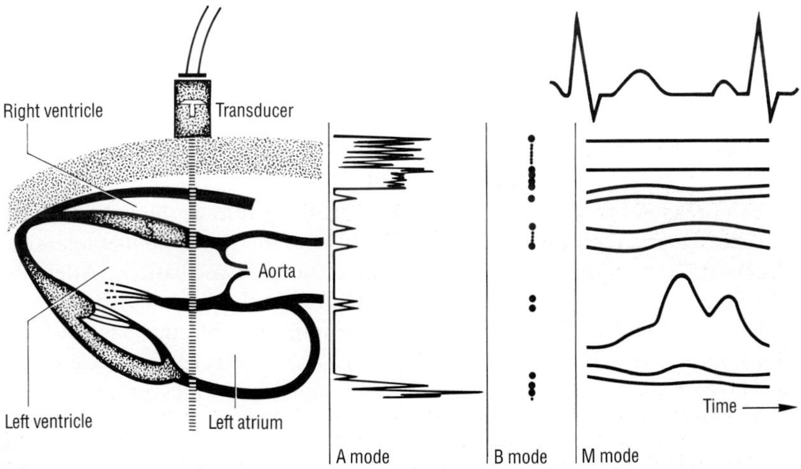

Fig. 11.6 A, B, and M mode displays of the heart

is displayed as a function of depth. Boundary surfaces moving in the body can be recognized by the backwards and forwards movement of the corresponding echo amplitudes.

M mode (M for time motion) is obtained in a similar manner to the A image, i.e. with a stationary transducer. The difference is that the echoes are displayed in B mode (B for brightness modulation): the echoes are imaged as pixels whose light density on the screen or their blackening on photographic paper depends on the height of the echo amplitudes.

By juxtaposing successive echo lines in the image memory or on UV-sensitive paper (M recorder), the time motion in the object can be recognized and evaluated.

In the 2-dimensional B image method, the body is scanned line by line; the echo signals obtained are displayed as a 2-dimensional sectional image. As the designation B image expresses, the echoes are described in the B mode, i.e. as light density modulated pixels, or in a similar manner as with the M mode.

The main disadvantage of beaming from one direction, whether A, M or B, is that the contours of the organ boundaries – in general not perpendicular to the direction of sound – are only poorly displayed or not at all. So-called compound methods, which emit sound waves toward the region from several directions, can help here. Because of the long scanning times of a few seconds, these methods are only suitable for regions with little motion, which in addition must have access free of air and bones over a large angular range.

The different methods for acquiring fast sectional images (so-called real-time images) are described in section 11.2. It should be noted that today the image information is totally reproduced in accordance with television standards. With the digital memories and scan converters necessary for this, user-friendly presentation and documentation systems are provided.

11.1.4 Doppler methods

In the ultrasound diagnostic systems considered up to now, the amplitude of the echo signals received by the transducer was evaluated. A source for extra information is the frequency content of the ultrasound oscillations. Attempts have been continually made to exploit the effect of the frequency-dependent attenuation of human tissue as a means of identification, but this has not been totally satisfactory. On the other hand, there are various methods based on the Doppler effect which have matured to standard methods or are on the brink of this.

The principle is based on the physical effect of the frequency shift of a moving signal source discovered by Doppler. In ultrasound diagnostics, these signal sources are reflecting parts of tissue which move relative to the ultrasound transducer.

The components of the movement which lie in the direction of sound propagation contribute to the Doppler signal. If the movement is directed towards the transducer, a signal with higher frequency is received and vice versa. What is especially interesting diagnostically is the total blood circulation of the heart and the peripheral vessels (see also section 6.2.1). In order to assess the blood flow, the weak back-scattering of the sound energy from the blood particles must be evaluated. Here, the most stringent requirements must be made on the signal dynamics of the equipment.

Two basic methods are:

a) continuous wave methods (CW Doppler) and
b) pulse wave methods (PW Doppler).

In CW Doppler, a transducer with two elements is used. One is used as the transmitter and the other as the receiver. The receiving frequency is shifted with respect to the transmission frequency, f_0, by the difference or Doppler frequency, Δf:

$$\Delta f = 2 f_0 \frac{v}{c} \cos \varphi .$$

where

v is the speed of the reflector
c is the velocity of sound and
φ is the angle between the directions of sound propagation and movement of the reflector.

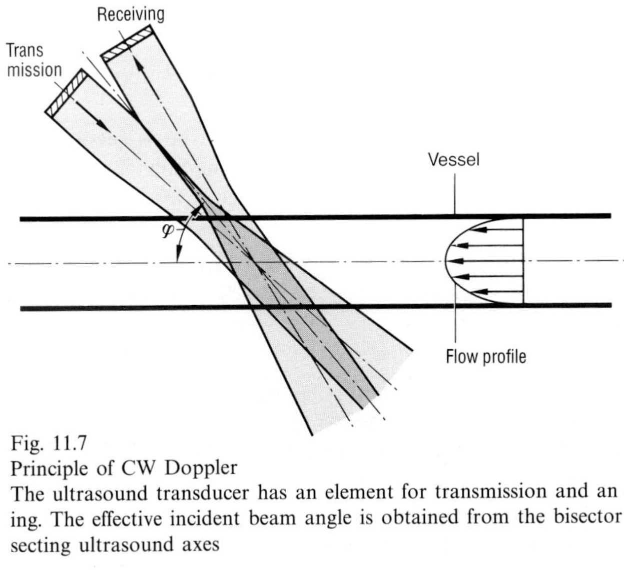

Fig. 11.7
Principle of CW Doppler
The ultrasound transducer has an element for transmission and an element for receiving. The effective incident beam angle is obtained from the bisector of the two intersecting ultrasound axes

There are practically no restrictions on the speed of movement of the reflector, i.e. of the tissue, since this is always small compared to the velocity of sound. However, it is a disadvantage that this method does not contain any depth information. Reflectors lying behind each other in the ultrasound path are taken together.

In this case, the PW Doppler method provides assistance. Since pulses are employed, the transducer can consist of a single element which transmits and receives successively.

In order to be able to evaluate information from a desired depth, a gate is set by the user and opened for a time which can be selected. The unit then only processes these signals which enter this time gate.

The advantage of the axial resolution in pulsed Doppler is however at the cost of restrictions in the measurement range of the speeds and accuracy. For a given pulse repetition frequency f_A, the limit for the speed of movement, v_{max}, is:

$$v_{max} = c \frac{f_A}{4 f_0}, \quad \text{if } \varphi = 0.$$

With increasing pulse repetition frequency, higher speeds can therefore be measured. This is also possible if the transmission frequency is selected lower, but then the resolution falls off. If the object speeds are higher than allowed by the measurement conditions, ambiguities occur in determining the frequency (frequency aliasing). Ambiguities in the depth determination occur if the pulse repetition frequency is too high compared to the gate position.

Apart from direct display of the speeds, recording of the Doppler frequency spectrum also gives information on vascular flow dynamics. For this, fast Fourier transforms (FFT) are used [11.17].

A new development is the processing of flows in a total cross section and their color-coded display in anatomical ultrasound sectional images. For this method, called CFI (color flow imaging), mainly phased array equipment is used.

11.2 Scanner designs

In ultrasound diagnostics, scan means the regular scanning of a plane of the body region of interest with ultrasound pulses according to a certain scan format in a predefined time sequence. Here, the echoes of the tissue structures encountered by the sound pulse and also the geometrical reference points distance (sound transit time) and direction (instantaneous transducer position) belonging to every reflection position are the raw scanning data.

In its initial phase, ultrasound diagnostics was dominated by mechanical scan methods. Apart from the manually operated compound scanner (Fig. 11.8), mechanical real-time scanners with parallel scanning (Fig. 11.9) and with sector scanning (Fig. 11.10) were used.

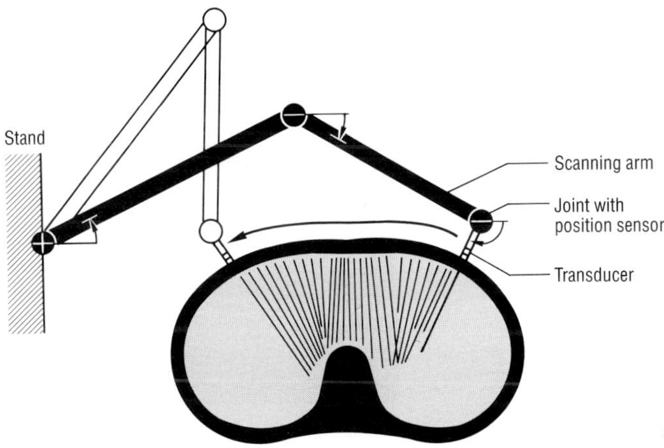

a)

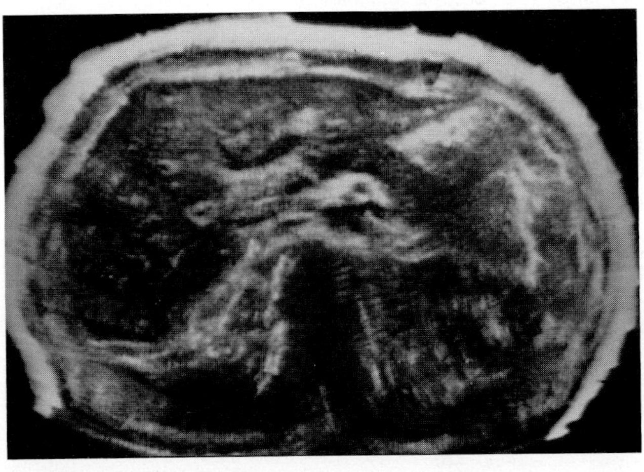

b)

Fig. 11.8
Compound scanner. Basic representation of the transducer guide and determination of the coordinates (a) and example (b): whole-body cross section

The common characteristic of these systems is the use of an individual transducer (also, if necessary, several in succession though only one transducer is activated at any time). With this transducer, usually one scan of the investigation plane is carried out automatically, with subsequent repetition of the cycle.

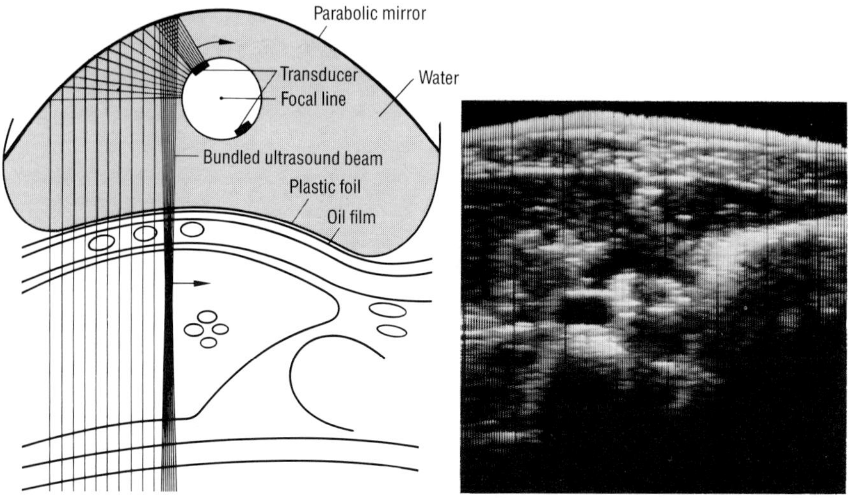

a) b)

Fig. 11.9
VIDOSON 635 Mechanical linear scanner with parallel scanning. Principle (a) and example (b): cross-section of the upper abdomen with right and left liver lobes, pancreas, vena cava and aorta

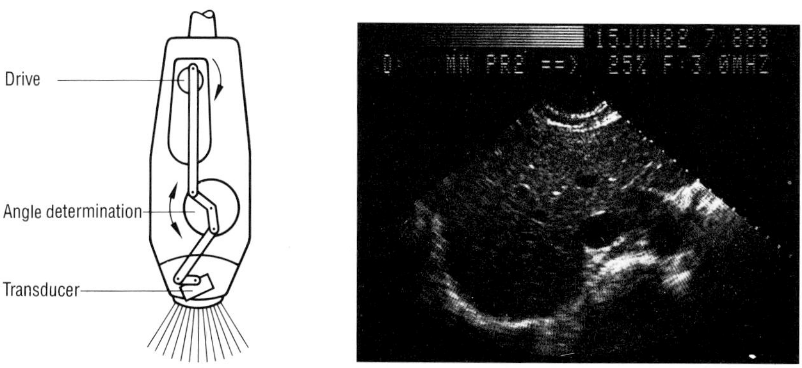

a) b)

Fig. 11.10
Mechanical sector scanner based on the wobbler principle. Mechanical design of the scanner (a) and example (b): cross section of the right liver lobe

Since the introduction of array technology in 1974, these mechanical methods have fallen more and more into disuse. The main reasons for this are the maintenance-free operation and resulting increase in reliability, the flexibility (simultaneous display of different operating modes, e.g. B and M) and the user friendliness of the array system.

An array is the name given for an arrangement in rows of the individual transducers (linear or curved), whereby the transducers are so small that they do not exhibit any marked directional characteristics.

The desired directional characteristic is only produced by simultaneous stimulation of a group of individual elements. Here, a scanning operation can be carried out purely electronically, both in rectilinear coordinates (linear array) and in polar coordinates (phased array or curved array). Array systems provide additional possibilities of improving image quality, such as dynamic focussing and dynamic aperture (see section 11.2.2).

Two basic scanning formats have become widespread:

1. Scanning in rectilinear coordinates, where practically only the linear array is used as a scanner (see Fig. 11.22).
2. Scanning in polar coordinates (sector). Here, mechanical systems and array systems (phased array, curved array) are in use (Fig. 11.11).

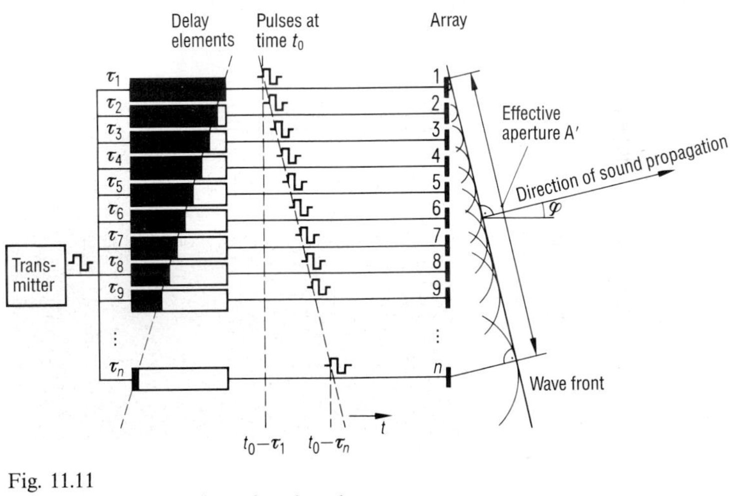

Fig. 11.11
Schematic representation of a phased array
The scanning angle is controlled by time-delayed excitation (τ_1 to τ_n) of the individual elements of the array (transmission case)

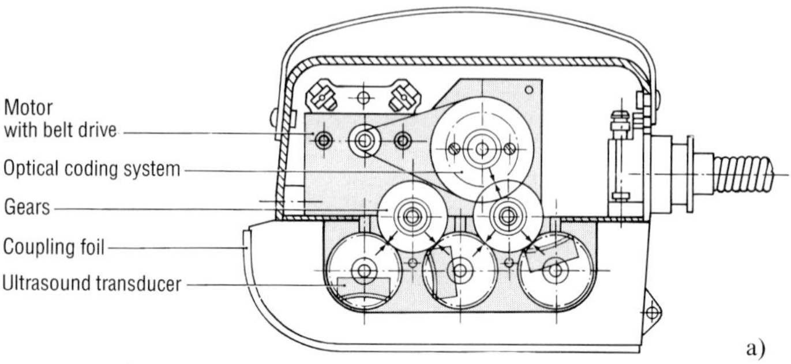

a)

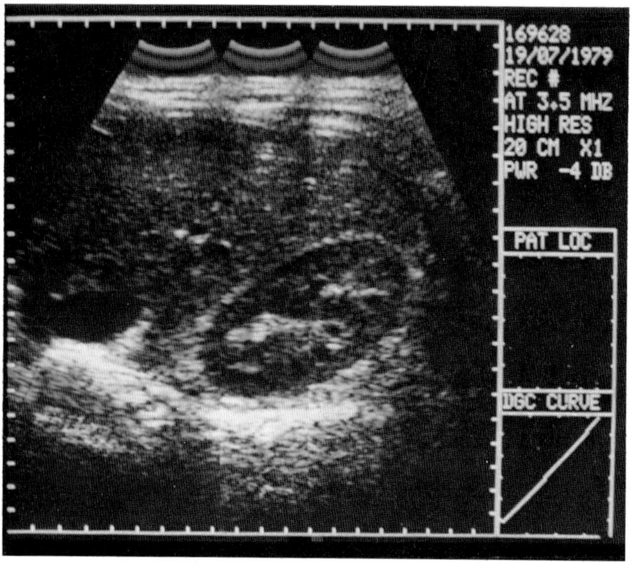

b)

Fig. 11.12
Design of a mechanical trapezoidal scanner with multi-transducer system (a) and example (b): longitudinal section through the right liver and kidneys

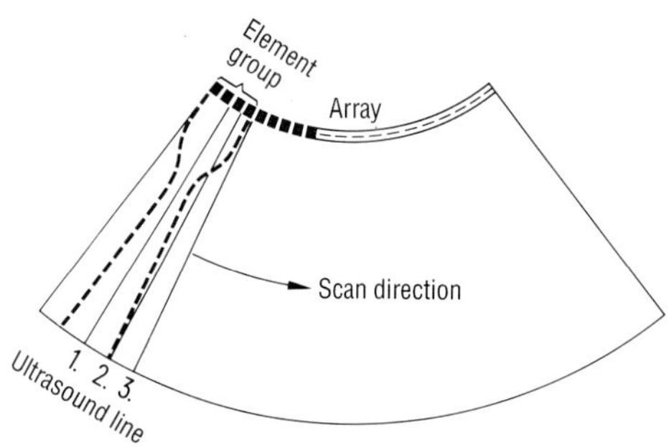

Fig. 11.13
Principle of a curved array (convex array)

Apart from these basic forms of scanning formats, there are also hybrid forms, of which the trapezoidal format and the ring segment (curved array) are the most common (Figs. 11.12 and 11.13).

The type of application essentially determines which scanning format will be used. Certain examinations in which acoustic access to the body region concerned is difficult are best carried out with sector systems, because these only have small acoustic coupling surfaces and can be very flexibly handled in terms of the direction of the sectional plane. Preferred areas of application for this type of scanner are examinations of the heart, the skull of a baby (fontanella), the pancreas, and also intraoperative applications.

For examination of regions in which a certain display width is already required by the body surface, preference is given to linear scanning formats or hybrid formats, such as in the display of the liver, perinatal examinations or in the examination of the thyroid glands and the female breast.

The specific properties of the individual scanning procedures are given in more detail in the following sections.

11.2.1 Mechanical sector scanners

Out of the large number of mechanical scanning systems, the only one which has survived in competition with electronic scanning array systems is the mechanical sector scanner. It will continue to be important in the future.

In the first instance, the reason for this is the price-performance ratio. By contrast with electronic sector scanners, the requirements for signal processing are relatively low. Due to the symmetric construction of the transducer, the image quality is already very good without dynamic focussing (fixed focus). A further increase in image quality can be expected with extra dynamic focussing for receiving (annular array). From today's point of view, annular arrays cannot be discussed except in the context of mechanical scanning systems.

Scanning principles

A circular single transducer is arranged so that it can be rotated or swung about an axis, so that for a predefined angular movement it scans a defined section of a circular plane, a sector, in polar coordinates about this axis with its ultrasound beam. This already defines the most important geometric pixel parameters, the distance r and the scanning angle φ. The distance r (for a predefined velocity of sound) depends on the transit time of the echo. The angle of the sound beam relative to a predefined reference line is provided by an electronic angle generator connected to the transducer (Fig. 11.14).

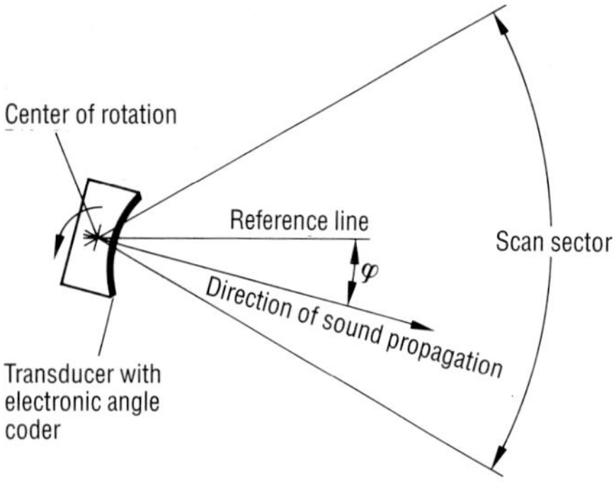

Fig. 11.14
Principle of a mechanical sector scanner

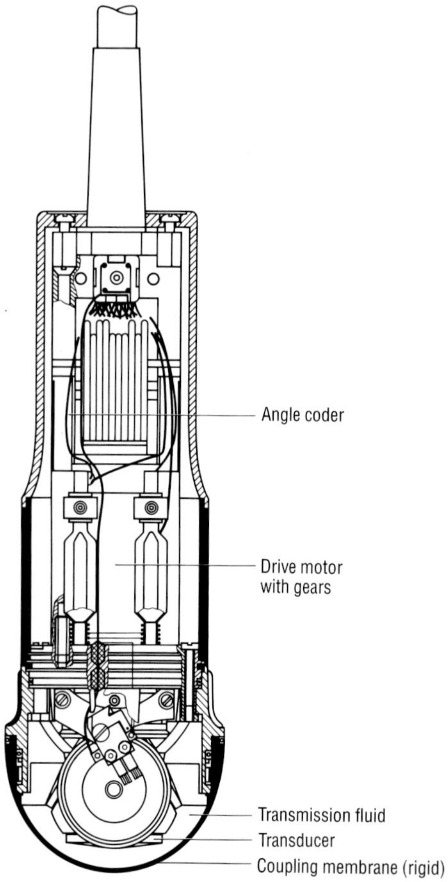

Fig. 11.15
Design of a mechanical sector scanner

The transducer is usually accommodated in a closed chamber filled with a suitable fluid. The coupling to the patient is carried out by a sound-permeable membrane. This membrane can be rigid; in this case, effects of the transmission fluid and the membrane material on the ultrasound field (refraction, reflection) can be compensated. In order to facilitate the coupling it can also be made flexible; in this case, the acoustic properties of the membrane and of the transmission fluid must be adapted to the corresponding parameters (density, velocity of sound) of biological tissue. Otherwise, there are unavoidable image distortions. The "rigid" window is predominant (Fig. 11.15).

With the mechanical scanners in use today, two different scanning principles are used:

1. The rotor principle
2. The wobbler principle.

Rotor principle

Instead of the above-mentioned individual transducer, several (3–5) transducers of the same type are arranged at equal angular intervals (72° to 120°) on the circumference of a rotating carrier. This carrier is made to rotate at constant angular speed with a suitable drive mechanism which is normally accommodated in the grip of the applicator. Only the transducer turned towards the sector concerned is activated. An angle coder provides the instantaneous position of the transducer (image coordinate) and also an identification for the transducer which is just to be activated (Fig. 11.16).

The output signal of the angle coder is usually used besides the image coordinate generation as an actual value in a control loop to achieve a defined angular speed or a defined hold position (M mode, Doppler). At constant angular speed,

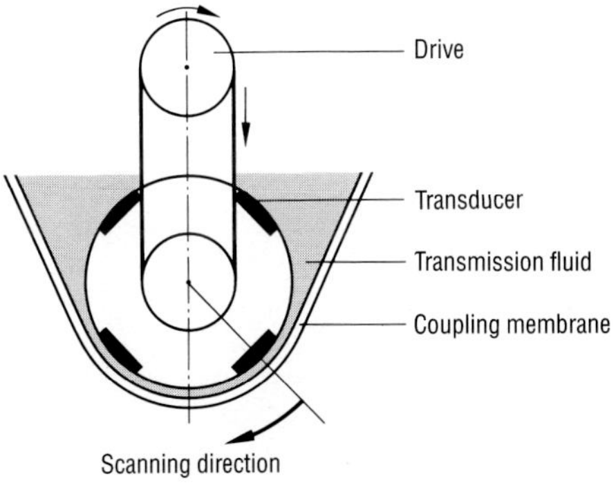

Fig. 11.16 Design of a mechanical scanner based on the rotor principle

there are no interfering mechanical moments of inertia in this system. The image sequence is not limited by the mechanical scanning principle and the line density is also constant for a constant pulse train.

Rotor systems place very high demands on the individual transducer systems in terms of their sensitivity and their adjustment of the ultrasound axes and on the angular determination itself. Even small deviations can lead to image distortions (flickering) due to differences in brightness or coverage errors of the individual partial images.

The sector angle of a rotor system is constant. The image frequency is variable over measurement depth and line density within certain limits.

Wobbler principle

Continuous scanning over a limited sector angle is also possible with only one transducer if the transducer is moved in a swinging movement around the axis (Fig. 11.17). The high demands on the rotor in terms of sensitivity and adjustment no longer apply in this case, since only one transducer is involved in the image display.

In contrast to the rotor, the sector angle is not a predefined quantity; sector angle and image frequency or line density are interchangeable within limits.

However, these advantages are offset by greater demands on the driving mechanism. The mechanical moments of inertia of the system can no longer be neglected in this operating mode: reversal of the direction of movement. A certain reduction in image frequency due to the dead times at the point of reversal must therefore be accepted.

There are more stringent requirements on the control loop of the drive mechanism for achieving an approximately constant angular speed of the scanning

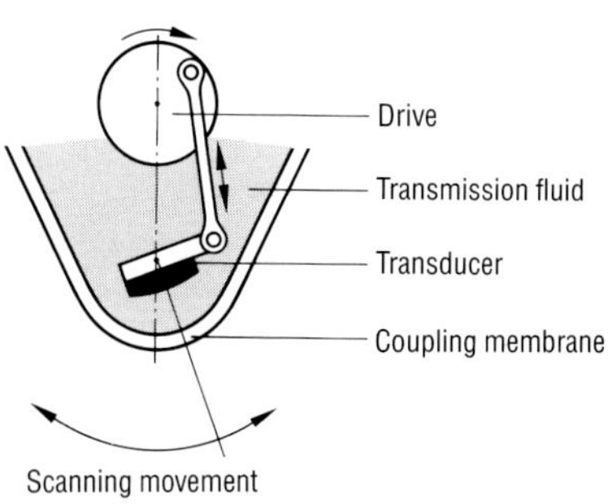

Fig. 11.17 Design of a mechanical scanner based on the wobbler principle

movement (accuracy of angle determination, drive performance). Mechanical vibrations and running noises can increase.

The individual images from the two scanning directions are not exactly identical, because the velocity of sound is finite compared to the scanning speed. An additional image compensation is therefore necessary.

A number of different drive mechanisms are used for the wobbler: the most important are a crank mechanism, reversing drive motor or purely magnetic drives.

Comparison of the scanning principles

Rotor and wobbler systems have equal merits, although wobbler systems are preferred for cardiac diagnostics because, in such applications, the free choice of the sector angle offers certain advantages. In particular, with mechanical scanners which are intended for use with transducers having a large aperture and thus high lateral resolution (annular array), wobbler systems are preferred. The geometrical dimensions can therefore be kept smaller and the signal transmission problem (number of channels!) can be overcome. In high-resolution systems, the line density must be increased. This reduces the scanning frequency. It is easier to deal with the effect of the moments of inertia of the oscillating mass in this design.

However, all mechanical scanning systems have the disadvantage of low flexibility. In particular, it is impossible to rapidly change modes, e.g. from the B image to the M or Doppler display, because of mechanical inertia. Simultaneous display of a real-time B image and M or Doppler display is therefore not possible in general, so that this remains an area of application for array systems.

Nevertheless, it is possible to obtain a display in several modes in an approximate manner with mechanical scanners if instead of the real-time B image, reference is made to a stored B image during the Doppler or M display with this image being refreshed at certain intervals in time (a few seconds).

This disadvantage can be further overcome with Duplex scanners (see section 11.2.3), which are a combination of a real-time scanner with a separate Doppler system.

Design of the transducer

Usually, individual transducers with circular symmetry and fixed focussing are used in mechanical sector scanners (see also section 11.1.2). This focussing can be carried out with the help of a spherical dome or by means of a cemented acoustic lens, allowing for the additional ultrasound field parameters resulting from the transmission fluid and (rigid) coupling membrane (Fig. 11.18).

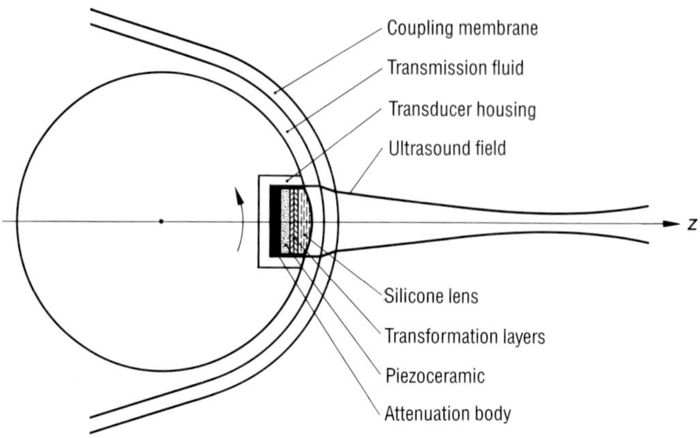

Fig. 11.18 Design of the acoustic part of a mechanical sector scanner

This type of transducer design only requires single channel signal processing and is thus economic.

The image quality is very good, in particular in the area of medium image depth (focus position); the rotation-symmetric design is the ideal configuration here in terms of focussing and side lobe distance.

The image quality is constant over the entire scanning angle.

In general, the resolution is reduced in the far field and in the extreme near region. Multiple echoes can interfere.

Annular array

The image quality and thus the diagnostic capability of an ultrasound system, apart from the value of the ultrasound frequency which is predefined by the necessary penetration depth, is essentially given by the axial and lateral resolution parameters (see also section 11.1.2).

The axial resolution, which is determined by the duration of the emitted ultrasound pulse, is in general better than the lateral resolution. An improvement in image quality can therefore be obtained in the first instance by increasing the lateral resolution.

The lateral resolution of an ultrasound system can be influenced by the degree of focussing, i.e. the ratio of the active transducer diameter (the aperture) to the focal distance, z_0.

Fig. 11.19 shows that, with increasing degree of the focussing, the lateral resolution in the focussing region (focus distance $z_0 \approx R$) decreases, but at the same time the useful depth acuity region becomes smaller and smaller.

Thus, for every distance z a different radius of curvature R and, if the lateral resolution has to remain constant over the entire imaging range, an aperture 2a increasing with the distance z should be chosen with the ratio of $z/2a$ (F number) being constant.

Fixed focus transducers as described in the previous sections fall far short of attaining the maximum possible focussing. In these systems, a compromise has

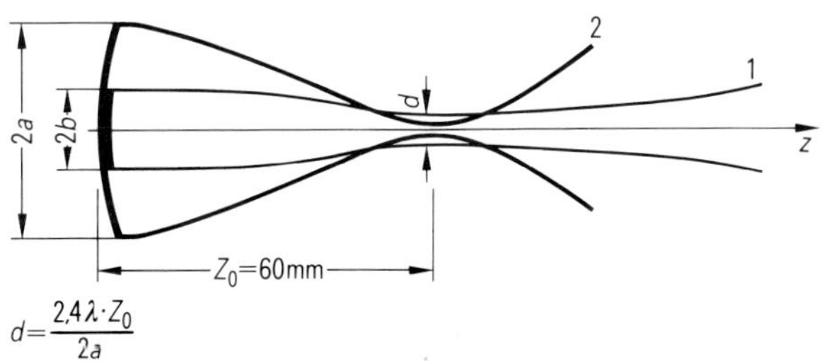

Fig. 11.19
Resolution and depth acuity as a function of degree of focussing.
Comparison of the ultrasound fields of two transducers of 3.5 MHz focussed at 60 mm with different apertures ($2a=15$ mm and $2a=40$ mm)

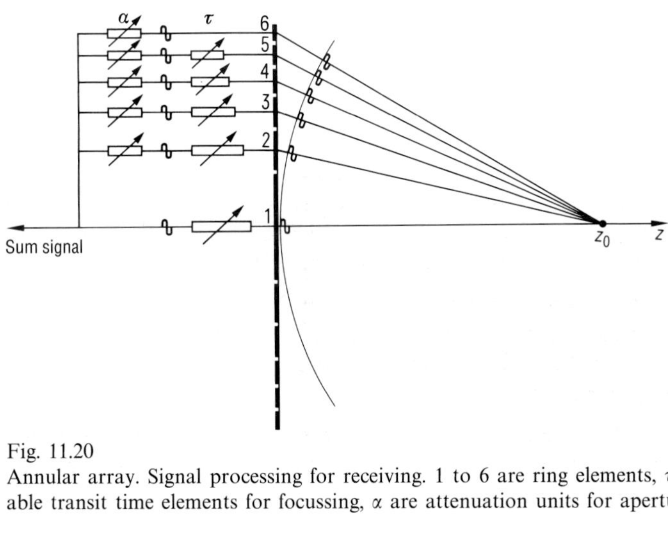

Fig. 11.20
Annular array. Signal processing for receiving. 1 to 6 are ring elements, τ are controllable transit time elements for focussing, α are attenuation units for aperture weighting

to be made between depth acuity and degree of focussing, so that the image quality can be kept more or less constant over the entire imaging range. The maximum possible resolution, in the last analysis limited by the ultrasound frequency, is never attained at all.

This hurdle of reduced depth acuity can be largely overcome at least during receiving using the method of electronic dynamic focussing (Fig. 11.20).

The transducer is divided into a number of concentric rings, for which the number and diameter graduations are determined in line with a predefined lateral resolution. The overall diameter of this arrangement of transducers is considerably larger than that of the usual fixed focus transducer.

The signals received for the individual rings pass through controllable delay stages and also controllable attenuating units; they are combined to produce a summed signal at their outputs.

The delay times of these devices can be adjusted electronically in sufficiently fine graduations in the microsecond range.

In order to achieve dynamic focussing, the delay times τ_1 to τ_n should be adjusted for every distance z so that the sum of the transit time of the signal from the point of reflection as an acoustic signal to the corresponding transducer ring, as well as in the form of an electric signal from the transducer ring via the electrical delay unit to the summing point, is equally large for all channels. In this case, all partial signals are added together in phase to a sum signal of maximum amplitude.

The delay times τ' necessary for every distance z can be calculated from simple geometrical relationships and controlled in a time sequence, so that the receiving focus of the system exactly tracks the echoes from increasing distance, also

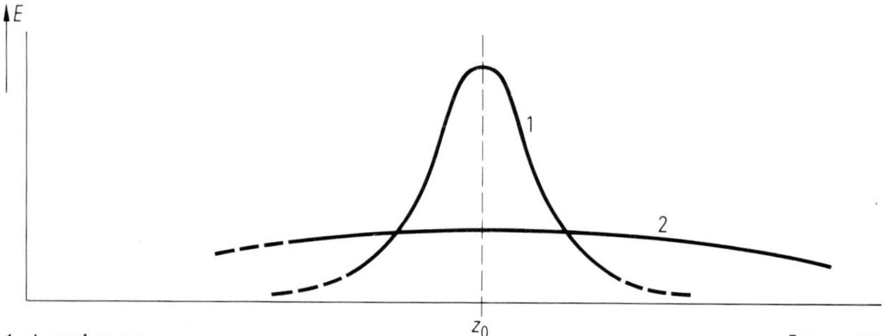

1 Annular array
2 Fixed focus system (focussed on z_0)

Fig. 11.21
Echo sensitivity, E, for point targets as a function of distance, z (qualitative)

in order of time. The original disadvantage of the low depth acuity of a high-focussing system is overcome to a large extent in this way.

The fact that the sensitivity of such a system rapidly decreases for distances of $z \neq z_0$ for a given focal distance z_0 (in contrast to fixed focus systems) leads to an additional suppression of multiple echoes; the image quality is therefore further enhanced (Fig. 11.21).

The requirement of a depth-dependent aperture can be satisfied by dynamic weighting of the parts of the individual ring elements via a depth-dependent modification of attenuation units α_2 to α_n.

From today's point of view, the highest possible image quality is to be expected from annular arrays with dynamic focussing and dynamic aperture for receiving.

The use of annular arrays is at present inextricably linked with a mechanical scanning system. Electronically scanning annular arrays, although physically feasible, essentially fail because of the high number of channels necessary.

11.2.2 Electronic scanners

The method is based on the following idea: the required scanning width (image width) is covered by a large number of identical individual transducers. Suppose that during one transmit-receive cycle only one transducer is activated, with the information from one line being obtained in the direction of sound propagation. The cycle time is proportional to the required penetration depth, because of the approximately constant velocity of sound in soft tissue. After this time, the adjacent transducer is switched on, etc. In this way, the entire sectional image is produced line for line without any mechanical movement. The image frequency possible only depends on the transit time of the echo. A further advantage is that the transducer is stationary during the entire receiving time.

Of course, the model as presented here has been greatly simplified. In practice, many narrow strip elements are arranged next to each other. The name array has become common for this. In such arrays, apart from a few exceptions, an entire group of neighboring elements (Fig. 11.22) is combined during a transmit-receive cycle (switched on electronically). This group is only shifted in the scanning direction by one element. Only this measure makes it possible to produce the required scanning density. Furthermore, the aperture of the antenna can be easily varied with the group size in the scanning direction.

With a special stepping procedure, the number of lines can be further doubled if two groups with different group sizes are acceptable (Fig. 11.23): first, a group is addressed with m elements. It transmits and receives as a unit. Then a further element is added without disconnecting another. This group now has $m+1$ elements. The central axis of the second group $(m+1)$ is shifted by half the element spacing in the scanning direction, compared with the first group (m). After another transmit-receive cycle the first element is disconnected. The third again has group m elements and its central axis has also moved on by a half element spacing. For the fourth group, a new element is added, etc.

Piezoceramic materials are used as electroacoustic transducers (see section 6.1.4). As with other echo transit time methods, the transducers are stimulated by electrical pulses to thickness oscillations. The piezoceramic itself tolerates field strengths up to above 1 kV/mm and is thus not the limiting element in the generation of adequate sound intensities.

The transmitter voltages applied range from 5 V to a few hundred volts. Many units have operating controls for adjusting the transmission intensity, so that it is possible for the user to work in his area of application with minimum transmission power.

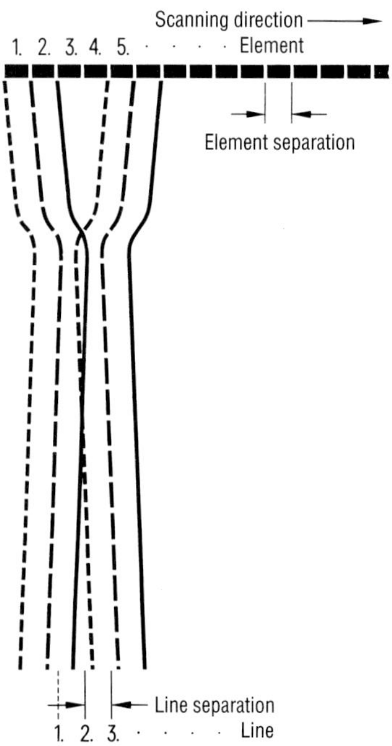

Fig. 11.22
Principle of the parallel scan
(line separation is the element separation)

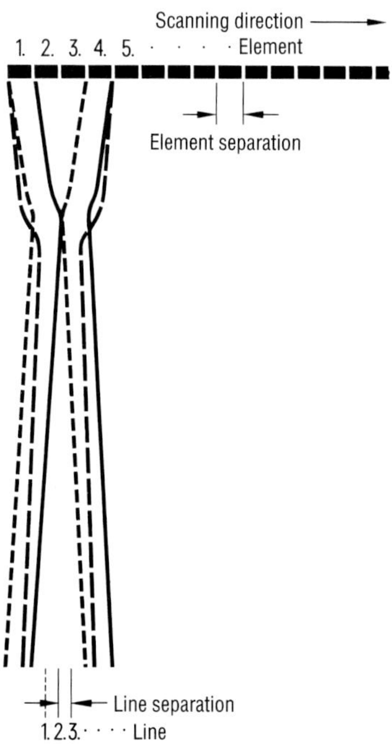

Fig. 11.23
Principle of group stepping with doubling of the line density

Electronic focussing

As described in section 11.1.2, the ultrasound field of a transducer is strongly determined by its focussing. In individual ultrasound transducers, the focussing is performed by curvature of the surface or by an acoustic lens attached to it. In the array, the ultrasound field can be focussed by means of electronic aids.

We will first look at the receive case for the elements of a group, using Fig. 11.24: echoes which come from a target from the point called the focus first arrive at the array element "0", since here the transit path is shortest. If these echo signals for the element "0" are delayed by a time τ_0, it is possible to add them to the echo signals in time and in phase which are received at the elements "5" and "5′":

$$\tau = \frac{s}{c}.$$

where

s is the maximum path difference
c is the velocity of sound in the tissue.

If the signals are also delayed corresponding to the transit path difference at the other elements, all elements supply coherent signal components, i.e. the addition of the delayed signals produces the best possible echo display for the focus point.

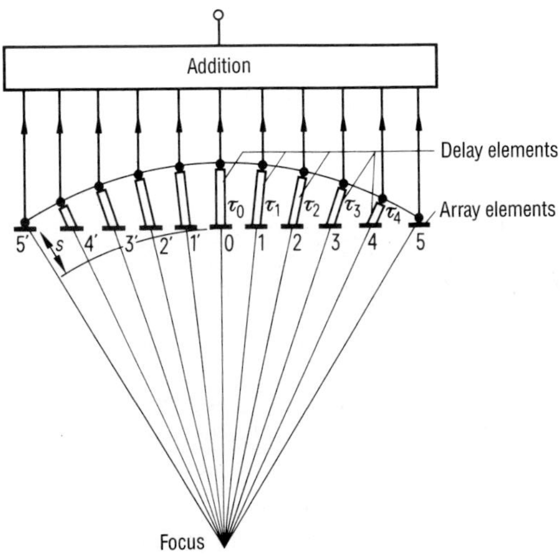

s Path in the tissue

Fig. 11.24
Electronic receive focussing

If the delay times are changed during receiving of the echo signals, it is always possible to place the focus at the depth from which the echoes arrive. For this, the focus should be allowed to travel to the depth. This is why we speak of a dynamic focussing.

Fig. 11.25 shows an example for an ultrasound field consisting of four focus positions which are selected corresponding to the depth. The more focus positions used, the fewer transitions appear. If only a few focus positions are used (e.g. three focus positions), then the delay times are to be switched over discretely, and the transitions would have more of a disturbing effect in the image. In this case, "soft switching" is used for the transition zones (Fig. 11.26).

In principle, by corresponding delay of the stimulation pulse of the array, the ultrasound field can also be focussed for transmission. However, only one focus

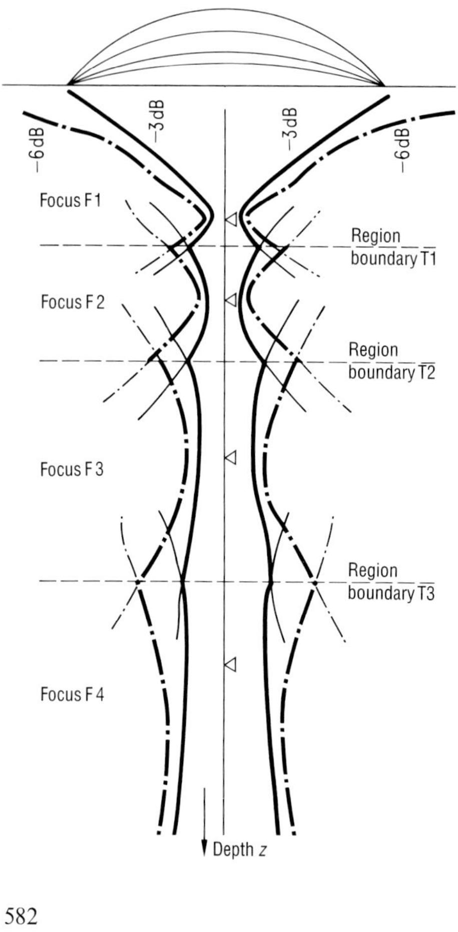

Fig. 11.25 Dynamic focussing

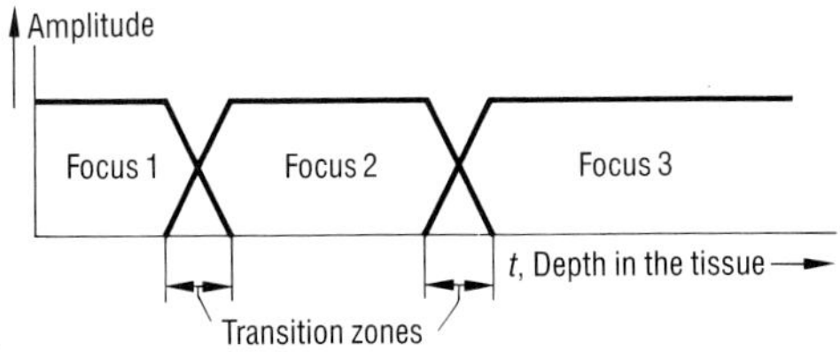

Fig. 11.26 Reception focussing with soft switching

position can be produced for every transmission pulse. If several transmission foci are to be used, then several ultrasound lines need to be used one after the other in the same scanning position.

Linear and curved arrays

Linear and curved arrays can be distinguished from sector scanners through their relatively large body entry areas.

Linear array

Typical values:

Total number of elements, n	60 to 120
Element width, b	1 to 4λ
Group width $B = m \cdot b$	8 to 32 elements
Frequencies, f	3.5 to 7.5 MHz
Length of ceramic L	2 to 11.5 cm
Scanning length (image width) $S \approx L - B$	2 to 10 cm
Width of ceramic	6 to 14 mm

Scanning mode:

Parallel scan by means of electronic scanning

Applications:

Entire abdomen
Gynecology
Thyroid gland
Superficial vessels
Special applications, such as intracavitary applications and ultrasound-guided puncture

The ultrasound field of the linear array is defined by the rectangular shape of the transmit and receive group [11.8].

Natural focussing:

Near field length $N \approx 1.3\ B^2/4\ \lambda$

In the scanning direction, the ultrasound field is improved by electronic transmit and receive focussing. A fixed focussing is usually present perpendicular to the scanning direction through an acoustic lens.

Advantages:

▻ No moving parts

▻ Large body entry surface

▻ Good displays of superficial regions

▻ Dynamic focussing

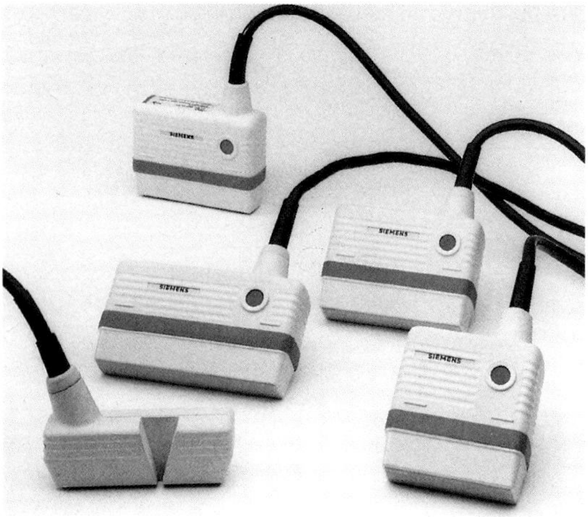

Fig. 11.27
Different standard linear array probes, a biopsy array

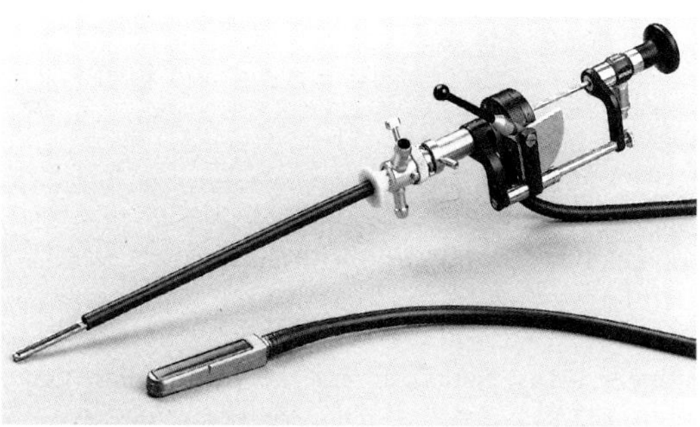

Fig. 11.28
Intracavitary and transurethral array probe

Disadvantages:

▻ Relatively large array lengths (scanning length + group width)

▻ Varying lateral resolution in and perpendicular to the scanning direction

▻ Increased interference and formation of side lobes, compared to the circular transducer (mechanical sector scanner)

Disturbances due to the element geometry

Piezoceramic transducers, apart from the thickness oscillation, also undergo parasitical transverse oscillations which are produced as a result of Poisson transverse contraction and the components of the piezo effect lying vertical to the poling direction. In the linear array, the dimensions of the individual element with its rectangular element geometry are such that low-frequency interference oscillations can be produced.

However, these effects can be eliminated in the design. A very effective measure is to divide the elements into subelements, for which the width is smaller than the thickness of the ceramic (fine graduation). The subelements are completely separated mechanically from each other and electrically connected in parallel. Due to this fine division, the parasitic transverse oscillations have a higher frequency relative to the useful oscillation and thus no longer interfere with the ultrasound field.

Image artifacts

Image artifacts which can be ascribed to interference can have various causes and are superimposed as a rule onto the tissue image, making them difficult to analyze. However, they can be easily provoked with a suitable test object and clearly displayed. Such a test object consists of a metal rod in water, which is placed vertically to the scanning plane. The sectional image of this rod must produce a point. The metal rod has a very high reflection factor in water. In this way, the interference patterns – some of which are only very weak – are clearly revealed.

Fig. 11.29 shows different image artifacts. The vertical ghost image pointing downwards is produced by oscillations inside the brass rod and is therefore not important here.

The hyberbolic image artifact B (Fig. 11.30) is the result of lack of lateral resolution and ambiguities due to so-called grating lobes. These are side lobes which occur additionally with periodically divided antenna. The horizontal artifact with constant distance to the array is caused entirely by the inadequate blocking attenuation of the element switches for transmission and receiving. The artifact C can be observed with inadequate blocking attenuation of the element switches during transmission (non-selected elements also transmit).

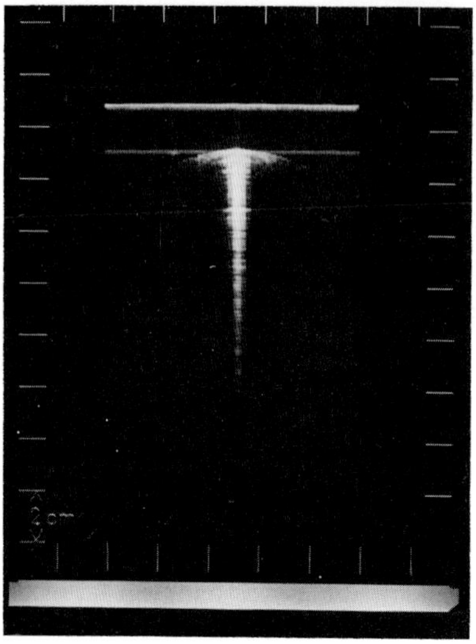

Fig. 11.29
Image artifacts generated with a brass rod (3 mm diameter) in water, 3.5 MHz array

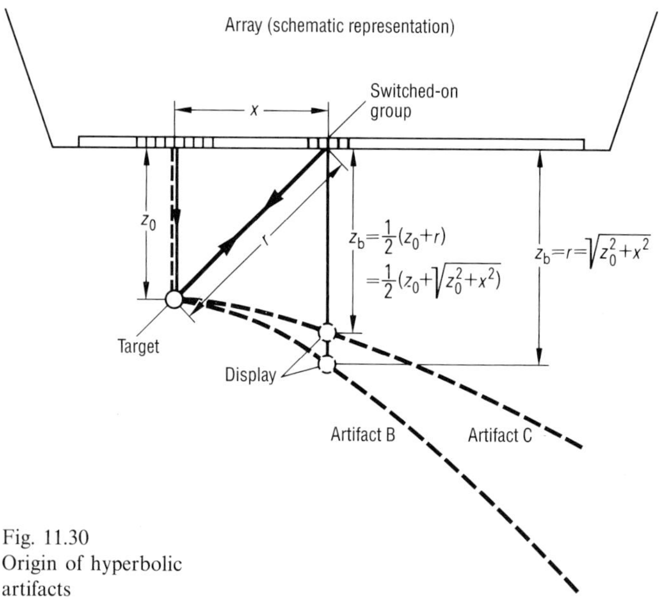

Fig. 11.30
Origin of hyperbolic artifacts

Curved arrays

A curved array should be regarded as a modification of the linear array. The difference is that the curved array is not straight, but bent. The scan is produced as with the linear array, by electronic switching or by shifting an element group.

As can be seen from Fig. 11.31 the curved array produces a sector scanning of the tissue.

Advantages:

▻ Sector scanning without moving parts and without having to use phase control electronics (see phased array)

▻ Smaller coupling surface than with the linear array

▻ Curved coupling surface, permitting easy coupling to many points on the body

Disadvantages:

▻ Greater coupling surface than with the phased array for the same effective aperture

Applications:

Mainly abdominal applications

Typical values:

Radius of curvature R	40 to 80 mm
Frequency f	3.5 to 5 MHz
Total number of elements n	>100
Group width B	16 to 32 elements

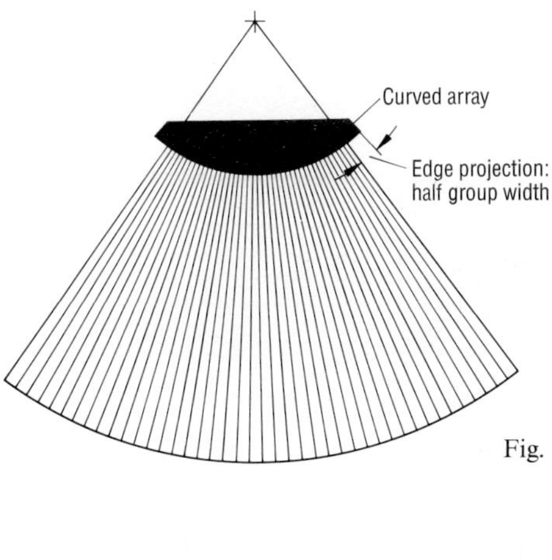

Fig. 11.31 Scan format of a curved array

Phased arrays

With phased arrays, a sector scan of the tissue is performed. A relatively small array serves as the probe. All elements of the array are used at the same time for transmitting and receiving. The sector scan is obtained by electronic beam steering [11.4 and 11.5].

As can be seen from Fig. 11.11, the transmit pulse is not directly applied to the individual array elements, but via a suitable delay electronic unit. If τ_1 is greater than τ_n, then the transmit pulses arrive first at element n and last at element 1. In the ideal case, every element can be regarded as the starting point for a cylindrical wave (if the element is sufficiently small). The superposition of the cylindrical waves forms a wave front. If, as shown in Fig. 11.11, a linear delay is predefined and τ_1 is the maximum delay time, then the wave produced at element n has already traversed a path

$$s = (\tau_1 - \tau_n) \cdot c$$

($c = 1540$ m/s, velocity of sound in the tissue).

The same applies to the elements lying in between. The result is a propagation of a swivelled wave front. The effective aperture A' for the swivelled sound field is:

$$A' = A \cdot \cos \varphi$$

(A is the aperture of the array without swivel).

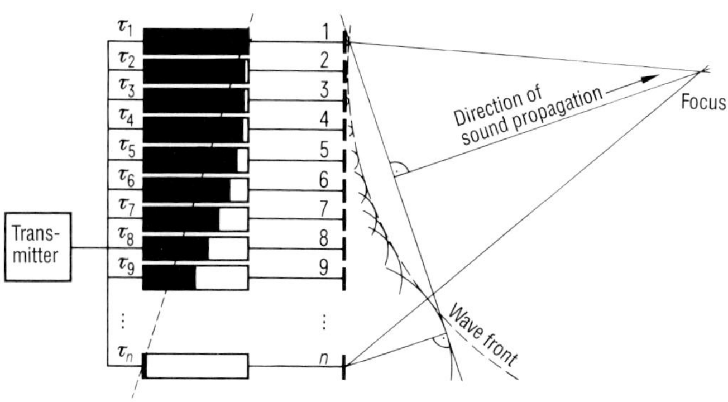

Fig. 11.32
Generation of a swivelled and curved wave front

With suitable delay times, a curved wave front can also be generated which is focussed on a point (Fig. 11.32).

The same applies to the receive case (Fig. 11.33). The echo signal at element 1 originating from a target placed on the scanning line is delayed until the associated echo signal has arrived at element *n*.

The measures for electronic focussing already described are used in addition to the swivel, for both transmit and receive. In the reception case, the focussing can also be carried out dynamically.

The delay time required for maximum beam steering is longer than the delay time required for focussing by a factor of 10 to 20.

The phased array has relatively demanding electronics requirements, since a separate controllable transmission and receive delay channel must be present in the unit for every element. The number of elements lies between 48 and 128.

High demands are also made of the transducer in the phased array. The directional characteristic of the elements determines the swivel angle which can be used. For common sectors with 90° (swivel ±45°), an approximately cylindrical characteristic is necessary. This is only possible with very narrow elements, of the order of magnitude of half a wavelength.

Typical values:

Maximum swivel angle	40 to 45°
Aperture (array length)	14 to 28 mm (3.5 MHz array)
Receive channels (number of elements)	48 to 128
Frequency	2.5 to 7 MHz

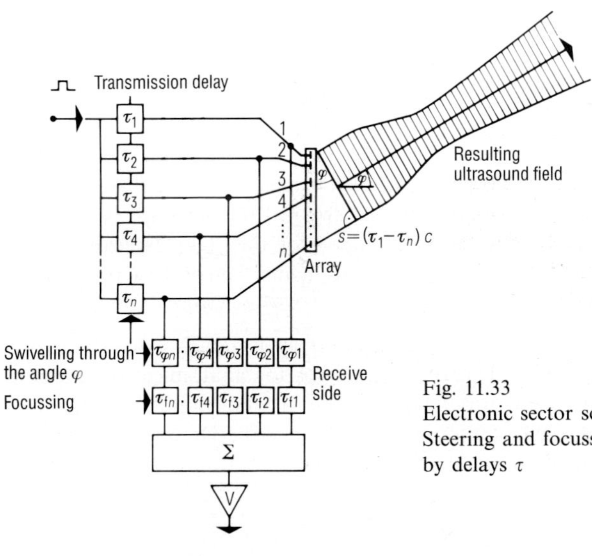

Fig. 11.33
Electronic sector scanner.
Steering and focussing of the sound beam by delays τ

Applications:

- ▻ Echocardiography, small arrays (14 mm aperture) for precordial access to the heart (only through the small acoustic window between the ribs) [11.18].
- ▻ All applications for which sector scanners are used (abdomen, neurosonology, gynecology, etc.)
- ▻ Special applications, oesophageal, transrectal, transvaginal probes

Advantages:

- ▻ Sector scan without moving parts
- ▻ Small probes
- ▻ Application with small coupling surface; similar to the mechanical sector scan
- ▻ Special probes allow access paths to the body which otherwise could not be used for ultrasound
- ▻ Simultaneous display of B image, Doppler and time motion possible

Disadvantages:

- ▻ Ultrasound field of a transducer with rectangular base area (see linear array)
- ▻ Dependence of the effective aperture A' on the scan angle (see Fig. 11.1) (in contrast to the mechanical sector scanner), i.e. worse resolution and lower sensitivity around the edges of the sector image
- ▻ Demanding electronics requirements

11.2.3 Duplex scanners

One-dimensional ultrasound examinations with A and M mode or Doppler require that the user have sufficient anatomical knowledge. In difficult situations, such as pulsed Doppler, where a gate has to be placed at a defined position in a vessel, a simultaneous display of the anatomical relationships is essential. So-called duplex scanners have been developed for this. Duplex scanners are probes with two independent transducer arrangements. One of these transducers produces a sectional image and the other serves for M or Doppler images.

Fig. 11.34 shows an example. Here, a linear array is rigidly connected to a transducer for CW Doppler. The B image serves for anatomical orientation. A line is superimposed onto this image on the viewing monitor to make it possible to estimate at what point and at what angle the Doppler information is taken.

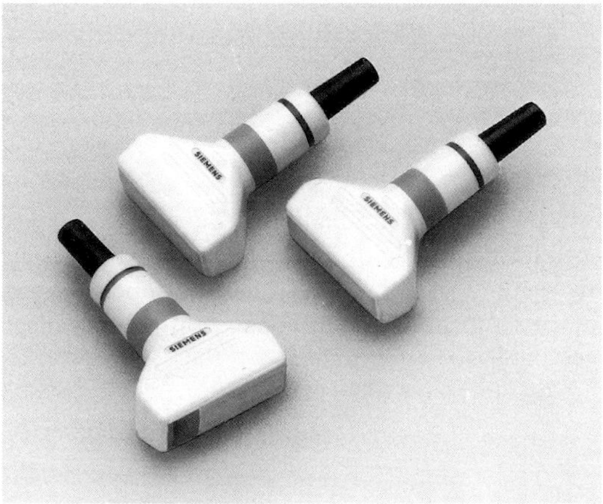

Fig. 11.34
Duplex (front left) and linear arrays for special applications

Every image probe principle can be used for the B image probe in duplex scanners, i.e. mechanical scanners, linear, curved and phased arrays.

A transducer for M mode and pulsed Doppler or a CW Doppler transducer can be used as the second transducer.

An example of application: in a Doppler examination on a vessel with pulsed Doppler, the position of the measurement point can be exactly located and if necessary corrected with the help of the B image.

This design with two specific transducer systems makes it possible to optimize the B image or Doppler properties. In this way it is possible to use different frequencies for the B image part (e.g. 5 MHz) and for the Doppler part (e.g. 3.5 MHz) with the same probe.

12 Biomagnetic diagnostics

Biomagnetism concerns the measurement and evaluation of the magnetic fields originating through sources of electrical activity in the human body, mainly the heart and the brain. This method may become clinically important for functional diagnosis and shows its full potential in connection with medical imaging, e.g. MR or CT images.

12.1 Biomagnetic fields

Activity of biological cells, such as nerves and muscle fibers, is of electrical origin. From a physical standpoint, excited cells can be considered as galvanic elements situated in a conductive medium. Often bundles of cells are active at the same time. These cells can be modelled as an equivalent current dipole, consisting of a current source and sink separated by a small distance. Different groups of simultaneously active cells distributed in a volume can be considered as multiple current dipoles or a distribution of current sources.

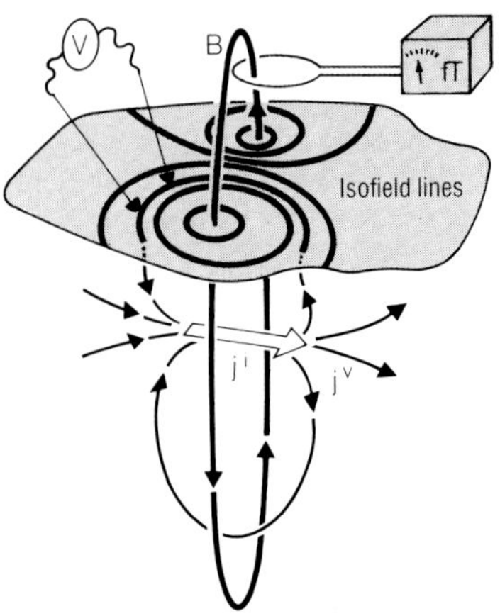

$$\frac{4\pi}{\mu_0}\vec{B} = \int \frac{\vec{j}^{\,i} \times \vec{R}}{R^3}\, dv - \sigma \int V \nabla\left(\frac{1}{R}\right) \times d\vec{s}$$

Figure 12.1 Electric dipole source
Volume currents and magnetic field of an electric source (current dipole) within the body. The flux density is a sum of two contributions: The first term arising from the impressed primary current j^i, the second from the volume currents j^v. The second term is transformed from the original Biot-Savart formula into a surface integral with the aid of Stokes' Law (electric conductivity σ) [12.1]

A current dipole, i.e. a small battery with an internal primary current, sends volume currents into the conductive surrounding tissue (Fig. 12.1). When these currents reach the surface of the body, electric potentials can be measured using electrodes. In medical diagnosis this is routinely done on the head with the electroencephalogram (EEG) and on the heart with the electrocardiogram (ECG). The EEG and ECG give information on the variation with time of the current sources in the body.

The strength of these electric fields depends on the strength of the source and on the position of the electrodes with respect to the source. Since the conductivities of the different tissues normally are not known, localization of a current source in the body is only possible if the electrodes are brought very close to the location of the electrical activity. To analyze the origin of electric activity in the brain or the heart, one has to work with depth electrodes or catheters, an invasive procedure.

It is well known that every electric current is surrounded by a magnetic field, which is for the most part not influenced by the electric properties of the tissue. Research in localizing current sources from magnetic fields was performed as early as 1963 [12.2]; recording the magnetic field from the head is referred to as the magnetoencephalogram (MEG) and from the heart as the magnetocardiogram (MCG). The magnetic field, generated by current dipoles in the human body and measured outside the body, consists of two terms: one originating from primary currents and one from the volume currents. While the influence of the first term can easily be calculated from the Biot-Savart law, the second term again depends on the paths of the currents in the body. The influence of the volume currents can be quantitatively taken into account if the geometry of the body is known [12.3, 12.4].

Theoretical and experimental investigations have shown that, in contrast to electric fields, volume currents contribute to the magnetic fields much less than the current dipole itself [12.5]. This is the reason why biomagnetic localization in many cases yields satisfactory results even if the shape and conductivity of the human body is only approximately taken into account.

12.2 Measurement of biomagnetic fields

Biomagnetic fields at the surface of the body are six to eight orders of magnitude smaller than the earth's magnetic field, as shown in Table 1.

Evoked cortical activity	50fT
MEG spontaneous activity ($\alpha \cdot \delta$)	1pT
MCG (R-wave)	50pT
Magnetized lung contaminants	1nT
Geomagnetic activity	0.1nT
Urban noise	10-100nT
Earth's magnetic field	50μT

Table 1
Magnitudes of biomagnetic and noise fields

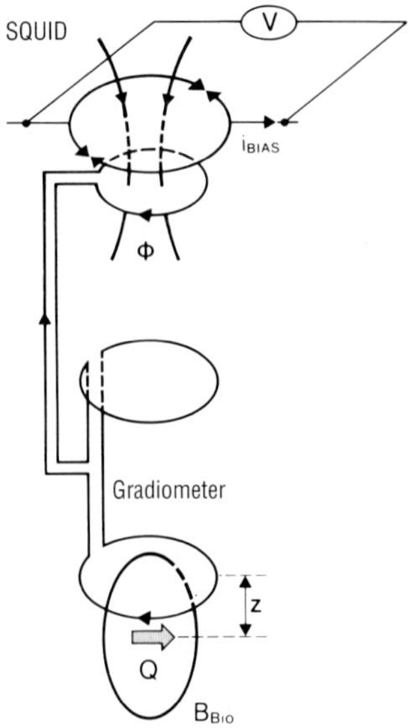

Figure 12.2
Measurement of biomagnetic fields
Axial 1st order gradiometer, consisting of a superconductive pickup coil and a counterwound compensation coil.
The induced current is measured by its magnetic flux coupled into a SQUID (superconducting quantum interference device)

Their measurement requires considerable effort to suppress interfering external fields and to reach the necessary sensitivity. Measurement is performed with superconducting induction coils connected to superconducting quantum interference devices (SQUIDs), which are magnetic flux sensors of extreme sensitivity [12.6] (Fig. 12.2).

To localize current sources with reasonable accuracy, the distribution of the magnetic field has to be known. With current dipoles as sources one observes a north pole where the magnetic field lines leave the body and a south pole where they enter again. The current dipole lies between those poles, the depth being determined by their separation: The further the two poles are apart, the deeper the dipole is situated.

Since recently research in biomagnetism had to be performed with only one or a few sensors [12.7,12.8]. Sequential measurements were necessary to record the magnetic field distribution: Investigations could last from several hours to several days and spontaneous and sporadic electrical activity could hardly be investigated. Multichannel systems, however, register the complete magnetic field distribution in one acquisition. An investigation takes only a couple of minutes and even spontaneous events are accessible.

12.3 Technical realization

The KRENIKON (from Greek krene [source or spring] and ikon [image]) is a biomagnetic multichannel system [12.9] for the investigation of the brain and the heart (Fig. 12.3 and 12.4). Biomagnetic field distributions are acquired by 37 superconductive sensor coils arranged on a circular plane 19 cm in diameter.

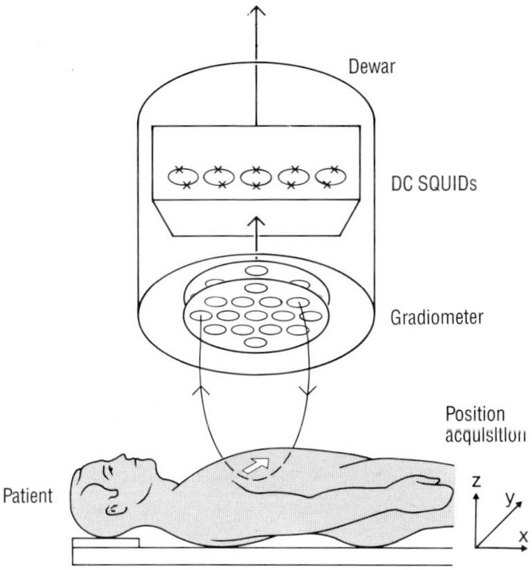

a) Sensor system

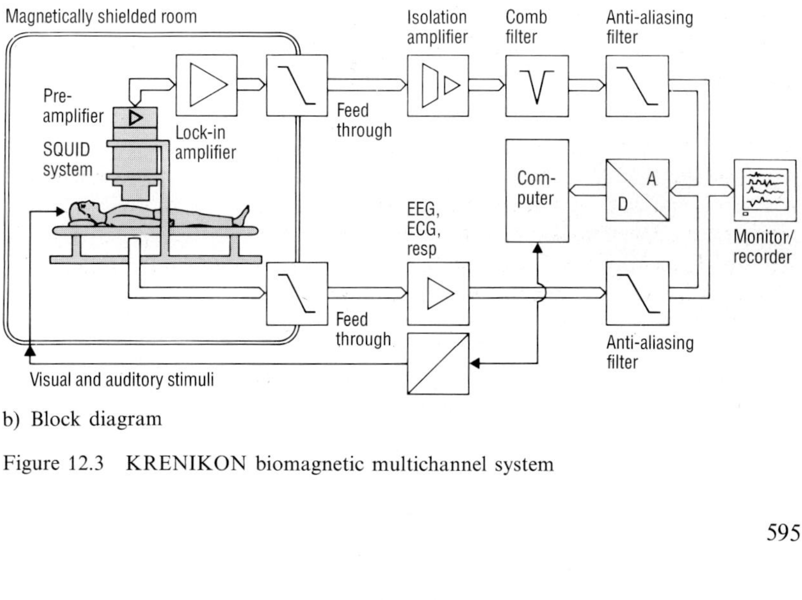

b) Block diagram

Figure 12.3 KRENIKON biomagnetic multichannel system

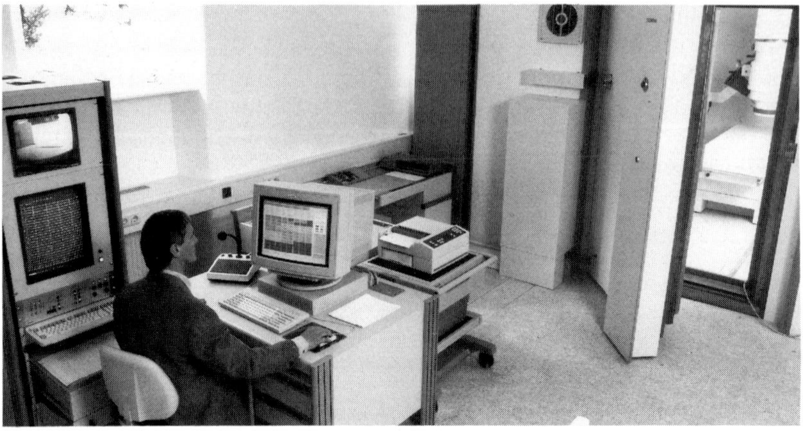

Figure 12.4
KRENIKON biomagnetic multichannel system
View towards shielded room and operator's console. Installation at the University of Erlangen-Nürnberg

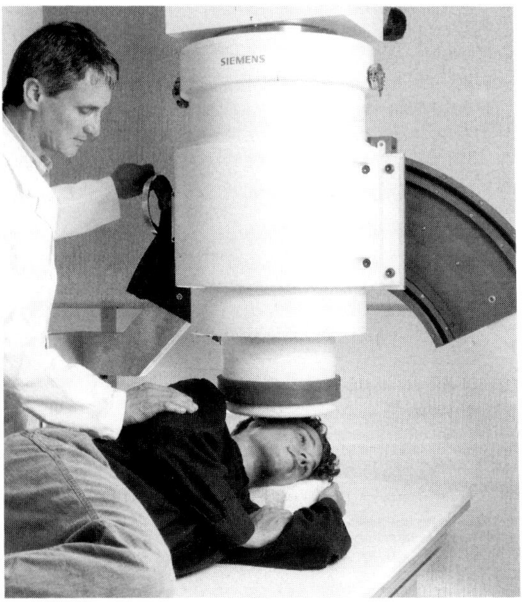

Figure 12.5
Application of the KRENIKON biomagnetic multichannel system
Gantry with dewar vessel containing the multichannel sensor. Position for lateral MEG measurement from one hemisphere. Installation at the University of Erlangen-Nürnberg

To allow clinical operation in a normal urban environment, measurements are performed inside a shielded room, which is made of two layers of soft magnetic material (Mumetal®, Vacuumschmelze Hanau) with one layer of aluminum in between. Mechanical vibrations, which could cause intolerable interfering signals, are avoided by mounting the shielded room and the support of the measurement system on a specially designed concrete foundation.

The sensor is located in a cryostat (dewar vessel) filled with liquid helium (Fig. 12.5). Interfering signals not yet sufficiently suppressed in the shielded room are further reduced by the application of superconducting first-order gradiometers: compensating coils are arranged 7.1 cm above the 37 pickup coils. While the biomagnetic field rapidly decays and is therefore seen only by the sensor coils close to the source, interfering fields penetrate both the pickup and the compensating coils; since the coils are counterwound, the signals from both coils cancel. These gradiometers are coupled to dedicated silicon chips, each comprising 10 DC-SQUIDs [12.10], which are operated in the flux locked loop [12.10] and act as very sensitive current amplifiers.

Within the shielded room, an every day noise of 10 $fT/\sqrt{Hz}$ at frequencies above 10 Hz results.

Electric signals (EEG with surface or depth electrodes, ECG), other physiological signals (e.g. respiration), and trigger signals can be recorded in parallel with the magnetic fields, if special nonmagnetic electrodes and sensors are used.

The signals are further processed with notch filters to prevent interference from the line frequency and with high-pass and anti-aliasing filters to improve the signal-to-noise ratio. Data are digitized with 400-1,000 Hz (depending on the application) and system operation, and data evaluation is performed with a workstation.

The patient is examined in a relaxed, reclining position on an adjustable couch. Using a light marker, the cryostat can be adjusted vertically and tilted in two directions for access to any part of the body. Due to the large sensitive sensor area, no repositioning is necessary during an examination.

The diagnostic value of biomagnetically determined locations can be significantly improved if they can also be examined with reference to human anatomy and morphology (Fig. 12.6). A combination of biomagnetic evaluation with MR imaging is well suited, because this modality provides three-dimensional images. To fuse biomagnetic localizations with MR images, common reference coordinates have to be established. With an MEG investigation this is achieved by fixing the patient's head to a support with aid of a silicon rubber impression of the upper teeth. The removable support is mounted on the patient couch and is used during the MR examination as well. The biomagnetic sensor coordinates are defined with respect to the support, and water-filled markers allow identification of reference points in the MR images.

For MCG measurements, the patient's position is determined either from reference points on the chest (e.g. the jugular notch of the sternum) or by using a system of calibration coils fixed to the patient's body. During MR imaging these coils are replaced by contrast medium-filled markers. Coordinate transfor-

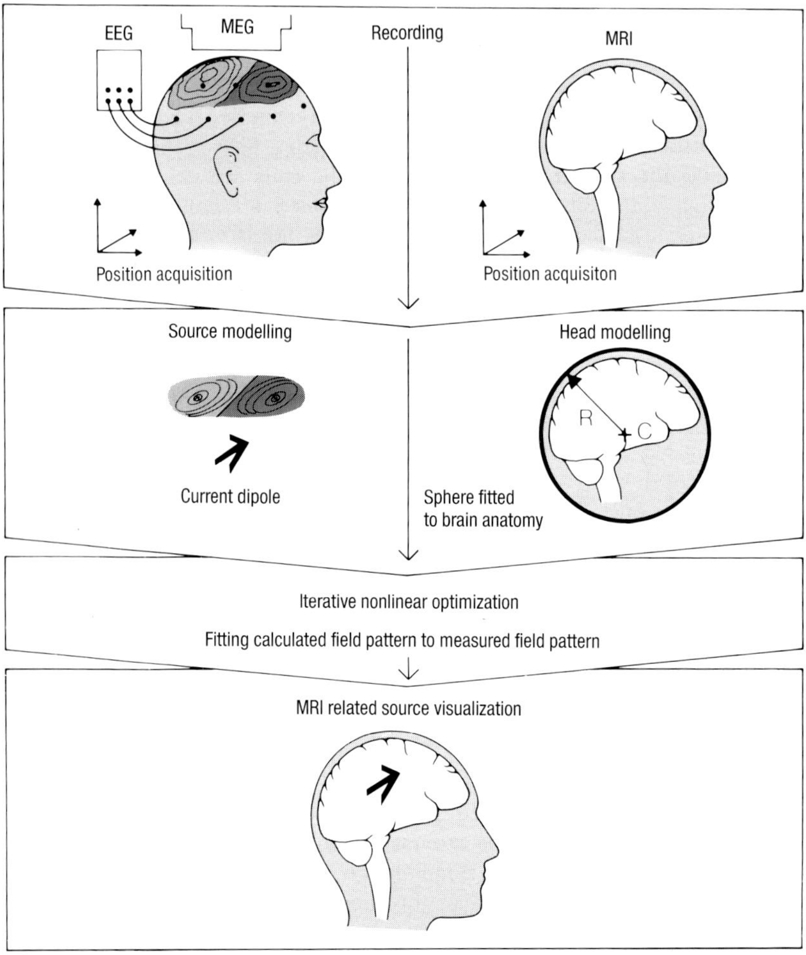

Figure 12.6 Evaluation scheme for biomagnetic source localization in the head
The brain is considered to be a sphere with homogeneous conductivity, and the electrical source to be localized is assumed to be a current dipole. The center of the sphere is fitted to a 3D image set obtained with MR. During the biomagnetic and MR investigations the patient's head is fixed to the same support, so that the measurements can be described within the same coordinate system

mation is performed with the use of coils and markers as common reference points. Combination of results with other anatomic images, e.g. from CT, is also feasible.

12.4 Source localization

While a given configuration of current sources has a unique electric and magnetic field distribution, the inverse problem, i.e. the determination of the location and strength of sources from a given field distribution, in principle has an infinite number of solutions. Only by restricting oneself to models is it possible to obtain solutions, the simplest being the current dipole in a homogeneous sphere or the infinite halfspcace. These structures permit analytical treatment of the volume currents. We remark that neither the electric conductivity nor the radius has to be known; only the center of the sphere is of importance. Also, current dipoles perpendicular to the surface do not produce any magnetic fields outside the body. The human skull is most simply modelled as a sphere, and the chest as an infinite halfspace [12.11].

Determination of current dipoles in three dimensions from the measured external magnetic field distribution is performed by a nonlinear, iterative procedure [12.11] (Fig. 12.6): The field distribution is calculated based on a first estimate of the dipole position; the deviation from the measured field is then compared and the locus of the dipole altered until a minimum deviation is reached. This final result is then considered as the location of the electric source.

The validity of the source localization can be checked by prior knowledge: Especially when source localization is performed over a complete time interval, such as ictal or interictal activity in epileptics, physiological knowledge can help to exclude false localizations; the combination of the following five criteria has proven to be a valuable tool:

- ▻ The deviation of the measured field distribution from the distribution produced by the reconstructed source must not exceed a predefined threshold.
- ▻ The location of the reconstructed source must be within anatomically defined limits, e.g. within the brain in MEG evaluations.
- ▻ The distance between successive source locations has to be within the limits of the electric conductance velocity of the activated tissue.
- ▻ A reconstructed source location or sequence of locations has to stabilize within a time interval typical for the action or generator potentials of the type of cells unter consideration.
- ▻ Upper and lower limits for the strength of the reconstructed source can be defined from electrophysiology. Furthermore, an upper limit for the rate of change of the source strength can be defined.

12.5 Application

Biomagnetism is now applied to functional studies of the brain and the heart. In neurology, examinations of patients with pharmacoresistant partial epilepsy [12.12] (Fig. 12.7) demonstrated localized primary and secondary foci from interictal activity.

Brain function can be studied with magnetic fields generated by auditory, visual, or somatosensory stimulation, or by mental tasks [12.7]. Localization accuracy in the outer cortex reaches a few millimeters; in deeper regions 1 to 2 cm are typical.

In cardiology biomagnetic investigations allow the noninvasive localization of the accessory bundle in WPW syndrome [12.13]. Centers of pathologic excitation, like ventricular ectopic areas of activity causing extrasystoles, have been successfully localized (Fig. 12.8).

Besides information about geometric locations, quantitative information about strength of cardiac sources, e.g. in patients with cardiac hypertrophy [12.13], can also be obtained and used for diagnosis and follow up.

Biomagnetism is still in its infancy. One can expect, however, that now with the availibilty of multichannel systems a phase starts, where the clinical relevance is rapidly investigated and further applications are found. It has already been demonstrated that functional information with high temporal resolution becomes accessible as with no other method.

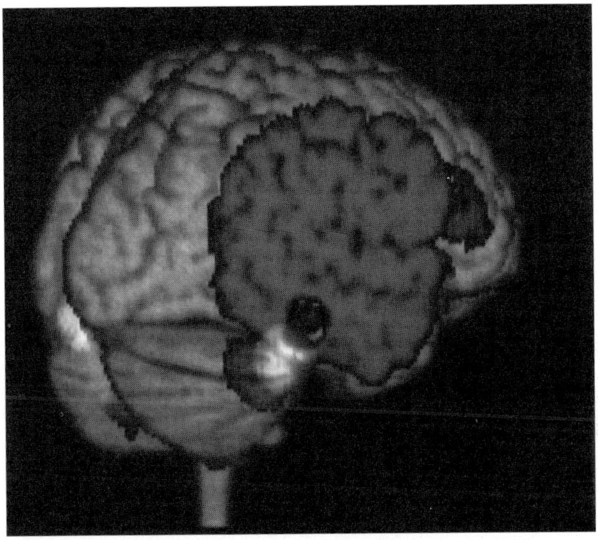

Figure 12.7 Clinical application of the MEG
3D MR view of a patient with an angioma causing epileptic seizures. Intericatal electric activity has been localized biomagnetically and the respective regions have been highlighted.(By courtesy of Prof. H. Stefan, Department of Neurology of the University of Erlangen-Nürnberg)

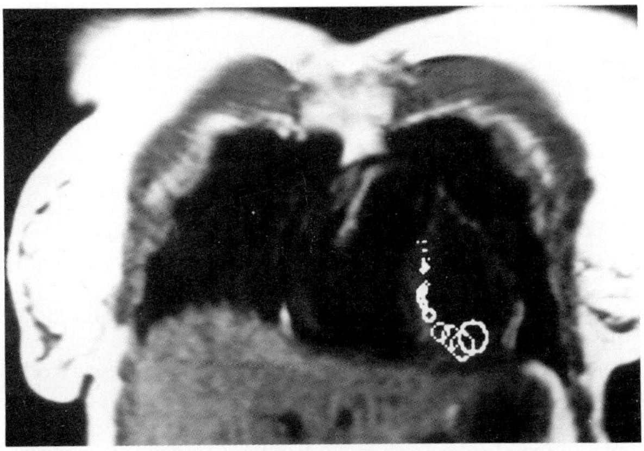

Figure 12.8 Clinical application of the MCG
Frontal MR projection with localization of ectopic activity from the MCG of a patient with parasystoly: The origin of ventricular extrasystole is found at the proximal interventricular septum, from where it propagates towards the apex while area of the depolarized myocardium increases (2 ms time interval between points, diameter of circles indicates dipole strength). (By courtesy of Dr. W. Moshage, Medical Department II (Cardiology) of the University of Erlangen-Nürnberg (Director: Prof. K. Bachmann))

References

1 Physiology of vision

[1.1] Keidel, W.D.: Sinnesphysiologie, Teil 1. Heidelberger Taschenbücher, Bd. 97. Berlin, Heidelberg, New York: Springer-Verlag 1971

[1.2] Keidel, W.D.: Kurzgefaßtes Lehrbuch der Physiologie. Informationsverarbeitung, Abschnitt 16, S. 3. 4. Aufl. Stuttgart: Georg Thieme Verlag 1975

[1.3] Finkelnburg, W.: Einführung in die Atomphysik, S. 46. Berlin, Göttingen, Heidelberg: Springer-Verlag 1964

[1.4] Rohen, J.W.: Handbuch der mikroskopischen Anatomie. Bd. 3/4. Springer-Verlag 1964

[1.5] Trendelenburg, W.: Lehrbuch der Physiologie. Der Gesichtssinn, Grundzüge der physiologischen Optik. 2. Aufl. Berlin, Göttingen, Heidelberg: Springer-Verlag 1961

[1.6] Graff, Th.: Die Akkommodation beim Sehen durch das Nahbrillenglas. Mbl. Augenheilkunde 121 (1952) S. 205

[1.7] Fuortes, M.G.F.: Handbook of sensory physiology, Vol. VII/2. Physiology of photoreceptor organs. Berlin, Heidelberg, New York: Springer-Verlag 1972

[1.8] Dartnall, H.J.A.: Handbook of sensory physiology, Vol. VII/1. Photochemistry of vision. Berlin, Heidelberg, New York: Springer-Verlag

[1.9] Baumgartner, G.: Physiologie des zentralen Sehsystems. In: Sehen Sinnesphysiologie III, S. 276 und 277. München, Wien, Baltimore: Urban & Schwarzenberg 1978

[1.10] Gebauer, A.; Lissner, J.; Schott, O.: Das Röntgenfernsehen. 2. Aufl. Stuttgart: Georg Thieme Verlag 1974

[1.11] Ranke, O.F.: Sinnesorgane. In: Handbuch der gesamten Arbeitsmedizin, Bd. 1 (Hrsg.: Lehman, G.) München, Berlin: Urban & Schwarzenberg 1961

[1.12] Stange, G.: Rankes Streulichttheorie bei Blendung. Z. f. Verkehrssicherheit 9 (1963) S. 50 bis 55

[1.13] Keidel, W.: Rankes Adaptionstheorie. Z. f. Biol. 112 (1961) S. 411 bis 425

[1.14] Starkiewicz, W.: Physiologische Grundlagen der Helligkeits- und Farbempfindungen. Leipzig: VEB Georg Thieme 1970

[1.15] Commichau, R.: Adaptionszustand und Unterschieds-Schwellenenergie für Lichtblitze. Z. f. Biol. 108 (1956) S. 145 bis 160

[1.16] Rohen, W.: Funktionelle Anatomie des Nervensystems. Stuttgart, New York: K.F. Schattauer Verlag 1976

[1.17] Schober, H.: Das Sehen. Leipzig: Fachbuchverlag 1958

[1.18] Zusne, L: Visual perception of form. New York, London: Academic Press 1970

[1.19] Kienle, G.: Wahrnehmungsstörung und die nicht euklidische Struktur des Sehraums. Stuttgart: Georg Thieme Verlag 1968

[1.20] Hensel, H.: Allgemeine Sinnesphysiologie. Hautsinne, Geschmack, Geruch. Berlin, Heidelberg, New York: Springer-Verlag 1966

[1.21] David, E. (Hrsg.): Grundlagen der Sportphysiologie. Erlangen: Perimed-Verlag 1986

2 Quantitative assessment of image quality

[2.1] Normenreihe DIN 6814 Teil 1 bis 14: Begriffe und Benennungen in der radiologischen Technik – Abbildende Systeme

[2.2] Angerstein, W.; Stargardt: Über die Bildgüte in der Radiologie. Röntgenprax. 20 (1967) S. 241 bis 246 und 278 bis 290; 21 (1968) S. 1 bis 15, S. 41 bis 49, S. 67 bis 73, S. 117 bis 121, S. 132 bis 139, S. 191 bis 196 und S. 209 bis 218

[2.3] Wittmann, F.; Röhler, R.: Vergleichende Messungen der Kontrastübertragungsfunktion mit Sinusgittern und Rechteckgittern. Optik 19 (1962) S. 243 bis 249

[2.4] Altar, W.: Westinghouse research memorandum 60-944110-14-19

[2.5] Coltman, J.W.: The specification of imaging properties by response to sine wave input. J. of the optical Soc. America 44 (1954) S. 468 bis 471

[2.6] Stahnke, J.; Heinrich, H.: Die Modulations-Übertragungsfunktion einer elektronenoptischen Röntgen-Bildverstärker-Röhre. Optik 23 (1965/66) S. 251 bis 267

[2.7] Kuhn, H.: Bildrauschen bei Film-Folien-Systemen: seine Ursachen und Komponenten. Electromedica 51 (1983) Heft 2, S. 46

[2.8] Goodenough, D.J.; Rossmann, K.; Lusted, L.B.: Radiographic Applications of Receiver Operating Characteristic (ROC) Curves. Radiology 110 (1974) S. 89 bis 95

[2.9] Linke, G.; Brunner, J.; Geyer, H.: Objektives Verfahren zur Bestimmung des Kontrast-Detail-Diagramms in der Computer-Tomographie. Röntgenblätter 38 (1985) S. 190 bis 192

3 X-ray and gamma radiation

[3.1] Flügge, S.: Handbuch der Physik. Bd. XXX. Berlin, Göttingen, Heidelberg: Springer-Verlag 1957

[3.2] Dietz, H.; Dietz, K.; Geldner, E.: Einfluß der Reichweite der Elektronen im Anodenwerkstoff und der Umlauffrequenz auf die zulässige Belastung von Röntgendrehanoden. Siemens Forsch.- und Entwickl.-Ber. 10 (1981) S. 188 bis 193

[3.3] Vieten, H. (Hrsg.): Handbuch der medizinischen Radiologie, Teil 1, Berlin, Heidelberg, New York: Springer-Verlag 1968

[3.4] Dietz, K.: Altes und Neues über Röntgenröhren. Stuttgart: S. Hirzel Verlag 1964

[3.5] Evans, R.D.: The Atomic Nucleus. McGraw-Hill Book Comp. 1955

[3.6] Hubbel, J.A.: Atomic form factors, incoherent scattering functions, and photon scattering cross sections. J. of phys. and chem. Reference Data 4 (1975) S. 431 bis 538

[3.7] Johns, H.E.; Cunningham, J.R.; Thomas, C.G.: The physics of radiology publishers. Charles C. Thomas, Publisher. Springfield, Illinois (USA): 1969

[3.8] Storm, E.; Israel, H.I.: Photon cross sections from 0,001 to 100 MeV for elements 1 throught 100. Clearinghouse for Federal Scientific and Technical Information, LA 3753 MC 34, Physics TID-4500 (1967)

[3.9] Ter-Pergossian, M.M.: The physical aspects of diagnostic radiology. Hoeber Medical Division, Harper & Row 1967

[3.10] Kalender, W.A.: Determination of the intensity of scattered radiation and performance of grids in diagnostic radiology by Monte Carlo methods. University of Wisconsin, Madison (USA) Thesis (1979)

4 X-ray computed tomography

[4.1] Stieve, F.-E.: Bevorzugte Darstellung einzelner Körperschichten. In Handbuch der medizinischen Radiologie, Bd. III: Allgemeine Röntgendiagnostische Methodik. Hrsg. H. Vieten. Berlin, Heidelberg, New York: Springer-Verlag. 1967, S. 716 bis 1041

[4.2] Vieten, H.: Verfahren zum röntgenographischen Darstellen eines Körperschnittes. Deutsche Patenschrift Nr. 672518 (1939)

[4.3] Gebauer, A.; Schauen, A: Das transversale Schichtverfahren. Stuttgart: Georg Thieme Verlag 1955

[4.4] Frank, G.: Verfahren zur Herstellung von Körperschnittbildern mittels Röntgenstrahlen. Deutsche Patentschrift Nr. 693374 (1940)

[4.5] Takahashi, S.: Rotation radiography. Tokyo: Maruzen 1957

[4.6] Gajewski, H.; Linke, G.: Altes und Neues über das Transversalschichtverfahren. Radiol. clin. et biol. 40 (1971) S. 463 bis 473

[4.7] Cormack, A.M.: Representation of a function by its line integrals, with some radiological applications. J. of appl. Phys. 34 (1963) S. 2722 bis 2727

[4.8] Cormack, A.M.: Representation of a function by its line integrals, with some radiological applications. II. J. of appl. Phys. 35 (1964) S. 2908 bis 2913

[4.9] Radon, J.: Über die Bestimmung von Funktionen durch ihre Integralwerte längs gewisser Mannigfaltigkeiten. Ber. d. math.-phys. Kl. Sächs. Gesell. Wiss. 59 (1917) S. 262 bis 277

[4.10] Hounsfield, G.N.; Ambrose, J.; Perry, J., et al: Computerized transverse axial scanning (tomography). Parts 1, 2, 3. Brit. J. of Radiol. 46 (1973) S. 1016 bis 1051

[4.11] Ambrose, J.A.: Computerized transverse axial tomography. Brit. J. of Radiol. 46 (1973) S. 401

[4.12] Groedel, F.M.; Wachter, R.: Unter welchen Voraussetzungen ist die röntgenologische Qualitätsdiagnose der Lungentuberkulose praktisch möglich? Beitr. zur Klin. d. Tuberk. u. spezif. Tuberk.-Forsch. 69 (1928) S. 192 bis 208

[4.13] Führer, K.; Liebetruth, R.; Linke, G., et al.: SIRETOM – ein Schädel-Transversalschichtgerät mit Computer. Electromedica 43 (1975) S. 48 bis 55

[4.14] Pfeiler, M.; Schwierz, G.; Linke, G.: Modellvorstellungen zur Bildaufzeichnung bei der Computertomographie (Computerized axial tomography). Electromedica 44 (1976) S. 19 bis 25

[4.15] Linke, G.: Technische Grundlagen der Computertomographie. Röntgenprax. 30 (1977) S. 159 bis 180

[4.16] Jaß, W.; Linke, G.; Schwierz, G.: SOMATOM – Ein schneller Ganzkörper-Computertomograph mit unmittelbarer Bildwiedergabe. Electromedica 45 (1977) S. 118 bis 122

[4.17] Petersilka, E.; Pfeiler, M.: Zur Technik der Computertomographie. Röntgenber. 6 (1977) S. 233 bis 257

[4.18] Schittenhelm, R.; Schwierz, G.: Das Computertomogramm: Seine Erzeugung und sein Bildcharakter. Medizintechn. 18 (1978) S. 87 bis 94

[4.19] Alexander, J.; Kalender, W.; Linke, G.: Computertomographie: Bewertungsmerkmale, Gerätetechnik, Anwendungen. Berlin, München: Siemens Aktiengesellschaft 1985

[4.20] Gordon, R.: A tutorial on ART (algebraic reconstruction techniques). IEEE Trans. on Nucl. Sci. NS–21 (1974) S. 78 bis 93

[4.21] Radon, J.: Über die Bestimmung von Funktionen durch ihre Integralwerte längs gewisser Mannigfaltigkeiten. Ber. d. math.-phys. Kl. Sächs. Gesell. Wiss. 59 (1917) S. 262 bis 277

[4.22] Bracewell, R.N.; Riddle, A.C.: Inversion of fan-beam scans in radio astronomy. Astronom. J. 150 (1967) S. 427 bis 434

[4.23] Cormack, A.M.: Representation of a function by its line integrals, with some radiological applications. J, of appl. Phys. 34 (1963) S. 2722 bis 2727

[4.24] Ramachandran, G.N.; Lakshminarayanan, A.V.: Three-dimensional reconstruction from radiographs and electron micrographs: Application of convolution instead of Fourier-transform. Proc. of the nat. Acad. Sci. USA 68 (1971) S. 2236 bis 2240

[4.25] Shepp, L.A.; Logan, B.F.: The Fourier reconstruction of a head section. IEEE Trans. on nucl. Sci. NS-21 (1974) S. 21 bis 43

[4.26] Gajewski, H.; Linke, G.: Altes und Neues über das Transversalschichtverfahren. Radiol. clin. et biol. 40 (1971) S. 463 bis 473

[4.27] Jaß, W.: Transformation von Parallelstrahl-Koordinaten zu Fan-Beam-Koordinaten. Persönliche Mitteilung

[4.28] Rosenfeld, A.; Kak, A.C.: Digital picture processing, Chapter 4. New York: Academic Press 1976

[4.29] Schwierz, G.; Härer, W.: Patent VPA 77 P 5049 BRD

[4.30] Rührnschopf, E.P.; Kalender, W.A.: Artefakte durch nichtlineare Teilvolumen und Aufhärtungseffekte bei der Computertomographie. Electromedica 2 (1981) S. 96 bis 105

[4.31] Ludwig, D.: The radon transform of euclidean space. Commun. on pure and appl. Math. XIX (1966) S. 49 bis 81

[4.31] Frank, G.: Verfahren zur Herstellung von Körperschnittbildern mittels Röntgenstrahlen. Deutsche Patentschrift Nr. 693374 (1940)

[4.32] Takahashi, S.: Rotation radiography. Tokyo: Maruzen 1957

[4.33] Gajewski, H.; Linke, G.: Altes und Neues über das Transversalschichtverfahren. Radiol clin. et biol. 40 (1971) S. 463 bis 473

[4.34] Cormack, A.M.: Representation of a function by its line integrals, with some radiological applications. II. J. of appl. Phys. 35 (1964) S. 2908 bis 2913

[4.35] Hounsfield, G.N.; Ambrose, J.; Perry, J., et al.: Computerized transverse axial scanning (tomography). Parts 1, 2, 3. Brit. J. of radiol. 46 (1973) S. 1016 bis 1051

[4.36] Ambrose, J.A.: Computerized transverse axial tomography. Brit. J. of Radiol. 46 (1973) S. 401

[4.37] Groedel, F.M.; Wachter, R.: Unter welchen Voraussetzungen ist die Röntgenologische Qualitätsdiagnose der Lungentuberkulose praktisch möglich? Beitr. zur Klin. d. Tuberk. u. spezif. Tuberk.-Forsch. 69 (1928) S. 192 bis 208

[4.38] Führer, K.; Liebetruth, R.; Linke, G., et al.: SIRETOM – ein Schädel-Transversalsichtgerät mit Computer. Electromedica 43 (1975) S. 48 bis 55

[4.39] Pfeiler, M.; Schwierz, G.; Linke, G.: Modellvorstellungen zur Bildaufzeichnung bei der Computertomographie (Computerized axial tomography). Electromedica 44 (1976) S. 19 bis 25

[4.40] Linke, G.: Technische Grundlagen der Computertomographie. Röntgenprax. 30 (1977) S. 159 bis 180

[4.41] Jaß, W.; Linke, G.; Schwierz, G.: SOMATOM – Ein schneller Ganzkörper-Computertomograph mit unmittelbarer Bildwiedergabe. Electromedica 45 (1977) S. 118 bis 122

[4.42] Petersilka, E.; Pfeiler, M.: Zur Technik der Computertomographie. Röntgenber. 6 (1977) S. 233 bis 257

[4.43] Schittenhelm, R.; Schwierz, G.: Das Computertomogramm: Seine Erzeugung und sein Bildcharakter. Medizintech. 18 (1978) S. 87 bis 94

[4.44] Gordon, R.: A tutorial on ART (algebraic reconstruction techniques). IEEE Trans. on nucl. Sci. NS-21 (1974) S. 78 bis 93

[4.45] Radon, J.: Über die Bestimmung von Funktionen durch ihre Integralwerte längs gewisser Mannigfaltigkeiten. Ber. d. math.-phys. Kl. Sächs. Gesell. Wiss. 59 (1917) S. 262 bis 277

[4.46] Bracewell, R.N.; Riddle, A.C.: Inversion of fan-beam scans in radio astronomy. Astronom. J. 150 (1967) S. 427 bis 434

[4.47] Cormack, A.M.: Representation of a function by its line integrals, with some radiological applications. J. of appl. Phys. 34 (1963) S. 2722 bis 2727

[4.48] Ramachandran, G.N.; Lakshminarayanan, A.V: Three-dimensional reconstruction from radiographs and electron micrographs: Application of convolution instead of Fourier-transform. Proc. of the nat. Acad. Sci. USA 68 (1971) S. 2236 bis 2240

[4.49] Shepp, L.A.; Logan, B.F.: The Fourier reconstruction of a head section. IEEE Trans, on nucl. Sci. NS-21 (1974) S. 21 bis 43

[4.50] Gajewski, H.; Linke, G.: Altes und Neues über das Transversalschichtverfahren. Radiol. clin. et biol. 40 (1971) S. 463 bis 473

[4.51] Jaß, W.: Persönliche Mitteilung

[4.52] Rosenfeld, A.; Kak, A.C.: Digital picture processing, Chapter 4. New York: Academic Press 1976

[4.53] Schwierz, G.; Härer, W.: Schichtgerät zur Herstellung von Transversalschichtbildern. Patent VPA 77 P 5049 BRD

[4.54] Rührnschopf, E.P.; Kalender, W.A.: Artefakte durch nichtlineare Teilvolumen und Aufhärtungseffekte bei der Computertomographie, electromedica 2 (1981) S. 96 bis 105

[4.55] Ludwig, D.: The radon transform of euclidean space. Commun. on pure and appl. Math. XIX (1966) S. 49 bis 81

[4.56] Schwierz, G.; Härer, W.; Rührnschopf, E.-P.: Principles of image reconsruction in X-ray computer tomography. Siemens Forsch.- u. Entwickl.-Ber. 7 (1978) S. 196 bis 203

[4.57] Krumme, H.J.: Ein neues Schädel-Computertomographiegerät: SIRETOM 2000. electromedica 45 (1977) S. 123 bis 128

[4.58] Linke, G.; Pauli, K.; Pfeiler, M.: Zur Strahlenbelastung des Patienten bei der Computertomographie (Computerized axial tomography). electromedica 44 (1976) S. 15 bis 18

[4.59] Pfeiler, M.: Auswertung und Archivierung von CT-Bildern. Vortrag bei den »2. Journees Montpellieraines de Radiodiagnostic«, Montpellier, 1978

[4.60] Scharl, P.; Weckesser, W.-D.; Peter, F.: Einfluß verschiedener Bilddarstellungen auf die Qualität von Computer-Tomogrammen. Vortrag auf dem XIV. Internationalen Röntgenkongreß, Rio de Janeiro, Okt. 1977

[4.61] Weckesser, W.-D.; Scharl, P.; Krumme, H.J.: CT-Bilddokumentation – Stand und Aussichten. electromedica 46 (1978) S. 122 bis 127

[4.62] Schlegel, W.; Scharfenberg, H.; Müller, W., et al.: Computereinsatz zur Bearbeitung und Auswertung von CT-Aufnahmen. electromedica 45 (1977) S. 189 bis 196

[4.63] Huffman, D.A.: A method for the construction of minimum-redundancy codes. Proc. of the IRE 40 (1952) S. 1098 bis 1101

[4.64] Keller, H.U.; Anliker, M.; Rüegsegger, P.: Bildmanipulation in der Computertomographie. Fachtagung Medex 76 Basel (Schweiz) Biomed. Tech. Bd. 21 – Ergänzungsband Juni 1976

[4.65] Weckesser, W.-D.; Pfeiler, M.: Verzeichnungsprobleme bei der Sekundärschnittrekonstruktion in der Röntgen-Computertomographie. Vortrag auf dem IV. Europäischen Kongreß für Radiologie, Hamburg, Sept. 1979

5 Magnetic resonance imaging

[5.1] Abragam, A.: The principles of nuclear magnetism. Oxford University Press 1961

[5.2] Farrar, T.C.; Becker, E.D.: Pulse and Fourier transform NMR, introduction to theory and methods. Academic Press 1971

[5.3] Michel, D.: Grundlagen und Methoden der kernmagnetischen Resonanz. Berlin: Akademie Verlag 1981

[5.4] Pauli, W.: Naturwiss. 12 (1924) S. 741

[5.5] Bloch, F.; Hansen, W.W.; Packard, M.: The nuclear induction experiment. Phys. Rev. 70 (1946) S. 474

[5.6] Bloembergen, N.; Purcell, E.M.; Pound, R.V: "Relaxation effects in nuclear magnetic resonance absorption". Phys. Rev. 73 (1948) S. 679

[5.7] Bottomley, P.A.; Foster, T.H.; Argersinger, R.E.; Pfeifer, L.M.: A review of normal tissue hydrogen NMR relaxation times and relaxation mechanisms from 1–100 MHz: Dependence on tissue type, NMR frequency, temperature, species, excision and age. Med. Phys. 11 (1984) S. 425

[5.8] Hahn, E.: Spin echos. Phys. Rev. 80 (1950) S. 580

[5.9] Carr, H.Y.; Purcell, E.M.: Effects of diffusion on free precession in nuclear magnetic resonance experiments. Phys. Rev. 94 (1954) S. 630

[5.10] Meiboom, S.; Gill, D.: Modified spin-echo method for measuring nuclear relaxation times. Rev. Sci. Instrum. 29 (1958) S. 688

[5.11] Hoult, D.I.; Lauterbur, P.C.: The sensitivity of the Zeugmatographic experiment involving human samples. J. Magn. Reson. 343 (1979) S. 425

[5.12] Brunner, P.; Ernst, R.R.: Sensitivity and performance time in NMR imaging. J. Magn. Reson. 33 (1979) S. 83

[5.13] Damadian, R.; Minkoff, L.; Goldsmith, M.; Scanford, M.; Koutcher, J.: Field focusing NMR (FONAR): Visualization of a tumor in a live animal. Science 194 (1976) S. 1430

[5.14] Gordon, R.E.; Hanley, P.E.; Shaw, D.; Gadian, D.G.; Radda, G.K.; Styles, L.; Bore, P.J.; Chan, L.: Localization of metabolites in animals using ^{31}P TMR. Nature 283 (1980) S. 167

[5.15] Hoult, D.I.: Zeugmatography: A criticism of the concept of a selective pulse in the presence of a field gradient. J. Magn. Reson. 26 (1977) S. 165

[5.16] Lauterbur, P.C.: Image formation by induced local interaction: Examples employing nuclear magnetic resonance. Nature 242 (1973) S. 190

[5.17] Cooley, J.W.; Tukey, J.W.: An algorithm for machine calculation of complex Fourier series. Math. Computation 19 (1965) S. 297

[5.18] Kumar, A.; Welti, D.; Ernst, R.: Imaging of microscopic objects by NMR Fourier Zeugmatography. Naturwiss. 62 (1975) S. 34

[5.19] Dennis, P.M.; Bene, G.J.; Exterman, R.C.: Arch. Sci. 5 (1952) S. 32

[5.20] Maudsley, A.A.; Oppelt, A.; Ganssen, A.: Rapid measurement of magnetic field distributions using nuclear magnetic resonance. Siemens Forsch.- u. Entwickl.-Ber. 8 (1979) S. 326

[5.21] Dixon, W.T.: Simple proton spectroscopic imaging. Radiology 153 (1984) S. 189

[5.22] Hore, P.J.: Solvent suppression in Fourier transform nuclear magnetic resonance. J. magn. Reson. 55 (1983) S. 283

[5.23] Hoult, D.I.: Rotating frame Zeugmatography. J. Magn. Reson. 33 (1979) S. 183

[5.24] Cox, S.J.; Styles, P.: Towards biochemical imaging. J. Magn. Reson. 40 (1980) S. 209

6 Ultrasonic techniques

[6.1] Auenbrugger, L.: Inventum novum ex percussione thoracis humani ut signo. Typis Joannis Thomae Trattner, Vindobonae (1761). S. 127, S. 178 bis 180

[6.2] Langevin, P.: French Patent, 505, 703 (1918); British Patent, 145, 691 (1921)

[6.3] Firestone, F.: U.S. Patent, 2,280,226 (1942)

[6.4] Ludwig, G.D.; Struthers, F.W.: Project N.M. 004, 001, report 4, U.S. Naval Medical Research Institute, S. 1 (1949)

[6.5] Wild, J.: The use of ultrasonic pulses for measurement of biologic tissues and the detection of tissue density changes. Surgery 127 (1950) S. 183 bis 188

[6.6] Leksell, L.: Echo-encephalography. I. Detection of intragranial complications following head injury. Acta chirurgica scandinave 110 (1955/56) S. 301

[6.7] Sokolov, S.: Zur Frage der Fortpflanzung Ultraakustischer Schwingungen in verschiedenen Körpern. Elektr. Nachr.-Tech. 6 (1929) S. 454 bis 461

[6.8] Dussik, K.T.: Possibility of using mechanical high frequency vibrations as a diagnostic aid. Z. f. Neurol. Psychiatr. 174 (1942) S. 153 bis 168

[6.9] Reid, J.; Wild, J.: Application of echo ranging techniques in determination of structure of biological tissues. Sci. amer. 115 (1952) S. 153 bis 168

[6.10] Howry, D.; Bliss, W.: Ultrasonic visualization of soft tissue structures of the body. J. lab. and clin Med. 40 (1952) S. 579 bis 592

[6.11] Meyer, E.; Neumann, E.-G-: Physikalische und Technische Akustik. Braunschweig: Friedr. Vieweg & Sohn 1967

[6.12] Skudrzyk, E.: Die Grundlagen der Akustik. Wien: Springer-Verlag 1954

[6.13] Bergmann, L.: Der Ultraschall. 6. Aufl. Stuttgart: S. Hirzel-Verlag 1954

[6.14] Krautkrämer, J.; Krautkrämer, H.: Werkstoffprüfung mit Ultraschall. Berlin, Heidelberg, New York: Springer-Verlag 1975

[6.15] Fry, F.J.: Ultrasound: its applications in medicine and biology. Amsterdam, Oxford, New York: Elsevier Scientific Publishing Company 1978

[6.16a] Kresse, H.: Kompendium Elektromedizin. Grundlagen, Anwendungen, Geräte. 3. Aufl. Berlin, München: Siemens AG 1982

[6.16b] Kresse, H.: Anwendungsmöglichkeiten der Ultraschalldiagnostik. Teil I. Grundlagen der Ultraschalldiagnostik. Röntgenprax. 26 (1973) S. 228 bis 239

[6.17] Wells, P.: Physical principles of ultrasonic diagnosis. London, New York: Academic Press 1969

[6.18] Erikson, K.R.: Ultrasound in medicine – a review. IEEE Trans. on Sonics and Ultrasonics B21 (1974) S. 144

[6.19] Kresse, H.: Kompendium Elektromedizin. Grundlagen, Anwendungen. 2. Aufl. Berlin, München: Siemens AG 1978

[6.20] Gore, J.C.; Leeman, S.: Ultrasonic backscattering from human tissue: A realistic model. Phys. in Med. and Biol. 22 (1977) S. 317 bis 326

[6.21] Kresse, H.: The physical principles in the use of the ultrasound echo method. Proc. in echo-encephalography. Berlin, Heidelberg, New York: Springer-Verlag 1968

[6.22] Gregg, E.C.; Palagallo. G.L.: Acoustic impedance of tissue. Invest. Radiol. 4 (1969) S. 357ff.

[6.23] Tarnoczy, T.: Sound focussing lenses and waveguides. Ultrasonics 3 (1965) S. 115ff.

[6.24] Grolis, J.: An analysis of the ultrasonic zone lens. IEEE Trans. on Sonics and Ultrasonics Vol. SU-15 (1968) S. 105ff.

[6.25] Mole, L.A.; Hunter, J.L.; Davenport, J.M.: Scattering of sound by air bubbles in Water. J. of the Acoustical Soc. of America (1970) S. 837ff.

[6.26] Shung, K.K.; Sigelmann, R.A.; Reid, J.M.: Scattering of ultrasound by blood. IEEE Trans. on biomed. Engng. 23 (1976) S. 460ff.

[6.27] Chivers, R.C.: The scattering of ultrasound by human tissues – some theoretical models. Ultrasound in Med. and Biol. 3 (1977) S. 1 bis 13

[6.28] Welton, P.J.; Frey, H.G.; Moore, P.: Experimental measurements of the scattering of acoustic waves by rough surfaces. J. of the Acoustical Soc. America (1972) S. 1553ff.

[6.29] Zemanek, J.: Beam behavior within the nearfield of a vibrating piston. J. of the Acoustical Soc. America (1971) S. 181ff.

[6.30] Weyns, A.: Radiation fields of Pulsed ultrasonic transducers plane square, plane annular and spherical radiators. 3rd European Congress an Ultrasonics in Medicine, Bologna, 1978. Edizioni centro minerva medica, S. 497ff.

[6.31] Schwarz, R.: Digital computer simulation of a piezoelectric thickness vibrator. J. of the Acoustical Soc. America 62 (1977) S. 463ff.

[6.32] Rhyne, T.L.: An improved interpretation of Mason's model for piezoelectric plate transducers. IEEE Trans. on Sonics and Ultrasonics SU 25 (1978) S. 98 bis 103

[6.33] Desilets, C.S.; Fraser, J.D.; Kino, G.S.: The design of efficient broad-band piezoelectric transducers. IEEE Trans. on Sonics and Ultrasonics SU 25 (1978) S. 115 bis 125

[6.34] Foster, F.S.; Hunt, J.W.: The design and characterization of short pulse ultrasound transducers. Ultrasonics (1978) S. 116ff.

[6.35] Kossoff, G.: The effects of backing and matching on the performance of piezoelectric ceramic transducers. IEEE Trans. on Sonics and Ultrasonics SU 13 (1966) S. 20ff.

[6.36] Penttinen, A.; Luukkala, M.: The impulse response and pressure nearfield of a curved ultrasonic radiator. J. of Phys. D, Appl. Phys. 9 (1976) S. 1547 bis 1557

[6.37] Yao, S.T.: Ultrasound in the transcutaneous assessment of blood flow. British J. of Hosp. Med. (1972) S. 521ff.

[6.38] Gosling, R.G.; King, D.H.: Continuous wave ultrasound as an alternative and complement to X-rays in vascular examinations. Cardiovascular appl. of ultrasound 74, S. 266ff.

[6.39] Kresse, H.; Beck, N.: Erste Mitteilung über ein gefäßdiagnostisches Bildverfahren mit Ultraschall. Biomed. Tech. 18 (1973) S. 152 bis 154

[6.40] Mozersky, D.J.; Hokanson, D.E.; Sumner, D.S., et al.: Ultrasonic visualization of the arterial lumen. Surgery 72 (1972) S. 253 bis 259

[6.41] Fish, P.J.; Kakkar, V.V.; Corrigan, T. et al.: Arteriography using Ultrasound. Lancet 10 (1972) S. 1269 und 1270

[6.42] O'Donnell, M.; Jaynes, E.T.; Miller, J.G.: Relationship between ultrasonic attenuation and dispersion. Abstracts book of 3rd Int. Symp. on Ultrasound Imaging and Tissue Characterisation, Washington NBS 1978

[6.43] Barber, F.E.; Baker, D.W.; Nation, A.W., et al.: Ultrasonic duplex echo-Doppler scanner. IEEE Trans. on biomed. Engng. BME-21 (1974) S. 109 bis 113

[6.44] Green, P.S.; Taenzer, J.C.; Ramsey, S.D.; Holzemer, J.F.; Suarez, J.R.; Marich, K.W.: A real-time ultrasonic omaging system for carotid arteriography. Ultrasound in Med. and Biol. 3 (1977) S. 129 bis 142

[6.45] Kresse, H.: Anwendungsmöglichkeiten der Ultraschalldiagnostik. Teil II. Diagnoseverfahren und ihre technische Realisierung. Röntgenprax. 26 (1973) S. 286 bis 295

[6.46] de Vlieger, M.: Handbook of clinical ultrasound. New York, Chichester, Brisbane, Toronto: John Wiley & Sons 1978

[6.47] Hassler, D.: Einführung in physikalische und technische Grundlagen der diagnostischen Ultraschallverfahren. Klinikarzt (1977) S. 414 bis 419

[6.48] Holbrooke, D.R.; McCurry, E.M.; Richards, V.; Shibata, H.: Through transmission ultrasonic imaging of intrauterine and fetal structures using acoustical holography. 2nd World Congress of Ultrasonics in Medicine, Rotterdam, 1973

[6.49] Green, P.S.; Schaefer, L.F.; Jones, E.D.; Suarez, J.R.: A new high-performance ultrasonic camera. Acoustical Holography Vol. 5, S. 493ff.

[6.50] Green, P.S.; Marich, K.W.: Potential of real-time orthographic ultrasonic imaging for cardiovascular diagnosis. Cardiovascular Imaging and Image Processing, Theory and Practice 72 (1975)

[6.51] Zatz, L.M.; Marich, K.W.; Green, P.S.; Lipton, M.J.; Suarez, J.R.; Macovski, A.: Real-time imaging with a new ultrasonic camera: Part I, In vitro experimental studies on transmission imaging of biological structures. Part II, Preliminary studies in normal adults. J. of clin. Ultrasound 3 (1975) S. 5 bis 22

[6.52] Glover, G.H.; Sharp, J.C.: Reconstruction of ultrasound propagation speed distributions in soft tissue: time-of-flight tomography. IEEE Trans. on Sonics and Ultrasonics SU 24 (1977) No. 4

[6.53] Carson, P.L.; Ougthon, T.V.; Dick, D.E.; Kubitschek, J.E.; Scherzinger, A.L.; Kitson, F.L.; Johnson, M.L.; Lambert, P.A.; Moore, G.: Preliminary characterization of breast tissue in vivo with ultrasonic computed tomography of attenuation. Abstracts book of 3rd Int. Symp. on Ultrasound Imaging and Tissue Characterisation. Washington NBS 1978

[6.54] Greenleaf, J.F.; Johnson, S.A.: Measurements of spatial distribution of refractive index in tissues by ultrasonic computer assisted tomography. Ultrasound in Med. and Biol. 3 (1978) S. 327 bis 339

[6.55] Glover, G.H.: Computerized time-of-flight ultrasonic tomography for breast examination. Ultrasound in Med. and Biol. 3 (1977) S. 117 bis 127

[6.56] Becker, R.: Bildgüte bei schnellen Ultraschallabtastverfahren am Beispiel des Ultraschall-Scanners „Vidoson“ der Firma Siemens. Diplomarbeit, Universität Karslruhe (1976)

[6.57] Hassler, D.; Hönig, D.: Resolution of B-scanners: widening of conception and corresponding demonstration with a second kind of test phantom. 3rd European Congress on Ultrasonics in Medicine, Bologna, 1978

[6.58] Papoulis, A.: The Fourier integral and its applications. New York, San Francisco, London, Toronto: McGraw-Hill Book Company 1962

[6.59] Maginness, M.G.: Gray scale performance of displays for dynamic ultrasound imaging. J. of clin. ultrasound 5 (1977) S. 329ff.

[6.60] Foster, F.S.; Hunt, J.W.: The focussing of ultrasound beams through human tissue. Abstracts book of 3rd Int. Symp on Ultrasound Imaging and Tissue Characterisation, Washington NBS 1978

[6.61] Kresse, H.: Der Einfluß des Einfallswinkels bei der Ultraschall-Echo-Diagnostik. Elektromedizin-Sonderausgabe (1968)

[6.62] Goldman, D.E.; Hueter, T.F.: Tabular data of the velocity and absorption of high-frequency sound in mammalian tissues. J. of the Acoustical Soc. America 28 (1956) S. 35ff.

[6.63] Kresse, H.: Wirkungen und Nebenwirkungen medizinischen Ultraschalles. Atomkernenerg. Bd. 21 (1973) S. 269 bis 273

[6.64] Fry, F.J.; Erdmann, W.A.; Johnson, L.K.; Baird, A.I.: Ultrasonic toxicity study. Ultrasound in Med. and Biol. 3 (1978) S. 351 bis 366

[6.65] Wells, P.N.T.: Absorption and dispersion of ultrasound in biological tissue. Ultrasound in Med. and Biol. Vol. 1 (1975) S. 369 bis 376

[6.66] Fung, A.K.; Leovaris, A.: Frequency dependence of ultrasonic scatter from statistically known rough surfaces. Wescon Technical Papers (1968) S. 1 bis 4

[6.67] Hill, C.R.: Manual on health aspects exposure to non ionizing radiation. Chapter: Ultrasound. WHO Regional Office for Europe (1977)

[6.68] Billy, M. de; Doucet, J.; Quentin, G.: Angular dependence of the backscattered intensity of acoustic waves from rough surfaces. Conference Proceedings. Ultrasonics International (1975)

[6.69] Eaglesfield, C.C.: The angular dependence of scattering by nearly polished surfaces. Proc. Phys. Soc., Vol. 80 (1962) S. 947 bis 951, Vol. 82 (1963) S. 406 bis 411

[6.70] Goss, S.A.; Johnston, R.L.; Dunn, F.: Comprehensive compilation of empirical ultrasonic properties of mammalian tissues. J. of the Acoustical Soc. America 64(2) (1978) S. 423 bis 457

[6.71] Anliker, M.; Casty, M.; Friedli, P.; Kubli, R.; Keller, M.: Cardiovascular flow dynamics and measurement. Baltimore: University Parks Press 1977 S. 43 bis 88

[6.72] Hassler, D.: DBP 2461 264,4 vom 23.12.1974

[6.73] Hassler, D.: DBP 2724 437,7 von 1979

[6.74] Keidel, W.D.: Sinnesphysiologie Teil 1. Berlin, Heidelberg, New York: Springer-Verlag 1971

[6.75] Biedermann, K.; Borcke, E.; Buchmann, F.; Frieser, H.; Munker, H.; Schober, H.; Schott, O.; Stieve, F.E.; Wiedemann. L.: Über Kontrastbegriffe in der Radiologie und ihre Definitionen. Röntgenblätter 20 (1967) S. 131 bis 147

[6.76] Dillenburger, W.: Einführung in die Fernsehtechnik Bd. 1. Berlin: Fachverlag Schick und Schön 1964

[6.77] Zagzebski, J.A.; Banjavic, R.A.; Jutila, R., White, D.: Ultrasonic transducer sensitivity in attenuating and scattering material. Ultrasound in Medicine 3. New York, London: Plenum Press 1976

[6.78] Shegal, Chandra M.; Greenleaf, James F.: Scattering of Ultrasound by Tissues. Ultrasonic Imaging 6 (1984) S. 60 bis 80

[6.79] Parker, Kevin J.: Ultrasonic Attenuation and Absorption in Liver Tissue. Ultrasound in Med & Biol. Vol. 9 (1983) S. 363 bis 369

[6.80] Hassler, D.: Einführung in die Systemtheorie der Puls- Dopplertechnik zur Blutflußmessung. Ultraschall in der Med. 8 (1987) S. 102 bis 107, 152 bis 154, 192 bis 196

[6.81] Hassler, D.; Köhl, W.: Beitrag zur Systemtheorie der Ultraschall-Puls-Echo-Technik. Ultraschall 5 (1984) S. 44 bis 55

[6.82] Nyborg, W.L.; Steele, R.B.: Temperature Elevation in a Beam of Ultrasound. Ultrasound in Med & Biol. Vol. 9 (1983) S. 611 bis 620

[6.83] Holländer, H.-J.; Hackelöer, B.-J.; Hassler, D.; Rott, H.D.; Vandenberghe, K.: Die Ultraschalldiagnostik in der Schwangerschaft. 3. Aufl. Urban & Schwarzenberg 1984

7 X-ray diagnostics

[7.1] Eichmeier, J.: Moderne Vakuumelektronik. Berlin, Heidelberg, New York: Springer-Verlag 1981

[7.2] Reiprich, S.; Seppelfeld, E.: Mammographie-Röntgenröhre (MBM60). NTG-Fachberichte 95 (1986) S. 248 bis 251

[7.3] Bouwers, A.: Über den Temperaturverlauf an der Anode einer Röntgenröhre. Z. f. techn. Phys. 8 (1927) S. 271 bis 277

[7.4] Oosterkamp, W.J.: The heat dissipation on the anode of an X-ray tube. Part I, Philips Res. Rep. 3 (1948) S. 49 bis 59; Part II, Philips Res. Rep. 3 (1948) S. 161 bis 173

[7.5] Dietz, H.; Geldner, E.: Temperature distribution in X-ray rotating anodes. Part I, Physical principles. Siemens Forsch.- und Entwickl.-Ber. 7 (1978) S. 18 bis 23

[7.6] Baumann, W.; Dietz, H.; Geldner, E.: Temperature distribution in X-ray rotating anodes. Part 2. Mathematical computation for compound anodes. Siemens Forsch.- u. Entwickl.-Ber. 7 (1978) S. 111 bis 117

[7.7] Baumann, W.; Dietz, H.; Geldner, E.: Temperature distribution in X-ray rotating anodes. Part 3: Comparison of various types of anode. Siemens Forsch.- und Entwickl.-Ber. 8 (1978) S. 239 bis 246

[7.8] Wolter, I.: Loadix – ein System zur thermischen Überwachung von Röntgenstrahlern. Electromedica 45 (1977) S. 73 bis 76

[7.9] Dietz, H.; Fenner, E.; Geldner, E.; Schnitger, H.: Intensity distribution in the focal spot an X-ray tube and its influence on loadability and image quality. Int. Congr. Series No. 339 – Radiology, Vol. 2, Proc. of the XIII Intern. Congr. of Radiology Madrid (1973) S. 392 bis 396

[7.10] Fenner, E.: Lochkamera-Aufnahmen der Brennflecke von Röntgenröhren. Elektronik 5 (1956) S. 257 bis 260

[7.11] Elsas, A.; Zimmer, Th.: Höhere Belastung von Drehanodenröhren durch Verwendung von legierten Anoden. Fortschr. auf dem Geb. d. Röntgenstrahlen u. d. Nuklearmedizin 97 (1962) S. 511 bis 514

[7.12] Geldner, E.; Schreiner, H.: Gefügeeinfluß auf mechanische Eigenschaften von WRe5- und WRe10-Legierungen. High Temp. High Pressures 6 (1974) S. 435 bis 441

[7.13] Schnitger, H.; Dietz, H.; Geldner, E.: Focal spot intensity distribution and its influence on loadability an geometrical image blurring. Proc. of photo-optical Instrument. 56 (1974) medical X-ray photo-optical Syst. Eval. S. 181 bis 183

[7.14] Meredith, W.J.; Massey, J.B.: Fundamental physics of radiology. Bristol: John Wright & Sons Ltd. 1968, Abschnitt 2/10

[7.15] Reiß, K.H.; Steinle, B.: Tabellen zur Röntgendiagnostik. Teil II. Siemens AG, Bereich Medizinische Technik (1973)

[7.16] Reiß, K.H.: Scattered radiation and characteristic film curve. Radiol. 80 (1963) S. 663 bis 667

[7.17] Gajewski, H.; Müller, D.: Die Abstandstechnik zur Verminderung des Streustrahlenanteils bei Röntgenaufnahmen. Strahlentherapie 138 (1969) S. 689 bis 695

[7.18] Dick, C.E.; Soares, C.G.; Motz, J.W.: X-ray scatter data for diagnostic radiology. Phys. in Med. and Biol. 23 (1978) S. 1076 bis 1085

[7.19] DIN 6826. Röntgen-Streustrahlenraster: Kenngrößen. September 1980

[7.20] Schubert, W.: Der Einfluß der Konstruktion und des Herstellungsverfahrens auf die Wirksamkeit von Streustrahlenrastern. Röntgenprax. 18 (1965) S. 277 bis 288

[7.21] Boldingh, W.H.: Quality and choice of Potter Bucky grids. Acta Radiol. 55 (1961) S. 230

[7.22] Boldingh, W.H.: The rational choice of an X-ray grid. Medica mundi 6 (1960) S. 115 bis 121

[7.23] Reiß, K.H.: Die physikalischen Grenzen der Beseitigung von Röntgenstrahlen durch Rasterblenden. Z. f. angew. Phys. 11 (1959) S. 184 bis 188

[7.24] Jaffe, C.; Webster, E.W.: Radiographic contrast improvement by means of slit radiography. Radiol. 116 (1975) S. 631 bis 635

[7.25] Barnes, G.T.: Cleare, H.M.: Brezovich, I.A.: Reduction of scatter in diagnostic radiology by means of a scanning multiple slit assembly. Radiol. 120 (1976) S. 691 bis 694

[7.26] Rudin, St.; Bednarek, D.R.: Improved contrast in special procedures using a rotating aperture wheel (RAW) device. Radiol. 137 (1980) S. 505 bis 510

[7.27] Levy, M.: Über die Abkürzung der Expositionszeit bei Aufnahmen mit Röntgenstrahlen. Fortschr. auf dem Geb. d. Röntgenstrahlen 1 (1897) S. 75

[7.28] Edison, Th.A.: Nature (1896) S. 470; Electr. Rev. 38 (1896) S. 508

[7.29] Gasper, J.: Modulation transfer function and efficiency of transparent luminescent materials. J. of the Optical Soc. America 63 (1973) S. 714

[7.30] Hamaker, H.C.: Radiation and heat conduction in light-scattering material. Philips Res. Rep. 2 (1947) S. 55

[7.31] Doi, K., et al.: MTF's and Wiener Spectra of Radiographic Screen-Film-Systems, Vol. II. U.S. Department of Health and Human Services, March 1986, HHS Publication FDA 86-8257

[7.32] Kuhn, H.: Bildrauschen bei Film-Folien-Systemen: seine Ursachen und Komponenten. electromedica 51 (1983) S. 46

[7.33] Mirandé, W.; Hoeschen, D.: Wiener Spektren von Röntgenfilm-Folien-Kombinationen. Röntgen Bl. 38 (1985) S. 81

[7.34] Buchanan, R.A.; Solon, I.; Finkelstein, M.D.; Wickersheim, K.A.: X-ray exposure reduction using rare-earth oxysulfide intensifying screens. Radiol. 105 (1972) S. 185

[7.35] Fearon, Th. et al.: A comparative evaluation of Rare-Earth Screen-Film systems. Investigative Radiol. 21 (1986) S. 654

[7.36] Aichinger, H.: Gesichtspunkte und Folgerungen bei der automatischen Belichtung von Schichtaufnahmen. electromedica 39 (1971) S. 36 bis 43

[7.37] Meiler, J.: Die in der Röntgendiagnostik verwendeten Spannungskurvenformen und ihr Einfluß auf Bildqualität und Röhrenbelastung. Fortschr. auf d. Geb. d. Röntgenstrahlen (vereinigt mit Röntgenpraxis). 72 (1949) H 2, S. 222 bis 241

[7.38] Berger, A.: Zum Problem der Bewegungsunschärfe im Röntgenbild der Lunge und des Herzens. Röntgenblätter 14 (1961) H. 12, S. 369 bis 380

[7.39] Ammann, E.: Ein neuer Röntgengenerator für hohe Leistung bei sehr kurzer Belichtungszeit. Dissertation, Technische Universität Stuttgart (1974)

[7.40] Schmitmann, H.; Ammann, E.: PANDOROS OPTIMATIC – ein Röntgengenerator mit neuen Möglichkeiten. electromedica 41 (1973) S. 177 bis 181

[7.41] Kühnel, W.: Der Schwingkreiswechselrichter mit Gegenspannungslast zur Versorgung von Verbrauchern mit gepulstem Gleichstrom. Dissertation, Technische Fakultät der Universität Erlangen-Nürnberg (1986)

[7.42] Hoxter, E.A.: Röntgenaufnahmetechnik. Grundlagen, Anwendungen. Berlin, München: Siemens AG (1982) S. 23

[7.43] Laubenberger, T.: Leitfaden der medizinischen Röntgentechnik. Köln: Deutscher Ärzte-Verlag GmbH 1975

[7.44] Brody, W.R.: Digital radiography. New York: Ravenpress 1984

[7.45] Wolter, I.: LOADIX – ein System zur thermischen Überwachung von Röntgenstrahlern. electromedica 45 (1977) S. 42

[7.46] DIN 6814: Begriffe und Benennungen in der radiologischen Technik. Teil 3: Dosisgrößen und Dosiseinheiten (Entwurf Nov. 1983). Blatt 6: Technische Mittel zur Erzeugung von Röntgen- und Elektronenstrahlung. Berlin, Köln: Beuth Verlag 1963

[7.47] Coltmann, J.W.: Fluoroscopic image brightening by electronic means. Radiol. 51 (1948) S. 359 bis 367

[7.48] Gebauer, A.; Lissner, J.; Schott, O.: Das Röntgenfernsehen. 2. Aufl. Stuttgart: Georg Thieme Verlag 1974

[7.49] Greschat, W.; Heinrich, H.; Römer, P.: Quantum yield of Cs_3Sb photocathodes as a function of thickness and angle of incidence. Advances in Electron. and electron Phys. 40A (1976) S. 397 bis 408

[7.50] Schwierz, G.: Berechnung elektronenoptischer Kenngrößen von Röntgenbildverstärkern. Dissertation. Universität Erlangen (1972)

[7.51] Fenner, E.: Elektronenoptischer Röntgenbildverstärker – Kennwerte und Einsatz in der Röntgendiagnostik. Siemens-Z. 41 (1967) S. 749 bis 755

[7.52] Hofmann, F.W.: Röntgenbildverstärker mit verbesserter Bildqualität. Röntgenbl. 25 (1972) S. 198 bis 205

[7.53] Haendle, J.; Horbaschek, H.: Die hochauflösende Röntgenfernsehkette. Röntgenprax. 29 (1976) S. 95 bis 108

[7.54] Meyer-Ebrecht; Spiesberger, D.W.: Neue Verfahren in der medizinischen Röntgendiagnostik – eine Herausforderung für die industrielle Röntgenprüftechnik. Materialprüfung 19 (1977) S. 10

[7.55] Delgambe, R.: La troisieme generation des amplificateurs de brillance. H. Belge Radiol. 58 (1975) S. 101 bis 105

[7.56] Haendle, J.; Horbaschek, H.; Alexandrescu, M.: Das hochauflösende Röntgenfernsehen und die hochauflösenden Videospeicher. Electromedica 45 (1977) S. 83 bis 91

[7.57] Lissner, J.; Marhoff, P.: Fortschritte der Bildverstärker-Fernsehtechnik. Klinische Erfahrungen, Vortrag auf dem Deutschen Röntgenkongreß. Essen. 1976

[7.58] Pfeiler, M.; Jooß, B.: Zum Zeitverhalten eines Bildübertragungssystems am Beispiel des Röntgenfernsehens. Nachr.-Techn. Z. 22 (1969) S. 88 bis 92

[7.59] Haendle, J.: Entwicklungsstand des Röntgenfernsehens. Radiol. diagnost. 20 (1979) S. 554 bis 569

[7.60] Dümmling, K.: Die Trägheitseigenschaften von Röntgenbildübertragungsanlagen. Siemens Forsch.- u. Entwickl.-Ber. 1 (1971) S. 50 bis 57

[7.61] Arp, F.: Die Bildabtastung als Transformation einer zweidimensionalen Bildsystemcharakteristik in eine eindimensionale Funktion. Arch. f. Elektron. u. Übertr.-Tech. 17 (1963) S. 207 bis 216

[7.62] Kruger, R.A.; Mistretta, Ch.A., et al.: Computerized fluoroscopy in real time for noninvasive visualization of the cardiovascular system. Diagn. Radiol 130 (1979) S. 49 bis 57

[7.63] Heintzen, P.H.: Review on the research and some aspects upon the modern development of densitometry, particularly roentgen-video-computer-techniques. Ann. de Radiol. 21 (1978) S. 343 bis 348

[7.64] Höhne, K.H.; Nicolae, G.C.; Pfeiffer, G.: Functional imaging – a new tool for X-ray. Functional Diagnostics. DESY DV-78/01. (May 1978)

[7.65] Hoxter, E.A.: Röntgenaufnahmetechnik. Grundlagen. Anwendungen. Berlin, München: Siemens AG 1982

[7.66] Laubenberger, T.: Leitfaden der medizinischen Röntgentechnik. Deutscher Ärzte-Verlag GmbH 1975

[7.67] Aichinger, H.: Gesichtspunkte und Folgerungen bei der automatischen Belichtung von Schichtaufnahmen. Electromedica 39 (1971) S. 36 bis 43

[7.68] Wolter, I.: LOADIX – ein System zur thermischen Überwachung von Röntgenstrahlern. Electromedica 45 (1977) S. 73 bis 76

[7.69] Schmitmann, H.; Noske, E.; Sladek, W.: TRIDOROS – OPTIMATIC – ein neues Generatorsystem. Electromedica 39 (1971) S. 83 bis 86

[7.70] Schmitmann, H.; Ammann, E.: PANDOROS OPTIMATIK – ein Röntgengenerator mit neuen Möglichkeiten. electromedica 41 (1973) S. 177 bis 181

[7.71] Steiner, K.; Brundin, B.; Sladek, W.: Das OPTIMATIC-System. electromedica 41 (1973) S. 182 bis 187

[7.72] Grim, S.: Die programmierte Aufnahmetechnik bei der direkten Angiographie. electromedica 41 (1973) S. 162 bis 164

[7.73] Franke, K.: Die neue Generation der Röntgengeneratoren und ihr Einfluß auf die optimale Bildqualität. Radiol. Prax. I (1978) S. 24 bis 36

[7.74] Ammann, E.: Ein neuer Röntgengenerator für hohe Leistung bei sehr kurzer Belichtungszeit. Dissertation, Technische Universität Stuttgart (1974)

[7.75] Ahlbäck. S.O.: Skeletal radiography with Orbix. Siemens-Elema AB, MS 41/1198.101

[7.76] Rädberg, C.; Thibaut, A., et al.: Schädelaufnahmen am liegenden Patienten mit dem Orbix-Schädelaufnahmegerät. Siemens-Elema Ab, MS 41/1098

[7.77] Seitzer, D.: Elektronische Analog-Digital-Umsetzer. Verfahren, Bauelemente, Beispiele. Berlin, Göttingen, Heidelberg: Springer-Verlag 1977

[7.78] Tietze, U.; Schenk, Ch.: Halbleiter-Schaltungstechnik. 5. Aufl. Berlin, Heidelberg, New York: Springer-Verlag 1980

[7.79] Huffman, D.A.: A Method for the Construction of Minimum-Redundancy Codes. Proc. IRE 40 (1952) S. 1098

[7.80] Phelps, M.E.; Hoffman, E.J.; Ter-Pogossian, M.M.: Attenuation coefficients of various body tissues, fluids and lesions at photon energies of 18 to 136 keV. Radiology 117 (1975) S. 573 bis 583

[7.81] Mika, N.; Reiß, K.H.: Tabellen zur Röntgendiagnostik. Berlin, München: Siemens AG 1973

[7.82] Alvarez, R.E.; Macovski, A.: Energy-selective reconstructions in X-ray computerized tomography. Phys. Med. Biol. 21 (1976) S. 733 bis 744

[7.83] Lehmann, L.A.; Alvarez, R.E.; Macovski, A.; Brody, W.R.: Generalized image combinations in dual kVp digital radiography. Med. Phys. 8 (1981) S. 659 bis 667

[7.84] Brody, W.R.: Hybrid subtraction for improved arteriography. Radiology 141 (1981) S. 828 bis 831

[7.85] Keyes, G.S.; Riederer, S.J.; Belanger, B.F.; Brody, W.R.: Hybrid subtraction in digital fluorography. SPIE 347, Application of optical instrumentation in medicine X (1982) S. 34 bis 41.

[7.86] Foley, W.D.; Keyes, G.S., et al.: Work in progress: temporal energy hybrid subtraction in intravenous digital subtraction angiography. Radiology 148 (1983) S. 265 bis 271

[7.87] Höhne, K.H.; Böhm, M., et al.: Die Messung und differenzierte bildliche Darstellung der Nierendurchblutung mit der Computerangiographie. Fortschr. Röntgenstr. 129 (1978) S. 667 bis 672

[7.88] Böhm, M.; Höhne, K.H.: The processing and analysis of radiographic image sequences. In: Digital image processing in medicine. Höhne, K.H. (Ed.); Lecture notes in medical informatics 15 (1981) S. 15 bis 36

[7.89] Bürsch, J.H.; Hahne, H.J., et al.: Myocardial perfusion studies by digital angiography. Proc. Comp. Cardiol., IEEE Comp. Soc., Long Beach (1983) S. 343 bis 346

[7.90] Heintzen, P.H.; Brennecke, R., et al.: Quantitative analysis of structure and function of the cardiovascular system by roentgen-video-computer techniques. Mayo Clin. Proc. 57 (1982) S. 78 bis 91

[7.91] Ziedses des Plantes, B.G.: Serioskopie. Fortschr. a. d. Gebiet d. Röntgenstrahlen 57 (1938) S. 605 bis 616

[7.92] Dümmling, K.: Ein neues Verfahren zum Mehrfachschichten mit Hilfe von Fernsehspeichern. Der Radiologe 9 (1969) S. 37 bis 40

[7.93] Maravilla, K.R.; Murray, R.C.; Horner, S.: Digital tomosynthesis: technique for electronic reconstruction tomography. AJR 141 (1983) S. 497 bis 502

[7.94] Edholm, P.R.; Quiding, L.: Reduction of linear blurring in tomography. Radiology 92 (1969) S. 1115 bis 1118

[7.95] Pfeiler, M.; Marhoff, P.; Koch, R.: Das röntgentechnische Umfeld der Digitalen Radiographie. electromedica 53 (1985) S. 50 bis 57

[7.96] Shaw, C.-G.; Plewes, D.B.: Quantitative digital subtraction angiography: two scanning techniques for correction of scattered radiation and veiling glare. Radiology 157 (1985) S. 247 bis 253

[7.97] Röntgen, W.C.: Über eine neue Art von Strahlen. Sitzungsber. phys.-med. Ges. Würzburg (1895) S. 137ff.

[7.98] Seyferth, W.; Markhoff, P.; Zeitler, E.: Digitale Subtraktionsangiographie: Diagnostischer Stellenwert und Risiko. electromedica 50 (1982) S. 60 bis 80

[7.99] Seyferth, W.; Polster, W.: Pfadfindertechnik: eine Ergänzung der Digitalen Subtraktionsangiographie im fluoroskopischen Betrieb. electromedica 53 (1985) S. 39

[7.100] Chaussy, Ch.; Brendel, W.; Schmiedt, E.: Extracorporeally induced destruction of kidney stones by shock waves. Lancet 11 (1980) S. 1265 bis 1267

[7.101] Eisenmenger, W.: Elektromagnetische Erzeugung von ebenen Druckstößen in Flüssigkeiten. Akust. Beihefte (1962) S. 185 bis 202

[7.102] Reichenberger, H.; Naser, G.: Electromagnetic acoustic source for the extracorporeal generation of shock waves in lithotripsy. Siemens Forsch.- u. Entwickl.-Ber. 15 (1986) S. 187 bis 194

8 X-ray computed tomography

[8.1] Linke, G.; Pauli, K.; Pfeiler, M.: Zur Strahlenbelastung des Patienten bei der Computertomographie. electromedica 44 (1976) S. 15 bis 18

[8.2] Alexander, J.; Kalender, W.; Linke, G.: Computertomographie: Bewertungsmerkmale, Gerätetechnik, Anwendungen. Berlin, München: Siemens AG 1985

[8.3] Miller, D.; Dawes, A.T.; Cowie, J.W.: Routineuntersuchung des Felsenbeins mit Sekundärrekonstruktionen aus hochauflösenden 1-mm-Schnitten. electromedica 53 (1985) S. 2

[8.4] Luft, Ch.; Trenkler, J.; Hammer, B.; Valencak, E.: CT-gestützte Lokalisationsbestimmung bei intrakraniellen Prozessen. electromedica 54 (1986) S. 166

[8.5] Jescke, G.; Will, C.-H.: Quantitative Serien-Computertomographie: ein mathematisches Modell zur Bestimmung von Konversionskonstanten nach intravenöser Kontrastmittelapplikation. electromedica 53 (1985) S. 158

[8.6] Wermenski, K.; Majchrowski, M.: Ein mathematisches Rechenmodell des Dichte-Zeit-Diagramms bei nierenbedingter arterieller Hypertension. electromedica 53 (1985) S. 76

[8.7] Kalender, W.A.; Rettinger, G.; Süss, C.: Measurement of paranasal sinus ventilation by Xenon-enhanced dynamic computed tomography. Journal of Computer Assisted Tomography 9 (1985) H. 3

[8.8] Lackner, K.; Klotz, E.; Kalender, W.: Computergestützte Auswertung EKG-getriggerter CT-Aufnahmen des Herzens. electromedica 53 (1985) S. 113

[8.9] Bautz, W.; Kalender, W.A.: Materialselektive Bildgebung und Dichtebestimmung mit der Zwei-Spektren-Methode. Digitale Bilddiagnostik 7 (1987) S. 95 bis 103

[8.10] Kalender, W.A.; Klotz, E.; Süss, C.: Vertebral bone mineral analysis on integrated approach with CT. Radiol. 164 (1987) S. 419 bis 423

[8.11] Nagel, W.; Schmidt,M.; Alexander, J.; Drexler, J.: Neue klinische Ergebnisse zur Osteoporosse-Diagnose mit QCT. electromedica 55 (1987) S. 104

9 Nuclear medical diagnostics

[9.5] Faßbender, H.: Einführung in die Meßtechnik der Kernstrahlung und die Anwendung der Radioisotope. Stuttgart: Georg Thieme Verlag 1962

[9.6] Gelbke, W.: Nuklearmedizin. Funktionsdiagnostik (Hrsg. D. Emrich). Stuttgart: Georg Thieme Verlag 1971

[9.7] Rassow, G.: Fibel zur Nuklearmedizinischen Routinediagnostik. Berlin, München: Siemens AG 1970

[9.1] Prinzmetal, M., et al.: Radiocardiography, a new method for studying blood flow through chambers of the heart in humen beings. Sci. 108 (1948) S. 320

[9.2] Veall, N., et al.: A method for determination of cardiac output. 2nd Radioisotope Conference 1 (1954) S. 183

[9.3] Hundeshagen, H.: Kreislaufdiagnostik von Herz und Lunge mit radioaktiven Isotopen. Fortschr. auf dem Geb. d. Röntgenstrahlen. Sonderband Dtsch. Röntgenkongr. (1963) S. 243

[9.4] Hoffmann, G.; Kleine, N.: Die Methode der radiokardiographischen Funktionsanalyse. Nucl.-Med. 7 (1968) S. 350 bis 370

[9.8] Cassen, B., et al.: Instrumentation for I^{131} use in medical studies. Nucleonics 9 (1951) Heft 2, S. 46 bis 50

[9.9] Mayneord, W.V., et al.: A method of making visible the distribution of activity in a source of ionizing radiation. Nature 168 (1951) S. 762 bis 765

[9.10] Fucks, W.; Knipping, H.W.: Eine γ-Retina zur Bestimmung der raum-zeitlichen Verteilung radioaktiver Substanzen. Naturwiss. 42 (1955) S. 493

[9.11] Bender, M.A.: The digital autofluoroscope. Med. Radioisotope scanning. IAEA Wien (1964)

[9.12] Ter-Pogossian, M.M., et al.: An image tube scintillation camera for use with radioactive isotopes emitting low-energy photons. Radiol. 86 (1966) S. 463 bis 469

[9.13] Conrad, B.; Platz, W.: Das SCINTICON – eine neue Gammakamera. electromedica 41 (1973) S. 220 bis 225

[9.14] Anger, H.O.: Scintillation camera. Rev. of Sci. Instrum. 29 (1958) S. 27 bis 33

[9.15] Anger, H.O.: Instrumentation in nuclear medicine (Hrsg. G.J. Hine). I, S. 520. New York Academic Press 1967

[9.16] Keil, P.: Räumliches Auflösungsvermögen der Gammakamera SCINTICON. Siemens Forsch.- u. Entwickl.-Ber. 4 (1975) S. 152 bis 158

[9.17] Svedberg, J.B.: Computed intrinsic efficiencies and modulation transfer functions for gamma cameras. Phys. in Med. and Biol. 18 (1973) S. 658 bis 664

[9.18] Conrad, B.: Kamerasysteme in der Nuklearmedizin. Med. Physik (Hrsg. W.J. Lorenz) Bd. I, S. 51

[9.19] Beck, R.N.: The scanning system as a whole. In: A. Gottschalk, R.N. Beck: Fundamental problems in scanning. Springfield (USA): Charles C. Thomas publisher 1968

[9.20] Neumann, K.; Oberhausen, E.: Justierung der Angerkamera. Erstes Heidelberger Symposium über Kamera-Szintigraphie (Hrsg. K.E. Scheer) 1968

[9.21] Moretti, J.L., et al.: Comparative assays of scintillation cameras (type Anger). Nuclearmedicine Institute Cleveland (1974)

[9.22] Adams, A.; Zimmerman, D.: Methodes for calculating the deadtime of Anger camera systems. J. of nucl. Med. 14 (1973) S. 496

[9.23] Lange, D.; Kober, B.: Adressen-Pile-up in Szintillationskameras and Datenspeichern. Med. Physik (Hrsg. W.J. Lorenz) Bd. 2, S. 85

[9.24] Strand, S.-E.; Larsson, I.: Image artifacts at high photon fluence rates in single crystal NaI (Tl (Thallium)) scintillation cameras. J. of nucl. Med. 19 (1978) S. 407 bis 413

[9.25] Adam, W.E., et al.: Evaluation of left ventricular function by radionuclide angiography. Herz 2 (1977) S. 195

[9.26] Kuhl, D.E.; Edwards, R.Q.: Image separation radioisotope scanning. Radiol. 80 (1963) S. 653 bis 662

[9.27] Kuhl, D.E.; Edwards, R.Q.: Reorganizing data from transverse section scans of the brain using digital processing. Radiol. 91 (1968) S. 975 bis 983

10 Magnetic resonance imaging

[10.1] Loeffler, W.; Oppelt, A.; v. Wulfen, H.; Zimmermann, B.: An approach for selecting the best field strength for proton imaging. Proceedings of the SMRM (New York, 1984), S. 483
Hoult, D.I.; Chen, C.N.; Sank, V.J.: The field dependence of NMR imaging, II. arguments concerning on optimal field strength. Magn. Res. Med. 3 (1986) S. 730

[10.2] Jackson, J.D.: Classical Electrodynamics. (Chapter 6.1). London, New York. Wiley (1962)

[10.3] Bottomley, P.A.; Andrew, E.R.: RF magnetic field penetration, phase shift, and power dissipation in biological tissue: implications for NMR imaging. Phys. Med. Biol. 23 (1978) S. 630

[10.4] Bottomley, P.A.; Foster, T.H.; Argersinger, R.E.; Pfeifer, L.M: A review of normal tissue hydrogen NMR relaxation times and relaxation mechanisms from 1-100 MHz .... Med. Phys. 11 (1984) S. 425

[10.5] Wilson, M.N.: Superconducting Magnets. Oxford (U.K.): Clarington Press 1983

[10.6] Oxford Magnet Technology, "Magnets in clinical use", Oxford (UK): OMT Verlag (1983)

[10.7] Jahnke, E.; Emde, F.: Tafeln höherer Funktionen. Leipzig: Teubner Verlag 1952

[10.8] Hoult, D.I.; Lee, D.: Shimming a superconducting NMR imaging magnet with steel. Rev. Sci. Instr. 56 (1985) S. 131
Frese, G.; Pausch, G.; Ries, G.: Aspects of shimming a superconducting whole body MRI magnet. Proceedings of the 9. International Conf. on Magnet Technology, S. 249 (Zürich, 1985)

[10.9] Stetter, E.; Oppelt, A.: Image quality in NMR tomography. Proceedings of the world congress on medical physics and biomedical engineering. S. 24.10 (Hamburg, 1982)

[10.10] Wehrli, F.W.; McFall, J.R.; Glover, G.H.; Grigsby, N.; Haughton, V.; Johanson, J.: The dependence of NMR image contrast on intrinsic and pulse sequence timing parameters. Magn. Res. Imag. 2 (1984) S. 3

[10.11] Mansfield, P.; Chapman, B.: Active magnetic screening of gradient coils in NMR imaging. J. Magn. Res. 66 (1986) S. 573

[10.12] Meinke, H.; Gundlach, F.W.: Taschenbuch der Hochfrequenztechnik. Kap. U24, Berlin, Heidelberg, New York: Springer-Verlag 1968

[10.13] Hoult, D.I.: The NMR receiver: a description and analysis of design. Progress in NMR spectroscopy (Kap. 6.4) 12 (1978) S. 41
Shaw, D.: Fourier transform NMR spectroscopy (Kap.6.7). Amsterdam: Elsevier 1984

[10.14] Hayes, C.E.: Radio frequency coil for NMR. European Patent Application 0 151 745 (21.8.85)

[10.15] Krause, N.: Hochfrequenzfeldeinrichtung in einer Kernspinresonanzapparatur. German patent application 32 33 432 (3.3.83)

[10.16] Alderman, D., Grant, D.: An efficient decoupler coil design which reduces heating in conductive samples in superconducting spectrometers. J. Magn. Res. 36 (1979) S. 447

[10.17] Hoult, D.I.; Chen, C.N.; Sank, V.J.: Quadrature detection in the laboratory frame. Magn. Res. Med. 1 (1984) S. 339

[10.18] Heinzerling, J.: Technische Fortschritte in der NMR-Tomographie. Röntgenstrahlen 49 (1983) S. 34

[10.19] VAX/VMS User's Manual (Kap. 1.6.2). Digital Equipment Corp. Maynard (Massachusetts) 1986

[10.20] Champeney, D.C.: Fourier transforms and their physical applications (Kap. 2 und 3). London: Academic Press 1973

[10.21] Margosian, P.: Faster MR imaging – imaging with half the data. London: Proceedings of the SMRM (S. 1024) 1985

[10.22] Hahn, E.: Spinechos. Phys. Rev. 80 (1950), S. 580

[10.23] Graumann, R.; Oppelt, A.; Stetter, E.: Multiple spin echo imaging with a 2d Fourier method. Magn. Res. Med. 3 (1986) S. 707

[10.24] Stroebel, B.: German patent application 34 14 635 (24.10.85)

[10.25] Lampman, D.; Morich, M.: Artifact free multiple echo imaging in a single acquisition. Magn. Res. Imag. 4 (1986) S. 102
Crawley, A.P.; Henkelman, R.M.: Errors in T2 estimation using multislice multiple echo imaging. Magn. Res. Med. 4 (1987) S. 34

[10.26] Ernst, R.R.; Anderson, W.A.: Application of Fourier transform spectroscopy to magnetic resonance. Rev. Sci. Instr. 37 (1966) S. 93

[10.27] Haase, A.; Frahm, J.; Matthaei, D.; Hänicke, W.; Merboldt, K.D.: FLASH imaging. Rapid NMR imaging using low flip-angle pulses. J. Magn. Res. 67 (1986) S. 258

[10.28] Hinshaw, W.S.: Image formation by nuclear magnetic resonance: The sensitive point method. J. Appl. Phys. 47 (1976) S. 3709

[10.29] Freeman, R.; Hill, H.D.W.: Phase and intensity anomalies in Fourier transform NMR. J. Magn. Res. 4 (1971) S. 366
Matsui, S.; Kuroda, M.; Kohno, H.: A new method of measuring T2 using steady state free precession. J. Magn. Res. 62 (1985) S. 12

[10.30] Mansfield, P.: Multiplanar image formation using NMR spin echos. J. Phys. C10 (1977) S. L55

[10.31] Hennig, J.; Nauerth, A.; Friedburg, H.: RARE imaging: A fast imaging method for clinical MR. Magn. Res. Med. 3 (1986) S. 823

[10.32] Haacke, E.M.; Beardon, F.H.; Clayton, J.R.; Linsa, N.R.: Reduction of MR imaging time by the HYBRID fast scan technique. Radiol. 158 (1986) S. 521

[10.33] Deimling, M., et al.: Description of flow phenomena in magnetic resonance imaging. Diagn. Imag. 55 (1986) S. 37

[10.34] Moran, P.M.; Moran, R.A.; Karstaedt, N.: Verification and evaluation of internal flow and motion. True magnetic resonance imaging by the phase gradient modulation method. Radiol. 154 (1985) S. 433

11 Sonography

[11.1] Wells, P.N.T.: Physical principles of ultrasonic diagnosis. London, New York: Academic Press 1975

[11.2] Sutilov, V.A.: Physik des Ultraschalls. Wien, New York: Springer-Verlag 1984

[11.3] Krautkrämer, J.; Krautkrämer, H.: Werkstoffprüfung mit Ultraschall. Berlin, Heidelberg, New York: Springer-Verlag 1975

[11.4] Steinberg, B.D.: Principles of Aperture and Array System Design. Wiley-Interscience Publication, 1976

[11.5] Thurstone, F.L.; v. Ramm, O.T.: A new ultrasound imaging technique emploing two dimensional electronic beam steering. Acoustical Holography 5 (1974)

[11.6] Kossoff, G., et al.: Ultrasonic Two Dimensional Visualisation for Medical Diagnosis. J.A.S.A 44 (1968) Heft 5

[11.7] Zemanek, J.: Beam behavior within the nearfield of a vibrating piston. J.A.S.A 49 (1971) Heft 1

[11.8] Marini, J.; Rivenez, J.: Acoustical fields from rectangular ultrasonic transducers for nondestructive testing and medical diagnosis. Ultrasonics 12 (1974) S. 251 bis 256

[11.9] Weyns, A.: Radiation fields of pulsed ultrasonic transducers: plane square, plane annular and spherical radiators. Abstracts 3rd European Congress of Ultrasonics in Medicine, Bologne (1978) S. 497 bis 501

[11.10] Burckhardt, C.B.: Speckle in Ultrasound B-Mode Scans. IEEE Trans. on Sonics and Ultrasonics. SU 25 (1978) Heft 1

[11.11] Borburgh, J.; Feigt, I.; Zurinski, V.: Image artefacts in Linear Array Systems: Analysis of Phenomena and their Elimination. Abstract 2nd Meeting of WFUMB and 4th Congress on Ultrasonics in Medicine. Mijazaki, Japan (1979) S. 367

[11.12] Edler, I.; Hertz, C.H.: The use of ultrasonic reflectoscope for the continuos recording of the movements of heart walls. Kungl. Fysiografiska Sällskapet i Lund Förhandlingar 24 (1954) S. 5

[11.13] Krause, W.; Soldner, R.: Ultraschallbildverfahren (B-scan) mit hoher Bildfrequenz für medizinische Diagnostik. electromedica 35 (1967) Heft 4, S. 8 bis 11

[11.14] Braun, B.; Günther, R.; Schwerk, W.: Ultraschalldiagnostik, Lehrbuch und Atlas ab 1983 und Ergänzungen. Landsberg: ecomed-Verlag 1986

[11.15] Lutz, H.; Hackelöer, B.-J.; v. Kaick, G.; Räth, U.: Ultraschallanatomie. Berlin, Heidelberg, New York: Springer-Verlag 1986

[11.16] Köhler, E.: Klinische Echokardiographie. Stuttgart: Ferdinand Enke Verlag 1979

[11.17] Hatle, L.; Angelsen, B.: Doppler Ultrasound in Cardiology. Philadelphia: Lea & Febiger 1982

[11.18] Feigenbaum, H.: Echokardiographie. Erlangen: Perimed Verlag 1986

[11.19] Statement des "European Committee for Ultrasound Radiation Safety": Unbedenklichkeit des Ultraschalls zu diagnostischen Zwecken. Ultraschall 6 (1985) 172

[11.20] Rott, H.-D.: Ultraschall in der Medizin: Biologische Wirkungen und Sicherheitsaspekte. Deutsches Ärzteblatt 81 (1984) S. 1071 bis 1074

12 Biomagnetic diagnostics

[12.1] Tripp, J. H.: Physical concepts and mathematical models. In: Williamson SJ, Romani GL, Kaufmann L, Modena I, eds. Biomagnetism: an interdisciplinary approach. New York: Plenum, 1982; 101–139

[12.2] Baule G, McFee R: Detection of the Magnetic Field of the Heart. Am. Heart J. 1963, 66:95–96

[12.3] Peters MJ, Elias PJH. On the magnetic field and the electrical potential generated by bioelectric sources in an anisotropic volume conductor. Med Biol Eng Comput 1988; 11:617–623

[12.4] Purcell CJ, Stroink G, Horacek BM. Effect of torso boundaries on electric potential and magnetic field of a dipole. Trans Biomed Eng 1988; 35:671–678

[12.5] Mondt, J. P.: On the effects on source localization of volume currents in neuroelectric and neuromagnetic signals. Phys. Med. Biol. 1989; 34:1073–1088

[12.6] Zimmermann JE. Cryogenics. In: Williamson SJ, Romani GL, Kaufmann L, Modena I, eds. Biomagnetism: an interdisciplinary approach. New York: Plenum, 1982; 43–67

[12.7] Romani GL: Biomagnetism: An Application of SQUID Sensors to Medicine and Physiology. Physica 1984; 126B:70–81

[12.8] Kajola M, Ahlfors S, Ahonnen A, Hällström J, Knuutila J, Lounasmaa OV, Tesche C, Vilkman V: Low-Noise Seven-Channel DC-SQUID Magnetometer for Brain Research. In: Biomagnetism '87, Proc. 6 th Int Conf on Biomagnetism, Tokyo, August 27–20, 1987, ed. K Atsumi et al., Tokyo Denki University Press, Tokyo 430–433

[12.9] Hoenig HE, Daalmans G, Folberth W, Reichenberger H, Schneider S, Seifert H. Biomagnetic multichannel system with integrated SQUIDs and first order gradiometers operating in a shielded room. Cryogenics 1989; 29:809–813

[12.10] Clarke J, Goubau WM, Ketchen MW. Tunneljunction DC-SQUID: fabrication, operation, and performance. J Low Temperature Phys 1976; 28–99

[12.11] Cuffin BN, Cohen D: Magnetic Fields of a Dipole in Special Volume Conductor Shapes. IEEE Trans Biomed Eng 1977; BME 24:372–381

[12.12] Stefan H, Schneider S, Abraham-Fuchs K, Bauer J, Feistel H, Huk WJ, Neubauer U, Reichenberger H, Röhrlein G: Biomagnetic multichannel measurements in the pre-operative diagnostic evaluation of epilepsy. Electromedica 57 1989, 4:129–133

[12.13] Moshage W, Weikl A, Abraham-Fuchs K, Schneider S, Bachmann K, Reichenberger H: Magnetokardiographie (MKG): Technischer Fortschritt durch ein Vielkanal-SQUID-System. Klinische Anwendung bei Linkshypertrophie und WPW-Syndrom. Biomed.Technik 1989; 34:205–206.

Formula symbols

A	Focal spot area
	Focal spot size
	Gray level
	Mass number (number of protons + number of neutrons)
B	Magnetic flux density
B_0	Magnetic flux density of constant magnetic field
c	Specific heat
	Speed of light
	Sound propagation velocity
C_A	Distribution of gamma activity concentration
d	Object thickness
D	Self-diffusion coefficient
$\dot{D}$	Dose rate
e	Electron charge
	Electron mass
E	Electric field strength
	Energy
	Exposure intensity
	Modulus of elasticity
	Neural excitation
E'	Energy of recoil electron
E_M	Binding energy of electron shell M
E_{pot}	Potential (static) energy
E_{kin}	Kinetic energy
E_M	Specific evaporation energy
f_A	Acoustic repetition frequency
	Rotating anode drive frequency
f_0	Doppler transmission frequency
Δf	Doppler frequency difference
F_1	One-dimensional Fourier transform
F_2	Two-dimensional Fourier transform
G	Magnetic field gradient
h	Planck's constant
H	Hamiltonian operator
HU	Hounsfield units
I	Nuclear spin quantum number
I_A	Anode current
I_F	Filament current
I_S	Emitter surface saturation current
I_M	X-ray intensity behind object without contrast medium
I_0	X-ray intensity in front of the object
j_e	Emission current density
J	Acoustic intensity
	Radiation intensity behind the object
J_0	Radiation intensity at the same point in the absence of the object
k	Boltzmann constant ($1.38 \cdot 10^{-23}$ Ws/K)

K	Hooke‘s law constant
K_α	Characteristic radiation
K_β	Characteristic radiation
L	Line spread function
	Luminance (photometric light intensity)
m	Mass
m_0	Electron rest mass
M	Nuclear magnetization
MTF	Modulation transfer function
N	Frequency
	Number of quanta
N_v	Nuclear spin density
p	Acoustic pressure
p_i	Acoustic pressure of the incident wave
P	Electrical power
p_r	Acoustic pressure of the reflected wave
p_a	Intensity of scattered sound
p_φ	Fan-beam projection
$\hat{P}$	Peak value of acoustic pressure
Q	mAs product (electric charge)
R	Acoustic reflection coefficient
	Electrical resistance
	Stimulus intensity
R_0	Original stimulus intensity
	Radiation intensity
S	Gamma signal intensity
	Optical density (blackening)
t	Time
T	Exposure time
	Temperature
T_A	Anode Temperature
T_e	Echo time
T_N	Noise temperature
T_p	Transmission of primary radiation
T_r	Repetition time
T_s	Transmission of scattered radiation
T_1	Longitudional relaxation time
T_2	Transverse relaxation time
U	Tension, voltage
U_A	Anode voltage
v	Sound particle velocity
V	Bucky factor
	Volume
w	X-ray tube voltage ripple
W	Photoelectric work function
z_f	Acoustic focal distance
Z	Acoustic impedance
	Atomic number
	Electrical impedance

α	Conversion efficiency of x-ray quanta into light quanta
β	Acoustic absorption coefficient
γ	Gyromagnetic ratio
Σ	X-ray grid selectivity
δ	Dirac delta function Chemical shift
$\varepsilon(T)$	Specific emission capacity
ε_0	Electrical permittivity in a vacuum
η	Coil filling factor Efficiency Energy transfer coefficient
τ_{fl}	Coefficient for energy transfer to fluorescence quanta in photoelectric absorption
σ_s	Transfer coefficient for the energy of the scattered quanta in the Compton process
η_σ	Kinetic energy transfer coefficient in the Compton process
η_τ	Energy transfer coefficient for photoabsorption
ϑ_{max}	Maximum permissible temperature
λ	Thermal conductivity Wavelength
μ/ϱ	Mass absorption coefficient
ν	Radiation frequency Spatial frequency
ξ	Elongation
ϱ	Density
σ	Electrical conductivity Scattering coefficient Standard deviation
σ_c	Coefficient for incoherent scattering, Compton coefficient
σ_c^e	Compton scattering cross section per electron
$\sigma_{c,k}^e$	Cross section for energy transfer to Compton electrons for incoherent scattering per electron
σ_R	Coefficient for coherent scattering
σ_R^e	Coefficient for coherent scattering per electron
$\sigma_R^e\|_{th}$	Cross section for Thomson scattering
σ_τ^a	Cross section for photoabsorption per atom
σ_τ^e	Cross section for photoabsorption per electron
τ/ϱ	Mass photoabsorption coefficient
φ	Projection angle
χ	Pair production coefficient
ψ	Energy flux density (energy per unit surface and time)
ω_L	Larmor frequency
ω_0	MRI resonance frequency
$\Delta\omega$	Pulse bandwidth
μ	Linear attenuation coefficient for x-ray and gamma radiation
μ_0	Magnetic permeability in a vacuum
τ	Acoustic delay time Acoustic transmission coefficient Photoelectric absorption coefficient

Index